Excellence in dementia care

Excellence in dementia care

Research into practice

Edited by Murna Downs and Barbara Bowers

 Open University Press

Open University Press
McGraw-Hill Education
McGraw-Hill House
Shoppenhangers Road
Maidenhead
Berkshire
England
SL6 2QL

email: enquiries@openup.co.uk
world wide web: www.openup.co.uk

and Two Penn Plaza, New York, NY 10121—2289, USA

A catalogue record of this book is available from the British Library

ISBN-13: 978-0-33-5223756 (pb) 978-0-33-5223749 (hb)
ISBN-10: 0-33-5223753 (pb) 0-33-5223745 (hb)

Typeset by Kerrypress, Luton, Bedfordshire
Printed and bound in the UK by Bell and Bain Ltd, Glasgow.

The **McGraw·Hill** Companies

To Ian and Amanda

In memory of Bob and Leona

To Chris without whom. . .

In memory of Maureen and Tom Downs

Contents

Contributors

Kate Allan works as a freelance trainer and consultant. Her background is in clinical psychology and she previously worked as a researcher at the Dementia Services Development Centre, Stirling University. Her field is promoting communication, consultation and creativity with people with dementia, with particular interests in deafness and dementia, and the needs of people whose condition is very advanced.

Jesse F Ballenger is the author of *Self, Senility and Alzheimer's Disease in Modern America: A History* (Johns Hopkins University Press, 2006). He also co-edited with Peter J. Whitehouse and Konrad Maurer *Concepts of Alzheimer Disease: Biological, Clinical and Cultural Perspectives* (Johns Hopkins University Press, 2000), and is co-editing another book with Peter Whitehouse, Constantine Lyketsos, Peter Rabins and Jason Karlawish on the history and future of drug development for Alzheimer's disease, entitled *Do We Have a Pill for That? Interdisciplinary Perspectives on the Development, Use and Evaluation of Drug Treatment for Dementia*. He is Assistant Professor in the Science, Technology and Society programme at Pennsylvania State University, USA.

Clive Baldwin is Senior Lecturer with the Bradford Dementia Group, University of Bradford, where he is Course Leader for the MSc in Dementia Studies by distance learning. He was involved for many years in the field of community development in the voluntary sector in the UK. He was awarded his PhD from the University of Sheffield in 2000 for his thesis on narrative analysis and child abuse and then became a Research Fellow at the Ethox Centre, University of Oxford, where he was the principal researcher on a qualitative research project exploring the ethical issues faced by family carers of people with dementia. His publications cover the areas of ethics, family carers, personhood, technology, and narrative theory and methods.

Linda Boise is Associate Professor of Neurology and Director of the Education/Information Transfer Core for the Layton Aging and Alzheimer Disease Center at Oregon Health and Science University, Portland, Oregon. Over the past 15 years, she has been involved in education and research related to chronic illness and dementia. She has conducted numerous studies on family caregiving and primary care physician practices related to dementia. Her research interests include the development of interventions to enhance communication between clinicians and family caregivers, and family caregiver support, self-care, and self-efficacy. She holds a Master of Public Health degree from the University of North Carolina at Chapel Hill and a PhD in Urban Studies from Portland State University, Portland, Oregon.

Barbara Bowers is Associate Dean for Reasearch and Helen Denne Schulte Professor in the School of Nursing at the University of Wisconsin-Madison. She has an extensive record of research in aged care, specifically on the topics of care quality, the professional development of care staff, the implementation of new models of care, dissatisfaction and turnover of care staff in residential environments, and the impact of public policy on the aged care community. As the Director of the Center for Excellence in Long-term Care at the University of Wisconsin, Madison, USA, she has worked closely with state and federal government bodies to develop, implement and evaluate aged care public policies and new models of care.

Carol Brayne is Professor of Public Health Medicine in the Department of Public Health and Primary Care at the University of Cambridge. She is a medically qualified epidemiologist and public health academic. She graduated in medicine from the Royal Free Hospital School of Medicine, University of London, and went on to train in general medicine. After gaining membership she moved on to training in epidemiology with a training fellowship with the Medical Research Council. The research area for this fellowship was ageing and dementia. Since the mid-1980s her main research area has been longitudinal studies of older people following changes over time in cognition, dementia natural history and associated features with a public health perspective. She has been responsible for training programmes in epidemiology and public health for medical students and postgraduates during this time.

Dawn Brooker is Professor of Dementia Care Practice and Research at the Bradford Dementia Group, University of Bradford. She has twenty years academic and clinical experience of working in the field of dementia, during which her particular research interest has been the improvement of quality of life and of services for people with dementia.

Errollyn Bruce is a Lecturer in Dementia Studies with the Bradford Dementia Group at the University of Bradford, contributing to its modular undergraduate and postgraduate distance learning degrees in dementia care. Her research interests centre on quality of life for people with dementia and their families. Currently she is a co-investigator on a multi-centre trial of reminiscence funded by the National Institute for Health Research Health Technology Assessment programme. She has developed learning materials for family carers of people with dementia and for practitioners and professionals working with people with dementia. She was academic partner in a Wellcome Foundation Sciart project which made the short film *Ex Memoria* and produced the accompanying learning material for those working in dementia care. With Pam Schweitzer, she has co-authored *Remembering Yesterday, Caring Today, Reminiscence in Dementia Care: A Guide to Good Practice*.

Georgina Charlesworth is a Chartered Clinical and Health Psychologist (British Psychological Society) and has worked concurrently in National Health Service and university settings for the past 17 years. She is currently Lecturer in Clinical and Health Psychology of Old Age at University College London, and Honorary Consultant Clinical Psychologist at North East London Mental Health NHS Trust, working with older people. Her research work is with family carers of people with dementia, specializing in psychosocial interventions for carer support. Her current research work is on the impact of support from ex-carers for current carers of people with dementia. Her previous work includes a trial of long-term befriending for family carers of people with dementia (BECCA; http://www.hta.ac.uk/1233) and she was formerly an Alzheimer's Society Research Fellow working on the development and evaluation of a cognitive-behavioural therapy for clinically depressed carers of people with dementia.

Linda Clare is Professor of Clinical Psychology and Neuropsychology in the School of Psychology, University of Wales Bangor, and a practising clinical psychologist and neuropsychologist. She has pioneered the development of cognitive rehabilitation approaches for people with early-stage dementia, in the context of research aimed at understanding more about the subjective experience of dementia for all concerned and the awareness that people with dementia have of what is happening to them.

Jiska Cohen-Mansfield is the Head of the Herczeg Institute on Aging, and Professor and Chair of the Department of Health Promotion at the School of Public Health at Tel-Aviv University. She is Director of the Research Institute on Aging of the CES Life Communities and a Professor of Health Care Sciences and of Prevention and Community Health at the George Washington University Medical Center and School of Public Health. Her work focuses on improving quality of life for persons with dementia by understanding the perspective of the person with dementia, on end-of-life decision-making, and on health and mental health promotion in older persons. She has published numerous articles on the topic of agitation in the elderly, as well as addressing important issues for the elderly person such as sleep, religious beliefs, decisions regarding medical treatments, physical restraints, vision problems, depression, autonomy; and stress in nursing home caregivers. She has published over 200 publications in scientific books and journals, and has developed a number of assessment tools, which have been translated and used internationally. She is the recipient of several awards and is a highly cited researcher as listed by the ISI.

Karen Croucher joined the Centre for Housing Policy at the University of York in March 2000, after ten years in health consultancy and research in York Health Economics Consortium (YHEC). Karen's research interests include the interface between housing and health, with a particular interest in housing for later life. She was the main researcher on the 2000–2002 evaluation of the UK's first Continuing Care Retirement Community (CCRC). Most recently she has undertaken a systematic review of the literature relating to housing with care for later life for the Joseph Rowntree Foundation.

Sue Davies is an honorary Reader at the University of Sheffield. She has worked as a health visitor specializing in the needs of older people, and as a senior nurse in a unit providing continuing care for frail older people. Current research interests focus on quality of life and quality of care in care homes.

Murna Downs is Professor in Dementia Studies at Bradford University and Head of the Bradford Dementia Group, the Division of Dementia Studies. Her research interests focus on quality of life and quality of care for people with dementia and their families. She has published on a variety of topics including primary care and end of life care for people with dementia. Most recently she co-authorised *Living and Dying with Dermentia* (Oxford University Press, 2007).

Simon Evans is a Senior Research Fellow at the University of the West of England, Bristol. His research focuses on housing options for older people and recent projects include a study of extra care housing for people with dementia, an evaluation of a mixed tenure retirement village, a study of social well-being in extra care housing and an exploration of rehabilitation services for people with dementia. He is an Associate of Dementia Voice, a member of the Executive Committee of the British Society of Gerontology and Chair of his faculty research ethics committee.

Richard H Fortinsky is Professor of Medicine at the Center on Aging and Department of Medicine, University of Connecticut Health Center (UCHC). Professor Fortinsky holds the Physicians Health Services Endowed Chair in Geriatrics and Gerontology at the UCHC School of Medicine. He has authored or co-authored more than 80 peer-reviewed journal articles and book chapters, and invited publications on a range of health policy and practice-related topics in gerontology, geriatrics and long-term care. At present, his major research areas are: physician and family care for persons with dementia, patient outcomes and resource use in Medicare home health care, and evaluation of evidence-based community interventions to help prevent falls in older populations. He received his doctoral degree in Sociology in 1984 from Brown University, specializing in medical sociology and gerontology.

Jane Fossey is a consultant clinical psychologist working with older people's services for Oxfordshire and Buckinghamshire Mental Health Partnership NHS Trust. She has specialized in working with people with dementia and with care homes for over 15 years and has published a number of research studies into the quality of life in care homes. Her research interests include the effectiveness of psychosocial interventions on care practice and the therapeutic effects of animals for older people.

Katherine Froggatt trained as a nurse in London following completion of her geography degree in Durham. She worked in radiotherapy and the care of older people before moving into research in both higher education and hospital trusts, undertaking research and practice development in the areas of oncology and palliative care. Her interests in the care of older people and palliative care have led her to undertake several projects concerned with care homes. She currently holds a post-doctoral research fellowship, funded by The Health Foundation, at the School of Nursing and Midwifery at the University of Sheffield. The focus of this work is to develop end of life care in care homes involving older people, their relatives and staff. With Neil Small and Murna Downs she co-authored *Living and Dying with Dementia* (Oxford University Press, 2007).

Lynda Gatecliffe is a Senior Lecturer at the University of Bradford and Head of the Division of Health Care Studies. She currently teaches leadership and management development within the context of health and social care. Lynda has over twenty years experience in the NHS as a dietician, service manager and management developer.

Jane Gilliard is Social Care Lead, Older People's Mental Health Programme, Care Services Improvement Partnership. She worked first as a medical social worker, then with children and families and finally older people, and especially people with dementia. In 1990, she established an innovative service supporting the carers of people attending the Bristol Memory Disorders Clinic. In the mid-1990s she set up Dementia Voice, a regional dementia services development centre for the South-west and was the Director from 1997 to 2005.

Deborah Girling is consultant in old age psychiatry at Fulbourn Hospital in Cambridge, and Associate Lecturer in the Faculty of Clinical Medicine at the University of Cambridge. She provides consultant medical input to the older people's liaison mental health team at Addenbrooke's Hospital in Cambridge, UK.

Claire Goodman was appointed in October 2006 as Professor at the University of Hertfordshire, working in the Centre for Research in Primary and Community Care (CRIPACC). Before this she was Director of the Primary Care Nursing Research Unit UCL/KCL, a collaboration between two academic institutions, a primary care research network and a primary care trust. She has published widely on nursing and older people care in primary and community care settings. Current research focuses on the contribution of primary care nursing to promoting health and well-being to community dwelling older people and those with chronic disease, palliative care interventions for older people in care home settings, and the evaluation of new roles in primary care nursing.

Susan Green is an associate specialist in old age psychiatry in Cambridge. She provides medical input to the older people's liaison psychiatric service at Addenbrooke's Hospital in Cambridge, UK.

Julian C Hughes is a consultant in old age psychiatry in Northumbria Healthcare NHS Foundation Trust. He is also an Honorary Clinical Senior Lecturer in the Institute for Ageing and Health, Newcastle University. His interests lie in the fields of ethics and philosophy in relation to dementia and ageing. He has a particular clinical interest in palliative care in dementia.

Neil Hunt worked for many years in social care before joining the NSPCC, where he became director of child protection, chiefly responsible for the leadership of the charity's core service programme. He was seconded to the civil service to work on a range of projects in the Home Office and the Department of Education and Skills, prior to taking up the post of chief executive of the Alzheimer's Society in September 2003.

John Killick has a background in teaching and writing, particularly poetry and criticism. He began writing work with people with dementia in 1993, and since then has also promoted communication through the arts generally. His recent activities have explored the potential of photography and video, and communication with people with very advanced dementia. He has presented, written and broadcast widely on these subjects.

Rachael Litherland developed and managed the 'Living with Dementia' programme for the Alzheimer's Society, between 2000 and May 2006, to increase the involvement and support of people with dementia nationally in the organization. She supported people with dementia in the production of accessible information, service development, campaigning and self-advocacy. She also set up innovative projects with people with dementia including computer clubs and networking communities and ran the first national conference for and by people with dementia. With a background in psychology and advocacy for older people, she is now working on a freelance and research basis in the dementia field.

Esme Moniz-Cook is a consultant clinical psychologist in the National Health Service and Professor of Clinical Psychology and Ageing at the Institute of Rehabilitation, University of Hull, UK. She is Chair of Interdem, a pan-European multidisciplinary network of applied researchers interested in early psychosocial interventions for people with dementia (http://interdem.alzheimer-europe.org/). She has published numerous papers on psychosocial aspects of living with, and caring for, people with dementia.

Gail Mountain is Professor of Occupational Therapy Research at the Centre for Health and Social Care Research, Sheffield Hallam University. She has experience of working with people with dementia as a practitioner and as a researcher. She is particularly interested in how people with dementia can be assisted to self-manage.

Mike Nolan is Professor of Gerontological Nursing at the University of Sheffield. He has long-standing interests in the needs of family carers and of vulnerable older people in a range of care environments and has published extensively in these areas. He has worked in the field of gerontology for over 20 years.

Kimberly Nolet is a researcher in the School of Nursing at the University of Wisconsin-Madison. She has been engaged in research related to the professional development of care staff in residential aged care and home care and has investigated the implementation of new educational models and new models of care. Ms Nolet has worked with a variety of government agencies, private foundations and care organizations in her work across long-term care settings.

Jan Oyebode is a clinical psychologist specializing in work with older people. She is Senior Lecturer and Director of the Clinical Psychology Doctorate Course at the University of Birmingham and spends one day a week in clinical practice with Birmingham and Solihull Mental Health NHS Trust. Her particular interests are in psychological adaptation to late life events including dementia and bereavement.

Alison Phinney is an Assistant Professor in the School of Nursing and a research associate of the Centre for Research on Personhood in Dementia at the University of British Columbia in Vancouver, Canada. She conducts research in the area of Alzheimer's disease and related dementias, seeking to understand what it is like for people to live with this disease over time, what it means to them to have a dementing illness, and how individuals and families cope with the many changes brought into their everyday lives. She is currently conducting a study funded by the Social Sciences and Humanities Research Council and the

Canadian Institutes of Health to understand the significance of meaningful activity in the everyday lives of people with dementia.

Chris Rewston is a clinical psychologist working with older people at the Humber Mental Health NHS Teaching Trust. His role is to provide psychological care to alleviate distress in later life in people both with and without dementia. He has published on worry and rumination in older people.

Tonya Roberts is a pre-doctoral trainee in the School of Nursing at the University of Wisconsin-Madison. Her research is related to improving the quality of life for residents and the quality of the work environment for staff in long-term care settings. She has had extensive experience caring for older people and persons with dementia, holding both direct care and administrative positions in long-term care facilities prior to her graduate studies.

Steven R Sabat is Professor of Psychology at Georgetown University. He earned his PhD at the City University of New York, where he specialized in neuropsychology. The main focus of his research for the past 25 years has been the intact cognitive and social abilities of people with Alzheimer's disease in the moderate to severe stages, the subjective experience of having the disease, and the ways in which communication between people with Alzheimer's disease and their caregivers may be enhanced. In addition, his interests include issues surrounding the basis of our understanding of the effects of brain injury. He has explored all of these issues in depth in numerous scientific journal articles, in his book *The Experience of Alzheimer's Disease: Life Through a Tangled Veil* (Blackwell, 2001) and in his co-edited book *Dementia: Mind, Meaning, and the Person* (Oxford University Press, 2006).

Pam Schweitzer has many years experience developing reminiscence work both in the UK and internationally. In the 1980s, she founded Age Exchange Theatre Trust and Reminiscence Centre and remained its Artistic Director until 2005. For the last decade she has been actively developing reminiscence projects for people with dementia and their carers, including developing and coordinating a Europe-wide project, *Remembering Yesterday, Caring Today*. In 2000, she was awarded an MBE for services to Reminiscence and she continues to direct the European Reminiscence Network. She is an Honorary Research Fellow of Greenwich University and continues to lecture, train and write on all aspects of reminiscence. Her book *Reminiscence Theatre: Making Theatre from Memories* merited special acclaim in the Society of Theatre Research awards. With Errollyn Bruce, she has co-authored *Remembering Yesterday, Caring Today, Reminiscence in Dementia Care: A Guide to Good Practice*.

Blossom Stephan is a post-doctoral research associate in the Department of Public Health and Primary Care at the University of Cambridge. She graduated with a PhD from the University of Sydney. Her research interests lie in the field of ageing, mild cognitive impairment and dementia. She has been awarded the European Research Area in Ageing: Future Leaders of Ageing (FLARE) Fellowship (2008–2010).

Fiona Thompson is Specialist Registrar in Old Age Psychiatry at the Julian Hospital, Norwich. She is a specialist registrar in general, old age and liaison psychiatry. She has worked in both the general adult and older people's liaison mental health teams at Addenbrooke's Hospital in Cambridge, UK.

Sarah Vallelly is Housing 21's research manager. She has over seven years research and policy experience in the specialist older people's housing sector. She is one of the authors of '*Opening Doors to Independence*' and managed the research project which resulted in the publication. More recently she has co-written articles on end-of-life care for people with dementia and the role of specialist housing. Housing 21 is a national specialist in providing services to older people. They are a leader in the developing role of extra care housing.

Clare Wai is Liaison Mental Health Nurse based at Fulbourn Hospital in Cambridge. She is a specialist mental health nurse in liaison psychiatry for older people. She provides specialist nursing input to the older people's liaison mental health team at Addenbrooke's Hospital in Cambridge, UK.

Daphne Wallace is a retired consultant psychiatrist for older people having worked in Leeds since 1979. She has been involved in private practice (mostly psychotherapy). She has been a Medical Member of the Mental Health Review Tribunal since 1996 and a member of the Alzheimer's Society since the 1980s. She served as National Trustee from 1994 to 2006. She is a member of the Dementia Group of Christian Council on Ageing, serving as its Chair for almost ten years. She was diagnosed with early small vessel vascular dementia in August 2005.

Jane Wilcock is a research fellow with a background in psychology and health education and health promotion. Her specific research interests are in improving dementia care, older persons' perceptions of health care and unmet need, palliative care and development of educational materials with an emphasis on using new technologies. Jane is based at the Centre for Research in Primary and Community Care at the University of Hertfordshire and The Centre for Ageing Population Studies, University College London.

John Young has over twenty years experience as a consultant geriatrician. He is Professor of Elderly Care, University of Leeds and Head of the Academic Unit of Elderly Care and Rehabilitation, Bradford Teaching Hospital Trust. His research interests focus on stroke rehabilitation, intermediate care services and delirium for which he has received major grants from the Stroke Association, the NHS RandD Programme, PPP Health Care Trust, the MRC and the Department of Health. He is currently involved in evaluations of two intermediate care schemes in West Yorkshire, leading a collaborative multi-centre community hospital trial, developing a primary care-based model for stroke, and has initiated national work for delirium prevention. He has published over 100 scientific articles including major papers on stroke rehabilitation in the *British Medical Journal* and *The Lancet*.

Judy M Zarit is a clinical psychologist in private practice in State College, Pennsylvania. She specializes in neuropsychological assessment of dementia and clinical interventions with older adults. She also provides consultation services to nursing homes and assisted living facilities.

Steven H Zarit is Professor and Head of the Department of Human Development and Family Studies at Pennsylvania State University, and is also Adjunct Professor at the Institute of Gerontology at Jönköping University, Jönköping, Sweden. He has conducted research on a variety of late-life issues, including family caregiving and adaptation in very late life. He has written numerous papers and several books on family carers' experience.

Foreword

'Our job as human beings and healers is to preserve the quality of life unto its end as best we can.' So said Professor Peter Whitehouse while writing about 'the end of Alzheimer's disease' in 2006.

We know that dementia can have a significant impact on quality of life; for people with dementia and for the people around them. The compelling need to provide optimal support and services for people affected obliges us to draw on any available research and scholarship that will help us achieve this. Promoting quality of life and care for people with dementia and their families is at the heart of this new book by leading academics, researchers and practitioners.

When the bicentenary of Alzheimer's disease is marked in 2106 in the UK, the time between 2007 and 2008 will be observed to have been a critical tipping point for people with dementia and their carers. Momentum for improvement in care was created with the NICE Clinical Guideline on Dementia in 2006, the Alzheimer's Society UK Dementia Report in 2007, the National Audit Office report on dementia in 2007, and culminated in 2008 with the House of Commons Public Accounts Committee report *Improving Services and Support for People with Dementia* and the government's announcement of the creation of a *national dementia strategy* in England. At last the key role of health and social care in preventing the potentially devastating consequences of this condition was recognized.

England has now joined the small but growing number of countries, including Australia, France and Norway, who have professed a serious commitment to dementia in the form of strategies, plans and proposals. Expectations for achieving excellence in dementia care will be high following the publication of the forthcoming National Dementia Strategy for England. This has been tasked with prioritizing three areas: public and professional awareness, early diagnosis and support; and quality of care. This book offers this new era of dementia care a wealth of material on which to draw. It provides important insights into the many and complicated aspects of dementia and dementia care, the debates and controversies as yet unresolved, and compelling evidence for effectiveness of basing our policies and practices on the available science.

The key to this new era of dementia care must be informing, inspiring, educating and training the diverse workforce that delivers care and services to people with dementia and their carers. Yet the 'curriculum' for dementia in the UK has evolved 'like Topsy'. National Vocational Qualification Level 2 was the basic entry point for the majority of frontline care workers in residential homes invariably caring for people with dementia. More recently we have seen the production of a useful 'knowledge set' for dementia by Skills for Care, the Social Care Workforce Strategy Board for England. They will be used by service providers when developing in-house training or making decisions when buying training packages.

The growing field of academic study in dementia care requires some basic principles and perspectives to be laid down as foundations. Readers will be challenged and rewarded by a careful study of the individual chapters in this book. Taken as a whole they provide a contemporary overview of the foundations of dementia care. While at present we lack a coherent process or plan to educate and train the health and social care workforce in dementia, this book will make a significant contribution to the knowledge and skills of the workforce – no matter where or how educated.

The Alzheimer's Society expects to continue to develop and play its part. Ultimately, our vision is of a radically improved world for people with dementia, and excellence in dementia care will be the cornerstone. This book sets out an ambitious path which will guide our course.

Neil Hunt

Chief Executive

Alzheimer's Society

Reference

Whitehouse, P.J. (2006) The end of AD Part 3. *Alzheimer's Disease and Associated Disorders*, 20(4): 195–8.

Preface

Having worked for many years as a professional psychiatrist with people with dementia and now sharing the early experience dementia myself, I found this book accessible, informative and exciting. Much of what it says is reinforcing the ideas and experience I had in my work of supporting people with dementia. Now, as someone with dementia, I feel even more strongly that these ideas and principles are vital if we are to ensure humane care which is affirmative and supportive of the individual. In the year when the National Dementia Strategy for the UK is to be launched, this book could not be more welcome nor more timely with its comprehensive coverage of many important areas of current thinking in relation to dementia care.

The recognition of the importance of the person with dementia and their individual needs, together with explorations into the theoretical background to understanding the experience of dementia, are well outlined. Although some of the ideas are not new, for many people with dementia and their carers there seems to be NO understanding of the experience, and thus needs of those concerned, evident in those working in the services to help them. Only with training can one hope for this understanding in professional care staff.

Difficult philosophical and psychological ideas are presented with great clarity of exposition, making the chapters easily read by those with no background in the particular disciplines. I found this book helpful in putting my present and past experiences in context. In my time as a consultant psychiatrist for older people many of my ideas and practices were in tune with the ideas outlined but I had not formulated them fully. It is good to read them presented academically. At that time, however, when early diagnosis was less common, the views and experiences of those with dementia were not well known. I now understand the feelings which my patients tried to share and it is good to find the views of people with dementia and their carers included in this book. This can only increase the understanding and empathy of those professionally involved.

Ethical dilemmas are not shied away from and the need for flexibility is well expressed. A person with dementia will have ideas and thoughts about their future care which should inform care plans. They have a right to be consulted. In the past too often it has been assumed that they have lost the ability to have an opinion or feelings. People are infinitely different and this needs to be acknowledged. This book is concerned with the rights of people with dementia, whatever their age or degree of illness, paying attention to communication needs, help with cognition, and above all maintenance of maximum possible quality of life. Good quality of life is seldom cheap to achieve and failure to understand the individual's needs and rights may result in solutions to suit the providers rather than the receivers of care. Excellence in dementia care is not easily achieved in times of financial restraint or lack of resources. Many parts of the world without prior experience of the problems of significant numbers of people with dementia will be helped by this book towards a humane and person-centred care system. It is therefore valuable to have these issues and ideas expressed so clearly and in an academic context. It is good to see the emphasis in this book on consultation and recognition of individual differences. The policy aspects and the need for consultation with people with dementia and their carers, particularly with regard to quality of life issues, are now recognized as essential for good dementia care.

It needs to be recognized that there are many skills necessary in the care of people with dementia and their carers at different stages of the different types of dementia. Starting with assessment, not only leading to diagnosis but also to the understanding of particular problems, there are valuable accounts in this book by people who have been pioneering in their work to recognize the need for these skills. A person with dementia needs to feel that the professional who is advising and helping them is aware of current knowledge and skills in working with the different aspects of the illness. Problems will almost always arise and need sympathy and understanding. No one likes to be treated as a non-person and many with dementia have experienced this in the past. Much care in the past has worked on the premise that advanced dementia renders a person incapable of appreciating their environment and unable to communicate with other human beings. Recent work exploring communication with people with dementia has revealed that, as should have been realized before, human beings communicate in several modalities, not just by the spoken word. I have always been a 'talker' and I dread the day when I really have difficulty in verbal communication. I already have difficulties that I recognize in myself due to my vascular disease and I know that I will want people to recognize non-verbal communication as well as speech as my illness progresses. Psychological therapies do have a place in helping people to cope with this condition, whatever their diagnosis or symptomatology. In this book the people who inspire carers and professionals when they speak about their work are now able to reach a larger audience.

The issues that arise for all involved during the journey through the experience of dementia need to be explored. In this book, early support, often neglected, is outlined and then different contexts are discussed. Particular issues and how to deal with them are looked at, by people who have made valuable studies of the issues involved and are sharing their experiences, also by listening to those with dementia and their families and friends. We are all individuals with infinitely variable preferences and needs. This book not only emphasizes these points throughout, but also includes contributions from people with dementia and their carers. No one can deny the power of these chapters.

How to put theory and research evidence into practice is an important aspect of this book. Throughout there is a modular structure designed to facilitate learning and encourage further exploration. When I was grappling with setting up services for older people, many of them with dementia, I would have been greatly helped by this book. The most important basic concept for me is the simple one expounded by Tom Kitwood in 1997: 'We need to see the *person* with dementia, not the person with *dementia*.' All too often the disease model has predominated whether in a medical, social or psychological context. The experiences of many people who have thought long and hard over these issues are available here to guide those who recognize the need to revolutionize previous beliefs and practice. The increasing understanding of dementia from all perspectives informs and drives the improvement in all aspects of person-centred dementia care and I am sure that this book will provide an invaluable tool in the search for the excellence in dementia care of its title.

As a retired professional in the field I am only too well aware of the scarcity in the past of the material covered in this book. As a person with early dementia I am also keen that the knowledge and understanding that do exist are disseminated as swiftly and widely as possible. For too long, care of people with dementia has been viewed as unpopular and unrewarding. Those who strive to work in the ways outlined in this book know that the reverse is true, despite the difficulties of working in an unsympathetic culture and economically deprived area of care.

Throughout this book technical expertise is combined with sensitive and intuitive understanding of the situation and needs of people with dementia. A concern with quality of life pervades the book and is given a priority that will be welcomed by anyone with dementia. This book will prove to be a valuable training manual for those aiming to provide person-centred care for people with dementia, or indeed for those in any dependent caring situation.

Daphne Wallace

March 2008

Acknowledgements

Thanks to:

Rachel Roiland for her diligent editing and formatting, and her assistance in finding references to ensure the book draws on an international literature.

Luann Lawrence for her careful attention to omissions and redundancies in referencing, a monumental and tedious task.

Professor Dawn Brooker for her early involvement with the book.

Rachel Crookes and Jack Fray at the Open University Press.

All our contributors for being so patient with us.

In addition, the Authors and Publishers would like to thank Lippincott, Williams & Wilkins for permission to reproduce extracts from the following articles:

Cohen-Mansfield, J. (2000) Theoretical frameworks for behavioural problems in dementia. *Alzheimer's Care Quarterly*, 1(4): 8–21.

Cohen-Mansfield, J. (2000) Non-pharmacological management of behaviour problems in people with dementia: The TREA model. *Alzheimer's Care Quarterly*, 1(4): 22–34.

Cohen-Mansfield, J. (2005) Non-pharmacological interventions for persons with dementia. *Alzheimer's Care Quarterly*, 6(2): 129–45.

Introduction

Dementia is a global issue of concern to both developed and developing nations. There are approximately 24 million people with dementia in the world, with an additional four and a half million newly identified every year (Ferri *et al.* 2005). This number is expected double every 20 years, reaching approximately 81 million by 2040. Apart from the growth in numbers of people with dementia, dementia is of concern because of the degree of impairment and disability with which it is associated.

While dementia is most common in those over 80, a significant minority of people develop the condition before the age of 65. People with dementia experience impairments in cognition (including processing information, retaining memory for recent events and using verbal language) and difficulties in social, occupational and day-to-day self-care activities (Clare 2007). As dementia is a progressive brain disease, people who live long enough will eventually lose life-sustaining functions, including the ability to swallow. Living with dementia, and its associated impairments, is best supported by communities and care environments which accommodate these changed abilities and facilitate the expression of remaining capacities.

The quality of care for people with dementia and their family carers is a pressing concern throughout the world. There is now an almost universal recognition of the need to improve care practices and services for people with dementia and their families. By the time this book is published, the Department of Health in England will be implementing its National Dementia Strategy (House of Commons Committee of Public Accounts 2008). In Australia, dementia has been considered a public health priority since 2005. President Sarkozy has backed calls for a European dementia convention.

In the past 30 years we have come a long way from thinking about dementia as a 'living death' (Woods 1989), which merited little beyond custodial care. In contemporary times we recognize that while dementia is a progressive and life-limiting condition, there is life to be lived. Indeed we now recognize that the aim of care and support services is to optimize life with dementia. A variety of forces have come together to reinstate the person as someone who actively copes with the functional, psychological and social consequences of this condition. Due recognition is now being given to families, both in terms of their role in supporting their relative to live with dementia and as having entitlements for support in their own right. Such support is provided by practitioners and professionals who themselves need supportive work environments and government policies in order to maximize their potential.

People with dementia represent one of the most stigmatized and marginalized groups of older people (Graham *et al.* 2003). Nowhere are they more discriminated against than in the provision of health and social care. In the UK, the House of Commons Committee of Public Accounts (2008) openly acknowledges that, despite its significant human and financial impact, dementia, unlike other diseases such as cancer and coronary heart disease, has not been a priority for the Department of Health nor for the National Health Service.

It is now time to bring all the wealth of evidence we have to bear on achieving excellence in dementia care. Expectations about what is possible for people with dementia have been raised. Professionals and practitioners require improved levels of knowledge about the potential for a quality life with dementia (House of Commons Public Accounts Committee 2008). Competent and compassionate dementia care requires improved levels of awareness, knowledge and skills. It is now essential that we provide the workforce with a portfolio of education and training opportunities drawing on the evidence of what works, both in terms of how we care for people with dementia and how we embed such care in mainstream practice.

Aim of the book

The aim of the book is to make excellence in dementia care a part of everyday care practice and integral to services for people with dementia and their families. The book pays particular attention to the role of practitioners, professionals and service systems in promoting quality of life for people with dementia and their families. It addresses the need to support staff in order to achieve excellence in dementia care through the provision of training and education alongside leadership and organizational policies.

Drawing on current thinking, practice and policy from the English-speaking Western world, primarily the UK and the USA, it does the following:

1   Provides comprehensive coverage of a range of evidence about quality dementia care including user and family carer experience, practice wisdom, and research evidence.

2   Synthesizes the diverse range and multidisciplinary nature of evidence to guide professional practice and further academic work in this area.

3   Stimulates critical appraisal of existing systems, services and supports with respect to the extent to which they address the rights and diversity of needs of people with dementia and their families.

4   Provides strategies for developing sustainable working practices that actively promote health and well-being for people with dementia and their families.

Guide to the parts

Part One, Principles and Perspectives, presents the reader with key principles which set the context for best practice in understanding and supporting people with dementia and their families. The section includes a discussion of prevalence of dementia (Stephan and Brayne), subjective experience of dementia (Phinney), diversity and dementia (Boise), bio-psycho-social understanding of dementia (Sabat) and family carer perspectives (Zarit and Zarit), concluding with a discussion of philosophical (Hughes), including ethical (Baldwin), perspectives.

Part Two, Knowledge and Skills for Supporting People with Dementia, looks at the requisite knowledge and skills to provide effective and empathic support for people with dementia. No text can hope to cover the full range of knowledge and skills that practitioners and professionals need when working with people with dementia. We focus on the many ways we can improve quality of life for people with dementia. These include appropriate assessment (Mountain), supporting cognition (Oyebode and Clare), communication and social inclusion (Bruce and Schweitzer), understanding the language of behaviour (Cohen-Mansfield), promoting physical health and well-being (Killick and Allan), alleviating emotional distress (Young) and working with the life history (Rewston and Moniz-Cook).

Part Three, Journeys through Dementia Care, highlights and discusses specific points of intersection with services and supports along people's journey through the condition. People with dementia are cared for in a range of settings throughout their journey with dementia. This includes a discussion of how they first come to the attention of service systems (Fortinsky), the kinds of support available for living in one's own home (Charlesworth), hospitals (Thompson *et al.*) and nursing homes (Fossey). This part includes discussion of end-of-life care (Wilcock *et al.*) and grief and bereavement (Oyebode). Throughout there is a recognition that excellence in dementia care requires multidisciplinary and multiprofessional input. In this part the full potential of an effective service system is elucidated.

The final part, Embedding Excellence in Dementia Care examines the challenges of ensuring excellence in dementia care and outlines approaches to meeting them. The complex interrelationships between personal and organizational competencies and structures are discussed and the wider political and historic context provided. The part includes discussion of service user involvement (Litherland), a trained and supported workforce (Bowers), addressing the needs of all stakeholders (Davies and Nolan), management and leadership (Nolet *et al.*), the person's perspective on quality (Brooker), the historical context (Ballenger) and the policy context (Gilliard *et al.*).

Who the book is for

This book is intended for practitioners, professionals and academics working or volunteering in health and social care with people in dementia. It will serve as a core resource for those involved in training and education in dementia care and will be of use to undergraduate and postgraduate students in applied dementia studies and dementia care, gerontology, disability studies, medicine, nursing, occupational therapy, physiotherapy, psychiatry, psychology and social work. It is also relevant to students of organizational behaviour and management with an interest in organizations and systems designed for service delivery, and to future public policy workers who wish to understand how policies affect the lives of individuals and systems. The book will also be of interest to people with dementia or their advocates, family members, charity and voluntary sector organizations, policy-makers and those in senior positions in health care management.

Distinctive features of the book

The book adopts a modular structure so that each chapter can be read in sequence or in isolation from another.

Each chapter has the same structure including:

● learning objectives which let the reader know what to expect from each chapter

● text exercises which encourage readers to actively engage with the material presented

● debates and controversies in the field

● conclusion

● organizations established for a purpose relevant to the chapter topics.

The editors

Murna Downs is Professor in Dementia Studies at Bradford University and Head of the Bradford Dementia Group, the Division of Dementia Studies. Her research interests focus on quality of life and quality of care for people with dementia and their families. She has published on a variety of topics including primary care and end of life care for people with dementia. Most recently, she co-authored *Living and Dying with Dementia* (Oxford University Press, 2007).

Barbara Bowers is Associate Dean for Research and Helen Denne Schulte Professor in the School of Nursing at the University of Wisconsin-Madison. She has an extensive record of research in aged care, specifically on the topics of care quality, the professional development of carers, the implementation of new models of care, dissatisfaction and turnover of carers in residential environments, and the impact of public policy on the aged care community. As the Director of the Center for Excellence in Long-term Care at the University of Wisconsin, Madison, USA, Professor Bowers has worked closely with state and federal government bodies to develop, implement and evaluate aged care public policies and new models of care.

The contributors

Excellence in dementia care requires input from a range of disciplines and professionals. We are fortunate to have represented in this book contributions from the full range of professionals and disciplines concerned with the care of people with dementia. These include geriatric medicine, nursing, philosophy, psychology, occupational therapy, old age psychiatry, social work and sociology. In this book we have embraced the diversity of language and terminology presented to us by contributing authors. Biographical sketches of each of the authors can be found above.

What is omitted

As in all projects such as this one, there is much that cannot be included. We acknowledge that several important areas have been omitted. We are most aware of the following areas as not having received particular attention: younger people with dementia who merit a volume of their own; the physical environment and dementia; technology and dementia; creative arts; spirituality; and dementia care in developing nations.

References

Clare, L. (2007) *Neuropsychological Rehabilitation and People with Dementia*. London: Taylor & Francis Psychology Press.

Ferri, C.P., Prince, M., Brayne, C., Brodaty, H., Fratiglioni, L., *et al.* (2005) Global prevalence of dementia: a Delphi consensus study. *Lancet*, 366: 2112–17.

Graham, N., Lindesay, J., Katona, C., Bertolote, J.M. *et al.* (2003) Reducing stigma and discrimination against older people with mental disorders: a technical consensus statement. *International Journal of Geriatric Psychiatry*, 18: 670–8.

House of Commons Committee of Public Accounts (2008) *Improving Services and Support for People with Dementia*. London: The Stationery Office.

Woods, R.T. (1989) *Alzheimer's Disease: Coping with a Living Death*. London: Souvenir Press.

PART ONE

Principles and perspectives

1

Prevalence and projections of dementia

Blossom Stephan and Carol Brayne

Learning objectives

By the end of this chapter you will be able to:

- explain the implications of the ageing of our population for the prevalence and incidence of dementia
- describe the different types of dementia and the difficulty in distinguishing between them
- summarize the incidence and prevalence of dementia, regionally and worldwide
- identify risk factors for the development of dementia
- explain that dementia is associated with both disability and mortality

---

Introduction

In the next decades large numbers of people will enter the ages when the incidence rates of dementing diseases are the highest. People 60 years and over make up the most rapidly expanding segment of the population: in 2000, there were over 600 million persons aged 60 years or over worldwide, comprising just over 10% of the world population and by 2050 it is estimated that this figure will have tripled to nearly two billion older persons, comprising 22% of the world population (United Nations 2007).

This ageing epidemic, while once limited to developed countries, is expected to become more marked in developing countries (see Figure 1.1: Population pyramids high income countries). Population ageing poses the greatest threat to Japan and Continental Europe, where falling birth rates and increases in life expectancy are expected to have wide-ranging economic and social consequences especially with regard to health and long-term care. Yet in light of this, population ageing also has positive consequences. The elderly population make a valuable contribution to the society through volunteer work, providing informal care to grandchildren, families and communities, in addition to an accumulation of wisdom, experience and skills that can be passed to younger generations.

The change in population age structures will influence both the prevalence and incidence of age-related conditions such as dementia. In the United Kingdom alone, the percentage of older people (aged 65 and over) increased from 13% of the total population in 1971, to 16% in 2003 (Office for National Statistics 2003). It is estimated that of those individuals aged 65 and over, 6% will be suffering from dementia, with those in their eighties having

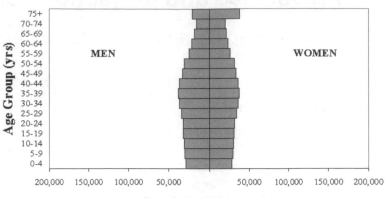

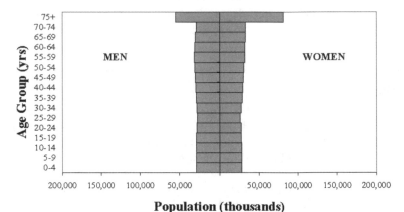

Figure 1.1   Population pyramid 2000 and 2040 (Source: The World Bank Group, http://devdata.worldbank.org/hnpstats/dp1.asp).

more than a 30% chance (Peters 2001). Worldwide the proportion of very elderly people (85 years and above) is also projected to grow (Table 1.1). Developing regions, particularly China, India and Latin America, which are set to dominate world ageing, will show the greatest increase in disease burden (Prince 2000). It is predicted that by 2040 there will be as many people with dementia in China as combined in the developed world (Ferri *et al.* 2005). The consequences of this ageing, epidemic will depend on how ageing is viewed in each culture and the mechanisms in place to anticipate and cope with demographic change.

The identification of modifiable risk factors that prevent or delay dementia onset is a major public health priority. It was concluded from a systematic review on dementia, cognitive impairment and mortality in persons aged 65 and over living in the community that there is an increased risk of mortality for even moderate levels of cognitive impairment and that at more severe levels the risk increases two-fold (Dewey and Saz 2001). In addition to increased mortality is increased dependence. The high dependency of patients with dementia means that any new information on aetiology would be an important addition to public health services not only for the potential sufferers and carers but also, financially, for future service planning. Indeed, the economic cost of dementia is already higher than that of heart disease and cancer together.

Table 1.1 Estimated changes in the world population age structure of the elderly (over 65 and over 80)

Population	2000	2025	2050
65 and over (%)	6.9	10.5	16.2
80 and over (%)	1.1	1.9	4.4
TOTAL (millions)	6055	7823	8900

Source: United Nations Population Division (2007)

In the past twenty years there has been a large advance in our understanding of the epidemiology of dementia and its subtypes. Epidemiological studies have been carried out with three principal aims. The first is to describe the frequency and distribution of disease. This informs health services planning and public health priorities. The second is to identify risk factors responsible for disease in order to guide treatment and ultimately prevention. These, along with evidence of change, feed a third aim which is to assess the possible impact of protective action in future populations. It is assumed that the clinical expression of dementia is to some extent environmentally modifiable so that its clinical manifestations can be delayed or prevented and its signs and symptoms alleviated.

Defining dementia and its subtypes

The term dementia defines a group of syndromes characterized by progressive decline in cognition of sufficient severity to interfere with social and/or occupational functioning, caused by disease or trauma, and often associated with increasing age. To date, over 200 subtypes have been defined, each characterized by differences in course and subtle variations in pattern of expression and neuropathology. The main subtypes include Alzheimer's disease (AD), vascular dementia (VaD), dementia with Lewy bodies (DLB), frontal lobe dementia, Pick's disease and alcohol-related dementia. Each is briefly described in Table 1.2.

Table 1.2   Summary of the main dementia types

	Primary impairments/disability/ symptoms	**Pathology/causes**
Alzheimer's disease	Memory, language and functional disability	Neuritic plaques (proteinaceous extra-cellular deposits consisting mainly of amyloid-beta peptide fragments) and neurofibrillary tangles (twisted fibres of a protein called tau)
Vascular dementia	Poor concentration and communication and physical symptoms such as paralysis or weakness in limbs	Problems of circulation of blood to the brain – related to stroke, high blood pressure (hypertension), diabetes and heart problems
Dementia with Lewy bodies	Hallucinations, spatial disorientation, impaired recent memory and fluctuations in mental performance	Presence of Lewy bodies which refer to abnormal structures within nerve cells of the brain
Frontal lobe dementia	Changes in personality and behaviour, and emotional and language dysfunction. No dysfunction in memory	Frontal lobe degeneration
Pick's disease	Impairment in emotional and social functioning	Abnormalities in Pick's bodies. Focal damage in the frontal and temporal lobes
Alcohol related dementia – Korsakoff's syndrome	Impaired memory, planning, organizing, judgement, social skills and balance	Chronic/excessive alcohol intake

AD is the most prevalent subtype, accounting for approximately 70% of all cases (Barberger-Gateau and Fabrigoule 1997; Cowan *et al.* 2000; Nour-hashemi *et al.* 2000). AD is characterized by a steady and progressive loss of memory and cognitive faculties including language deterioration, impaired visuospatial skills, poor judgement and an attitude of indifference. AD has a distinct neuropathological pattern of amyloid plaques and neurofibrillary tangles predominately in the neocortex, but becoming more widespread with disease progression. The second most common cause of dementia is VaD, accounting for 10–20% of all cases (Barberger-Gateau and Fabrigoule 1997; Ladislas 2000). VaD represents a heterogeneous group of conditions that includes all dementia syndromes that result from ischaemic, anoxic or hypoxic brain damage. Similar to AD, onset is progressive and life expectancy poor although for VaD the disease course can be highly variable. The exact prevalence of DLB is not known although some estimates suggest that it may be as common as VaD.

The risk of developing dementia increases with age. Indeed, results from the Medical Research Council Cognitive Function and Ageing Study (MRC CFAS) found that for those individuals aged 65–69 years at death, 6% had dementia while for those aged 95 years and above at death, 58% had dementia. This pronounced increase in dementia with age has been interpreted as an increase in the rates of AD, as shown in Figure 1.2. In contrast, rates for clinically diagnosed VaD remain relatively constant across age. This has implications for the optimum health care strategy for different age groups, and raises the question of whether the effect of dementia risk manipulation on the prevalence estimates of dementia and its subtypes is constant across age groups.

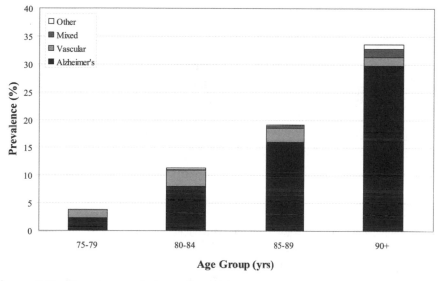

Figure 1.2 Prevalence of dementia subtypes
Data from the Cambridge City Over-75s Cohort Study (CC75C).

The distinction between subtypes has been questioned. Considerable overlap in pathology suggests that mixed forms may be more common (Peters 2001). Increased levels of amyloid plaques and neurofibrillary tangles characteristic of AD pathology have been found in hypertensive subjects post-mortem and it has been suggested that vascular pathology may play a role in the development of amyloid plaques (Peters 2001). Furthermore, both AD and VaD share similar risk factors (e.g. advancing age and poor cardiovascular health), overlapping clinical symptoms and cerebro-microvascular pathology (Skoog 1998). Yet, a steady progressive decline is still considered characteristic of AD while a stepwise deterioration characterized by periods of sharp decline alternating with plateaus or periods of minimal decline is characteristic of VaD (Peters 2001). Novel neuroimaging strategies coupled with careful clinical and pathologic examinations may provide the answers needed to determine whether VaD is really mixed dementia or AD alone.

Diagnosis of dementia depends on the defining criteria and sampling method. Different diagnostic criteria can produce up to a ten-fold variation in prevalence (O'Connor *et al.* 1996). For example, the WHO International Classification of Diseases, 10th revision (ICD-10) sets a higher threshold for dementia diagnosis compared to the widely used Diagnostic and Statistical Manual of Mental Disorders (DSM-IV-TR) criteria. Dementia variation can also be related to culture or diagnostic applicability (e.g. views of ageing and validity of instruments). When applying criteria it is also necessary to distinguish dementia from other disorders such as poor physical health, depression, anxiety, sensory difficulties, language barriers and education level, all of which can reduce cognitive scores.

Prevalence and incidence of dementia

Table 1.3 Prevalence and incidence

	Description
Prevalence	The total number of individuals with a disease in the population at a particular time point
Incidence	The rate of occurrence of new cases with a given disease during a specific time period

Variation in the incidence and prevalence of dementia across populations may provide insight into the aetiology and prevention of the disease. Although there have been few large population-based studies of dementia internationally or in multiethnic communities, a consistent pattern has emerged of decreased incidence and prevalence in: (1) Asian nations compared to Europe and North America; (2) rural compared to urban areas; and (3) developing rather than developed countries (White 1992; White *et al.* 1996). These differences have been linked to various factors including diet, genetics, mortality and criteria for case selection. We will first look at the challenges inherent in conducting research of this kind.

Methodological issues when studying prevalence and projections

For no other disorder associated with old age are the methodological issues of conducting community-based studies so complex. The lack of a unique pattern of clinical symptoms for dementia and its subtypes, for example, only reflects a mixture of underlying aetiologies and pathogenetic mechanisms. Population-based studies of incident disease where risk factors are identified before disease onset and individuals followed up longitudinally to document change are powerful tools for the identification of risk factors and modifiable strategies. However, these studies are expensive, time-consuming and are only now being conducted. Furthermore, differences in methodology and sample population lead to inconsistencies in findings, making comparative research difficult.

All epidemiological research depends on the definition of a 'case', that is, who is identified as having that particular condition. When evaluating dementia research, the following must be considered:

- *Observation bias* as individuals with dementia often are unable to provide their own past medical and social histories and the information has to be supplied by surrogate informants who may have variable amounts of knowledge about these factors.

- *Selection bias* through the choice of population source as the percentage of persons with AD, for example, living in institutions varies widely from place to place but may exceed half of all cases with severe AD. Exclusion of institutionalized persons would result in an underestimation of prevalence rates.

- *Response rate* as it is likely that response is affected by cognitive status so that more impaired individuals are less likely to have complete data and typically refuse further testing. This affects prevalence estimates and it is hard to guess in what direction they may have been biased because non-response can cause over- as well as under-estimation.

Exercise 1.1 Identifying the number of people with dementia in a given geographic area

Steve is a new commissioner of services for people with dementia in Edinburgh. In order to understand the extent of need for services, he is interested in finding out the number of people with dementia in the city. He has decided to send a survey to all day centres in the area asking them to tell him the number of people with dementia they serve. Based on replies to this survey he feels he will have a good sense of the number of people with dementia in the city.

Consider the above information and complete the following:

- List three reasons that Steve may be misled by his findings.

- Suggest an alternative approach to finding out the number of people with dementia in Edinburgh.

Prevalence of dementia

It is currently estimated that there are 24 million people with dementia worldwide and if mortality, prevention and treatment strategies remain unchanged this number will double every 20 years to an estimated 42 million by 2020 and 81.1 million by 2040 (Ferri *et al.* 2005). However, increases are not uniform across the world. A 100% increase is predicted in developed countries from 2001 to 2040, while more rapid changes in life expectancy in developing countries is estimated to result in a more marked effect, with the number of people with dementia in China and India likely to rise over 300% over this time period. In Latin America and Africa, depending on region, prevalence is estimated to either double or triple (Ferri *et al.* 2005). Projected increases across the 17 sub-regions of the world as defined by the World Health Organization (WHO) are shown in Figure 1.3.

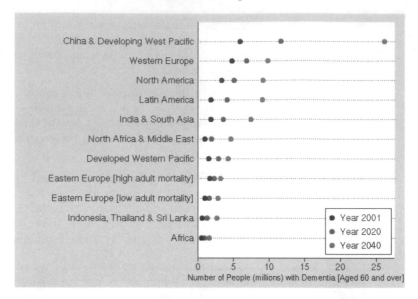

Figure 1.3 Dementia prevalence 2001, 2020, 2040 by WHO Region
Source: Ferri *et al.* (2005).

Where available, cross-national comparisons using similar methodology have highlighted this variation: lower prevalence of AD in rural India (28 villages in the Ballabgarh district of the state of Haryana in northern India) compared to a predominately Caucasian community cohort in the USA (Pennsylvania; MoVIES Project) (Chandra *et al.* 1998), lower prevalence of overall dementia in Malays compared to Singapore Chinese (Kua and Ko 1995) and lower prevalence of overall dementia and AD in Nigerians (Yoruba Nigerians) compared to African Americans in Indianapolis (2.4 times higher) (Hendrie *et al.* 2001).

Sub-type prevalence (AD and VaD) is also variable. In North America, AD accounts for approximately two-thirds of all cases. In Japan prior to 1990 VaD was found to be more common than AD, although more recent data suggest a Westernization in trend with AD now nearly twice as prevalent as VaD (Shigeta 2004). Similar trend changes have also been observed in Korea (Seoul) (Lee *et al.* 2002) and Taiwan (Liu *et al.* 1995, 1998) linked to urbanization, industrialization and lifestyle changes (e.g. alcohol use). In China, VaD is more common in northern regions, with AD more prevalent in the south (Chiu and Zhang 2000). Different reasons have been given including over-diagnosis of VaD and differences in case definition, vascular risk association and relative number of the young-old and oldest-old (Ineichen 1998).

Cross-ethnic comparisons from the UK, the USA and Canada have also found differences in rates between ethnic groups sharing the same territory (Ineichen 1998). In the USA, VaD is significantly more prevalent in individuals of African American and Hispanic origin (vs. Caucasian Americans) (Miles *et al.* 2001). In Washington and Hawaii, although individuals of Japanese origin were found to show similar AD estimates to those reported in European-ancestry populations, prevalence was found to be lower when a Japanese diet was adhered to (Hatada *et al.* 1999; White *et al.* 1996). Furthermore, although the prevalence of VaD was slightly lower in Japanese Americans than that reported in Japan, it was higher than that reported in European-ancestry populations (White *et al.* 1996). However, there were differences in diagnostic approaches between countries that may have confounded this finding. In Canada, the prevalence of all dementias was found to be significantly lower in Cree Indians compared to Caucasians (0.5% vs. 3.5%, respectively) (Hendrie *et al.* 1993); while in the UK, VaD has been found to be more prevalent than AD in individuals of African Caribbean origin vs. British Caucasians (Livingston *et al.* 2001; Richards *et al.* 2000).

Age-specific estimates of dementia have been more consistent worldwide with a predicted exponential rise in dementia with age. Prevalence studies indicate that dementia doubles approximately every 5 years after the age of 65 (Jorm *et al.* 1987). This increase is more marked for females for whom prevalence is higher in the oldest-old compared to males. Collapsed across studies from Europe, North America, Australasia and Japan, prevalence rates for the five-year age groups from 65 years to 85 and over were found to be 1.4, 2.8, 5.6, 11.1, 23.6, respectively (Jorm *et al.* 1987). A pooling of results from European studies found similar figures (Hofman *et al.* 1991). Findings from three meta-analyses, the Medical Research Council Cognitive Function and Ageing Study (MRC CFAS) (Matthews and Brayne 2005), and the most recent estimates from Knapp *et al.* (2007) are reported in Table 1.4.

Table 1.4 Prevalence rates of dementia from age-specific prevalence meta-analyses, MCR CFAS and latest estimates from Knapp *et al.* (2007)

	Jorm *et al.* 1987	Ritchie *et al.* 1992	Hofman *et al.* 1991	Matthews and Brayne 2005	Knapp *et al.* 2007
60–64	0.7	–	–	–	–
65–69	1.4	1.3	1.4	1.5	1.3
70–74	2.8	2.4	4.1	2.6	2.9
75–79	5.6	4.4	5.7	6.3	5.9
80–84	10.5	8.1	13.0	13	12.2
85–89	20.8	14.9	21.6	25.3	20.3
90–94	38.6	27.3	32.2		28.6
95+	–	50.2	–		32.5

Prevalence estimates for the oldest-old (90 years and over) remain controversial. Age-specific models, although appearing to hold well for certain age groups (65–85 years), assume that prevalence increases at an exponential rate over time, across all ages (Matthews and Brayne 2005). Very high prevalence rates estimated at 77.6% (Jorm *et al.* 1988), 61.6% (Jorm *et al.* 1987), and 39.3% (Ritchie *et al.* 1992) have been reported in the 95-year-old and over age group. However, this is not consistent with other findings of stability in trend for this age group (Ritchie *et al.* 1992; Wernicke and Reischies 1994). This could result from older individuals not living as long with dementia as younger individuals with dementia, or the fact that the survivors into late old age are relatively resistant to developing dementia. Smaller sample sizes and decreased response rate in this age group may also influence findings.

Incidence of dementia

Incidence of dementia rises rapidly with age. Generally, in people younger than 65 years dementia is rare: early-onset dementia (prior to the age of 65 years) is typically observed between 40 and 50 years of age and is very uncommon prior to this, and is generally linked to genetic risk factors (e.g. defect on chromosome 14 and Down's syndrome). The incidence of old-age dementia increases exponentially in individuals aged 65 and older (Barberger-Gateau and Fabrigoule 1997; Cowan *et al.* 2000). This trend, hypothesized to continue with advancing age is found in some, but not all studies (Matthews and Brayne 2005). Incidence of AD increases from approximately 0.2% between 60–69 years old, 1% for people who are 70 years old to 3% for people who are 80 years old to approximately 8% for people who are older than 85 (Barberger-Gateau and Fabrigoule 1997; Patterson and Gass 2001). In contrast, incidence of VaD does not appear to show an age effect (Brayne *et al.* 1995).

Gender effects on incidence are controversial. Some studies suggest that female sex is associated with increased risk. Up to 2000, the number of people with dementia was estimated at about 25 million people worldwide (approximately 0.5% of the whole worldwide population), of which 59% of cases were female (Hofman *et al.* 1991). More recent findings suggest a somewhat stronger pattern of 65% (70% in developed regions and 60% in developing regions) (Fratiglioni *et al.* 2000). One meta-analysis found a subtype difference indicating that women were at a higher risk of AD (Black *et al.* 2001; Dartigues *et al.* 2000; Jorm and Jolley 1998). Another concluded that women had a higher risk of AD at older ages (above 80 years) and that men had a higher risk of VaD at younger ages, but any differences in overall age-specific incidence rates were small (Copeland *et al.* 1999). Cohort studies in the UK and the USA have consistently reported no gender differences in the incidence or prevalence of dementia or AD (Edland *et al.* 2002; Matthews and Brayne 2005). Increased longevity, increased survival with disease and some increase in intrinsic vulnerability probably all play a part in female predominance in some estimates.

Cross-cultural studies reveal lower incidence estimates in Asian populations compared to North American and European populations, particularly for AD. However, more recent findings suggest greater convergence in line with prevalence findings.

In early studies looking at secular changes in the incidence of dementia, no time trends were detected. In a study based in Rochester, Minnesota, incidence rates of AD and dementia were stable between 1960 and 1984, except for a slight increase in the very old (Kokmen *et al.* 1993). Re-analysis incorporating more recent data for the period 1975–1985 confirmed previous findings of absence of a secular trend (Rocca *et al.* 1998). In the Lundby Study in Sweden incidence rates for multi-infarct dementia (caused by multiple strokes) and senile dementias (which typically consist of a group of diseases including Alzheimer's disease and vascular dementia) remained stable from 1947 to 1972.

However, more recent data suggest that rates of dementia in the USA have increased from 1984–1990 to 1991–2000 and that this increase was more marked in persons with stroke compared to the stroke-free population (Ukraintseva *et al.*, 2006).

Variation across regions

Given cultural, demographic and ethnic variability in incidence and prevalence, there is a need for further cross-national and cross-cultural epidemiological studies in indigenous as well as migrating populations. At present it is difficult to establish to what extent findings are merely an artefact of methodology (e.g. sampling procedures and diagnostic criteria), differential exposure to risk factors (e.g. education, health care, cardiovascular disease), demographic changes (e.g. increased numbers of the oldest-old), cultural views on ageing (status of dementia as a 'devastating disease'), response rates or survival trends (Fratiglioni *et al.* 1999). It is also conceivable that differences reflect real geographical and ethnic variations. A marked geographical dissociation in Europe between the north and south, linked to differences in vascular risk factors has been proposed to account for the higher incidence rates in the oldest-old of north-western countries (Finland, Sweden, Denmark, the Netherlands, and the United Kingdom) compared to southern countries (France and Spain) (Fratiglioni *et al.* 2000). This division is further supported by north–south regional findings of differences in MRI-detected white matter lesion (WML) pathology (Launer *et al.* 2006). Greater WML pathology linked to progression of dementia has been observed in southern Europe relative to northern and central European countries. However, this differential based on vascular risk was not replicated in MRC CFAS. Here comparison of incidence across five sites (urban and rural settings) in England and Wales associated with different patterns of vascular risk and mortality failed to find cross-site variation (Matthews and Brayne 2005).

Risk factors

The pathological origin and aetiology of dementia remain unknown. Treatment and prevention will largely depend on the level of understanding of the underlying biological and environmental factors associated with increased risk both in current, as well as future cohorts of older people. Although methodological factors do contribute importantly to reported variations in prevalence, it is also thought that variability could reflect factors relevant for disease pathogenesis or expression in various populations or subgroups (Corrada *et al.* 1995). Conclusions from previous studies have determined that dementia is a complex, multi-factorial process that is essentially under genetic control (Salib 2000). However, there is also compelling evidence for a predominantly acquired (environmental) form of AD. Indeed, Kumar *et al.* (1991) reported detailed neuroanatomical, neuropsychological and neuropathological examination of three monozygous twin pairs containing an individual with onset of AD disease between ages 50 and 60 years. All three twins remained well and each disease-free pair had been AD-free for over a decade. While this does not rule out the operation of genetic influences in the affected members of the pairs, this finding suggests that any such predisposition would have been exaggerated substantially by environmental variation between twin pairs that accelerate disease onset.

Age

Age is the strongest risk factor for dementia. The incidence of dementia has been found to rise exponentially from 65 to 90 years of age (Jorm and Jolley 1998). Beyond this, controversy remains as to whether this trend continues: if dementia is an inevitable consequence of ageing or whether risk plateaus so that some individuals over a reasonable lifespan would never develop the disease (Goa *et al.* 1998; Matthews and Brayne 2005). Age findings are complicated by the lack of consensus as to exactly what cognitive changes occur as a function of the normal ageing process and where the boundary between normal and pathological ageing lies. Furthermore, the extent to which age is responsible for disease, rather than as serving as a proxy for as yet unidentified age-related factors which lead to disease is unclear.

Family history and genetics

Dementia risk can increase two- to four-fold among individuals who have at least one first degree relative with dementia (Devi *et al.* 1999; van Duijn *et al.* 1991). This effect is stronger for those where a relative had early onset and with increased longevity. Risk increases from 5% up to the age of 70, to 33% up to the age of 90 years (Lautenschlager *et al.* 1996). However, while the familial occurrence of dementia may reflect shared environmental factors, there is strong evidence to support a genetic link (Black *et al.* 2001). In very rare cases (less than 5%), AD can be inherited in an autosomal dominant pattern. This occurs when a single abnormal gene on one of the first 22 non-sex chromosomes is inherited. Disease onset is typically in the beginning of middle age (Bird 1994). By the age of 40 almost all individuals with Down's syndrome have neuropathological changes consistent with AD, although onset can be modified by gender and apolipoprotein (ApoE) (Prasher *et al.* 1997; Schupf *et al.* 1998). Furthermore, mutations on the presenilin genes on chromosome 14 (PSI) and chromosome 1 (PSII), which have been found to alter the production or deposition of beta-amyloid in the brain (Selkoe 2001), have been linked to autosomal dominant familial Alzheimer's disease. Phenotypic heterogeneity reflects differences in site and nature of mutation, with PSI linked to early onset and complete penetration, and PSII linked to variable onset and incomplete penetration (Boteva *et al.* 1996; Levy-Lahad *et al.* 1995; Rogaev *et al.* 1995). These risks are most important in the early onset dementia groups, also including Huntington's disease.

Perhaps the clearest genetic risk associated with dementia, particularly AD is the apoliproprotein E (ApoE) gene. This is a plasma protein involved in cholesterol transport and neuronal repair. ApoE has three common variants, the E2, E3 and E4 alleles. Individuals can inherit any combination of these. The E4 allele is a risk factor for Alzheimer's diseases (AD). Within a lifetime the estimated risk of developing AD is 15% for the general population with an increase to 29% for those possessing an E4 allele (Seshadri *et al.* 1995, 1997).

Lifetime risk also increases with the number of E4 alleles: homozygous carriers are at a greater risk than heterozygous carries or those who do not carry the E4 variant. However, these findings are modified by age, gender and ethnicity: risk differentials diminish after the age of 70, in some (Farrer *et al.* 1997; Osuntokun *et al.* 1995), but not all studies (Brayne *et al.* 1996), and the effect is weak in Hispanics, Africans, African Americans and Chinese (Farrer *et al.* 1997). Whether this is a result of differences in the population distribution of ApoE alleles or due to differences in the environmental impact on gene expression is unclear. While this association is strong in many non-population-based studies, it is not always found in population settings and instead appears to be related to specific aspects of cognition (Small *et al.* 2004; Yip *et al.* 2002).

While the relationship between dementia and specific mutations including PSI, PSII, and Down's syndrome is definitive, the relationship between ApoE and dementia is less clear. Exactly how ApoE is involved in the pathogenesis of AD is still not known: ApoE E4 is neither necessary nor sufficient for dementia and rather appears to operate as a risk modifier. The clinical role of ApoE testing remains unclear and therefore is not recommended for routine testing in susceptible individuals (Patterson *et al.* 2001).

Exercise 1.2 Is dementia inherited?

Someone hears you are working with people with dementia and approaches you with deep concern on their face. 'My mother, aunt, uncle and grand-mother all had dementia. Is it inevitable that I too will get it?'

How would you reply?

List three sources of evidence to suggest that the person is at an increased risk of developing dementia.

List three sources of evidence to suggest that they are not.

Lifestyle risk factors

Risk findings for alcohol and smoking are not consistent. Alcohol has been found to have a protective effect in moderate drinkers with a five-fold increase in dementia in both abstainers and those who drink heavily (Anttila *et al.* 2004; Orgogozo *et al.* 1997). However, Orgogozo *et al.* (1997) found a link between increasing alcohol consumption and VaD. With regard to smoking, after adjusting for age, ApoE, education, cardiovascular and respiratory factors, Tyas *et al.* (2003) found an increased risk of AD with medium and high levels of smoking, but not for very heavy levels of smoking. Smoking is known to cause cardiovascular and respiratory diseases which are both risk factors for AD. For heavy smokers it could be that they are not living long enough to develop dementia. In some studies alcohol and smoking (never, past and current) are neither strongly protective nor predictive (Doll *et al.* 2000), while in others both have been associated with an increase in the age-specific onset rate of AD (Brayne 2000). Conflicting results as to the direction of association between smoking and AD may be due to survival bias and methodological differences across studies. Yet, if smoking and drinking do confer increased risk of dementia, educational programmes on prevention and cessation will become important public health priorities.

Healthy diet spanning across life may have a protective effect. A role for dietary antioxidants (from foods containing vitamin E especially vegetables, beta-carotene, omega-3 and vitamin C) in preventing or delaying dementia has been found (Engelhart *et al.* 2002). Higher adherence to a Mediterranean diet (high in fruit and vegetables, grain, and unsaturated fats, and low in meat and dairy products) has recently been found to significantly lower the risk of developing AD, even after adjusting for age, gender, ethnicity, education, caloric intake, weight, smoking and comorbid conditions (Scarmeas *et al.* 2006). However, these findings have not been replicated, particularly in clinical trials (the most rigorous form of clinical research to determine the impact of an intervention). Inconsistency in findings and questions regarding the accuracy of diet measurement suggests that no definitive evidence exists for dietary recommendations for the prevention of dementia beyond general exhortation of healthy diet and lifestyle to minimize vascular risk.

Vascular factors

Vascular factors and conditions, including history of stroke or transient ischaemic attack (TIA), diabetes mellitus, hypertension, congestive heart failure and obesity are major risks for cognitive decline and dementia by accelerating Alzheimer-type changes in the brain. Indeed, vascular disease is thought to reduce blood flow to the brain and hypoperfusion (decreased blood flow through an organ) has been found to cause oxidative stress, neurodegeneration and cognitive decline (de la Torre 2002). The hypothesis that both the clinical expression and severity of dementia (including AD and VaD) are mediated at least in part by the presence of cerebrovascular disease is supported by imaging findings where individuals with lacunar infarcts in the basal ganglia, thalamus or deep white matter have a higher prevalence of dementia compared to those without infarcts (Snowdon *et al.* 1997). Stroke and hypertension accelerate atrophy and degenerative changes resulting from neuronal shrinkage or loss (de la Torre 2002). The aggregation of risk factors is suggested to have a greater impact on the development of dementia than each factor independently. Furthermore, the relationship between vascular factors and dementia has been found to be moderated by various genetic and non-genetic factors including ApoE and age. Attention to these modifiable risk factors will have important implications for reducing the incidence and prevalence of dementia.

Exercise 1.3   Can we prevent dementia?

Health promotion and prevention of chronic illness in later life are now common approaches in the government's approach to health care. Get a hold of last week's newspaper and leaf through looking for examples of health promotion in relation to chronic health conditions including dementia.

List all the examples that you find.

How many of the examples have to do with dementia?

What do you think is the reason for this?

Hypertension and anti-hypertensives

Mid-life hypertension (high blood pressure) has been associated with impaired cognitive function even in otherwise healthy individuals. It has been suggested that for every 10 mmHg rise in blood pressure the risk of impairment to cognitive function rises 7% (Peters 2001) although some studies have found no association between high blood pressure, its reduction and cognitive function. Traditionally it is VaD that has been considered affected by hypertension and the alleviation of it. However, recent data suggest that vascular factors may influence the clinical expression of AD although the extent to which this reflects a true increase in the risk of AD rather than the combination of AD and small strokes is not clear (Bennett 2000). Nonetheless, hypertensive treatment has been found to reduce the incidence of AD (Peters 2001) although it is currently difficult to separate the effects of blood pressure reduction and/or the direct action of the anti-hypertensives themselves on the preservation of cognitive function. For example, while some medications (e.g. diuretics) may have adverse effects on cognitive function, others (e.g. some angiotensin converting enzyme (ACE) inhibitors) are known not to have a deleterious effect (Peters 2001).

Mild cognitive impairment

Clinical criteria dictate that the onset of dementia is preceded by a prodromal state of mild cognitive decline and, unsurprisingly, individuals with mild cognitive impairment (MCI) have been found to be at increased risk of dementia conversion compared to normal unimpaired individuals (5–15% per year versus 1–3%, respectively). However, although defined as a risk factor for AD, the clinical course of MCI is not always pathological. While in some studies impairment has been associated with increased risk of progression to AD, in others, individuals remain stable or even show improved cognitive functioning at follow-up (Portet *et al.* 2006). Variability is probably due to population selection, threshold for impairment, follow-up interval and operationalization of criteria. Indeed, rates of conversion to dementia are generally highest among clinic-based samples and for definitions of MCI where a memory impairment predominates. Yet the diagnosis of MCI remains difficult. Many forms have been identified (Stephan *et al.* 2007). Due to a lack of standardized diagnostic criteria the prevalence in older populations has varied widely between studies (3–36%) with an incidence of 8–58% per thousand per year (Busse *et al.* 2003). Furthermore, defining what distinguishes this condition from normal age-associated changes, early dementia and dementia itself is unclear. Whether this condition is distinct from early AD has been questioned and there is growing evidence that this, and related systems, are unstable in population-based studies.

Education

People who have less than six years of formal education are reported to have a higher risk of developing dementia, particularly AD (Black *et al.* 2001). Education as a protective factor has been linked to the ability to compensate for cognitive decline, thus delaying the diagnosis of dementia (Mortimer 1988). It has also been hypothesized that this effect may be mediated by brain reserve/size (Schofield *et al.* 1997). Whether it is education itself that makes a difference or other related factors such as occupational status and income level that can account for these effects is unclear.

Head injury

Head trauma with loss of consciousness is a risk factor for dementia in some but not all studies (Bennett 2000; Haan and Wallace 2004; Salib 2000). Several hypotheses have been offered to explain the association, including neuronal damage, which reduces neuronal reserve and causes release of amyloid (Bennett 2000). An interaction between head injury and ApoE E4 has also been reported (Bennett 2000; Kukull and Ganguli 2000) with the potential explanation that the E4 allele is associated with inadequate neuronal repair and deposition of beta-amyloid after injury (Kukull and Ganguli 2000). The hypothesis of head trauma as a risk factor for AD comes from the observation of neurofibrillary tangles, indistinguishable from those seen in AD in the brains of boxers with dementia pugilistica (Breteler *et al.* 1992). However, the possibility that head trauma may be a consequence of an early stage of the dementia cannot be excluded. For example, although an association has been consistently found in case-control studies, there is considerable opportunity for recall bias for events that occurred long before disease onset and the association has not also been confirmed in population-based studies.

Other risk factors

Other risk factors include brain tumour, kidney failure, liver disease, thyroid disease, vitamin deficiencies (B12, folic acid, thiamine), chronic inflammatory conditions (such as certain forms of arthritis), a history of episodes of clinical depression, stress, inadequate mental exercise, exposure to aluminium, pesticides and other toxins (see van der Flier and Scheltens (2005) for an overview). The unique risk associated with each and the timing of their effect are still yet to be determined. Furthermore, there is no age cut-off at which the major risk factors for disease become insignificant.

Summary of risk

A number of risk and protective factors for dementia, in particular AD, have been reported in the literature. The general conclusion is that the pathophysiology of dementia is very complex and may include genetic, physiologic, psychological, as well as lifestyle elements, some of which may be linked. In fact, the multi-environmental and genetic risk factors for dementia suggest that it is a clinical syndrome analogous in aetiology to cancer (Jones 1997). The heterogeneous genetic influences on dementia have probably contributed substantially to difficulties in the detection of host or environmental factors associated with modified disease. There is a need to better understand both the genetic and environmental mechanisms that may modify these effects. These alleged linkages offer the basis for potential intervention for the prevention or the slowing down of those processes that lead to disease (Nourhashemi *et al.* 2000). Because of the number of people who are expected to be affected by dementia, just shifting the prevalence curve slightly to the right could have a huge impact on numbers and a substantial effect on health care costs depending on the extent to which survival is lengthened.

Studies that combine clinical and pathological assessment have a special role in the search for potential risk factors. A small number of ongoing longitudinal epidemiological studies include a post-mortem brain donation programme (e.g. the Nun Study, the Religious Orders Study, the Baltimore Longitudinal Study on Aging, the Medical Research Council Cognitive Function and Ageing Study, the Cambridge City Over-75s Cohort Study (CC75C); the Vantaa 85+ Study, the Cache County Study). This provides researchers with an opportunity to examine the neuropathology and molecular biology underlying the changes associated with dementia and link risk factors directly to brain pathology to understand how risk factors lead to clinical disease.

Disability and mortality associated with dementia

Disability

Dementia is one of the leading causes of non-fatal disability in the developed world and by 2030 it is predicted that dementia will be the third leading cause of years of life lost due to death and disability (measured using the concept of disability adjusted life years (DALYs) which combines a measure of the average years of life lost due to disease with the years lived with disability) in high-income countries (Mathers and Loncar 2006). Indeed, in developed countries dementia accounts for more than half of all DALYs in the domain of burdensome neuropsychiatric disorders (Murray and Lopez 1996). In the WHO Global Burden of Disease (GBD) report (WHO 2003), it was estimated that the disability from dementia is higher than almost all conditions with the exception of spinal cord injury and terminal cancer. The World Health Organization Report 2003 estimated that for people aged 60 years and over dementia contributed 11.2% of all years lived with disability, while stroke contributed 9.5%, musculoskeletal disorders 8.9%, cardiovascular disease 5.0% and all forms of cancer 2.4%. With increasing pressure on health care budgets, accurate estimations of the type and distribution of dementia in addition to the burden it causes are necessary to help quantify health care needs and highlight areas for future research into curative and preventative strategies.

The disability associated with dementia is unevenly distributed across the world and is greater in developed countries. Furthermore, it is also related to age and gender, being greater in females and in the oldest-old. However, increases in male life expectancy and a shift in the age demographic of developing countries are predicted to result in an increased number of elderly individuals and non-communicable diseases, such as dementia, in these groups.

Mortality

It is estimated that in the high-income countries AD and other dementias are the seventh leading cause of death, accounting for 3.6% of total deaths. Studies from developed countries report a median survival time after the onset of dementia symptoms ranging from 5.0 to 9.3 years (Walsh *et al.* 1990), while in developing countries the reported median survival is 3.3 years for all demented individuals and 2.7 years for those with AD (Chandra *et al.* 1998). Overall, individuals with dementia have poorer survival and a shorter life expectancy than those without, with the risk of mortality greater the earlier the disease onset.

Debates and controversies

To what extent do classification concepts of mild cognitive impairment (MCI) accurately capture those at risk of progressing to dementia? The clinical course is not always pathological: while in some studies impairment has been associated with increased risk of progression to AD, in others, individuals remain stable or even show improved cognitive functioning at follow-up. The lack of consistency in definition may explain the resulting discrepancy conversion rates.

Diagnostic criteria for Alzheimer's disease and for vascular dementia are mutually exclusive. Yet mixed forms are common. Do we not need accepted criteria for mixed dementia?

Should the same factors (e.g. life expectancy and diet) be taken into consideration when estimating prevalence of dementia across the developed and developing world? How accurate are our calculations and what assumptions are we making?

What are the risk and protective factors for dementia? Question of the risk associated with exposure to aluminium and the role of genetic and environmental factors (e.g. alcohol, smoking, diet) in moderating risk.

Conclusion

Dementia is set to become a worldwide epidemic. Accurate estimates of both prevalence and incidence are necessary not only as a foundation for health and social policy but also to generate awareness. Of particular importance is a focus on developing countries where there is to be a more rapid demographic shift resulting in an increase in the number of elderly individuals and non-communicable diseases. The global challenge to policy makers is two-fold: (1) to implement immediate policy and infrastructure for the future provision and health care for the older population in all regions of the world; and (2) development of preventative strategies and treatment to delay disease onset and progression. Application of these measures is critical in less-developed countries which have a shorter timeframe to adjust to an ageing population. Findings from developed countries show that the prevalence of chronic diseases and level of disability can be ameliorated with appropriate health care and prevention strategies. Opportunities missed by developing counties may have devastating economic and social consequences.

Further information

The **Cognitive and Functional Ageing Study** (CFAS) is a large longitudinal multi-centre population-based study of cognitive decline and dementia in people aged 65 and over living in the UK.

The **World Health Organization** is the directing and coordinating authority for health within the United Nations system.

The **Alzheimer Research Forum** is an independent non-profit-making organization. Its website reports on the latest scientific findings, from basic research to clinical trials; creates and maintains public databases of essential research data and reagents, and produces discussion forums to promote debate, speed the dissemination of new ideas, and break down barriers across the numerous disciplines that can contribute to the global effort to cure Alzheimer's disease.

Alzheimer's Disease International is an umbrella organization of national Alzheimer Associations around the world.

The **Alzheimer's Research Trust** is a research charity for dementia in the UK. It is dedicated to funding scientific studies to find ways to treat, cure or prevent Alzheimer's disease, vascular dementia, Lewy Body disease and fronto-temporal dementia.

The report of the **United Nations Department of Economic and Social Affairs,** Population Division, entitled *World Population Ageing 2000*, presents the current assessment of the status of the world's older population and prospects for the future. It provides a description of global trends in population ageing and includes key indicators of the ageing process for each of the major areas, regions and countries of the world.

References

Anttila, T., Helkala, E., Viitanen, M., Kareholt, I., Fratiglioni, L. *et al.* (2004) Alcohol drinking in middle age and subsequent risk of mild cognitive impairment and dementia in old age: a prospective population based study. *British Medical Journal*, 329: 539.

Barberger-Gateau, P. and Fabrigoule, C. (1997) Disability and cognitive impairment in the elderly. *Disability Rehabilitation*, 19: 175–93.

Bennett, D.A. (2000) Part I. Epidemiology and public health impact of Alzheimer's disease. *Disease of the Month*, 46: 657–65.

Bird, T.D. (1994) Clinical genetics of familial Alzheimer disease. In R.D Terry, R. Katzman and K.L. Bick (eds) *Alzheimer Disease*. New York: Raven Press, pp. 65–74.

Black, S.E., Patterson, C. and Feightner, J. (2001) Preventing dementia. *Canadian Journal of Neurology Science*, 28 (Suppl 1): S56–66.

Boteva, K., Vitek, M., Mitsuda, H., de Silva, H., Xu, P.T. *et al.* (1996) Mutation analysis of presenillin 1 gene in Alzheimer's disease. *Lancet*, 347: 130–1.

Brayne, C. (2000) Smoking and the brain. *British Medical Journal*, 320: 1087–8.

Brayne, C., Gill, C., Huppert, F.A., Barkley, C., Gehlhaar, E. *et al.* (1995) Incidence of clinically diagnosed subtypes of dementia in an elderly population. Cambridge Project for Later Life. *British Journal of Psychiatry*, 167: 255–62.

Brayne, C., Harrington, C.R., Wischik, C.M., Huppert, F.A., Chi L.Y. *et al.* (1996) Apolipoprotein E genotype in the prediction of cognitive decline and dementia in a prospectively studied elderly population. *Dementia*, 7: 169–74.

Breteler, M.M., Claus, J.J., van Duijn, C.M., Launer, L.J. and Hofman, A. (1992) Epidemiology of Alzheimer's disease. *Epidemiologic Reviews*, 14: 59–89.

Busse, A., Bischkopf, J., Riedel-Heller, S.G. and Angermeyer, M.C. (2003) Mild cognitive impairment: 1 prevalence and predictive validity according to current approaches. *Acta Neurologica Scandinavica*, 108: 71–81.

Chandra, V., Ganguli, M., Pandav, R., Johnston, J., Belle, S. *et al.* (1998) Prevalence of Alzheimer's disease and other dementias in rural India: the Indo-US study. *Neurology*, 51: 1000–8.

Chiu, H.F.K. and Zhang, M. (2000) Dementia research in China. *International Journal of Geriatric Psychiatry*, 15: 947–53.

Copeland, J.R., McCracken, C.F., Dewey, M.E., Wilson, K.C., Doran, M. *et al.* (1999) Undifferentiated dementia, Alzheimer's disease and vascular dementia: age- and gender-related incidence in Liverpool. The MRC-ALPHA Study. *British Journal of Psychiatry*, 175: 433–8.

Corrada, M., Brookmeyer, R. and Kawas, C. (1995) Sources of variability in prevalence rates of Alzheimer's disease. *International Journal of Epidemiology*, 24: 1000–5.

Cowan, L.D., Leviton, A. and Dammann, O. (2000) New research directions in neuroepidemiology. *Epidemiology Review*, 22: 18–23.

Dartigues, J.F., Letenneur, L., Joly, P., Helmer, C., Orgogozo, J. *et al.* (2000) Age specific risk of dementia according to gender, education and wine consumption. *Neurobiology of Aging*, 21: 64.

de la Torre, J.C. (2002) Alzheimer disease as a vascular disorder: nosological evidence. *Stroke*, 33: 1152–62.

Devi, G., Ottman, R., Tang, M., Marder, K., Stern, Y. *et al.* (1999) Influence of APOE genotype on familial aggregation of AD in an urban population. *Neurology*, 53: 789.

Dewey, M.E. and Saz, P. (2001) Dementia, cognitive impairment and mortality in persons aged 65 and over living in the community: a systematic review of the literature. *International Journal of Geriatric Epidemiology*, 16: 751–61.

Doll, R., Peto, R., Boreham, J. and Sutherland, I. (2000) Smoking and dementia in male British doctors: prospective study. *British Medical Journal*, 320: 1097–102.

Edland, S.D., Rocca, W.A., Petersen, R.C., Cha, R.H. and Kokmen, E. (2002) Dementia and Alzheimer disease incidence rates do not vary by sex in Rochester, Minn. *Archives of Neurology*, 59: 1589–93.

Engelhart, M.J., Geerlings, M.I., Ruitenberg, A., van Swieten, J.C., Hofman, A. *et al.* (2002) Diet and risk of dementia: Does fat matter? The Rotterdam Study. *Neurology*, 59: 1915–21.

Farrer, L.A., Cupples, L.A., Haines, J.L., Hyman, B., Kukull, W.A. *et al.* (1997) Effects of age, sex, and ethnicity on the association between apolipoprotein E genotype and Alzheimer disease: A meta-analysis. APOE and Alzheimer Disease Meta Analysis Consortium. *Journal of the American Medical Association*, 278: 1349–56.

Ferri, C.P., Prince, M., Brayne, C., Brodaty, H., Fratiglioni, L. *et al.* (2005) Global prevalence of dementia: a Delphi consensus study. *Lancet*, 366: 2112–17.

Fratiglioni, L., de Ronchi, D., Aguero-Torres, H. (1999) Worldwide prevalence and incidence of dementia. *Drugs Aging*, 15: 365–75.

Fratiglioni, L., Launer, L.J., Andersen, K., Breteler, M.M., Copeland, J.R. *et al.* (2000) Incidence of dementia and major subtypes in Europe: a collaborative study of population-based cohorts. Neurologic Diseases in the Elderly Research Group. *Neurology*, 54: S10–15.

Goa, S., Hendrie, H., Hall, K. and Hui, S. (1998) The relationships between age, sex, and the incidence of dementia and Alzheimer's disease: A meta-analysis. *General Psychiatry*, 55: 809–12.

Haan, M.N. and Wallace, R. (2004) Can dementia be prevented? Brain aging in a population-based context. *Annual Review of Public Health*, 25: 1–24.

Hatada, K., Okazaki, Y., Yoshitake, K., Takada, K. and Nakane, Y. (1999) Further evidence of Westernization of dementia prevalence in Nagasaki, Japan, and family recognition. *International Psychogeriatrics*, 11: 123–38.

Hendrie, H.C., Hall, K.S., Pillay, N., Rodgers, D., Prince, C. *et al.* (1993) Alzheimer's disease is rare in Cree. *International Psychogeriatrics*, 5: 5–14.

Hendrie, H.C., Ogunniyi, A., Hall, K.S., Baiyewu, O., Unverzagt, F.W. *et al.* (2001) Incidence of dementia and Alzheimer disease in 2 communities: Yoruba residing in Ibadan, Nigeria, and African Americans residing in Indianapolis, Indiana. *Journal of the American Medical Association*, 285: 739–47.

Hofman, A., Rocca, W.A., Brayne, C., Breteler, M.M.B., Clarke, M. *et al.* (1991) The prevalence of dementia in Europe: a collaborative study of 1980–1990 findings. *International Journal of Epidemiology*, 20: 736–48.

Ineichen, B. (1998) The geography of dementia: an approach through epidemiology. *Health and Place*, 4: 383–94.

Jones, R.W. (1997) Dementia. *Scottish Medicine Journal*, 42: 151–3.

Jorm, A.F. and Jolley, D. (1998) The incidence of dementia: a meta-analysis. *Neurology*, 51: 728–33.

Jorm, A.F., Korten, A.E. and Henderson, A.S. (1987) The prevalence of dementia: a quantitative integration of the literature. *Psychiatrica Scandinavica*, 76: 465–79.

Jorm, A.F., Korten, A.E. and Jacomb, P.A. (1988) Projected increases in the number of dementia cases for 29 developed countries: application of a new method for making projections. *Acta Psychiatrica Scandinavica*, 78: 493–500.

Knapp, M., Comas-Herrera, A., Somani, A. and Banerjee, S. (2007) *Dementia: International Comparisons*. PSSRU, LSE, www.pssru.ac.uk/pdf/dp(2418)pdf (accessed 12 April 2008).

Kokmen, E., Beard, C.M., O'Brien, P.C., Offord, K.P. and Kurland, L.T. (1993) Is the incidence of dementing illness changing? A 25-year time trend study in Rochester, Minnesota (1960–1984). *Neurology*, 43: 1887.

Kua, E.H. and Ko, S.M. (1995) Prevalence of dementia among elderly Chinese and Malay residents of Singapore. *International Psychogeriatrics*, 7: 439–46.

Kukull, W.A. and Ganguli, M. (2000) Epidemiology of dementia: concepts and overview. *Neurologic Clinics*, 18: 923–49.

Kumar, A., Schapiro, M.B., Grady, C.L., Matocha, M.F., Haxby, J.V. *et al.* (1991) Anatomic, metabolic, neuropsychological, and molecular genetic studies of three pairs of identical twins discordant for dementia of the Alzheimer's type. *Archives of Neurology*, 48: 160–8.

Ladislas, R. (2000) Cellular and molecular mechanisms of aging and age related diseases. *Pathology and Oncology Research*, 6: 3–9.

Launer, L.J., Berger, K., Breteler, M.M., Dufouil, C., Fuhrer, R. *et al.* (2006) Regional variability in the prevalence of cerebral white matter lesions: an MRI study in 9 European countries (CASCADE). *Neuroepidemiology*, 26: 23–9.

Lautenschlager, N.T., Cupples, L.A., Rao, V.S., Auerbach, S.A., Becker, R. *et al.* (1996) Risk of dementia among relatives of Alzheimer's disease patients in the MIRAGE study: What is in store for the oldest old? *Neurology*, 46: 641–50.

Lee, D.Y., Lee, J.H., Ju, Y.S., Lee, K.U., Kim, K.W. *et al.* (2002) The prevalence of dementia in older people in an urban population of Korea: The Seoul Study. *Journal of the American Geriatrics Society*, 50: 1233–9.

Levy-Lahad, E., Wasco, W., Poorkaj, P., Romano, D.M., Oshima, J. *et al.* (1995) Candidate gene for the chromosome 1 familial Alzheimer's disease locus. *Science*, 269: 973–7.

Liu, C.K., Lai, C.L., Tai, C.T., Lin, R.T., Yen, Y.Y. *et al.* (1998) Incidence and subtypes of dementia in southern Taiwan: impact of socio-demographic factors. *Neurology*, 50: 1572–9.

Liu, H.C., Lin, K.N., Teng, E.L., Wang, S.J., Fuh, J.L. *et al.* (1995) Prevalence and subtypes of dementia in Taiwan: a community survey of 5297 individuals. *Journal of the American Geriatrics Society*, 43: 144–9.

Livingston, G., Leavey, G., Kitchen, G., Manela, M., Sembhi, S. *et al.* (2001) Mental health of migrant elders: the Islington Study. *British Journal of Psychiatry*, 179: 361–6.

Mathers, C.D. and Loncar, D. (2006) Projections of global mortality and burden of disease from 2002 to 2030. PLoS Med 3: e442.

Matthews, F. and Brayne, C. (2005) The incidence of dementia in England and Wales: findings from the five identical sites of the MRC CFA Study. PLoS Med 2: e193.

Miles, T.P., Froehlich, T.E., Bogardus, S.T. and Inouye, S.K. (2001) Dementia and race: Are there differences between African Americans and Caucasians? *Journal of the American Geriatrics Society*, 49: 477–84.

Mortimer, J.A. (1988) Do psychosocial risk factors contribute to Alzheimer's disease? In A.S. Henderson and J.H. Henderson (eds) *Etiology of Dementia of Alzheimer's Type*. New York: Wiley, pp. 39–52.

Murray, C.J.L. and Lopez, A.D. (eds) (1996) *The Global Burden of Disease: A Comprehensive Assessment of Mortality and Disability from Diseases, Injuries and Risk Factors in 1990 and Projected to (2020)*. Cambridge, MA: Harvard University Press.

Nourhashemi, F., Gillette-Guyonnet, S., Andrieu, S., Ghisolfi, A., Ousset, P.J. *et al.* (2000) Alzheimer disease: protective factors. *American Journal of Clinical Nutrition*, 71: 643S–649S.

O'Connor, D.W., Blessed, G., Cooper, B., Jonker, C., Morris, J.C. *et al.* (1996) Cross-national interrater reliability of dementia diagnosis in the elderly and factors associated with disagreement. *Neurology*, 47: 1194–9.

Office for National Statistics (ONS) (2003) *Living in Britain: Results from the 2002 General Household Survey*. London: TSO.

Orgogozo, J.M., Dartigues, J.F., Lafont, S., Letenneur, L., Commenges, D. *et al.* (1997) Wine consumption and dementia in the elderly: a prospective community study in the Bordeaux area. *Revue Neurologique* (Paris), 153: 185–92.

Osuntokun, B.O., Sahota, A., Ogunniyi, A.O., Gureje, O., Baiyewu, O. *et al.* (1995) Lack of an association between apolipoprotein E epsilon 4 and Alzheimer's disease in elderly Nigerians. *Annals of Neurology*, 38: 463–5.

Patterson, C. and Gass, D.A. (2001) Screening for cognitive impairment and dementia in the elderly. *Canadian Journal of Neurological Sciences*, 28: S42–51.

Patterson, C., Grek, A., Gauthier, S., Bergman, H., Cohen, C. *et al.* (2001) The recognition, assessment and management of dementing disorders: conclusions from the Canadian Consensus Conference on Dementia. *Canadian Journal of Neurological Sciences*, 28: 3–16.

Peters, R. (2001) The prevention of dementia. *Journal of Cardiovascular Risk*, 8: 253–6.

Portet, F., Ousset, P.J., Visser, P.J., Frisoni, G.B., Nobili, J. *et al.* (2006) Mild cognitive impairment in medical practice: critical review of the concept and new diagnostic procedure. Report of the MCI Working Group of the European Consortium on Alzheimer's disease (EADC). *Journal of Neurology, Neurosurgery, and Psychiatry*: http://jnnp.bmj.com/cgi/content/abstract/jnnp.2005.085332v1 (accessed 12 April 2008).

Prasher, V.P., Chowdhury, T.A., Rowe, B.R. and Bain, S.C. (1997) ApoE genotype and Alzheimer's disease in adults with Down syndrome: meta-analysis. *American Journal of Mental Retardation*, 102: 103–10.

Prince, M. (2000) Dementia in developing countries: a consensus statement from the 10/66 Dementia Research Group. *International Journal of Geriatric Psychiatry*, 15: 14–20.

Richards, M., Brayne, C., Dening, T., Abas, M., Carter, J. *et al.* (2000) Cognitive function in UK community-dwelling African Caribbean and white elders: a pilot study. *International Journal of Geriatric Psychiatry*, 15: 621–30.

Ritchie, K., Kildea, D. and Robine, J.M. (1992) The relationship between age and prevalence of senile dementia: a meta-analysis of recent data. *International Journal of Epidemiology*, 21: 763–9.

Rocca, W.A., Cha, R.H., Waring, S.C. and Kokmen, E. (1998) Incidence of dementia and Alzheimer's disease: A reanalysis of data from Rochester, Minnesota, 1975–1984. *American Journal of Epidemiology*, 148: 51–62.

Rogaev, E.I., Sherrington, R., Rogaeva, E.A., Levesque, G., Ikeda, M. *et al.* (1995) Familial Alzheimer's disease in kindreds with missense mutations in a gene on chromosome 1 related to the Alzheimer's disease type 3 gene. *Nature*, 376: 775–8.

Salib, E. (2000) Risk factors for Alzheimer's disease. *Elder Care*, 11: 12–15.

Scarmeas, N., Stern, Y., Tang, M.X., Mayeux, R. and Luchsinger, J.A. (2006) Mediterranean diet and risk for Alzheimer's disease. *Annals of Neurology*, 59: 912–21.

Schofield, P.W., Logroscino, G., Andrews, H.F., Albert, S. and Stern, Y. (1997) An association between head circumference and Alzheimer's disease in a population-based study of aging and dementia. *Neurology*, 49: 30–7.

Schupf, N., Kapell, D., Nightingale, B., Rodriguez, A., Tycko, B. *et al.* (1998) Earlier onset of Alzheimer's disease in men with Down syndrome. *Neurology*, 50: 991–5.

Selkoe, D.J. (2001) Alzheimer's disease: Genes, proteins, and therapy. *Physiology Review*, 81: 741–66.

Seshadri, S., Drachman, D.A. and Lippa, C.F. (1995) Apolipoprotein E epsilon 4 allele and the lifetime risk of Alzheimer's disease: What physicians know, and what they should know. *Archives of Neurology*, 52: 1074–9.

Seshadri, S., Wolf, P.A., Beiser, A., Au, R., McNulty, K. *et al.* (1997) Lifetime risk of dementia and Alzheimer's disease: The impact of mortality on risk estimates in the Framingham Study. *Neurology*, 49: 1498–1504.

Shigeta, M. (2004) Epidemiology: rapid increase in Alzheimer's disease prevalence in Japan. *Psychogeriatrics*, 4: 117–19.

Skoog, I. (1998) Status of risk factors for vascular dementia. *Neuroepidemiology*, 17: 2–9.

Small, B.J., Rosnick, C.B., Fratiglioni, L. and Backman, L. (2004) Apolipoprotein E and cognitive performance: a meta-analysis. *Psychology and Aging*, 19: 592–600.

Snowdon, D.A., Greiner, L.H., Mortimer, J.A., Riley, K.P., Greiner, P.A. *et al.* (1997) Brain infarction and the clinical expression of Alzheimer disease: The Nun Study. *Journal of the American Medical Association*, 277: 813–17.

Stephan, B.C.M., Matthews, F.E., McKeith, I., Bond, J., Brayne, C. *et al.* (2007). Early cognitive change in the general population: how do different definitions work? *Journal of the American Geriatrics Society*, 55(10): 1534–40.

Tyas, S.L., White, L.R., Petrovitch, H., Webster Ross, G., Foley, D.J. *et al.* (2003) Mid-life smoking and late-life dementia: the Honolulu–Asia Aging Study. *Neurobiology of Aging*, 24: 589–96.

Ukraintseva, S., Sloan, F., Arbeev, K. and Yashin, A. (2006) Increasing rates of dementia at time of declining mortality from stroke. *Stroke,* 37(5): 1155–9.

United Nations Department of Economic and Social Affairs, Population Division (2007) *World Population Ageing 2000.* http://www.un.org/esa/population/publications/WPA2007/ES-English.pdf (accessed 12 April 2008).

United Nations Population Division (2007) *World Population Prospects.* New York: United Nations. Available at: http://esa.un.org/unpp (accessed 14 April 2008).

van der Flier, W.M. and Scheltens, P. (2005) Epidemiology and risk factors of dementia. *Journal of Neurology, Neurosurgery, and Psychiatry*, 76: 2–7.

van Duijn, C.M., Hendriks, L., Cruts, M., Hardy, J.A., Hofman, A. *et al.* (1991) Amyloid precursor protein gene mutation in early-onset Alzheimer's disease. *Lancet*, 337: 978.

Walsh, J.S., Welch, H.G. and Larson, E.B. (1990) Survival of outpatients with Alzheimer-type dementia. *Annals of Internal Medicine*, 113: 429–34.

Wernicke, T.F. and Reischies, F.M. (1994) Prevalence of dementia in old age: clinical diagnoses in subjects aged 95 years and older. *Neurology*, 44: 250–3.

White, L.R. (1992) Towards a program of cross-cultural research on the epidemiology of Alzheimer's disease. *Current Science*, 63: 456–69.

White, L., Petrovitch, H., Ross, G.W., Masaki, K.H., Abbott, R.D. *et al.* (1996) Prevalence of dementia in older Japanese-American men in Hawaii: The Honolulu-Asia Aging Study. *Journal of the American Medical Association*, 276: 955–60.

World Health Organization (WHO) (2003) *Global Burden of Disease (GBD) Report*. Geneva: WHO.

Yip, A.G., Brayne, C., Easton, D. and Rubinsztein, D.C. (2002) An investigation of ACE as a risk factor for dementia and cognitive decline in the general population. *Journal of Medical Genetics*, 39: 403–6.

2

Toward understanding subjective experiences of dementia

Alison Phinney

Learning objectives

By the end of this chapter, you will be able to:

- explain how people with dementia may experience the impact of the illness on their everyday activities and social involvements
- explain how people with dementia use both active and emotion-focused strategies to cope with the challenges they face in their everyday lives
- evaluate the methods that researchers have used to elicit the views of people with dementia

---

Introduction

Excellence in dementia care begins with an understanding of what it is like to live with dementia. To develop best practices that meet the needs of people with dementia while building on their enduring skills and strengths, it is necessary to have insight into how they themselves perceive their needs and strengths. However, it has long been assumed that people with dementia cannot reliably report their subjective experiences, and as a result their voices have not been heard until very recently.

Preliminary reports of studies conducted to explore the subjective experiences of people with dementia began to appear in the early 1990s (Cotrell and Schulz 1993; Downs 1997; Woods 2001). Over the past 15 years, this body of work has grown slowly but steadily, to the point where there now exists enough evidence to provide a basis for a beginning answer to the question 'What it is like to live with dementia?'

Current research exploring the experiences of people with dementia provides some preliminary direction in terms of understanding the impact of this illness on people's lives and how they manage the many challenges they face. Everyday activities become increasingly difficult to accomplish and people find themselves ever more disconnected from the social world. They feel angry, frightened and despondent as they lose confidence and a sense of their own self-worth. But at the same time, people may find ways to manage the effects of this illness so their life can continue to be satisfying and worth living. They use a variety of problem-solving approaches to conquer everyday challenges and they find ways to think about their illness that allow them to overcome feelings of hopelessness and despair. The aim of this chapter is to review and summarize this work to better understand what people with dementia are saying about their experience.

Impact of dementia on everyday life

It should come as no surprise that living with dementia is difficult. Certainly the enormous literature on caregiver burden would suggest as much. It is well known that people with dementia experience multiple losses and require increasing assistance with simple everyday tasks as the disease progresses. But it is important to listen carefully to what people with dementia are themselves saying about what it is like to live with this every day.

Difficulty taking part in activities

One consistent theme in the research literature relates to how people with dementia find it difficult to take part in various activities. They report being less able to do the things they used to do, and as a result, everyday life becomes hard work. Activities that had once been easy and taken for granted now require careful thought and attention (Imhof 2003; Nygard and Borell 1998). For example, a retired schoolteacher explained how he could no longer knot his tie in the morning without a great deal of repeated effort. 'I had to practice my tie not long ago. I had to go and get my tie out, put it on and take it off again, put it on, take it off. It's the familiar moves I'm supposed to not have to practice' (Phinney 2000).

Whether it is sorting though the mail, adjusting a thermostat, or potting a plant, this need to think things through and practise activities that were once routine has the effect of slowing down the pace of everyday life (Phinney and Chesla 2003). Getting through an activity simply takes longer, often to the point where people find themselves lost in time itself. Their sense of passing time has become less reliable and they are no longer sure of when something occurs or how long it takes (Nygard and Johansson 2001).

People with dementia usually explained their problems with activity as being the result of their poor memory, saying things like 'I can't remember anything at all about what I do' (Gillies 2000: 368; see also Clare 2002; Imhof 2003; Ostwald *et al.* 2002; Parsons 2005; Pearce *et al.* 2002; Snyder 2001). In a study exploring how people with dementia adapt to their changing abilities, one person explained the dilemma as follows: 'Now I have to think so hard. And my head is no good for thinking since there is not much left in it' (Nygard and Ohman 2002: 75).

While cognitive changes were the most common explanation, a few studies have reported that people with dementia may attribute their problems with activity to visual perception problems (Snyder 2001). They describe looking at something but not being able to understand what they see. These are uncanny experiences that they find difficult to describe. Their world has become strangely unfamiliar and everyday activities are more challenging as a result. As one woman explained, 'I try to go out and walk every day just to see if things have changed that much. But they do ... I can see the same things I've seen for years, and they're different. Everything is different. I can't explain it' (Phinney 1998: 12).

Losing social connectedness

In addition to finding everyday activities more difficult, people with dementia also find themselves increasingly isolated and detached from the world around them, losing a sense of social connectedness and belonging. Svanstrom and Dahlberg (2004) described it as an experience of 'homelessness'.

In part, this happens because of communication difficulties stemming from the dementia itself. People have trouble expressing themselves and they find it more difficult to follow along in conversations (Clare 2002; Holst and Hallberg 2003; Phinney and Chesla 2003; Snyder 2001). As one gentleman explained: 'Things don't come to me that fast, and it takes me a little time to think about what I want to say. So it isn't like you carry on a conversation and everything falls into place all the time. Sometimes it doesn't' (Phinney 2002b: 64). It is also harder to get out in the world when people are no longer able to drive and fear getting lost, which may leave them with fewer opportunities to connect with others. It is simply easier to stay at home alone.

While communication difficulties contribute to some of the social isolation experienced by people with dementia, more often they perceive their social losses as being the result of how they are perceived by others. Morhardt *et al.* (2003) found that members of an early diagnosis support group felt that they were treated as if they were somehow 'slipping away', in part because others saw them as being dependent. In some cases dependence was even forced on them. Other studies have reported people with dementia feeling 'invisible', despairing of their lack of involvement in decisions about their care (Beattie *et al.* 2004; Tyrrell *et al.* 2006). People with dementia report that others misjudge them, assuming they will say or do something wrong. Friends often drift away, leaving people feeling isolated and excluded (Graneheim and Jansson 2006; Harris and Keady 2004; Katsuno 2005; Snyder 2001).

People with dementia also find themselves living on the margins because of their loss of social roles. When people cannot live up to previously held roles, or those roles are taken away from them, they are less able to contribute to their families and communities, despite their strong desire to remain involved (Clare 2003; Droes *et al.* 2006; Harris and Keady 2004; Morhardt *et al.* 2003; Pearce *et al.* 2002). As one man explained: 'I am losing the temper of the world – that people are in activities that I don't participate in' (Phinney *et al.* 2007).

Exercise 2.1   Including people with dementia in service evaluation

'Keeping Up' is a newly developed activity programme for people with mild to moderate dementia. The programme serves 15 participants who attend two afternoons a week. They are a socially and culturally diverse group of nine men and six women, aged 57–84 years. Each session is led by a recreation therapist with the assistance of two volunteers. On Mondays, everyone takes part in small group and individual activities (e.g. games, crafts, discussion groups), while on Thursdays they go on field trips (e.g. art gallery, museum, swimming pool).

Imagine you are the coordinator of Keeping Up and you have been asked to evaluate its effectiveness. Consider how you would include the programme participants in this evaluation.

Which aspects of their experience would interest you?

What kind of information would you gather?

Impact of dementia on how people feel about themselves

The profound impact of dementia on everyday life naturally has a significant effect on how people feel about themselves and their situation. In their words, we also hear how emotionally devastating it can be not to be living up to deeply held socio-cultural values regarding autonomy and productivity.

Negative feelings

Most people living with dementia experience a variety of negative feelings in response to their illness and its impact on their life; intense anger and frustration are very common (e.g. Aggarwal *et al.* 2003; Gillies 2000; Holst and Hallberg 2003; Nygard and Ohman 2002). While these feelings are sometimes directed toward others, especially in response to feeling misunderstood and excluded (Beattie *et al.* 2004; Harman and Clare 2006; Snyder 2001), more often, the anger and frustration are self-directed when people feel they have failed themselves. They describe it as feeling 'violent to myself' (Clare 2003) or having 'inward anger' (Katsuno 2005). One woman explained how she is often disappointed in herself, even saying out loud 'You forgot this, Christina. How could you forget this? And I scold myself' (Phinney 2000). Those who are in the earliest stages of the illness may be more likely to direct anger toward themselves, although exactly how emotional responses change over time remains poorly understood (Ostwald *et al.* 2002).

Fear and sadness are also common feelings experienced by people with dementia (e.g. Aggarwal *et al.* 2003; Clare 2003; Harris and Keady 2004; Harris and Sterin 1999; Ostwald *et al.* 2002; Snyder 2001). People are fearful about what their future will bring, about 'getting worse', and 'going completely out of their heads' (Pearce *et al.* 2002: 183). They are also fearful in those moments of confusion and uncertainty when they find themselves to be a complete blank, unsure of where they are, or even who they are. One woman explained: 'It's scary. Yeah it's scary. I suppose in a way it's like being in a fog, and you can't find your way out of it. I mean, not knowing is frightening' (Phinney and Chesla 2003: 294). People feel deep sadness as they consider the hopelessness of their situation. 'Somehow you've got to get right to the bottom – it's a matter of feeling reality, not kidding yourself or making excuses' (Clare 2003: 1024). They express sorrow for all that they have lost, and regret for being a burden on their loved ones (Harris and Keady 2004; Ostwald *et al.* 2002).

Losing confidence and self-esteem

With the many challenges people face in their daily lives, they are often left feeling insecure and lacking in self-confidence. Experiences of uncertainty are so frequent and profound that people with dementia often feel they cannot fully trust themselves any longer. They are often unsure of where they are (Phinney 2002b), of what they have said or done (Phinney 1998), and even who they are (Harris and Sterin 1999; Phinney 2002a). People often feel embarrassed when their problems are witnessed by others (Aggarwal *et al.* 2003; Gillies 2000; Imhof 2003; Offord *et al.* 2006; Ostwald *et al.* 2002). They do not want people thinking that they are not competent, nor do they want others to feel uncomfortable in their presence. One man explained how he keeps quiet in conversations because: 'I would sound kind of foolish if I say something that has no relation to what they've been talking about.' When asked if he was concerned he if would embarrass himself, he nodded and said, 'Or embarrass them too. They're friends, so I am a little leery' (Phinney 2002b: 65).

In addition to their insecurity, people with dementia often feel that that their capacity for self-determination is slipping and that they are losing control over their lives (Droes *et al.* 2006; Graneheim and Jansson 2006; Nygard and Borell 1998). As a result, they are losing their sense of themselves as competent, independent persons. A 77-year-old woman stated: 'I get very frustrated, resentful and despondent. Don't forget, I ran the show, when you take that away from me, what have I got left?' (Harris and Sterin 1999: 246).

As difficult as it can be to bear witness to these difficult feelings, what may be most unsettling for care providers is recognizing the extent to which living with dementia can affect people's self-esteem. Again and again, people with dementia tell of how they feel useless and unproductive, incompetent, or quite simply, foolish and crazy. People perceive themselves as being a burden to others (Gillies 2000; Harris and Keady 2004; Ostwald *et al.* 2002). They feel unproductive and unimportant, unable to live up to their previous roles in life (Clare 2003; Gillies 2000; Harris and Keady 2004; Harris and Sterin 1999). Knowing their diagnosis does not stop people from feeling inadequate and disappointed in themselves. They say things like: 'You think, "Am I just somebody that's going a bit stupid or what?" ' (Offord *et al.* 2006: 179).

Responding to challenges: how people with dementia cope and adapt

From a practical perspective, it is important not only to know how people with dementia perceive the challenges in their lives, but also how they cope with or adapt to these challenges in order to maintain continuity and prevent further decline. Evidence from the research literature provides preliminary ideas as to what people find most helpful, which might ultimately provide direction for the development of supportive interventions and services (Werezak and Stewart 2002).

Active strategies

People with dementia become very creative in identifying active coping strategies, often working with family members and others to find approaches that work best in different circumstances (Nygard and Ohman 2002).

Working harder

What is perhaps the most common strategy used by people with dementia is facing their challenges head on by simply working harder at things (Clare 2002; Harris and Sterin 1999; Parsons 2005; Pearce *et al.* 2002). One man reported his wife's reaction to her dementia: 'Daily life is a burden. She says it and she means it and I agree with her. [It is] hard work' (Phinney and Chesla 2003: 288). People are willing to take this on because as much as possible, they want to be self-sufficient. One woman explained very simply: 'I don't ask my daughter to do anything for me. I'm an independent person and I do things for myself' (Ward-Griffin *et al.* 2006: 134).

Working harder is not just about exerting more effort; people also develop particular strategies to help them overcome the challenges they face as a result of the dementia. In the earlier stages of the illness, most people employ various kinds of memory aids, including making notes and writing lists (Aggarwal *et al.* 2003; Clare *et al.* 2005; Gillies 2000; Gilmour and Huntingdon 2005; Nygard and Ohman 2002; Preston *et al.* 2007; Van Dijkhuizzen *et al.* 2006). They try to stay organized, keeping items they need close at hand, or developing 'systems' to help them maintain a sense of order and control (Clare 2002; Nygard and Johansson 2001; Preston *et al.* 2007; Van Dijkhuizzen *et al.* 2006). They plan and practise ahead of time, and try to stay focused and attentive (Nygard and Ohman 2002; Phinney and Brown 2004).

Reducing demands

People also try to find easier ways of doing things (Imhof 2003; Nygard and Ohman 2002; Phinney 2006). Simply slowing down and allowing themselves sufficient time to complete a task is one approach (Nygard and Ohman 2002; Snyder 2001). People may find it helpful to 'clear out' their daily schedule so there are fewer demands being made on their time (Nygard and Johansson 2001). Maintaining routine is also a valuable strategy that effectively reduces the complexity of everyday life (Clare 2002; Harris and Sterin 1999). Familiar places and activities allow people to rely on their embodied skills, a kind of 'automatic pilot' that requires less explicit effort on their part (Nygard and Ohman 2002; Phinney and Chesla 2003; Van Dijkhuizzen *et al.* 2006). People also try to reduce the demands they make on themselves in terms of their own performance, focusing on what matters most to them and putting less pressure on themselves to 'do it all' (Nygard and Johansson 2001; Pearce *et al.* 2002). A retired musician explained how he could still perform, but he no longer tried to remember his medications, figuring that his wife could look after those kinds of details (Phinney 2006).

Avoiding challenging situations

Sometimes, rather than trying to cope or adapt to a challenging situation, people prefer to avoid the situation altogether. Some may try to cover up their difficulties (Aggarwal *et al.* 2003; Clare *et al.* 2005). 'It's quite an art really,' explains one gentleman, 'trying to behave socially normally without letting on that you've forgotten that person's name' (Clare 2002: 143). Others admit to 'taking a break' or withdrawing when they are faced with challenging circumstances (Aggarwal *et al.* 2003; Gillies 2000; Ostwald *et al.* 2002; Pearce *et al.* 2002; Werezak and Stewart 2002). Sometimes people with dementia purposely retreat from social situations as a way of protecting themselves, admitting that they feel more comfortable when not forced to live up to others' expectations (Ostwald *et al.* 2002; Phinney 2002a; Snyder 2001).

Seeking and accepting help

It can be difficult for people with dementia to find themselves increasingly dependent on others, and some prefer to keep their needs to themselves as a result (Ward-Griffin *et al.* 2006). However, most people recognize that seeking and accepting help from others is an important coping strategy. Sometimes this involves concrete assistance with everyday activities like doing laundry or going shopping, or taking medications. People may allow others to do things for them, or they may prefer to accept guidance and direction (Nygard and Ohman 2002; Phinney 2006). More often, however, help is most beneficial when it involves emotional support. People maintain connection with friends and family so they might feel 'loved and cherished' (Surr 2006: 1726). They draw sustenance from the knowledge that others care for them and are willing to help (e.g. Clare 2002; Droes *et al.* 2006; Gillies 2000; Nygard and Ohman 2002; Ostwald *et al.* 2002; Pearce *et al.* 2002; Phinney 2000; Van Dijkhuizzen *et al.* 2006).

As important as it is for people with dementia to have support, little is known about what this experience is like for them. For some, seeking and accepting help may be a simple matter, while for others it is only tolerable if they can control the amount and type of help they receive, or if they can 'work together' with others to achieve their goals in a collaborative way (Offord *et al.* 2006; Ward-Griffin *et al.* 2006). What determines these different responses is poorly understood. Moreover, most studies have only reported how people perceive support from family and friends (Droes *et al.* 2006; Phinney 2006; Surr 2006; Ward-Griffin *et al.* 2006). Less is known about how people with dementia seek and receive help through more formal channels (Aggarwal *et al.* 2003; Train *et al.* 2005; Tyrrrell *et al.* 2006).

Being active

Being active and involved is an important way for people with dementia to feel that they are managing their illness, preventing further decline and getting pleasure and meaning out of life (Aggarwal *et al.* 2003; Nygard and Ohman 2002; Ostwald *et al.* 2002). It is through their activities that people find their life to have meaning and purpose (Phinney *et al.* 2007; Van Dijkhuizzen *et al.* 2006; Werezak and Stewart 2002). They live up to previous social and work roles, and have a sense that they are 'giving back' by helping others and contributing to their family and community (Clare *et al.* 2005; Ostwald *et al.* 2002; Phinney *et al.* 2007, Surr 2006). A retired teacher commented: 'I certainly would like to help people … and I saw that as a way, taking those kinds of feelings and skills, and trying to turn this thing, and I've been working on that "What can I do? What can I be of value?" (Menne *et al.* 2002: 375). Maintaining involvement in activity also serves as an important distraction from negative feelings (Nygard and Ohman 2002), and gives people the sense that little has changed in their lives (Phinney *et al.* 2007).

Emotion-focused strategies

While active problem-solving strategies are common, equally important (if not more so) are emotion-focused coping strategies that people use to keep themselves from dwelling on their negative feelings. There seem to be two key strategies reported in the literature – 'minimizing difficulties' and 'keeping a positive outlook'. In one way or another, most people use both of these strategies to manage their emotional responses, thereby helping them maintain a sense that their lives are meaningful and worth living.

Minimizing difficulties

Perhaps the most common emotion-focused strategy for coping with dementia as reported in the literature is minimizing or downplaying the impact of the dementia. The most extreme example would be those who, even though they are well aware of their situation, either deny that anything is wrong (Harris and Sterin 1999; Ostwald *et al.* 2002), or choose to not think about it (Clare *et al.* 2005; Harman and Clare 2006; Van Dijkhuizzen *et al.* 2006). Others will consider their problems, but minimize the extent to which they are impaired, pointing out that they can remember when it is important to do so (Van Dijkhuizzen *et al.* 2006), or comparing themselves favourably to others who are more impaired (Phinney 1998). Normalizing is another common response, with people arguing, for example, that their memory loss is simply due to their age or the fact that they are slowing down toward the end of a busy active life (Clare 2002; Gillies 2000; Nygard and Ohman 2002; Pearce *et al.* 2002; Phinney 1998). Taken together, these minimizing strategies provide a way for people to feel as if they are unaffected by the dementia. For example, one gentleman was a musician who felt strongly that there was something deep in him that the dementia could not touch. He said: 'I can create music all right. That is just ingrained in me. I don't think that Alzheimer's is going to hurt that.' He later explained: 'I don't think [the Alzheimer's] is very deep. I can go all day and never think of it' (Phinney and Brown 2004: 6).

Keeping a positive outlook

Even when their lives are most difficult, people often try to maintain a positive outlook (Preston *et al.* 2007). They struggle to remain hopeful and they rely on humour and a sense of enjoyment to help them get through challenging situations (Clare 2002; Harris and Sterin 1999; Snyder 2001; Werezak and Stewart 2002). Most hope for the same thing – either a cure, or for something to halt the progression of their disease. But hope does not stop there. Even when people recognize the inevitability of their situation, some still face their future with a certain hopefulness that helps them feel more encouraged and less despairing. For example, more than anything, one person hoped that he would remain at home in the care of his family until the end, while another clung to the hope that she would continue to experience simple joys in her life as her cognitive capacities failed (Phinney 2000). Humour and enjoyment also serve to keep people oriented toward the positive aspects of their situation. People laugh at themselves and their 'crazy mistakes', making a point of enjoying themselves no matter what. One man explained: 'I make everybody laugh ... well, that's the only thing left for us ... if you haven't got a sense of humour you're dead ... you make people laugh and you laugh at yourself, and it works both ways. You do get something out of it' (Menne *et al.* 2002: 376).

Living in the moment has become something of a cliché to describe how people with dementia find meaning in their lives. But clichés always have some grounding in truth, and certainly in this case, people often take pleasure in simpler things as they slow down to 'enjoy what you can when you can' (Brennan 1996, cited in Snyder 2001: 18) or 'take things as they come' (Clare 2002: 142). Many people with dementia say that they have chosen to not worry about their future, but rather strive to appreciate and enjoy what they have today.

Exercise 2.2   Planning care based on strengths

Mrs Johansen is a 76-year-old woman with dementia who recently moved to a nursing home. She is a retired high school teacher who raised three sons on her own after her husband died in a car accident 35 years ago. She was first diagnosed with Alzheimer's disease at the age of 72 when her oldest son became concerned that she was starting to lose interest in her many volunteer activities. He had also noticed some memory lapses, although Mrs Johansen herself tended to laugh it off when confronted with what she called 'little slips'. Until six months ago, she had lived at home independently, and is described by her sons as a 'brilliant busy woman who never likes to ask for help'. Since moving into the nursing home, Mrs Johansen has been quiet, spending considerable time in her room. When asked about how she is feeling, she tends to report, 'Oh, I'm fine. I do miss my old friends and the things we used to do together, but I suppose I can't have everything now, can I?' Her sons tell you that she doesn't seem like her old self. 'She seems defeated' is how they describe it. You want to help Mrs Johansen feel less lonely and more satisfied with her days.

Describe how you would develop a care plan that builds on her unique coping strengths.

Methods used to research the experience of dementia: limitations and future directions

It is important to recognize that the knowledge base, while vastly improved over what existed 15 years ago, remains limited in important ways. Most of what is known is based on open-ended interviews conducted with people in the earlier stages of the disease. How the experience of dementia changes over the course of the disease remains poorly understood. A few studies have examined experiences of assessment and diagnosis (e.g. Moniz-Cook *et al.* 2006; Pratt and Wilkinson 2001; Robinson *et al.* 1997), but little is known about how people experience other key transitions in the disease trajectory. Little is known about later dementia, especially people's involvement in decisions regarding increasing care needs (Tyrrell *et al.* 2006) and their experience of events such as admission to a nursing home (Graneheim and Jansson 2006). While several studies have identified the importance of choice, there remains a need for further research to show how this can best be enacted to support the needs of those with dementia (Bamford and Bruce 2000; Graneheim and Jansson 2006; Train *et al.* 2005; Tyrrell *et al.* 2006).

Another important limitation of this work lies in its tendency to focus on exposing commonalities. While some research has examined the significance of age as a factor influencing people's experience of dementia (e.g. Beattie *et al.* 2004; Harris and Keady 2004), generally speaking, little attention has been paid to exploring difference, whether it be according to type of diagnosis, socio-cultural background, or gender. In part, this has happened because most of this research has been conducted with volunteers who are probably more similar than dissimilar to each other, with the end result being that study findings may be skewed, preferring certain kinds of experiences over others.

Certainly some of these limitations come from the fact that this work is difficult to do. While the research community has learned how to better involve people with dementia in research (Wilkinson 2002), it remains the case that most people with a dementing illness will have trouble completing questionnaires or taking part in interviews. In recognition of this fact, some researchers have experimented with different techniques for revealing experiences of those with dementia, but as noted earlier, most findings continue to be based on loosely structured interviews and conversations conducted with relatively articulate people in the earlier stages of disease. Moreover, study samples have tended to be small and relatively homogeneous, leading researchers to focus on the similarities rather than the differences across individuals. To develop a deeper and more nuanced appreciation of how it is to live with dementia, over time and in different situations, it is necessary to further develop and increasingly rely on other means of investigation and understanding.

While there has been some interest in developing quantitative strategies to understand the experiences and perspectives of those with dementia (e.g. Burgener *et al.* 2005; Katsuno 2005), most of the research in this field remains in the qualitative realm. Kitwood argued in 1997 that listening carefully to what people had to say about their experiences was critical, and certainly acknowledging the ability of people with dementia to participate meaningfully in a research interview has been an important methodological development.

However, relying exclusively on this single data source has limited the ability of researchers to move understanding forward. People's perception of their own experience remains a partial view; conducting interviews with other key informants would undoubtedly help enrich these interpretations. For example, asking those who know the person well to describe how they think the person is experiencing their world can provide an important context that in turn opens up new possibilities for understanding the experience of the person with dementia. Likewise, auto/biographical and literary accounts of dementia can provide yet another point of access for considering people's illness experiences (Basting 2003; Johnson 1999; Killick 1997; Soulsby 2006).

Observation is another important strategy for gaining different kinds of insight into the experience of dementia. There are many ways to do this. Structured observation of well-being, and participant observation of non-verbal communication are approaches that have been used in studies of people with advanced dementia (Brooker and Duce 2000; Hubbard *et al.* 2002; Schreiner *et al.* 2005). Kitwood himself suggested a more ecological approach, claiming the importance of 'attending carefully to what people with dementia say and do in the course of their ordinary life' (1997: 16). A creative example of this is found in a recent study by Sheehan *et al.* (2006), who were interested in 'wayfinding'. The researcher accompanied people during a walk outside, carefully observing while recording each individual's ongoing commentary describing what they were doing. Others have tried variations of this approach, sometimes using video to record the ongoing activity (e.g. Cook 2003; Offord *et al.* 2006; Palo-Bengtsson and Ekman 2002). The potential of video and other visual media is considerable given its capacity to draw on participants' non-verbal strengths and communicative capacity.

Exercise 2.3   Comparing experiences of dementia

Read one of the following autobiographical accounts of dementia:

Cary Henderson and Nancy Andrews (1998) *Partial View: An Alzheimer's Journal.* Dallas, TX: Southern Methodist University Press.

Diana Friel McGowin (1994) *Living in the Labyrinth: A Personal Journey through the Maze of Alzheimer's.* New York: Dell Publishing.

Thomas DeBaggio (2002) *Losing My Mind: An Intimate Look at Life with Alzheimer's.* New York: Free Press.

Consider the similarities and differences between the authors' experience and those described in the research literature.

Debates and controversies

Clearly, people with dementia can offer important insights into their experiences and it is important to listen to what they have to say. However, the extent to which the experiences described in the literature are typical of most people with dementia remains a contested point. To evaluate the significance of this work for practice, it is important to consider the findings in light of certain questions. For example, to what extent does this body of research draw on the views of very specific sub-groups, e.g. well-educated, Caucasian women with adequate social support? Are the experiences of those who face more barriers being included? While this work is often described as 'hearing the voices of dementia', are we in danger of satisfying ourselves that we have heard from people with dementia when we have only captured those voices representing the earliest stages of impairment? Is this model of subjective experience useful for understanding more advanced illness? Does this body of work tend to overlook the experiences of those who are having a difficult time coping with the challenges of their illness? Because these people may be far less likely to participate in a study, the literature may be overemphasizing the more positive aspects of people's experiences.

Conclusion

In answer to the question posed at the outset: 'What is it like to live with dementia?', the research literature presents an overall picture of people living with the continual stress of trying to overcome the profound challenges of dementia and its emotional impact, while at the same time trying to find meaning and quality of life within the disease. While much about dementia continues to be mysterious and difficult to grasp, this research offers some important insights into the experiences of people with dementia. As foundational knowledge, it potentially improves the capacity of carers to provide empathic support and provides people with the disease a sense that they are not alone, that many others share their experiences. This work also provides a basis for thinking about how better to serve the needs of people with dementia, directing services and interventions toward the challenges people find most difficult, and building on the strengths and skills that people already have for coping with and adapting to their illness.

Further information

The Dementia Advocacy and Support Network (DASN) is an international group of advocates for people with dementia. Over one-third of the members have dementia themselves. The website provides information and resources, as well as a link to an online support group for people with dementia.

Tom DeBaggio is the owner of a nursery in West Virginia who was diagnosed in 1999 with early onset Alzheimer's disease. National Public Radio has recorded several interviews with Tom in which he discusses the impact of the disease on his life.

Blogging has become more common among people with dementia as a way of sharing their experiences with others. See if you can find any online journals of people living with Alzheimer's disease.

A website called 'The Dementia Journey' has been developed by the local health authority in Vancouver, Canada. It includes links to stories told by people at various stages of dementia about their experience and feelings of living with this disease.

References

Aggarwal, N., Vass, A.A., Minard, H.A., Ward, R., Garfield, C. and Cybyk, B. (2003) People with dementia and their relatives: personal experiences of Alzheimer's and of the provision of care. *Journal of Psychiatric and Mental Health Nursing*, 10: 187–97.

Bamford, C. and Bruce, E. (2000) Defining the outcomes of community care: the perspectives of older people with dementia and their carers. *Ageing and Society*, 20: 543–70.

Basting, A.D. (2003) Looking back from loss: views of the self in Alzheimer's Disease. *Journal of Aging Studies*, 17: 87–99.

Beattie, A., Daker-White, G., Gilliard, J. and Means, R. (2004) 'How can they tell?': A qualitative study of the views of younger people about their dementia and dementia care services. *Health and Social Care in the Community*, 12: 359–68.

Brennan, T. (1996) Simple pleasures are best. *Perspectives – a Newsletter for Individuals with Alzheimer's Disease*, 1(3): 2.

Brooker, D. and Duce, L. (2000) Well-being and activity in dementia: a comparison of group reminiscence therapy, structured goal-directed group activity and unstructured time. *Aging and Mental Health*, 4: 354–8.

Burgener, S., Twigg, P. and Popovich, A. (2005) Measuring psychological well-being in cognitively impaired persons. *Dementia*, 4: 463–85.

Clare, L. (2002) We'll fight it as long as we can: coping with the onset of Alzheimer's disease. *Aging and Mental Health*, 6: 139–48.

Clare, L. (2003) Managing threats to self: awareness in early stage Alzheimer's disease. *Social Science and Medicine*, 57: 1017–29.

Clare, L., Roth, I. and Pratt, R. (2005) Perceptions of change over time in early stage Alzheimer's disease. *Dementia*, 4: 487–520.

Cook, A. (2003) Using video to include the experiences of people with dementia in research. *Research Policy and Planning*, 21(2): 23–32.

Cotrell, V. and Schulz, R. (1993) The perspective of the patient with Alzheimer's disease: a neglected dimension of dementia research. *The Gerontologist*, 33: 205–11.

Downs, M. (1997) The emergence of the person in dementia research. *Ageing and Society*, 17: 5976–7.

Droes, R., Boelens-van der Knoop, E., Bos, J., Meihuizen, L., Ettema, T.P., Gerritsen, D.L. *et al.* (2006) Quality of life in dementia in perspective. *Dementia*, 5: 533–58.

Gillies, B.A. (2000) A memory like clockwork: accounts of living through dementia. *Aging and Mental Health*, 4: 366–74.

Gilmour, J.A. and Huntingdon, A.D. (2005) Finding the balance: living with memory loss. *International Journal of Nursing Practice*, 11: 118–24.

Graneheim, U. and Jansson L. (2006) The meaning of living with dementia and disturbing behaviour as narrated by three persons admitted to a residential home. *Journal of Clinical Nursing*, 15: 1397–403.

Harman, G. and Clare, L. (2006) Illness representations and lived experience in early-stage dementia. *Qualitative Health Research*, 16: 484–502.

Harris, P.B. and Keady, J. (2004) Living with early onset dementia: Exploring the experience and developing evidence-based guidelines for practice. *Alzheimer's Care Quarterly*, 5: 111–22.

Harris, P.B. and Sterin, G. (1999) An insider's perspective: defining and preserving the self of dementia. *Journal of Mental Health and Aging*, 5: 241–56.

Holst, G. and Hallberg, I. (2003) Exploring the meaning of everyday life for those suffering from dementia. *American Journal of Alzheimer's Disease and Other Dementias*, 18: 359–65.

Hubbard, G., Cook, A., Tester, S. and Downs, M. (2002) Beyond words: Older people with dementia using and interpreting nonverbal behaviour. *Journal of Aging Studies*, 16: 155–67.

Imhof, L.B. (2003) Forgetfulness: an experience of elderly people and their significant others. Doctoral dissertation, University of California: San Francisco.

Johnson, B.P. (1999) Images of relational self: Personal experiences of dementia described in literature. Doctoral dissertation, University of Colorado Health Sciences Center.

Katsuno, T. (2005) Dementia from the inside: How people with early-stage dementia evaluate their quality of life. *Ageing and Society*, 25: 197–214.

Killick, J. (1997) *You Are Words: Dementia Poems*. London: Hawker Publications.

Kitwood, T. (1997) The experience of dementia. *Aging and Mental Health*, 1: 13–22.

Menne, H.L., Kinney, J.M. and Mordhart, D.J. (2002) 'Trying to do as much as they can do': theoretical insights regarding continuity and meaning in the face of dementia. *Dementia*, 1: 367–82.

Moniz-Cook, E., Manthorpe, J., Carr, I., Gibson, G. and Vernooij-Dassen, M. (2006) Facing the future. *Dementia*, 5: 375–95.

Morhardt, D., Sherell, K. and Gross, B. (2003) Reflections of an early memory loss support group for persons with Alzheimer's and their family members. *Alzheimer's Care Quarterly*, 4: 185–8.

Nygard, L. and Borell, L. (1998) A life-world of altering meaning: expressions of the illness experience of dementia in everyday life over 3 years. *Occupational Therapy Journal of Research*, 18: 109–36.

Nygard, L. and Johansson, M. (2001) The experience and management of temporality in five cases of dementia. *Scandinavian Journal of Occupational Therapy*, 8: 85–95.

Nygard, L. and Ohman, A. (2002) Managing changes in everyday occupations: The experience of persons with Alzheimer's Disease. *Occupational Therapy Journal of Research*, 22: 70–81.

Offord, R.E., Hardy, G., Lamers, C. and Bergin, L. (2006) Teaching, teasing, flirting and fighting: A study of interactions between participants in a psychotherapeutic group for people with a dementia syndrome. *Dementia*, 5: 167–95.

Ostwald, S.K., Duggleby, W. and Hepburn, K.W. (2002) The stress of dementia: View from the inside. *American Journal of Alzheimer's Disease and Other Dementias*, 17: 303–12.

Palo-Bengtsson, L. and Ekman, S.L. (2002) Emotional response to social dancing and walks in persons with dementia. *American Journal of Alzheimer's Disease and Other Dementias*, 17: 149–53.

Parsons, K.A. (2005) Losing one's memory: a phenomenological study of early Alzheimer's disease. Doctoral dissertation, Rush University, College of Nursing.

Pearce, A., Clare, L. and Pistrang, N. (2002) Managing sense of self: coping in the early stages of Alzheimer's disease. *Dementia*, 1: 173–92.

Phinney, A. (1998) Living with dementia from the patient's perspective. *Journal of Gerontological Nursing*, 24(6): 3–15.

Phinney, A. (2002a) Fluctuating awareness and the breakdown of the illness narrative in dementia. *Dementia: The International Journal of Social Research and Practice*, 1: 329–44.

Phinney, A. (2002b) Living with the symptoms of Alzheimer's disease. In: P.B. Harris (ed.) *The Person with Alzheimer's Disease: Pathways to Understanding the Experience*. Baltimore, MD: Johns Hopkins University Press, pp. 49–70.

Phinney, A. (2006) Family strategies for supporting involvement in meaningful activity by persons with dementia. *Journal of Family Nursing,* 12: 80–101.

Phinney, A. and Brown, P. (2004) Embodiment and the dialogical self in dementia. Symposium paper, Canadian Association of Gerontology Annual Scientific and Educational Meeting, Victoria, BC, October.

Phinney, A. and Chesla, C. A. (2003) The lived body in dementia. *Journal of Aging Studies*, 17: 283–99.

Phinney, A., Chaudhury, H. and O'Connor, D. (2007) Doing as much as I can do: the meaning of activity for persons with dementia. *Aging and Mental Health*, 11: 384–93.

Phinney, J.A. (2000) The persistence of meaning in the midst of breakdown: an interpretive phenomenological account of symptom experience in dementia. Doctoral dissertation, University of California, San Francisco.

Pratt, R. and Wilkinson, H. (2001) *Tell Me the Truth: The Effect of Being Told the Diagnosis of Dementia from the Perspective of the Person with Dementia.* London: Mental Health Foundation.

Preston, L., Marshall, A. and Bucks, R.S. (2007) Investigating the ways that older people cope with dementia: A qualitative study. *Aging and Mental Health*, 11: 131–43.

Robinson, P., Ekman, S., Meleis, A.I., Winblad, B. and Wahlund, L. (1997) Suffering in silence: the experience of early memory loss. *Health Care in Later Life*, 2: 107–20.

Sheehan, B., Burton, E. and Mitchell, L. (2006) Outdoor wayfinding in dementia. *Dementia*, 5: 271–81.

Schreiner, A.S., Yamamoto, E. and Shiotani, H. (2005) Positive affect among nursing home residents with Alzheimer's dementia: The effect of recreational activity. *Aging and Mental Health*, 9: 129–34.

Snyder, L. (2001) The lived experience of Alzheimer's: Understanding the feelings and subjective accounts of persons with the disease. *Alzheimer's Care Quarterly*, 2(2): 8–22.

Soulsby, M.P. (2006) Telling time of memory loss: narrative and dementia. In: J.A. Parker, M. Crawford and P. Harris (eds) *Time and Memory*. Leiden: Brill.

Surr, C.A. (2006). Preservation of self in people with dementia living in residential care: A socio-biographical approach. *Social Science and Medicine*, 62: 1720–30.

Svanstrom, R. and Dahlberg, K. (2004) Living with dementia yields a heteronomous and lost existence. *Western Journal of Nursing Research*, 26: 671–87.

Train, G.H., Nurock, S.A., Manela, M., Kitchen, G. and Livingston, G.A. (2005) A qualitative study of the experience of long-term care for residents with dementia, their relatives, and staff. *Aging and Mental Health*, 9: 119–28.

Tyrrell, J., Genin, N. and Myslinski, M. (2006) Freedom of choice and decision-making in health and social care. *Dementia*, 5: 479–502.

Van Dijkhuizzen, M. Clare, L. and Pearce, A. (2006) Striving for connection: appraisal and coping among women with early-stage Alzheimer's disease. *Dementia*, 5: 73–94.

Ward-Griffin, C., Bol, N. and Oudshoorn, A. (2006) Perspectives of women with dementia receiving care from the adult daughters. *Canadian Journal of Nursing Research*, 38: 120–46.

Werezak, L. and Stewart, N. (2002) Learning to live with early dementia. *Canadian Journal of Nursing Research*, 334: 67–85.

Wilkinson, H. (ed.) (2002) *The Perspectives of People with Dementia*. London. Jessica Kingsley Publishers.

Woods, R.T. (2001) Discovering the person with Alzheimer's disease: cognitive, emotional and behavioural aspects. *Aging and Mental Health*, 5(Suppl 1): S7–S16.

3

Ethnicity and the experience of dementia

Linda Boise

Learning objectives

By the end of this chapter you will be able to:

- identify social and structural factors which interact with ethnicity to influence how persons with dementia and their families experience dementia
- appreciate the diversity of understandings of dementia and help-seeking behaviour
- understand barriers that people of colour face when seeking help and support
- appraise the differences and similarities among people of colour in terms of their experience of dementia
- apply your understanding to the provision of culturally competent dementia care

---

Introduction

Ethnicity plays an important role in the experience of, beliefs about, and response to living with dementia. That said, there is considerable variation of experience within ethnic groups. Much of this diversity can be attributed to a host of factors which interact with ethnicity to influence how individuals and families experience dementia in their day-to-day lives. These include social and structural factors, such as economic disadvantage and health disparities, household and neighbourhood structures, education, literacy and health literacy, and concepts of family obligation. Such factors interact with ethnicity to affect lay beliefs and understandings about dementia and health and community service use. This multiplicity of factors makes it difficult to draw generalizations about how a specific individual or family will respond to dementia. To add to the challenge, much of the research on ethnic diversity considers similarities and differences among ethnic groups broadly defined, for example, Asians, African Americans, Latinos. Yet there is considerable variation within ethnic groups, and subgroups, in the underlying factors that influence the experience of dementia.

In this chapter, we review what is known about these factors' influence in diverse ethnic groups and consider the implications for providing culturally competent care. Our focus is on people of colour, that is, people other than those of Caucasian descent. We draw predominantly on research from the USA with some reference to research in the UK.

Social and structural factors which interact with ethnicity

Economic disadvantage and health disparities

Socioeconomic status is a major source of health disparities among diverse ethnic groups. It is widely known that people of colour in the USA and the United Kingdom have lower incomes and poorer health status than Caucasians (Nazroo, 2003; PEW Hispanic Center 2006; Townsend and Davidson, 1982). There is not, however, a consistent relationship between ethnicity, socioeconomic status and health. First, despite the lower average incomes among African Americans and Hispanics, there are many people from these ethnic groups with middle and higher incomes. Nearly 9 million African Americans 15 years or older in the USA have incomes above the median income for all people 15 years or older in the USA (US Census Bureau 2007). Asian immigrants in the USA are often viewed as an economically comfortable population group. As a group, Asian Americans have a higher average income than other ethnic groups (US Census Bureau 2007), but a number of studies have established that there is a bimodal pattern of socioeconomic and health characteristics and a substantial proportion of Asian immigrants have low incomes (Chen and Hawks 1995; Tanjasiri *et al.* 1995).

Another inconsistency between ethnic groups is the extent to which socioeconomic status affects health. In general, low socioeconomic status is associated with greater disability in older adults, more limitations in activities of daily living, and more frequent and rapid cognitive decline (Fiscella and Williams 2004; Kington and Smith 1997; Melzer *et al.* 2001). Yet, low socioeconomic status has a stronger effect on health status (lifetime morbidity) for black and American Indian/Alaska Native women than for white women and Hispanic women (Gold *et al.* 2006).

Physical health conditions in people with dementia are likely to have a significant impact on the experience of dementia. Since most people develop dementia over the age of 65, physical health conditions often co-exist with dementia (Artaz *et al.* 2006; Maslow 2004; Xie *et al.* 2008: Boddaert, Heriche-Taillandier, Dieudonne & Verny). For people with dementia from population groups of colour, the likelihood of living with dementia alongside co-morbidities may be even greater. African Americans and Hispanics have disproportionate rates of diabetes and cardiovascular conditions including stroke and hypertension when compared with whites (Mensah *et al.* 2005). These conditions are associated with an increased risk of dementia (Ritchie and Lovestone 2002) and they may also add to the challenges of caring for someone with dementia (Maslow 2004). Since most carers are also in older age groups, chronic illnesses that affect persons with dementia may also affect those who are carers. Arthritis, diabetes and cardiovascular illnesses in the carer may exacerbate the challenges of caring for someone with dementia.

Low socioeconomic status is also a barrier to accessing services for persons with dementia. For example, in the USA where many services require either insurance or direct payment, carers with low incomes have fewer options for support services such as home care, medical care, rehabilitation services and long-term care. African Americans and Hispanics have also been found to be more likely than white carers to reduce work hours to provide family care than whites (Covinsky *et al.* 2001), which may compound their economic disadvantage.

In the USA, access to services is affected by one's income, employment history, insurance coverage, and legal status. While most older adults in the USA are covered with health insurance through the federal Medicare (health insurance for people over 65 and with permanent disability) system, Medicare covers home care costs only for acute, short-term conditions. States and regions within states vary substantially in the kinds and extent of services offered: such as daycare, respite care, assisted living, home health and home maker services. For many older immigrants, many of whom come to the USA late in life and have minimal or no work history in the USA, Medicare is unavailable so access to health care is especially problematic. For persons under the age of 65, as some people with dementia and many carers are, health insurance is often unavailable. In 2004, 19.7% of African Americans and 32.7% of Hispanics were uninsured (Center on Budget and Policy Priorities 2005). A lack of health insurance plagues many working-age people in the USA as well: 20% of working adults in 2005 did not have health insurance (National Coalition on Health Care 2007). These gaps in health insurance coverage for people living in the USA cause substantial access barriers for health and community services and most acutely affect immigrant groups and persons with low incomes.

Exercise 3.1 Hard choices

Think of someone you know well who is over 75 years old.

What health problems do they have?

What health-related services are they using?

Think about how the absence of these services would affect them. Look at the services you have identified and reflect on what you would advise if they had only £50 per month to spend.

Which services would you advise them to keep and which would you advise them to do without?

How would the loss of those services affect their quality of life?

How would it affect the quality of life of those around them?

Household and neighbourhood structures

A key source of diversity of the experience of living with dementia is the person's household and neighbourhood structure. People with dementia and their family carers live within a family, household, neighbourhood and community structure. These sources of help and support can have a profound effect on carers' well-being. People from different ethnic groups tend to have differences in their household and neighbourhood structure (Wilmoth 2001). Although a surprisingly high number of people with dementia, as many as one-third overall, live alone (Nourhashemi *et al.* 2005); this may be less common for persons of colour with dementia. For example, in the USA, Asians, Blacks, and Hispanics are more likely than Caucasians to live in close proximity to extended family members and Hispanic elders are most likely to be cared for in multi-generational households (AARP 2001). African Americans are less likely than other ethnic groups to be married and more likely to be living in households headed by women (Stoller and Cutler 1992). Not surprisingly, African Americans with dementia are less likely to be cared for by a spouse than white carers and are more likely to be cared for by siblings, adult children, grandchildren and other non-spousal family members (Kosberg *et al.* 2007; Peek *et al.* 2000).

New immigrants often move to communities and neighbourhoods where others from their home country live. Such neighbourhoods can be valuable sources of support for families coping with illness. Nonetheless, the mere presence of extended family members is no assurance that they or their carers will receive the support they need. In a study of several Asian subgroups of carers in Britain (Sikh, Hindu, Bangladeshi and Pakistani), Katbamna *et al.* (2004) found that although these carers lived in neighbourhoods with other extended family members, they reported limited support from their social networks. The high rate of people of working age who are employed is likely to inhibit younger relatives (often caring for young children as well) from taking an older relative with dementia into their home. An additional problem for many families is that younger family members emigrate to Western societies in search of jobs or education; their parents or other older relatives may remain in their country of origin, relegating the emigrating members to the challenges of long-distance caring.

Education, literacy and health literacy

Another area of variation among diverse ethnic groups is education levels, literacy and health literacy. Understanding the meaning of dementia for people who are proficient in English is challenging enough. When one's preferred language is not the majority language, obtaining a clear understanding of dementia and its implications for care are so much more difficult. It is not just the ability to speak the language of the dominant culture that is important. How comfortable one is in conversing in that language can determine the extent to which the person with dementia and their family members understand the nature of the illness and caring needs. Although according to the 2006 American Community Survey of the US Census Bureau, only 19.7% of US residents aged 5 or older speak languages other than English at home, among foreign-born residents of the USA (13% of the total US population), 84% speak a language other than English at home and 52% report that they speak English less than 'very well' (US Census Bureau 2006). Many Hispanics and other immigrants in the USA have few years of formal education. Low education combined with a low level of English proficiency may have multiplier effects on the difficulties of managing serious chronic illnesses such as dementia by limiting access to health information and satisfactory interactions with health and service providers. In one study, members of African American, Latino and Asian groups often felt that medical staff judged them unfairly based on how well they spoke English (Johnson *et al.* 2004).

The ability to understand written and verbal information about dementia and caring is related to education and English language proficiency but these may not fully explain one's understanding of health information. Health literacy, that is, the ability to read and understand health information, is a related though distinct issue. In a study of the impact of health literacy on health, Howard *et al.* (2006) found that education and health literacy, both individually and separately, predicted self-reported health status of older adults. Roberts and colleagues at the University of Michigan found in an African American and Caucasian sample of mostly highly educated adults, that African Americans tended to have lower levels of knowledge about Alzheimer's disease, fewer information sources, and a lower perceived threat of this illness (Roberts *et al.* 2003).

Language and literacy may also affect the diagnosis of dementia. Manly, a neuropsychologist working in New York City, suggests that more sensitive measures of educational attainment, such as literacy rather than number of years of schooling, may be needed to accurately identify those who have dementia, particularly African Americans and other persons of colour (Manly and Espino 2004).

Degree of acculturation

An important source of variation within ethnic groups is the degree of acculturation. The extent of acculturation often influences how people blend traditional beliefs about illness and caring with Western medical beliefs and help-seeking. Mahoney *et al.* (2005), for example, found that Latinos often expressed fears that acculturation would end family home care. Manly and Espino (2004: 100) define acculturation as 'the level at which people participate in the values, language, and practices of their own ethnic community versus those of the dominant culture'. Acculturation may influence people's knowledge of community resources and their comfort in relating to service providers. Otilingam and Gatz (2005) found greater intention to seek help for a person with early stage dementia (presented as a vignette) for Asian Indian Americans who were more acculturated than for other Asian Indian Americans. Acculturation has also been associated with health outcomes and health risk behaviours (Manly and Espino 2004). Gonzalez *et al.* (2001) found among a sample of mostly Mexican-American Latinos that those who were less acculturated were at greater risk of depression. Acculturation has also been shown to affect the results of cognitive testing for blacks and Hispanics (Arnold *et al.* 1994; Artiola *et al.* 1998).

Filial obligation

> **Exercise 3.2** Education programmes: how transferable are they?
>
> Imagine that you want to start offering an education programme on dementia and dementia caring. You have a curriculum that was developed and used with white families.
>
> How would you go about implementing the programme for a group of carers from an immigrant community?
>
> Once the programme is implemented, how would you evaluate whether the programme is meeting the needs of the target group?
>
> What challenges might you have in developing, implementing and evaluating the programme?
>
> How would you address these challenges?

In discussing caring and other health-related programmes for people from diverse cultures, some researchers have questioned whether the models underlying interventions developed for whites can be applied to other groups. For example, researchers often describe the value-based beliefs in 'familism' present in Latino and Asian cultures (Dilworth-Anderson and Gibson 2002; Gallagher-Thompson *et al.* 1996; Gaugler *et al.* 2006; Luna *et al.* 1996). As defined by Luna *et al.*, 'familism' refers to 'the perceived strength of family bonds and sense of loyalty to family'; they point out that this conceptual frame 'undoubtedly relates to family members' propensity to provide care to elder relatives' (Luna *et al.* 1996: 267). Although this has not been examined with scientific rigour, values based on familism may conflict with concepts of self-efficacy in which many health and carer education programmes today are grounded. Self-efficacy-based programmes aim to increase not only knowledge but also people's confidence in handling the challenges they face. Whether self-efficacy, which is a uniquely individualistic concept, conflicts with familism, that is, values grounded in family responsibilities, is a question worthy of further examination.

Personal values and beliefs about dementia and family and community responsibilities grounded in one's cultural background may influence how families care for someone with dementia and how they choose to combine family and formal care. The degree of severity in cognitive impairment, the extent of challenging behaviours, and access to or unavailability of resources may affect families' need for and use of formal services, but their values and beliefs about family responsibilities may overlay carers' response to the demands of caring. Cox and Monk (1993) and Henderson and Guitierrez-Mayka (1992) identified a culturally-based expectation that Latino families provide needed care for their elderly relatives, especially when caring for someone with dementia. Youn *et al.* (1999) found that Korean families hold strong beliefs that daughters-in-law are expected to provided hands-on care to their husbands' parents, while sons are expected to have decision-making authority regarding parents' care. In general, Pinquart and Sörensen (2005) found that carers of colour provided more care than white carers and had stronger filial obligation beliefs about caring for older persons.

One question addressed in a number of studies is whether caring for someone with dementia is more or less stressful for people of colour than for people from the majority culture, Caucasians (see Chapter 5). Pinquart and Sörensen (2005) found in a review of research, that Hispanic and Asian American carers reported higher levels of depression than white carers. On the other hand, lower stress levels for African American carers than for Caucasian carers as well as less use of psychotropic medications were reported in a major study of dementia carers by Haley *et al.* (2004). This study also reported that African American carers rated memory and behaviour problems of their family member with dementia as less distressing than Caucasian carers and reported significantly higher appraisals of the benefits of caring. Given the challenges for many African Americans from lower average incomes and high levels of morbidity already described, these are surprising findings and ones that not all experts agree on. But if there is validity to them, it would be worth investigating the mechanisms by which African Americans successfully cope with the demands of caring. An interesting study of persons with functional disability by Gitlin *et al.* (2007) found that for whites, living alone, and for African Americans, low spirituality predicted higher levels of depression. Although this study is not specifically about caring, a review of research on dementia from 1980–2000 suggests that for African Americans, internal resources, such as appraisal and religious coping, may protect them from some of the negative consequences of caring (Dilworth-Anderson *et al.* 2002).

Understandings of dementia and their implications for service use

The social and cultural factors already discussed will interact with ethnicity to influence how people understand dementia. Dementia may be viewed as a disease, a consequence of old age or as a mental illness (Downs *et al.*, 2008; Henderson and Guitierrez-Mayka 1992; Jones *et al.* 2006). In some cultures, the symptoms of dementia may be thought to represent a religious or mystical experience (Downs *et al.* 2006; Mackenzie 2007; Mackenzie *et al.* 2005). Hinton *et al.* (2005) identified two distinct paradigms for understanding dementia, a 'biomedical model' that views dementia as a disease with underlying brain pathology and a 'folk model' that views the signs of dementia from a non-medical perspective, for example, as 'normal ageing', 'forgetfulness', 'difficult personality', or possibly as 'crazy'. In a qualitative study with a multiethnic sample of family carers, they found that many people from all cultural groups (African American, Latino, Asian American and Anglo) drew on explanations which combined folk and biomedical thinking. Carers from non-Caucasian ethnic groups and those with lower formal education were more likely to hold folk explanatory models of dementia or to combine both biomedical and folk models.

Service use

Lack of access to services places an extra burden on families when care needs exceed their ability to provide them (see Chapters 5 and 16). Even when services are available, however, variations exist in how receptive people are to using them. Boult and Boult (1995) found, in a study of older recently hospitalized Medicaid recipients in Minnesota, that being Asian (in a sample that was 76% Hmong) was strongly associated with infrequent doctor visits. Further, they found that Asian American carers used less formal supports than non-Hispanic white carers whereas African American and Hispanic carers used levels of services comparable to whites. In a random telephone sample of carers in California, however, Giunta *et al.* (2004) found that both Latin American and Asian/Pacific Islander carers were less likely than white or African American carers to use formal carer services.

There is abundant evidence that people of colour tend to have unsatisfactory experiences with health and social services more often than whites. In one study of African Americans, Latinos and Chinese in their experience of obtaining a diagnosis of dementia, the failure of physicians to recognize Alzheimer's disease or refer them to specialists was found to be more problematic than language barriers or specific ethnic differences (Mahoney *et al.* 2005). Johnson *et al.* (2004) reported that African American, Hispanic and Asian adults tend to believe that they would receive better medical care if they belonged to a different race or ethnic group. Both African Americans and Latinos have reported high levels of physician distrust (Armstrong *et al.* 2007). Differences have also been noted among diverse ethnic groups in their concerns regarding interaction with physicians: African Americans often report physician disrespect (Mahoney *et al.* 2005); Gallagher-Thompson *et al.* (1996) found that several Hispanic subgroups lacked access to culturally specific educational or clinical services and had limited awareness of available support services; and Chinese respondents reported concern about stigmatization. Asians also reportedly appreciate health care professionals who show an interest in the patient's total needs and who are open to non-Western medical practices (Ngo-Metzger *et al.* 2004).

Providing culturally competent care

> **Box 3.1** Case example
>
> Luisa had recently moved to the USA from Colombia with her mother, Isabella, to a small town in southern California. Many other Colombian families lived in the community, including Luisa's cousins. Isabelle spoke no English. Luisa's English was improving due to her work at a local restaurant where she worked days and evenings. One night after a long and hard shift, she arrived home at 2 a.m. to find her mother dressed, with hat and coat on and her handbag over her shoulder. Isabella told Luisa she was ready to go home. Naturally this was upsetting to Luisa but it wasn't the first time this had happened, so she wasn't surprised. In the past few months, her mother had begun to behave strangely. Luisa figured that this behaviour must be due to the stress of moving to the USA and possibly her worry about their financial situation which was anything but secure.
>
> A month earlier, Luisa had taken her mother to the local medical clinic. Luisa offered to go into the examining room with her mother but her mother did not want her to and the nurse told her that she spoke Spanish and would

take good care of her. Luisa tried to explain to the nurse, first in English and then in Spanish, about her mother's strange behaviour but had a difficult time finding the right words in either language to explain her concerns.

When the nurse returned with Isabella to the waiting room, the nurse told Luisa that her mother was doing very well physically, but gave her a referral for a psychiatrist in case she wanted to follow up on her mother's strange behaviour. Luisa did not follow up with the referral to the psychiatrist. She understood that psychiatrists treat people who are crazy. She worried that a psychiatrist might put her mother in a mental hospital. Luisa hoped that people in the community could help her figure out what to do, but so far, she had been unable to talk with anyone about her mother's strange behaviour.

Providing culturally competent dementia care is now recognized as integral to excellence in dementia care (Mackenzie *et al.* 2005). Despite the gaps in our knowledge about how ethnicity and culture affect people's experience of dementia, ethnicity and culture do matter. People's beliefs about the origins of dementia, expectations of family care, and access to informal and formal resources may all be influenced by their ethnicity and culture. Socioeconomic and structural factors as well as barriers related to language, English proficiency, health literacy, beliefs and education may affect access to quality dementia care. The goal in providing culturally competent services should be to promote optimal wellness and to enhance families' efficacy within the conceptual framework within which they understand the affected person's condition.

The first step toward developing culturally competent care and support is to acknowledge that culture and ethnicity guide and affect expectations and behaviour. Becoming aware of one's own cultural attitudes and beliefs can provide a conceptual basis for understanding how a person's life experiences may influence his or her beliefs about dementia and caring. Second, it is valuable to consider not only differences but the many similarities in how people from diverse cultures experience dementia. Across multiple ethnic groups, early signs of dementia are often interpreted initially as normal ageing. The explanations for why the person is forgetting or acting differently from how they previously behaved are likely to incorporate some elements of non-medical reasoning. Obtaining a diagnosis is often a lengthy and difficult process and for many people with dementia a clinical diagnostic work-up is never done. Families in every ethnic group have a sense of obligation and responsibility for caring for a relative with dementia, although how these play out in specific family and neighbourhood structures may vary. Regardless of beliefs about the origin and causes of dementia, coping with day-to-day care requires knowledge, skill and support. It is fair to assume that for many, probably most, carers of whatever ethnic or cultural background, caring for someone with Alzheimer's disease or other form of dementia is, at least at times, a stressful undertaking. For carers of colour, there is the added tension that may come from dissatisfaction with care they have received from physicians or other service providers.

Providing care for persons with dementia from diverse ethnic groups should be approached from a perspective of discovery. Taking into consideration the many factors that can influence the experience of dementia, the provision of care for persons with dementia and their families requires an individualized and flexible approach that seeks to understand and accommodate the many variations in carer and care receiver experience. In response to the needs of diverse ethnic groups, many health systems now provide guidance in delivering services for persons from diverse cultural and language groups.

Box 3.2 Developing a culturally responsive dementia care plan

The goal is to determine a mutually acceptable plan for treatment, care or support. Seek ways to collaborate with the person with dementia, his/her family members, health team members, healers and community resources. The plan may incorporate community resources, traditional medical care, alternative treatments, spirituality, other cultural practices and a variety of education approaches (e.g. written materials, one-on-one or group-based teaching).

Some questions to consider

'What language do you prefer to use when receiving medical care?'

'In what language do you prefer to receive your written materials?'

'What do you think has caused the dementia?' ('memory loss', 'Alzheimer's disease' or other term as appropriate)

'What kind of help (treatment) are you seeking? What results do you hope to achieve?'

'What have you done already to deal with your problem?'

'Have you sought advice from friends, alternative healers or other practitioners?'

'When you are ill, whom do you usually go to for help or treatment?'

'Are you taking any treatments, medicines or home remedies?'

'Who from your family should we involve in your care plan?'

In Box 3.2 are some questions to ask when developing a culturally responsive dementia care plan. As you gather information from a person with dementia and/or their family members, consider the following:

- Does he or she relate dementia symptoms to disease or to the inevitable progression of old age?

- Do the signs of dementia merit a clinical evaluation?

- Do the affected individual and members of that person's family and social network agree on these questions?

- Do they view behaviours associated with dementia as best kept hidden from neighbours, other family members and social groups?

- What are the strengths and abilities in the person with dementia?

- What decisions can the person with dementia participate in making?

- What kinds of formal help or assistance do the person with dementia and his or her family members desire and need?

Regardless of the primary language a person with dementia and his/her family speak, clear communication between patients and their doctors is essential. Seeking compassionate and effective ways to communicate with patients and their families when giving or explaining a diagnosis of dementia is more an art than a science (Boise and Connell 2005). It is important to acknowledge the unique perspectives of the individual and his or her family and to assist them in identifying their needs within their cultural frame. The challenge may be multiplied when the patient and his/her family members have varying levels of familiarity with the English language and levels of acculturation to Western society. Translation of complex medical information in ways that will helpfully guide families through the ever-unfolding path of dementia is needed. Professionals often warn against using a static stage-based approach to counselling families about the progression of dementia but finding ways to communicate with families about the anticipated transitions the person will go through, acknowledging and preparing people for the inevitable uncertainty of what lies ahead, require skill, sensitivity and tact.

Discussing with the person with dementia and with their family members or significant others how their culture affects their understanding of dementia, their values related to care, and their needs provides the opportunity to learn how best to provide culturally appropriate care. This may, at times, be challenging and even awkward for the provider. Manly, a neuropsychologist at Columbia University, whose clinical practice and research often require gathering detailed information about clients' cultural experiences and perspectives, offers helpful advice for interviewing clients or patients from diverse cultures:

> We have found that asking participants about their cultural and education experience can be weaved into a standard interview assessing demographic variables; however, the comfort level of the participant is largely determinant on the comfort level of the interviewers in discussing these issues. Like any other set of questions that are potentially sensitive, the interviewer must have had established good rapport with the interviewee, should spend time to provide sufficient explanation of why questions about educational history, literacy level and cultural background are being asked, ensure the participant that their responses will remain confidential, and welcome any feedback the interviewee may have about the questions.

(Manly 2006)

Given the high likelihood that people people of colour have had unsatisfactory experiences with service providers, providers should seek to build trust and respect when serving families from these ethnic groups. In recent years, a number of health and service providers have developed and adapted programmes to better serve diverse ethnic groups. Such programmes must address and respond to factors grounded in culture, language, literacy, deference to and/or distrust of medical providers and other persons in authority, health status and access barriers. One programme that promotes positive communication and partnering relationships between doctors and patients from diverse ethnic groups is the 'Partnering with your Doctor' programme offered by Alzheimer's Association chapters throughout the USA This programme, which aims to empower patients and family members to effectively communicate their concerns and needs to health providers, may have particular application for persons from diverse ethnic groups and is available in English and Spanish at: www.alz.org/we_can_help_partnering_with_your_doctor.asp

In the USA, many health education materials are available in Spanish and, to a lesser extent, in Chinese, Vietnamese, Korean, Russian and other languages. Written health materials are an important means of communication and federal laws require health care organizations to translate 'vital' documents for patients with limited English proficiency. Health and service providers are expected to provide professional translation services for patients and their carers, but translation alone may be insufficient to adequately address patients' and clients' needed. Given the wide variations in educational levels, socioeconomic status and comfort people have in group learning, Gallagher-Thompson *et al.* (1996) recommend that programmes should be presented with a multimodal approach consisting of oral, written, visual and interactive elements.

The Alzheimer's Association also has helpful consultation and educational materials for diverse ethnic groups particularly for African Americans, as well as materials in Spanish and Asian languages. The Northern California Chapter of the Alzheimer's Association has developed a programme 'Maximizing Your Memory' that is particularly useful for seniors from diverse ethnic groups, and is available in Chinese, Vietnamese, Spanish, as well as in English. This programme, geared to older adults with concerns about their memory, teaches strategies for maintaining one's memory and provides information about resources. Other programmes and resources may be found by searching the internet.

Many worthwhile programmes are available for family carers and persons with dementia but many of these have not been adapted for use with specific ethnic or cultural groups. A helpful strategy for using such programmes with diverse ethnic groups is to work with representatives of the groups to be served to explore ways in which these programmes can be adapted. Gonzalez and Lorig offer valuable recommendations for working with community members, including using case examples that are specific and relevant for the cultural group being served, creating explanations or descriptions that fit people's understandings of the key concepts, and incorporating a group's cultural beliefs and practices into the programme (1996: 160–1). Attention is also needed in how programmes serving diverse ethnic groups are publicized. These need to be sensitive to the words that best explain for the target group whom the programme is intended for and the nature of the programme. Many people, for example, will not respond to a programme for 'carers' (or the direct translation of that word in a language other than English), as they may view themselves as caring family members rather than as carers.

Providing culturally appropriate and responsive care for persons with dementia and their families is a responsibility that must be addressed at all levels of the social and health care system. The provision of care takes place within a complex system of individual, family, neighbourhood influences, and in health and social care systems supported by public and private sector resources. Training is needed to ensure that, regardless of the cultural attributes of patients and clients, providers will offer appropriate and sensitive care. Administrators must recognize that culturally responsive and sensitive care takes time and attention to the unique characteristics and needs of the individuals to be served.

Exercise 3.3   Building on strengths

Strengths for coping with dementia may come from a person's beliefs or values, e.g. in how he/she understands dementia or in his/her feelings of responsibility as a carer. Assets for coping with dementia may come in the form of actual help or support available from one's community.

Thinking about a person you know who is caring for someone with dementia, answer the following:

What strengths or assets does this person bring to their caring situation?

Are there ways in which his/her community, either local or distant, creates particular opportunities or challenges in caring for someone with dementia?

Training in culturally competent care is one important aspect of responsive care but attention to the way health care is delivered and how resources are allocated are equally important. Western societies have yet to eliminate the disparities that exist among cultures or to accomplish the goal of equitable care for all people regardless of their ethnicity or their culture. Even as we seek to redress these inequities, the values and needs of people from diverse cultural groups are likely to continually change over time. Changes in immigration patterns, global economies, and governmental policies are constantly in flux. New immigrant groups are arriving daily from regions of the world where health, health needs, and beliefs may be quite different from those of earlier immigrant groups. Subgroups within broad ethnic categories will have their own unique needs.

Debates and controversies

An area of debate within this field is the extent to which one can explain diversity of experience in terms of ethnicity. Are differences in the experience of dementia among people from diverse ethnic groups primarily due to socioeconomic status or to differences in family beliefs and attitudes about illness, dementia and caring? How do the migration experiences of families and their neighbourhood and social network characteristics affect the care and support available for people from diverse ethnic groups?

Another area of controversy is the degree to which simple translation of educational materials into the language of the minority ethnic group is desirable when resources are not available to develop culturally tailored materials. We know that the way one conceptualizes dementia may be influenced by one's membership of an ethnic group. For example, many government and policy documents suggest that culturally competent care relies on the provision of information in the language of that particular ethnic group. Such an approach fails to address the differences in conceptualizing dementia in these groups.

Conclusion

From this review of ethnicity and the experience of dementia, it is clear that ethnicity plays an important role in beliefs about, and response to, living with dementia. It should be equally clear that there is considerable variation within ethnic groups in terms of their degree of acculturation, education and literacy levels, socioeconomic status, and household and community structures. Differences in these variables interact with ethnicity to influence how dementia is experienced by individuals and their families. Thinking in terms of these broader and more fluid cultural factors rather than ethnicity may be a more fruitful approach to understanding the complexity of forces which influence how individuals understand and cope with dementia.

Further information

The **Family Caregiver Alliance** is a community-based non-profit-making organization in the USA addressing the needs of families and friends providing long-term care at home.

The **Alzheimer's Disease Education and Referral (ADEAR) Center** website provides information and resources about Alzheimer's disease. It is run by the National Institute on Aging (NIA) in the USA.

The **Alzheimer's Association** in the USA offers a wide range of consultative and education materials in English and other languages.

References

American Association of Retired Persons (AARP) (2001) *In the middle: A report on the Multicultural Boomers Coping with Family and Aging Issues.* A National Study Conducted for AARP, July.

Armstrong, K., Ravenell, K.L., McMurphy, S. and Putt, M. (2007) Racial/ethnic differences in physician distrust in the United States. *American Journal of Public Health,* 97: 1283–9.

Arnold, B.R., Montgomery, G.T., Castenada, I *et al.* (1994) Acculturation and performance of Hispanics on selected Halstead-Reitan neuropsychological tests. *Assessment,* 1: 239–48.

Artaz, M.A., Boddaert, J., Heriche-Taillandier, E., Dieudonne, B. and Verny, M. (2006) Medical comorbidity in Alzheimer's disease: baseline characteristics of the REAL.FR Cohort. *Revue de Médéciné interne,* 27(2): 91–7.

Artiola, I., Fortuny, L., Healton, R.K. and Hermosillo, D. (1998) Neuropsychological comparisons of Spanish-speaking participants from the US-Mexico border region versus Spain. *Journal of the International Neuropsychological Society,* 4: 363–79.

Boise, L. and Connell, C.M. (2005) Diagnosing dementia – What to tell the patient and family. *Geriatrics and Aging,* 8(5): 48–51.

Boult, L. and Boult, C. (1995) Underuse of physician services by older Asian-Americans. *Journal of the American Geriatrics Society,* 43: 408–11.

Center on Budget and Policy Priorities. (2005) The number of uninsured Americans continued to rise in 2004. 30 August. Available from: www.cbpp.org/8-3-05health.htm (accessed 24 November 2007).

Chen, M.S. and Hawks, B.L. (1995) A debunking of the myth of health Asian Americans and Pacific Islanders. *American Journal of Health Promotion,* 9(4): 261–8.

Covinsky, K.E., Eng, C., Lui, L., Sand, L.P., Sehgal, A.R., Walter, L.C., Wieland, D., Eleazer, G.P. and Yaffe, K. (2001) Reduced employment in carers or frail elders: Impact of ethnicity, patient clinical characteristics, and carer characteristics. *Journal of Gerontology: Medical Sciences,* 56: 707–13.

Cox, C. and Monk, A. (1993) Hispanic culture and family care of Alzheimer's patients. *Health and Social Work,* 18(2): 92–100.

Dilworth-Anderson, P. and Gibson, B.E. (2002) The cultural influence of values, norms, meanings, and perceptions in understanding dementia in ethnic minorities, *Alzheimer's Disease and Associated Disorders,* 16(Suppl 2): S56–S63.

Dilworth-Anderson, P., Williams, I.C. and Gibson, B.E. (2002) Issues of race, ethnicity, and culture in caring research: A 20-year review (1980–2000). *The Gerontologist,* 42(2): 237–72.

Downs, M., Clare, L. and Anderson, E. (2008) Dementia as a bio-psychosocial condition: implications for practice and research. In: R. Woods and L. Clare (eds) *Handbook of the Clinical Psychology of Ageing,* 2nd edn. Chichester: Wiley.

Downs, M., Mackenzie, J. and Clare, L. (2006) Understandings of dementia: Explanatory models and their implications for the person with dementia and therapeutic effort. In J.C. Hughes, S.J. Louw and S.R. Sabat (eds) *Dementia: Mind, Meaning and Person.* Oxford: Oxford University Press, pp. 235–59.

Fiscella, K. and Williams, D.R. (2004) Health disparities based on socioeconomic inequities: Implications for urban health care. *Academic Medicine,* 79(12): 1139–47.

Gallagher-Thompson, D., Talamantes, M., Ramirez, R. and Valverde, I. (1996) Service delivery issues and recommendations for working with Mexican American family carers. In: G. Yeo and D. Gallagher-Thompson (eds) *Ethnicity and the Dementias.* Washington, DC: Taylor & Francis, pp. 137–52.

Gaugler, J.E., Kane, R.L., Kane, R.A. and Newcomer, R. (2006) Predictors of institutionalization in Latinos with dementia. *Journal of Cross-cultural Gerontology,* 21: 139–55.

Gitlin, L.N., Hauck, W.W., Dennis, M.P. and Schulz, R. (2007) Depressive symptoms in older African-American and white adults with functional difficulties: the role of control strategies. *Journal of the American Geriatrics Society,* 55(7): 1023–30.

Giunta, N., Chow, J., Scharlach, A.E. and Dal Santo, T.S. (2004) Racial and ethnic differences in family caring in California. *Journal of Human Behavior in the Social Environment,* 9(4): 85–109.

Gold, R., Michael, Y.L., Whitlock, E.P. *et al.* (2006) Race/ethnicity, socioeconomic state, and lifetime morbidity burden in the Women's Health Initiative: A cross-sectional analysis. *Journal of Women's Health,* 15(10): 1161–72.

Gonzalez, H.M., Haan, M.H. and Hinton, L. (2001) Acculturation and the prevalence of depression in older Mexican Americans: Baseline results of the Sacramento area. Latino Study on Aging. *Journal of the American Geriatrics Society,* 49: 948–53.

Gonzalez, V. M. and Lorig, K. (1996) Working cross-culturally. In: K. Lorig (ed.) *Patient Education: A Practical Approach.* Thousand Oaks, CA: Sage Publications, pp. 151–71.

Haley, W.E., Gitlin, L.N., Wisniewski, S.R., Mahoney, D.F., Coon, D.W., Winter, L., Corcoran, M., Schinfield, S. and Ory, M. (2004) Well-being, appraisal, and coping in African American and Caucasian dementia carers: findings from the REACH study. *Aging and Mental Health,* 8(4): 316–29.

Henderson, J.N. and Guitierrez-Mayka, M. (1992) Ethnocultural themes in caring to Alzheimer's disease patients in Hispanic families. *Clinical Gerontologist,* 11: 59–74.

Hinton, L., Franz, C.E., Yeo, G. and Levkoff, S.E. (2005) Conceptions of dementia in a multiethnic sample of family carers. *Journal of the American Geriatrics Society,* 53: 1405–10.

Howard, D.H., Sentell, T. and Gazmararian, J.A. (2006) Impact of health literacy on socioeconomic and racial differences in health in an elderly population. *Journal of General Internal Medicine,* 21(8): 857–61.

Johnson, R.L., Somnath, S., Arbelaez, J.J., Beach, M.C. and Cooper, L.A. (2004) Racial and ethnic differences in patient perceptions of bias and cultural competence in health care. *Journal of General Internal Medicine,* 19: 101–10.

Jones R.S., Chow, T.W. and Gatz, M. (2006) Asian Americans and Alzheimer's disease: Assimilation, culture, and beliefs. *Journal of Aging Studies,* 20: 11–25.

Katbamna, S., Ahmad, W., Bhakta, P., Baker, R. and Parker, G. (2004) Do they look after their own? Informal support for South Asian carers. *Health & Social Care in the Community,* 12(5): 398.

Kington, R.S. and Smith, J.P. (1997) Socioeconomic status and racial and ethnic differences in function status associated with chronic diseases. *American Journal of Public Health,* 87: 805–10.

Kosberg, J.I., Kaufman, A.V., Burgio, LD, Leeper, J.D. and Sun, F. (2007) Family caring to those with dementia in rural Alabama: Racial similarities and differences. *Journal of Aging and Health*, 19(1): 3–21.

Luna, I., Torres de Ardon, E., Lim, Y.M., Cromwell, S.L., Phillips, L.R. and Russell, C.K. (1996) The relevance of familism in cross-cultural studies of family caring. *Western Journal of Nursing Research*, 18(3): 267–83.

Mackenzie, J. (2006) Stigma and dementia: South Asian and Eastern European family carers negotiating stigma in two cultures. *Dementia: The International Journal of Social Research and Practice*, 5: 233–48.

Mackenzie, J. (2007) Ethnic minority communities and the experience of dementia. In: J. Keady, C. Clarke and S. Page (eds) *Partnerships in Community Mental Health Nursing and Dementia Care*. Buckingham: Open University Press.

Mackenzie, J., Bartlett, R. and Downs, M. (2005) Moving towards culturally competent dementia care: Have we been barking up the wrong tree? *Reviews in Clinical Gerontology*, 15: 39–46.

Mahoney, D.F., Cloutterbuck, J., Neary, S. and Zhan, L. (2005) African American, Chinese, and Latino family carers' impressions of the onset and diagnosis of dementia: cross-cultural similarities and differences. *The Geriatrician*, 45(6): 783–92.

Manly, J.J. (2006) Deconstructing race and ethnicity: Implications for measurement of health outcomes. *Medical Care*, 44: S10–S16.

Manly, J.J. and Espino, D.V. (2004) Cultural influences on dementia recognition and management. *Clinics in Geriatric Medicine*, 20(1): 93–119.

Maslow, K. (2004) Dementia and serious co-existing medical conditions: a double whammy. *Nursing Clinics of North America*, 39(3): 561–79.

Melzer, D., Izmirlian, G., Leveille, S.G. and Guralnik, J.M. (2001) Educational differences in the prevalence of mobility disability in old age: the dynamics of incidence, mortality, and recovery. *Journal of Gerontology: Social Sciences*, 56: S294–301.

Mensah, G.A., Mokdad, A. H., Ford, E.S., Greenlund, K.J. and Croft, J.B. (2005) State of disparities in cardiovascular health in the United States. *Circulation*, 111(10): 1233–41.

National Coalition on Health Care (2007) Health Insurance coverage. Available at: www.nchc.org/facts/coverage.shtml (accessed 24 November 2007).

Nazroo, J.Y. (2003) The structuring of ethnic inequalities in health: economic position, racial discrimination, and racism. *American Journal of Public Health*, 93(2): 277–84.

Ngo-Metzger, Q., Legedza, A.T.R. and Phillips, R.S. (2004) Asian Americans' reports of their health care experiences: Results from a national survey. *Journal of General Internal Medicine*, 19: 111–19.

Nourhashemi, F., Amouyal-Barkate, K., Gillette-Guyonnet, S., Cantet, C. and Vellas, B. (2005) Living alone with Alzheimer's disease: cross-sectional and longitudinal analysis in the REAL.FR Study. *Journal of Nutrition, Health & Aging,* 9(2): 117–20.

Otilingam, P.G. and Gatz, M. (2005) Perceptions of dementia among Asian Indian Americans: Does acculturation matter? *Gerontologist,* 45 (Suppl): 348.

Peek, M.K., Coward, R.T. Peek, C.W. (2000) Race, aging and care: can differences in family and household structure account for race variations in family care? *Research on Aging,* 22(2): 117–42.

Pew Hispanic Center (2006) *2005 American Community Survey.*

Pinquart, M. and Sörensen, S. (2005) Ethnic differences in stressors, resources, and psychological outcomes of family caring: A meta-analysis. *The Geriatrician,* 45(1): 90–106.

Ritchie, K. and Lovestone, S. (2002) The dementias. *Lancet,* 360: 1759–66.

Roberts, J.S., Connell, C.M., Cisewski, D., Hipps, Y.G., Demissie, S. and Green, R.C. (2003) Differences between African Americans and whites in their perceptions of Alzheimer's disease. *Alzheimer's Disease & Associated Diseases,* 17(1): 19–26.

Stoller, J. and Cutler, R. (1992) The impact of gender on configurations of care among married elderly couples. *Research on Aging,* 14: 313–30.

Tanjasiri, S.P., Wallace, S.P. Shibata, K. (1995) Picture imperfect: Hidden problems among Asian Pacific Islander elderly. *The Gerontologist,* 35(6): 753–60.

Townsend, P. and Davidson, N. (1992) *Inequalities in Health* (the Black Report). Harmondsworth: Penguin.

Wilmoth, J.M. (2001) Living arrangements among older immigrants in the United States. *The Gerontooglist,* 41(2): 228–38.

US Census Bureau (2006) *2006 American Community Survey S0501: Selected Characteristics of Native and Foreign-born Populations.* Washington, DC: US Government Printing Office.

US Census Bureau (2007) *Current Population Survey (CPS): Annual Social and Economic (ASEC) Supplement.* Table PINC-01. Washington, DC: US Government Printing Office.

Xie, J., Brayne, C., Matthew, F.E. and MRC Cognitive Function and Ageing Study collaborators. (2008) Survival times and people with dementia – analysis from a population based cohort study with 14 year follow up. *British Medical Journal,* 336: 258–65.

4

A bio-psycho-social approach to dementia

Steven R Sabat

Learning objectives

By the end of this chapter, you will learn that people with dementia:

- are capable of learning new things
- can be sad about and embarrassed by their condition
- do not lose their selfhood
- can be powerfully affected by how they are treated by others

---

Introduction

In the coming decades, barring medical interventions that can prevent or reverse the occurrence of Alzheimer's disease and other types of dementia, the numbers of people affected directly and indirectly will reach into the tens of millions and the financial costs required to care for such people will be in the hundreds of billions of US dollars (ADRDA 2000) (see Chapter 1). It is of paramount importance in the absence of such interventions that we understand the effects of dementia in order to develop more effective means of treating and sustaining those who have been diagnosed. If we assume that dementia is the outcome of brain damage and that much of what a person does that can be seen as being 'abnormal' in one way or another (such as anxiety, agitation, anger, etc.) is directly caused by the brain damage, we are then left with the job of 'managing the patient' so as to make him or her more and more comfortable and less and less of a burden on caregivers. Management is often accomplished via the use of drugs, including anti-anxiety and antidepressant medication, in addition to drugs that may enhance synaptic transmission between neurons in the brain and thereby improve aspects of memory, such as the ability to recall recent events.

There is a very important assumption in the above paragraph: many, if not all, of the 'symptoms' of dementia are, in one or another way, the direct outcome of the neuropathology caused by the disease process. This assumption is the foundation of the purely biomedical approach that dominated our understanding of dementia for decades (Katzman *et al.* 1978). In the past two decades, Kitwood (1997, 1998) called attention to significant problems with a strictly biomedical approach and, increasingly, research has shown that a broader understanding of people with dementia is required, for the behaviour of such people is affected by at least four factors (Harris 2002; Killick and Allan 2001; Sabat 2001; Snyder 1999; Wilkinson 2002):

- brain damage
- the person's reaction to the effects of the brain damage
- the ways in which the person is treated by healthy others
- the reactions of the diagnosed person to the ways in which he or she is treated by others.

Kitwood (1990) captured some of these factors in the following formula:

$$SD = NI + MSP$$

where SD is senile dementia, NI is neurological impairment, and MSP is malignant social psychology.

Malignant social psychology was Kitwood's term for a style of interaction and relationship which had the effect of diminishing a person's personhood such as is seen in the depersonalizing treatment given to persons with dementia. In the quest for ways to sustain and care for people with dementia so as to enhance as much as possible their quality of life, it is important to examine closely each of the different factors so as to understand what people with dementia can and cannot do and under what conditions their abilities are facilitated as opposed to inhibited. It is important, in other words, to identify correctly what constitutes a symptom of neuropathology as opposed to an appropriate emotional reaction to an extremely undesirable situation or to dysfunctional social treatment. This chapter will examine the biological, the psychological, and the social domains, so as to develop a clear picture of a bio-psycho-social approach.

The biological domain

As described in Chapter 1 the biological and clinical aspect is different in the different types of dementia. Depletion of certain transmitter substances occurs in Alzheimer's disease, but not necessarily in vascular dementia. A person with a vascular dementia might not have damage to the hippocampus, but people with Alzheimer's disease do have that damage. In addition, people with multi-infarct dementia have had several small strokes, but people with Alzheimer's disease have not. As described in Chapter 1, Alzheimer's disease is a type of dementia said to involve a depletion of a variety of neurotransmitters as well as the purported development of senile plaques and neurofibrillary tangles (Gaines and Whitehouse 2006). Over the course of the disease, there is a significant loss of neurons in the brain. This section will focus on the relationship between damage to particular areas of the brain (damage includes the loss of neurons) and losses in particular cognitive abilities and skills associated with Alzheimer's disease.

Memory

Dementia involves brain damage that can affect a variety of cognitive abilities. Dementia of different types can affect different parts of the brain. One of the first areas of the brain that is affected by Alzheimer's disease is the hippocampus, and the effects of damage here involve defects in what is known as 'explicit' memory. Among the ways by which information can be retrieved from memory are explicit and implicit forms of retrieval (Squire 1994). Explicit memory involves the ability to recall consciously or to recognize specific pieces of information on demand. So, when we ask someone what today's date is, or what month it is, we are asking the person to recall in a conscious way a specific piece of information. Thus, when a person with Alzheimer's disease asks a question and we answer it and then, five minutes later, the person asks the same question again as if it were the first time he or she was asking, we are witnessing a failure of recall. If we then ask the person, 'What did I just tell you five minutes ago?' the person might say, 'I don't know', and that would be another example of the failure to retrieve information via recall.

In some instances, one may change the format of the question from 'What day of the week is it today?' (to which the person with Alzheimer's disease said, 'I don't know') to a multiple-choice format ('Is it Tuesday?', 'Is it Friday?', etc.) and with this format, the person might identify the day correctly. This can happen because recall is much more difficult than recognition, which is the method of retrieval being used with a multiple-choice format, and this phenomenon is seen in many people with Alzheimer's disease. Therefore, one should not assume that a person's failure to recall information means that the person cannot remember that information. Recall and remembering are not the same things. Recall is one way to remember, but there are other ways to do so, including recognition (Sabat 2001).

Another form of memory, apparently involving mechanisms of retrieval that are different than those used with explicit memory, is known as 'implicit' memory, and this is defined as a change in behaviour that can occur as a result of an experience that the person is not consciously aware of having had (Grosse *et al.* 1990; Howard 1991; Roedigger 1990; Russo and Spinnler 1994).

Box 4.1   Case example

In what is called a word-stem completion task, a person with a memory dysfunction, such as AD, is presented with a list of words including the word, 'defend'. The person's memory of the words on the list can be tested in different ways. In one format, testing explicit memory, the person can be given the word-stem, 'def —', and then asked to complete the blank so as to make a word that he or she studied on the list presented earlier. In a different format, testing implicit memory, the person would be asked to complete the blank so as to form the first word that comes to mind. Note that in this latter format, there is no mention of the list of words presented previously. When employing the first format, using explicit memory, it is not uncommon for the person being tested to respond by saying, 'What list?' By asking that question, the person with AD exhibits a dysfunction in explicit memory, specifically, recall. The same person who appears to have no memory of having studied the list of words will complete the word-stem correctly if asked to complete the blank so to make the first word that comes to mind. Note that there is a plethora of words that begin with 'def —', so that one could not be 'lucky' in guessing correctly simply because there are so few words that could be made by filling in the blank.

Such findings have been shown in people with AD in the mild to moderate stages (Randolph *et al.* 1995; Russo and Spinnler 1994). Thus, although the ability of a person with AD to recall information may be compromised, his or her ability to recognize the same information may be less compromised, and the ability to learn new information can be intact, even if the person does not recall having learned that information.

A specific version of the problem with recall is observed in what are called 'word-finding' problems. The person with AD, while speaking, has difficulty in finding the word or words that he or she wants to use. Again, however, although the person may have a severe problem recalling the words in question, it is often possible for him or her to recognize the sought after words if the healthy partner in conversation provides some possibilities.

Box 4.2 Case example

Person with dementia: 'I went to see the uh, the, the, person who takes care of me when I'm not well physically.'

Respondent: 'Do you mean the dentist?'

Person with dementia: 'Well, it could be, but not in this case.'

Respondent: 'Do you mean a physician?'

Person with dementia: 'Yes.'

(From Sabat 2001)

Organization of movement

Damage to 'association' areas of the parietal lobe of the brain may result in 'apraxia', or the inability to organize in the correct order a sequence of movements. Thus, although not paralysed, a person might not be able to:

- tie his or her shoelaces
- button a shirt
- sign his or her name
- use eating utensils correctly.

It is important in each case to establish that the person can identify correctly the object in question (the eating utensils, the shirt, the shoes and laces), because if he or she cannot identify the object, it would be incorrect to say that the person's inability to use the object was due to a problem with the organization of movement. Another form of apraxia may, from the point of view of Brown (1972), be seen in instances of speech sounds that are misplaced so that the order of the sounds is incorrect, interfering with the communicative process. Brown proposed that some fluent aphasias might be considered apraxias of speech production.

Visual identification of objects

Following damage to so-called 'association' areas of the occipital lobe of the brain, a person may see objects clearly but may be unable to identify them by name. This problem is known as visual agnosia and it can result from damage due to Alzheimer's disease and other dementias. A specific instance of this problem is 'prosopagnosia', or the inability to identify another person by sight, by looking at the person's face. Thus, a person might be able to see and even acknowledge all the details, or features, of an object, but will be unable to organize those features into a coherent whole and name the object or person as the case may be.

Exercise 4.1   Different ways of interpreting behaviour

Consider the following:

You are a staff member at a day centre that serves people including those diagnosed with dementia. You enter a room with a wardrobe containing participants' coats, and you see one of the participants who is diagnosed with dementia reaching into the pockets of one coat, looking at the contents, putting them back, and repeating this process with the next coat and the next. What do you assume about this behaviour and what do you do?

How might our different views of what influences behaviour affect how we interpret this behaviour?

If the staff member's understanding of people with AD is one that emphasizes such persons' defects, the staff member might well view this behaviour as a socially inappropriate 'symptom' and proceed to stop the person from continuing.

Imagine you did not choose to intervene but simply watched the participant move from coat to coat, looking at the contents of the pockets of each and replacing contents, until he came to one particular coat. When he looked at the contents of this particular coat's pockets, he replaced the contents in the coat pocket, but then took the coat off the hanger and put the coat on. And, most significantly, it was his coat. It is true that going through the pockets of coats that belong to others is inappropriate. It is the case, however, that the intention of the person with AD in this example was not to act inappropriately, to invade the property of others or violate their privacy. Rather, the man was simply trying to find his coat, which he could not recognize by sight, perhaps not recalling which coat he wore that day. He did know that his coat pockets contained his property and he knew, consciously or unconsciously, that he would recognize his belongings when he saw them. Thus, his behaviour was not simply some species of 'social disinhibition' resulting from brain damage caused by AD, but an adaptation to the effects of AD.

How might it feel for a person not to be able to recognize his own coat by sight, or not to be able to put on a shirt or a pair of trousers or to sign his or her name? This is very much a psychological issue and it is to such matters that we now turn.

The psychological domain

Understanding what Alzheimer's disease or another type of dementia does to a person psychologically requires more than simply observing his or her behaviour from afar or examining standard neuropsychological test results. Indeed, it requires that we engage that person as a person so as to understand what he or she is experiencing (Laing 1965; see Chapter 2). To assume that a person would not have any reactions to the loss of his or her ability to use eating utensils, to tie shoelaces, sign his or her name, recall what happened moments ago, spell simple words, would be to assume that the person in question was quite dysfunctional. To assume that depression, anxiety, agitation, so-called 'wandering', and the like, are symptoms of Alzheimer's disease in the same way that fever is a symptom of malaria, is to depersonalize the individual in question (Bender and Cheston 1997; Harris 2002; Kitwood 1997; Kitwood and Bredin 1992; Sabat 2001). What do we discover when we engage people with AD as people, even as partners in research?

Snyder (1999) interviewed people recently diagnosed with probable Alzheimer's disease and, in so doing, revealed much about their reactions to the symptoms, the diagnosis, and the ways in which others treated them. Some people reacted strongly and negatively to the treatment they received from the medical personnel involved in arriving at and communicating the diagnosis. For example, Bea described the neurologist who interviewed her:

> He was very indifferent and said it was just going to get worse ... If he had just shown a little compassion. He was there to diagnose my problem, but he wasn't there to understand my feelings. He had no feelings for me whatsoever. I've hated him ever since. Health care professionals need to be compassionate.
>
> (Snyder 1999: 18)

Another of Snyder's interviewees, Betty, a retired social worker and former faculty member at San Diego State University, discussed health care professionals whom she encountered during the process of being diagnosed:

> They're busy wanting to climb up to the next rung on the ladder. That's very human. I don't blame them. But they don't really accept the significance of illness for people. They know the diagnosis, but they don't take time to find out what it truly means for that person. This casualness with which professionals deal with Alzheimer's is so painful to see ...You have to really be willing to be present with the person who has Alzheimer's. But there are some people who don't want to learn, and it's the looking down on and being demeaning of people with Alzheimer's that is hard to watch.
>
> (Snyder 1999: 123–4)

Connell *et al.* (2004) have found these experiences to be similar in many ways to those reported by family caregivers.

Both women felt depersonalized by the health care professionals who informed them of their diagnosis, and who seemed to lack any interest in exploring with them what the diagnosis meant to them, how they felt, or in extending to them any human compassion or caring. Still, one should not assume that the professionals in question were callous, uncaring people. So why did they behave as they did? Among the possible reasons is how the professionals positioned Bea and Betty as well as how they positioned themselves (Harré and van Langenhove 1991). That is to say, the professionals understood their roles as being limited to communicating the facts of the diagnosis and nothing more. They did not think that there was any reason to discuss anything further with their patients, perhaps because there was nothing they could do to stop the disease from progressing toward its eventual conclusion. In a subtle way, though, they may have been incorrectly positioning Bea and Betty negatively as people who, because of their illness, would either have no particular reaction to the news, given that they have a form of dementia, or lack the ability to engage in any kind of discussion about what the news meant to them.

It would be incorrect to assume that interactions of this type occur in each and every situation between health care professionals and their patients, but it surely was true in these cases, as well as in the case of Dr B (Sabat 2001), whose internist commented that 'treating a person with Alzheimer's is like doing veterinary medicine'. Under these conditions, the person with Alzheimer's disease feels ignored, unworthy of being treated as a human being, and someone who is defined to a great extent, if not completely, by his or her diagnosis. Betty said, 'A person with Alzheimer's disease is many more things than just their diagnosis. Each person is a whole human being' (Snyder 1999: 123–4).

Once persons are positioned socially as nothing more than instantiations of a diagnostic category, their essential humanity, including their intellectual and emotional characteristics, needs, and their social personae beyond that of 'demented, burdensome patient' become more and more invisible and can ultimately be erased. When viewed in this way, the extent to which such people can enjoy any semblance of a good quality of life is correspondingly reduced and this, in turn, will require increasing expenditures of resources in order to 'manage the patients' instead of interacting with them as persons in ways that would not lead to conflict, disparagement, and the resulting need for 'management'.

Although Bea commented that she often felt 'nearly invisible' in social situations, she did perceive others' apparent discomfort about her diagnosis and her problems with aspects of memory as well as with organizing and directing bodily movements such as shaking hands. Others in her social milieu seemed to position her negatively as being far more disabled than she actually was, and treated her as if the negative positioning were actually valid, thereby creating a dramatic constriction of her social world to the point of her being isolated and increasingly dependent upon her husband. She was well aware of this entire dynamic: 'I'm isolating him as well as myself and I'm not being fair to him' (Snyder 1999: 24).

Feelings such as these, that arise from being negatively positioned by others and then treated in socially malignant ways such as being ostracized and banished (Kitwood 1998) create internal conflict within the person with AD and diminish the person's sense of self-worth.

It may seem strange that the two women who were quoted verbatim above could be treated as they were, given that they expressed themselves clearly, cogently, and with grace. Nothing in what they said or how they said it could conduce to the idea that they were cognitively compromised, yet they were still treated by healthy others in ways that could be described as 'dysfunctional' and 'malignant'. It is precisely this confluence of facts that underscores how powerful an influence a diagnosis can be. What is the foundation of this sort of treatment? Two possibilities spring to mind:

- There is a stereotypic view, promoted by professionals, the public press, entertainment media, and the like, that focuses on the defects that AD can ultimately cause, and simultaneously ignores the person's remaining intact abilities.

- There is the tendency for diagnostic overshadowing to occur such that all reported 'defects' in people thus diagnosed are due to the disease alone and not to the ways in which the people thus diagnosed are treated by others.

There is, however, the testimony of people in the moderate to severe stages of AD, who express appropriate anger, frustration, sadness and embarrassment regarding the losses that they have experienced. Dr M was very clear about this when she spoke about writing and typing, things that she once did with great facility: 'Now it is so miserable a chore that I avoid it as much as possible. And all these things take ridiculous amounts of time ... as to how my symptoms affect me, do not think I am just being frivolous if I say they drive me crazy' (Sabat 2001: 115).

Add to this the fact that others see the person with Alzheimer's disease principally in terms of what he or she cannot do and is it any wonder that such a person would feel depressed? Indeed, for a person not to feel depressed in such circumstances would be 'inappropriate' and worthy of being described as 'having no insight' into, or being 'blissfully unaware' of, one's problems. We could just as easily observe that to feel all of the above negative emotions in the face of the effects of Alzheimer's disease and the ensuing social treatment is, itself, evidence of the intact complex cognitive function that is required for a person to be a 'semiotic subject' – one whose behaviour is driven by the meaning that situations hold for him or her (Sabat and Harré 1994).

To summarize, negative positioning of people diagnosed with Alzheimer's disease is based on a medical view that every instance of seemingly 'abnormal' behaviour seen in the person diagnosed is due to brain damage, and that such people are immune to being treated in dysfunctional ways by others. So, for example, if a person with a diagnosis of probable Alzheimer's disease is treated in a way that would be humiliating and embarrassing to any reasonable, healthy person, and if the person with Alzheimer's disease reacts with anger or grief or by pulling away from others or avoiding them completely, the anger, grief, social isolation are viewed as symptoms of Alzheimer's disease instead of symptoms of dysfunctional social treatment, so as to validate the original malignant positioning of the person.

> **Exercise 4.2**   The importance of knowing the full context
>
> Consider the following:
>
> You are a staff member at a day centre that serves people including those diagnosed with dementia. The spouse of one of the participants tells you about his wife, 'Her Alzheimer's is getting worse; yesterday, after I picked her up from the day centre, she became irrationally hostile toward me, wouldn't speak to me or look at me at all during the evening.'
>
> What do you say?
>
> What do you think?
>
> Consider what you might think if you also knew the larger context of the scenario: When the husband arrived to pick up his wife, she was standing in the hallway conversing with others, including staff members. The husband joined in the conversation but, as his wife was talking, he began to tuck her turtleneck top into her trousers (she was wearing it outside of her trousers and it looked fine). As he did this in front of others, thinking (incorrectly) that she'd forgotten to do so herself, she was clearly humiliated, her eyes bulging out of their sockets, so to speak, but this went unnoticed by her husband. She reacted toward him later with anger, but the anger was anything but 'irrational'. Indeed, one could quite easily refer to her reaction as 'righteous indignation' instead of 'irrational hostility'.

The message in this case is clear: it is of tremendous importance to understand the larger social context in which a person acts; and not to assume that because a person with AD reacts in a way that is not immediately understandable to the caregiver, the behaviour in question is 'irrational' and a product of brain damage as opposed to dysfunctional social treatment.

People with AD live in a social world with others much of the time and it is to the social domain that we now turn.

The social domain

> **Box 4.3**   Case example
>
> Mrs R attended an adult day centre and, according to standard assessments, was in the moderate to severe stages of AD. Her husband commented that she did nothing around the house, save for watching television and walking around 'aimlessly', that she did not help with the household chores, that he did everything. At the day centre, however, Mrs R helped set tables prior to the lunch meal, acted almost as a volunteer (according to the staff members) by helping participants in wheelchairs navigate through doorways, by comforting others who were recovering from illness and by calling staff's attention to participants who needed a level of help that she could not provide (Sabat 2001). Although it is true that brain damage can result in increased variability in the performance of many tasks, there was no variability in Mrs R's behaviour: at home she did nothing, but at the day centre, she did a great deal, much of which she could have done at home as well, such as setting the table. Thus, one must look beyond the biological

level to find an explanation for this striking difference in her behaviour. In the past, Mrs R served as a volunteer in a variety of ways, from working in hospitals to caring for abandoned children in undeveloped countries. Being of service to others was an abiding aspect of her personality.

We can examine this as well as her situation at home and at the day centre by using a social constructionist approach (Harré 1991) as a heuristic device. Among the aspects of selfhood, there is the self of one's attributes, mental and physical, past and present. So, one's eye pigmentation, facility with languages, college degree, sense of humour, are all part of this aspect of selfhood (called Self 2). Also part of Self 2 are one's beliefs (political, religious, etc.) and one's beliefs about one's attributes: one can take pride in some of one's attributes, while viewing other attributes with disdain, even antipathy. People with AD even in the moderate to severe stages have made it clear that they view their losses as embarrassing, frustrating, even maddening. Also part of the selfhood of an individual is the multiple social personae (Self 3) that he or she constructs with the cooperation of others. Each of one's social personae is marked by a unique pattern of behaviour, so that the behaviour connected with being a loving spouse is quite different from that connected with being a devoted parent, a demanding supervisor at work, and a loyal friend, to name a few. We can examine Mrs R's situation at home as opposed to the day centre by examining the social dynamics required for the construction of the social personae of Self 3.

Recall that it is necessary to have the cooperation of at least one other person in order to construct (jointly) a particular social persona.

Box 4.4 Case example

It would be impossible to behave as a loving spouse if one's husband or wife did not recognize him or her as being a spouse. One cannot construct the persona of the devoted parent if one's child does not recognize one as being his or her mother or father. Mrs R could not construct the social persona of 'helpful spouse' at home because her husband did not allow her to engage in helping him with household jobs. He indicated his concern that she would fail to do what he would ask of her and so, according to him, he 'protected' her by doing everything himself. Conversely, at the day centre, the staff cooperated with Mrs R, allowing her to be of help to participants as well as to other staff members, thereby helping her in constructing the social persona of 'helpful participant/quasi volunteer'.

There have been reports of similar examples in recent years (Sabat 2003; Sabat *et al.* 2004). In many cases, it appears, the person with Alzheimer's disease is prevented from constructing a valued social persona due to: (a) the lack of cooperation from healthy others in the social milieu, and the intimately related (b) tendency of others to view the person with Alzheimer's disease increasingly in terms of his or her deficits. By viewing the person in question mainly in terms of his or her diagnosis and all the losses it entails, healthy others thereby ignore more and more the attributes in which the person in question takes pride. This dynamic serves to restrict the social persona of the individual with Alzheimer's disease to something that the person with Alzheimer's disease finds abhorrent, embarrassing, humiliating – 'the burdensome patient' or 'the defective patient' because others do not provide the necessary cooperation for the person to construct a worthy social persona. In this way, the person with Alzheimer's disease is confined to a social persona that is constituted of everything that is defective and embarrassing. Is it any wonder that Dr M, a retired university professor in the moderate to severe stage, commented about Alzheimer's, 'Is it even more embarrassing than a sexual disease?' (Sabat 2001: 115).

Exercise 4.3   How a person can be positioned malignantly by language

Consider the following:

You make a visit to the home of a married couple. The husband has been diagnosed with dementia. You are greeted by the wife who then introduces you to her husband by saying, 'This is my husband; he's the patient.'

Do you have a private reaction to this introduction, and if so, what is it?

Here we see a perfectly loving, devoted, respectful wife introducing her husband as 'the patient'. Of course, her husband had many other attributes that could have been used as part of an introduction, and it was clear that some of those attributes were positive and worthy of honour and respect. Yet, the wife focused on an attribute that he found abhorrent.

It is common to hear people described as 'patients'. Still, the plain fact is that people are patients only in relation to their physicians, nurses, dentists and other health professionals. In other social relationships, people can be many things, but they cannot be patients in the true sense of the social situations at hand. Why, then, are people with AD seen as being 'patients' regardless of the social situation of which they happen to be a part? In a sense, the restriction of a person's social persona to an attribute that the person loathes and is embarrassed by is a form of what Kitwood (1998) called 'malignant social psychology' because this type of treatment depersonalizes the individual and constitutes an assault on the person's sense of self-worth.

It is clear that people with Alzheimer's disease even in the moderate to severe stage of the disease can construct worthy social personae when given the necessary cooperation. It is clear also that those who live in residential settings for people with dementia can still enjoy and experience meaningful social interactions (Hubbard *et al.* 2003). It is extremely important to note, however, that such people are far more dependent on there being supportive environments and venues within which they can have the opportunities to engage in these kinds of interactions. Hence, people with Alzheimer's disease or other forms of dementia are far more vulnerable than they were during the balance of their adult lives because it is much more difficult for them to gain the cooperation they need in order to construct valued social identities. There is reason to emphasize strongly, therefore, that the measurement tools that are used to assess the so-called cognitive abilities of people with dementia, obviously do not predict or assess a person's capacity to enjoy meaningful social interactions with others. In other words, practitioners (a) should not assume anything at all about the social identity or potential social identity of a person with dementia on the basis of his or her standard test scores because (b) such tests make little, if any, contact with the combination of cognitive abilities that is required for a person to be a semiotic subject who can enjoy valued social relationships with others.

Box 4.5 Case example

A man to whom I was about to administer a battery of neuropsychological tests made what seemed to be a completely unsolicited (by me) comment: 'Doc, ya gotta find a way to give us purpose again.' Although he was in the moderate to severe stage of Alzheimer's disease, he possessed the ability (and the requisite functional brain systems) to discern the importance of having a purpose in life, that he lacked a meaningful purpose, and that he needed help from someone else in his quest to regain what he so strongly desired. A bio-psycho-social approach allows us to understand that:

1 Some of the losses he sustained had their roots in biological terms, but also simultaneously.

2 He was able to experience and articulate a completely appropriate reaction to those losses.

3 He understood what those losses meant to him personally and socially.

4 There are non-pharmaceutical ways to enhance his quality of life.

Debates and controversies

Within the domain of a bio-psycho-social approach to dementia, professionals in different disciplines still engage in debates around the issues:

- Does a purely biomedical approach to dementia provide a complete understanding of the person diagnosed?

- Are pharmaceutical treatments (drugs) all that are required to treat the person?

- Is it practical to try to understand and treat each person in the light of his or her unique history when each person is different? Is this possible in residential homes?

- What is the difference between understanding the disease a person has and the person the disease has?

Conclusion

The behavioural changes observed in people with dementia were, for decades, attributed solely to brain damage. More recently, it has become clear that, in addition to the effects of brain injury, people with dementia also have psychological reactions to their brain injuries, and these reactions affect what they say and do in relation to others. Furthermore, people with dementia are affected by the ways in which they are treated by healthy others in social situations. Although biological explanations are appropriate in explaining certain aspects of Alzheimer's disease, such as the relationship between damage to the hippocampus and defects in explicit memory, there are other effects that are not explainable in purely biological terms. Specifically, people with dementia are embarrassed by, angry about, and sometimes depressed about the problems caused by brain injury and they seek to avoid embarrassment and humiliation. Furthermore, they can retain aspects of selfhood, including worthy social personae, but the latter depends upon how they are treated by others. A bio-psycho-social approach is required for understanding people with AD and for the further evolution of good practice in the treatment and support of people with other types of dementia.

Further information

MedlinePlus provides information on-line about health conditions, including dementia. It brings together information from NLM, the National Institutes of Health (NIH), and other US government agencies and health-related organizations.

The Merck Manual of Geriatrics is available online and provides information about the care of older people.

The National Institute of Neurological Disorders and Stroke is part of the US National Institutes of Health. It has web pages devoted to dementia.

The **University of California at San Francisco Memory and Aging Center** has a web-site with useful information about dementia.

References

Alzheimer's and Related Disorders Association (ADRDA) (2000) *A Race Against Time*. Chicago, IL: ADRDA.

Bender, M.P. and Cheston, R. (1997) Inhabitants of a lost kingdom: a model of the subjective experiences of dementia. *Ageing and Society*, 17(5): 513–32.

Brown, J.W. (1972) *Aphasia, Apraxia, and Agnosia: Clinical and Theoretical Aspects*. Springfield, IL: C.C. Thomas.

Connell, C.M., Boise, L., Stuckey, J.C., Holmes, S.B. and Hudson, M.L. (2004) Attitudes toward the diagnosis and disclosure of dementia among family caregivers and primary care physicians. *The Gerontologist*, 44(4): 500–7.

Gaines, A.D. and Whitehouse, P.J. (2006) Building a mystery: Alzheimer's disease, mild cognitive impairment, and beyond. *Philosophy, Psychiatry, & Psychology*, 13(1): 61–74.

Grosse, D.A., Wilson, R.S. and Fox, J.H. (1990) Preserved word stem completion priming of semantically encoded information in Alzheimer's disease. *Psychology and Aging*, 5(2): 304–6.

Harré, R. (1991) The discursive production of selves. *Theory and Psychology*, 1(1): 51–63.

Harré, R. and van Langenhove, L. (1991) Varieties of positioning. *Journal for the Theory of Social Behavior*, 21(4): 393–408.

Harris, P.B. (ed.) (2002) *The Person with Alzheimer's Disease: Pathways to Understanding the Experience*. Baltimore, MD: Johns Hopkins University Press.

Howard, D.V. (1991) Implicit memory: An expanding picture of cognitive aging. In: K.W. Schaie (ed.) *Annual Review of Gerontology and Geriatrics* (Vol. 11). New York: Springer-Verlag, pp. 1–22.

Hubbard, G., Tester, S. and Downs, M.G. (2003) Meaningful social interactions between older people in institutional care settings. *Ageing and Society*, 23(1): 99–114.

Katzman, R., Terry, R.D. and Bick, K.L. (eds) (1978) *Alzheimer's Disease: Senile Dementia and Related Disorders*. New York: Raven Press.

Killick, J. and Allan, K. (2001) *Communication and the Care of People with Dementia*. Buckingham: Open University Press.

Kitwood, T. (1990) The dialectics of dementia: With particular reference to Alzheimer's disease. *Ageing and Society*, 10(2): 177–96.

Kitwood, T. (1997) *Dementia Reconsidered: The Person Comes First*. Philadelphia, PA: Open University Press.

Kitwood, T. (1998) Toward a theory of dementia care: Ethics and interaction. *Journal of Clinical Ethics*, 9(1): 23–34.

Kitwood, T. and Bredin, K. (1992) Towards a theory of dementia care: Personhood and well-being. *Ageing and Society*, 12(1): 269–87.

Laing, R.D. (1965) *The Divided Self*. Baltimore, MD: Penguin Books.

Randolph, C., Tierney, M.C. and Chase, T.N. (1995) Implicit memory in Alzheimer's disease. *Journal of Clinical and Experimental Neuropsychology*, 17(3): 343–51.

Roedigger, H.L. (1990) Retention without remembering. *American Psychologist*, 45(9): 1043–56.

Russo, R. and Spinnler, H. (1994) Implicit verbal memory in Alzheimer's disease. *Cortex*, 30(3): 359–75.

Sabat, S.R. (2001) *The Experience of Alzheimer's Disease: Life Through a Tangled Veil*. Oxford: Blackwell.

Sabat, S.R. (2003) Some potential benefits of creating research partnerships with people with Alzheimer's disease. *Research Policy and Planning*, 21(2): 5–12.

Sabat, S.R. and Harré, R. (1994) The Alzheimer's disease sufferer as a semiotic subject. *Philosophy, Psychiatry, and Psychology*, 1(1): 145–60.

Sabat, S.R., Napolitano, L. and Fath, H. (2004) Barriers to the construction of a valued social identity: A case study of Alzheimer's disease. *American Journal of Alzheimer's Disease and Other Dementias*, 19(3): 177–85.

Snyder, L. (1999) *Speaking Our Minds: Personal Reflections from Individuals with Alzheimer's*. New York: Freeman.

Squire, L.R. (1994) Declarative and nondeclarative memory: Multiple brain systems supporting learning and memory. In: D.L. Schacter and E. Tulving (eds) *Memory Systems*. Cambridge, MA: MIT Press, pp. 203–32.

Wilkinson, H. (ed.) (2002) *The Perspectives of People with Dementia*. London: Jessica Kingsley Publishers.

5

Flexibility and change: the fundamentals for families coping with dementia

Steven H Zarit and Judy M Zarit

Learning objectives

By the end of this chapter you will be able to:

- distinguish between primary and secondary stressors in caring
- discuss how carers' views affect their experience of caring
- describe the satisfactions and rewards of caring
- outline the steps carers can take to improve quality of life for themselves and their relatives with dementia

---

Introduction

As our population ages, more people develop disabilities that require assistance (see Chapter 1), and more family members are called upon to lend a hand. Families account for a majority of all the care received by older people, with paid help and institutional care providing a surprisingly small role often mainly near the end of life (Spillman and Black 2005). This commitment of families to their older relatives has remained strong, despite all the changes that have taken place during the past half century in family roles and relationships. Family carers provide this help, however, often at considerable risk to their own health and well-being. Studies have consistently found that providing care to a disabled elder is associated with increased rates of depression and other mental health symptoms (Aneshensel *et al.* 1995; Schulz *et al.* 1995). The health of carers can also suffer, either directly due to the stressors associated with care, or because carers do not take the time to attend to their own health needs (Schulz and Beach 1999).

In this chapter, we look at the adjustments and adaptations that occur within families caring for someone with dementia. We draw upon the research on caregiving, as well as our clinical experience and discussions with carers over the past 25 years. We consider both the main carer, as well as other family members who provide a portion of the help. We examine the stressors and challenges carers experience, as well as the satisfactions and rewards of caring for a relative with dementia.

Caregiving stressors and their impact

Much of the focus of research on caring has been on stressors and their consequences. Examination of stressors has been guided by a 'stress and coping' framework (Pearlin *et al.* 1990; Lazarus and Folkman 1984). From this perspective, stressful events lead to a mobilization of psychological and social resources for managing or coping with these events and their consequences. In the case of caregiving, stressors are not one-off events but are ongoing. How much impact particular stressors will have on carers' lives is influenced by:

- the meanings that people give to events
- their beliefs about their ability to manage the events
- the skills and resources they have.

From our clinical experience we know that for some carers even mild perturbations can overwhelm their poor coping resources, while other people can take on an exhausting routine without much difficulty. Of course, symptoms of dementia worsen over time, which can diminish the carer's coping resources. As discussed in Chapter 14, when people are unable to contain the effects of stressors, they will experience anxiety, depression or other psychological distress. Chronic stress also affects the body's hormonal and immune systems, and these changes can lead to an increased vulnerability to disease (Vitaliano *et al.* 2003).

Caregiving stressors can be divided into two main types: primary stressors or those events and challenges directly related to their relative's illness; and secondary stressors, the ways in which primary stressors may interfere with the carer's other roles, involvements and activities (Aneshensel *et al.* 1995; Pearlin *et al.* 1990).

Primary caregiving stressors

Primary stressors fall into three categories:

- changes in the person's cognition and abilities
- behavioural and emotional changes
- changes in the relationship between the carer and person with dementia, including a sense of loss.

Cognition and day–day abilities

Changes in cognition and abilities include being able to look after oneself and to initiate and engage in activities. We have observed that initially families typically respond to memory lapses with commonsense approaches that worked in the past, such as giving reminders or encouraging the person to remember on his/her own, but these strategies have limited utility for people experiencing dementia-related progressive memory loss. In addition, as discussed in Chapter 2 and Chapter 9, the person with dementia may have limited awareness of his/her limitations, or may deny having a problem.

For example, people with dementia may ask where their mother is, even though their mother may have died 20 or 30 years earlier. They may be concerned that their purse or wallet was stolen. In response families often contradict the person with dementia, saying 'I've already told you your mother died 20 years ago' or 'No one stole your wallet, it's under your bed.' While attempting to resolve their relative's concern, carers frequently ignite an argument instead.

Instead of trying to reason with or reorient the person with dementia, we encourage carers to take a two-step approach:

1   to think about why their relative would behave in this way

2   to think about what their relative might be feeling (Zarit and Zarit 2007).

For example, we encourage carers to consider why their relative would ask to see their mother. For one thing, the request suggests that the person's cognitive impairment is severe enough that he does not remember that his mother is dead. Presenting the fact that she is dead can sometimes produce a grief reaction. We suggest that it is better to focus on the underlying feeling, what emotions might underlie the request to see one's mother? The person may be seeking comfort and reassurance. A carer can respond by providing comfort, rather than directly challenging the request, for example, stating, 'Let's sit down and have a cup of tea and talk about your mother.' In other words, carers need to learn not to argue over the facts of a situation, but instead to identify the feelings that are embedded in these communications (see Chapter 12). Instead of trying to convince someone who has impaired cognitive abilities about the facts of a situation, it is far more productive to respond at a feeling level, providing comfort or reassurance, when needed.

As memory problems and other cognitive difficulties worsen, people with dementia gradually require assistance with a variety of daily tasks, as well as supervision to make sure that they do not get into difficulty, for example, by getting lost. Carers gradually begin helping the person with instrumental activities of daily living (IADL). They may give occasional reminders to dress or bathe, or a bit of help with complex activities, such as cooking or grocery shopping. Another complex area to negotiate is driving (Breen *et al.* 2007). Providing help with personal care can be difficult. The person with dementia may resist help, insisting they can look after themselves, or in other ways be uncooperative (Fauth *et al.* in press). In late stage dementia, carers may have to assist in transfers from bed to chair, and chair to standing. Depending on their strength and how much the person with dementia weighs, this can be quite challenging.

An often overlooked problem is that people with dementia become increasingly unable to initiate or sustain meaningful activities on their own (Perrin and May 1999). The lack of activity, combined with taking frequent naps during the day, can lead to a variety of other problems, including restlessness and not sleeping at night.

Behavioural and emotional changes

As mentioned above, as dementia progresses, the carer provides increasing assistance with activities of daily living such as dressing and bathing. This assistance can create anxiety for, or alarm in, the person with dementia. As discussed in Chapter 9 and Chapter 11, there are a variety of psychosocial approaches to providing such assistance which can prevent or minimize the occurrence of these reactions. The behaviour disturbances that occur when the carer is assisting with ADLs or in reaction to increasing inactivity are part of a larger constellation of problems that are typically experienced as the most stressful events by carers (Aneshensel *et al.* 1995). These problems, which constitute the second area of primary stressors, are called behavioural and psychological symptoms of dementia (BPSD) (Finkel *et al.* 1996; see Chapter 11). BPSD can include depressive symptoms, agitation and restlessness, angry or aggressive actions, and hallucinations and delusions. Additionally, people with dementia may have difficulty falling asleep and sleeping through the night. As a result, they may keep the carer awake.

Carers often feel helpless in the face of behavioural problems, a reaction which is confirmed by physicians who too often have limited knowledge of the strategies that are helpful. Medications, though sometimes useful, can have significant adverse effects (Ballard and Cream 2005). As an alternative or to complement medications, carers can learn to use simple behavioural strategies (Zarit and Zarit 2007), including those for help with sleeping (McCurry *et al.* 2005). One approach is to learn to identify antecedents (triggers) and consequences (reinforcements) of the behaviour and to make changes in these sequences. Carers can be encouraged to look for triggers in the environment that initiate and reinforcement which reward these behaviours.

Box 5.1   Case example

A person with dementia might become restless after a long period of inactivity (the antecedent), and the restlessness would be reinforced by the attention that the carer gives to the person. In that situation, carers could prevent restlessness by addressing the antecedent (i.e. inactivity) by engaging the person with dementia in meaningful activities. The carer could also direct attention (i.e. reinforcement) to the person with dementia at times when he/she is engaging in socially appropriate behaviour, in other words, reinforce adaptive rather than problem behaviour.

Relationship with carer

With improved diagnostic processes, there is now a trend toward early diagnosis, which makes it possible to engage both the carer and the person with dementia during the formative period of caregiving. These conversations can be very useful for everyone involved (Clare 2002; Clare *et al.* 2002; Kuhn 1998; Moniz-Cook *et al.* 1998; 2003; Whitlatch *et al.* 2006; Zarit *et al.* 2004). They can help the dyad to learn more about what lies ahead, and to begin making plans for the future. Carers also have the opportunity to hear about the preferences of the person with dementia. In turn, people with dementia who still have an awareness of their problem can talk about how they would like to be cared for without becoming overwhelmed or depressed. They may be able to help carers develop realistic plans by indicating that the carer does not have to provide all the help by him/herself (Whitlatch *et al.* 2006).

Living with dementia can change the relationship between the person with dementia and his/her carer. As discussed in Chapter 21, carers may grieve or experience a sense of loss as their relative loses cognitive and functional abilities. Some carers may also lose the tangible benefits they received from the relationship. For a spouse, the relationship probably provided companionship, affection and intimacy, as well as some division of labour around household tasks. Adult children may feel a loss of the support they received from a parent, including advice, assistance and affection.

The carer's reactions to these changes depend partly on his/her past relationship with the person with dementia. When that relationship has been positive, the carer may feel a greater sense of loss, but also have a strong commitment to providing the needed care. A relationship that has been more conflicted often leaves carers feeling ambivalent. They may have a sense of obligation, but may also resent or be angry over being put in this position. Wives who become carers sometimes feel that they have been cheated out of the benefits of retirement, such as opportunities to travel, and instead they must reassume the roles of homemaker and carer that they have played their whole lives. Children who are carers may similarly struggle with the ambivalence they feel toward a parent. Long-standing dysfunctional relationships in the family will be carried forward into caregiving and complicate the process of giving care and receiving help from others.

Another important source of stress is that the contributions that the person with dementia made to the family system are lost. This loss can have a considerable impact, for example, when the person with dementia previously functioned as kin-keeper, bringing everyone else in the family together.

From our experience, carers need opportunities to address their feelings of grief, loss and ambivalence (see Chapter 21). Carers who are grieving the loss of the person or their relationship with that person cannot do the planning needed or learn the skills that will help them manage other stressors effectively. They must first be able to get beyond their grief and reconceptualize their relationship with the person with dementia as one in which they have to take the initiative. Carers who do well are those who see themselves as maintaining continuity of the relationship through the help they are giving, even as that relationship is changing. Their role is an extension of the love and obligation they feel for the person with dementia, and they accept that these feelings cannot be reciprocated. Helping carers reach this understanding, of course, is not accomplished by pointing it out to them, but through open and non-judgmental discussions about the meaning the relationship holds for them and their goals in providing care.

In a similar fashion, carers who have ambivalent and conflicted feelings about providing care can benefit from opportunities to talk with a supportive person, such as a counsellor. One goal of these conversations is to help carers realize that they have a choice in the matter. They may decide to continue to providing care, or they can set limits on the amount of help they are willing to give. Helping carers restructure their commitment to a level that they are willing to make can reduce their ambivalence.

Exercise 5.1   Rating the stressfulness of care demands

For each area of primary stressors:

- changes in the person's cognition and abilities
- behavioural and emotional changes
- changes in the relationship between carer and person with dementia

identify one or two problems that would be relatively easy for you to manage, and one or two problems that you would find very difficult or stressful to manage.

For each problem, write down what makes it stressful or easy for you to manage.

Review the reasons that you found some problems easy to manage and some problems stressful. What coping strategies could you use for managing the problems you found stressful?

Secondary stressors: changes in the carer's life

Secondary stressors include:

- the impact of caring on the carer's usual activities, including work and leisure
- conflict or strain in family relationships and friendships
- economic strains.

The impact of caring on the carer's usual activities, including work and leisure

The increasing demands of caring can disrupt and absorb other activities. Eventually carers may find that they have little time for anything except giving care. They frequently describe themselves as trapped, and that caregiving has taken over their lives and identity (Aneshensel *et al.* 1995).

Leisure and social activities are often the first to go. Sometimes carers give up these activities because the person with dementia can no longer participate, or may behave in embarrassing or socially inappropriate ways. In some instances, friends and relatives feel uncomfortable around the person with dementia and decrease contact. Carers may also view leisure activities as discretionary, and so they decrease or eliminate them in order to devote more time to caregiving. Rather than just being discretionary, however, these activities often contribute to positive feelings and may prevent depression in the carer (Teri *et al.* 1997).

Carers may also decrease activities that support good health. They may no longer exercise regularly, may not eat a healthy diet, or may not go to the doctor when they have a health problem. Some carers increase maladaptive health behaviours, smoking or eating more or increasing alcohol intake. Not surprisingly, carers with more stress in their daily lives are less likely to engage in positive health behaviours (Son *et al.* 2007).

Many carers continue to work outside the home. For them, daily routines are a continuing challenge, juggling multiple responsibilities and hoping that the care arrangements that they have made for their relative will continue to be adequate. Working sometimes has a positive influence on the carer's well-being (Aneshensel *et al.* 1995; Edwards *et al.* 2002). Going to work gives carers time away from the person with dementia. Work may give them satisfaction and the feeling that they can accomplish something. Sometimes, the competing demands of working and caregiving are too great, leading to an erosion of well-being (Stephens *et al.* 2001). In the end, many carers are forced to choose between their work and continuing to provide care.

The carers that we have known who have been successful are those who maintain significant activities away from the person with dementia. One man who was caring for his wife worked for many years as a volunteer at a local radio station. The enjoyment and recognition he received from this weekly show helped carry him through the rest of the time. Other carers participate in sports, and some continue to work, either full or part-time. One woman derived considerable satisfaction from spending a couple of days a week doing the bookkeeping for the family business.

Conflict or strain in family relationships and friendships

In earlier times in the West and in contemporary times in other cultures, the person identified for the care role was prescribed by tradition and sometimes law (see Chapter 3). Today, in Western societies the individual most likely to become carer is the husband or wife of the person with dementia, if that person is married. When the person with dementia is widowed or single and has children, a daughter typically assumes the role of carer. A daughter or son who takes on the primary care role sometimes finds that siblings disagree with, or challenge, his/her decisions. They may argue over whether care is needed and how it should be provided. Resentment can even develop over which one of them is helping, as shown in Boxes 5.2 and 5.3.

Box 5.2   Case example

Lesley was the younger of the two children in her family. Her brother was an international businessman, who travelled extensively and was rarely at home. He had been doted upon by their mother when he was a child. Their father had died in his early 60s. When their mother began to show signs of dementia, Lesley sought help from the local public agency that provides help to older people. Her mother's financial resources were modest, and she qualified for some public help. Her brother, whose main contact with his mother was over the telephone, questioned the need for help, since she sounded fine to him when they talked. As the dementia progressed, there were repetitions of the following scenario. The brother would fly into town, spend time in the family home with their mother and then declare that she was 'just fine', and that he did not agree that she needed help. Of course, he was not listening carefully to the emptiness of her responses to him, nor did he challenge her memory at all. Instead he talked about himself, and she smilingly listened to him, which was a pattern in their relationship all along.

Another family we have worked with had a similar pattern of sibling tensions:

Box 5.3   Case example

Ruth, the eldest of three children, took on the care of her mother. She had two siblings, a sister who lived in another part of the country, and a much younger brother, who lived nearby. Ruth carefully researched her mother's problems and accompanied her to medical appointments. When the neurologist explained that her mother had dementia and would eventually need caretakers, Ruth initiated a family consultation with an elder law specialist, with all three children and her mother present. As her mother continued to deteriorate, the various provisions that had been agreed upon with the attorney were invoked, but at each step the two younger children opposed them. Ruth's brother did not see the necessity for paying for help in the home. He visited his mother frequently, but he minimized her problems until she was so far into her dementia that she could not live alone at all. The out-of-town sister was actually a nurse, but she, too, minimized her mother's problems. After their mother ended up in a personal care home for dementia patients, she would swoop in, criticize the care, get the staff defensive and agitated, then leave for another several months. After several years of this pattern of interactions, the relationships among the three children were severely strained.

These examples indicate the tensions that can emerge among siblings. These conflicts add considerable stress to the primary carer (Aneshensel *et al.* 1995) and, in the end, may erode the family's ability to provide care.

> **Exercise 5.2** Expectations about caring in your family
>
> This exercise is designed to help you understand the expectations in your family about caring. You can do the exercise if you are already in a caring relationship or in a hypothetical way if you are not.
>
> 1   Identify a person in your family currently receiving care, or an older relative who might need care in the future.
>
> 2   Identify the people in that individual's immediate family. These could include a spouse, children (including sons-in-law and daughters-in-law), grandchildren and anyone else who has a close relationship to the older person.
>
> 3   For each person, including yourself, write down the strengths and limitations of that person as a primary carer.
>
> 4   Who is, or who would probably become, the primary carer for this person? Why would that person be selected?
>
> 5   Review the strengths of everyone in the family network, and highlight those strengths that would be helpful to the primary carer.
>
> At this point, you have a plan for drawing on the available resources within the family network. This plan can help the main carer manage all the demands and responsibilities, while drawing upon positive qualities of the other people in the family. The limitations of each person are a reminder that families often have long-standing points of conflict or tension, but that it is possible in care situations to focus on what each person can contribute, rather than on their limitations.

From our experience, as carers become involved in a daily care routine, they may begin to receive help from family, friends, neighbours and other informal helpers. They may get assistance with daily living, such as errands, housework or transportation. Friends and family may also stay with the person with dementia or take that person out, which gives the carer an always-welcome break. The carer can benefit from emotional support, for example, having an understanding person to talk with in person or on the phone. It can also be helpful when friends or family participate with the carer in leisure activities, such as going out to dinner or the cinema. This type of support has the potential to relieve strain on the primary carer and help sustain him/her in the role (Aneshensel *et al.* 1995).

Support, however, is not always forthcoming. There can be conflict in the family over what help is needed and who should provide it. Sometimes, relatives decide what the carer or person with dementia needs, without discussing it with either of them. These helpers may be providing potentially useful assistance, but sometimes it leaves the carer feeling angry or frustrated, or that he/she has no control over the situation. Some family and friends offer only advice and criticism. Carers, however, are often more knowledgeable about dementia and its consequences than the rest of the family, and so do not need well-intentioned but often poorly-informed advice (Malone Beach and Zarit 1995). In some cases, friends and family wait to be asked to assist, or do not realize that the carer needs help. And finally, some carers have difficulty asking for the help that they need, or think that help should be forthcoming without their having to ask. All of these scenarios have the same result. Carers end up providing most of the help, and feel isolated and unsupported by family and friends.

The example in Box 5.4 describes problems that can develop around giving and receiving assistance.

Box 5.4   Case example

Marie had a mild vascular dementia when she and Phil moved back to her home town to be near her sister, Connie. Marie also had high blood pressure and was on several cardiac medications. As Marie's dementia progressed, Phil tried the medications that the neurologist prescribed for her memory problems, but Connie was very critical of this decision. She had worked in a doctor's office and she did not 'believe' in taking medication. She also thought that Phil was just using the medication to keep Marie docile. Tension developed between Connie and Phil, which was very upsetting to Marie.

Phil did a heroic job of keeping Marie independent in her activities of daily living (ADL), encouraging her and never accepting 'I can't do it' as an answer. Consequently, she surprised even her doctors with how much she continued to do for herself. Conversely, Phil had great difficulty accepting the fact the Marie could not control her symptoms. He thought that she should try harder to remember and that if she had a more positive attitude, she would be able to do more. Even as her memory and behaviour deteriorated, Phil held onto a belief that she could remember if he reminded her enough times, or if she would just rehearse things more. He would get frustrated and impatient at times and raise his voice at her, which in turn would cause her to cry.

The solution came from an outside source. One of the carers that Phil hired to help with Marie's physical care was a retired nurse who developed a true fondness for her patients. She spent enough time with Marie, Phil and Connie to observe all of the dynamics, and then took it upon herself to teach Marie to be assertive with both of them. She taught Marie that when Phil started to raise his voice, she should put her index finger to her lips and say, 'Shhh,' and that was the signal to him that he was too loud and he was upsetting her. Similarly, Marie learned to tell Connie that while she appreciated her concern, she was going to let her doctors decide which medications she should take. And with enough reminders, Marie was able to do just that.

Another source of misunderstandings and conflict over care and support is the lack of adequate communication between the primary carer and other family members. The main carer may believe that family members should offer help without being asked, while children and/or siblings are waiting to be asked, or may not even be aware of the carer's needs. Other carers may believe they cannot impose on children or other relatives, without asking children or other relatives.

To address these types of issues, we pioneered the use of a family meeting that brings everyone involved in the care together (Zarit and Zarit 1982, 2007;

Zarit *et al.* 1985). The family meeting does not address long-standing family conflicts, but instead addresses the current care needs of the person with dementia and answers everyone's questions. The counsellor leading the family meeting can usually present those needs, and then draw on the family's coping strategies to come up with a plan for providing help. In doing so, the counsellor must identify and avoid the pitfalls associated with long-standing conflicts, such as competition between siblings over who is giving more help, and hence who is giving less. Instead, the goal is to get everyone to help in some way, and to emphasize that all help is important.

Economic strain

Finally, caregiving may place considerable economic strain on the family. The carer, or, in some instances, the person with dementia, may leave the workforce, decreasing the income available. Medical and care-related expenses may place an increasing burden on the family budget. Families in the United States, in particular, are likely to find that many support services (e.g. respite) for their relative are not covered by insurance, and they may also have to make large payments for medical expenses.

Families can face different kinds of economic stress. If the person with dementia has few assets, the challenge is over where to find services and how to pay for them. Tensions can flare up when the carer expects children or siblings to pay a portion of the cost for care, but they are unwilling. Another problem is doing the paperwork to get public assistance. A spouse, in particular, may feel shame or humiliation when having to apply for public assistance. In the United States, there is usually a difference in the quality of care in private institutions compared to those that accept payment from the state. When a person with limited resources must move to a public facility, the carer may feel guilt or shame at not having been able to do more.

In cases when the person with dementia has financial assets, children may argue about the proper ways of using the money. Some children see their parent's estate as their rightful inheritance, and resent using assets to pay for care. If one or more of the children has financial pressures of their own and may have been dependent on the parent for assistance, they may continue to try to divert money for their own needs.

Box 5.5   Case example

Lesley did not have a large income herself, but assumed much of the financial burden of paying for home helpers in order to keep her mother in the family home as long as possible. Her brother had a much higher income, but contributed very little. Leslie did not resent spending the money, and did not really see any other choice. In some ways, she found compensation in how her mother responded to the care she gave. As her mother's dementia progressed and her brother visited less and less frequently, Lesley began receiving the attention she had always craved from her mother. Her mother enjoyed spending time with her and no longer compared her unfavourably to her brother.

Caring for a relative at the end of life

One of the more difficult problems for families are the decisions they must make at the end of their relative's life (see Chapter 20). The emotional burden is especially great when the dying person has dementia or other cognitive impairment. In that case, unless that person has written an advance directive or communicated his/her preferences, the family must guess about what their relative would have wanted. Before we examine the issues that families face, conduct Exercise 5.3 in which you examine your own preferences and values.

Exercise 5.3 Planning your end-of-life directive

For this exercise, plan your own advance directive for end-of-life care, addressing each of the following points:

1   What would you want to emphasize, prolonging life at any cost or maintaining your comfort?

2   If your condition were terminal, would you want to use any of these medical devices?

● feeding tube

● intravenous hydration

● respirator

3   What regimen of pain medication would you prefer, maximum dosage even though it might impair cognition, or minimal dosage to preserve awareness, but not fully control your pain?

4   Would you want heroic efforts to be made on your behalf, such as a surgical procedure, even though it would prolong life only a short while longer?

Although some people with dementia die during the early and middle stages of the disease, others live to a point where illness has caused significant damage to the brain, and consequently to everyday functioning. With the progression of the disease, patients gradually lose their ability to communicate verbally so that little or no conversation is possible, and they often have trouble recognizing familiar people. They also become increasingly frail, and may end up spending most or all of their time in bed. They are prone to infections, injury and aspirating food.

Late stage care poses four main challenges to the family:

● grappling with the definition of quality of life for the person with dementia

● deciding how to respond to the various medical crises that will arise

● deciding on the location for late stage care

● finding closure.

Quality of life for the person with dementia

With limited verbal communication, pleasure and discomfort often have to be discerned from non-verbal signs (see Chapter 27). Care at this stage should emphasize keeping the person comfortable, and to the extent possible, free from pain and other sources of discomfort. People at this stage of their life value contact with the people with whom they have been close, such as a spouse or child, even though it may not always be apparent that they recognize those people.

Deciding how to respond to the various medical crises that arise

In an optimal situation, the person with dementia would have previously prepared a living will and discussed it with the main carer long before the onset of the disease. When the patient's wishes about end-of-life decisions are well known, the choices for the family are simpler, although not without potential hazards. One dilemma for the family is in understanding the implications of the choices they are asked to make when there is a medical problem. A physician may present an intervention such as the use of an intravenous tube for hydration as addressing an immediate problem, yet it may be difficult to stop the procedure once it has been started. Thus, the person who did not want life prolonged artificially may now be headed down that pathway. In a way, the family need to decide something that physicians cannot tell them, that is, when the time has come to let go, so that they do not authorize further treatment. This decision becomes much harder when the person with dementia has not left a living will, or any other clear directives. The other dilemma is that whether or not there is a living will, some family members may dispute the decisions that the main carer makes. Often, the child or other relative who is pushing to prolong life at any cost holds magical beliefs that a cure will be found that restores the person to health. This type of conflict is very distressing for the primary carer.

Choosing the location for care for relatives with dementia at the end of their life

Some carers keep their relative at home through the whole course of the disease. They have observed that care gets easier in some ways when the person with dementia is no longer mobile. With some help in the home, they find they are able to provide highly personal care at the end of life. Institutions also provide care for people at the end of life. As with the traditional hospice, the emphasis is on comfort, not intervention. The staff in a good care facility will also be comfortable with letting a medical crisis run its natural course if that has been the preference of the person with dementia, instead of rushing the person to the emergency room or insisting on invasive treatment.

Finding closure

Carers have been involved for years by the time the end comes. They can take pride in the many ways they made the person's life better, and reminisce about the good times they spent together before the illness.

Satisfactions and rewards of caring

The rather bleak portrayal of carers that emerges from stress process models raises the question of why so many people help out an older relative with dementia or disability. In our experience their motivation is often a mixture of affection and obligation. Some carers embrace the role, and are willing to make sacrifices necessary to carry it out. We have seen carers provide help for as long as 20 years, which is well past the time when most people would have given up. Our discussions with these carers suggest that they are not acting out of guilt, but rather they have made considerable sacrifice because of a genuine commitment to the person for whom they are caring.

In addition to the stressors of caregiving, people can gain satisfaction from how they perform the role and also grow from their experiences. Positive emotions and experiences are an important factor in promoting adaptation and coping with a variety of chronic stressors (Folkman 1997; Fredrickson and Joiner 2002). People who experience positive emotions in the face of stressors are more likely to build resources and identify possible solutions to address the problems they are facing (Fredrickson 2001). Positive experiences and satisfaction have been found to act as a buffer to the many stressors faced by carers (Levesque *et al.* 1995; Riedel *et al.* 1998; Robertson *et al.* in press).

Many carers feel satisfied that they have been able to fulfil their obligation to a spouse or parent. They face many challenges and the effort they make can build self-esteem. Children who care for an ageing parent gain a sense that they are giving back to their parents for the care they received when they were children. In Box 5.5 when Lesley talks about what gives her satisfaction in her life, that her mother is happy is always the first thing she mentions. Her mother no longer knows her name, but always gives her a big smile and is happy to see her.

Debates and controversies

What should the obligation of families and government be to help older people with dementia? The increase in the older population throughout Europe, North America and parts of Asia raises a fundamental question of whether and to what extent government can afford to provide supportive services to families and, in turn, to what extent families will be expected to provide care for their older relatives. Should families be expected to help, either financially or by providing direct assistance? Should family help be a legal obligation, as it technically is in some states in the United States (though these laws are not enforced)? Or should families be guaranteed a certain level of support from government-funded programmes when they provide help to an older relative? Economic and demographic pressures suggest that these questions may be re-examined, even in countries that previously made a commitment to provide extensive services to their older population. In Sweden, for example, economic factors led to cut-backs in services to older people, which have shifted some types of assistance back to the family (Sundström *et al.* 2002). Should families be obliged that way out of necessity, or should help be completely voluntary?

How should we weigh the welfare of the carer compared to that of the person with dementia? As documented in this and other chapters in the book, there is extensive evidence that the interests of the carer and the person with dementia diverge. Carers will do better in some ways if they turn the care over to an institution, while the older person will usually function better at home (Aneshensel *et al.* 1995). Should public policy and the efforts of clinicians favour one person over the other? If a carer makes the commitment to provide help, whatever the cost, should that person be supported, or should clinicians encourage giving up the carer role?

Conclusion

The role of families is critical in the care of persons with dementia. Not only do people with dementia need assistance with daily tasks, but because of their cognitive impairment they also require that someone look out for their best interests, whether in everyday decisions, medical care or financial management. We know that dementia care can be very stressful, leading to harmful effects on health and well-being. From our understanding of the family carer's experience, we can make some observations that can guide the development of programmes and services to help carers as well as the person with dementia. First, caregiving stress is multidimensional. There is no single measure of stress or burden that can tell us what we need to know about a particular family. Rather, whether for planning services or conducting research, we need to assess the multiple stressors associated with care. Second, carers are characterized by a great deal of individual variability. There is no one pattern of stressors or adaptation, nor are there normative patterns. Carers should not be encouraged to act or feel in a certain way, because of our expectations that a particular type of adaptation is better. Rather, our goal should be to facilitate carers to find their own goals and make their own decisions. And third, toward that end, we can provide valuable information and tools for stress management that can help carers reach their goals more effectively, and thereby allow them to provide assistance for as long as they want without undue harm to themselves.

Further information

Carers UK is an organization of carers fighting for society and government to recognize the true value of carers' contribution to society so that carers get the practical, financial and emotional support they need. Their website has information about policy and campaigns.

The Family Caregiver Alliance is a pioneer in the development of programmes and services for carers of people with dementia and other brain disorders. The website contains extensive information on a wide range of topics.

The National Alliance for Caregivers is a coalition of organizations in the United States that focuses on issues of family caregiving. The website includes useful survey data that documents the extent of family involvement in caregiving, as well as resources for family carers.

References

Aneshensel, C.S., Pearlin, L.I., Mullan, J.T., Zarit, S.H. and Whitlatch, C.J. (1995) *Profiles in Caregiving: The Unexpected Career*. New York: Academic Press.

Ballard, C. and Cream, J. (2005) Drugs used to relieve behavioral symptoms in people with dementia or an unacceptable chemical cost? *International Psychogeriatrics*, 17(1): 12–22.

Breen, D.A., Breen, D.P., Moore, J.W., Breen, P.A. and O'Neill, D. (2007) Driving and dementia: A clinical review. *British Medical Journal*, 334: 1365–9.

Clare, L. (2002) We'll fight it as long as we can: Coping with the onset of Alzheimer's disease. *Aging and Mental Health*, 6(2): 139–48.

Clare, L., Wilson, B.A., Carter, G. and Hodges, J.R. (2002) Relearning face-name associations in early Alzheimer's disease. *Neuropsychology*, 16(4): 538–47.

Clare, L., Wilson, B.A., Carter, G. and Hodges, J.R. (2003) Cognitive rehabilitation as a component of early intervention in Alzheimer's disease: A single case study. *Aging and Mental Health*, 7(1): 15–21.

Edwards, A.B., Zarit, S.H., Stephens, M.A.P. and Townsend, A. (2002) Employed family caregivers of cognitively impaired elderly: An examination of role strain and depressive symptoms. *Aging and Mental Health*, 6(1): 55–61.

Fauth, E.R., Femia, E.E., Zarit, S.H. and Stephens, M.A.P. (In press) Behavioral and psychological symptoms of dementia in the context of personal activities of daily living: Prevalence and impact on caregivers. *The Gerontologist*.

Finkel, S.I., Costa de Silva, J., Cohen, G. *et al.* (1996) Behavioural and psychological signs and symptoms of dementia: A consensus statement on current knowledge and implications for research and treatment. *International Psychogeriatrics*, 8 (Suppl 3): 497–500.

Fredrickson, B.L. (2001) The role of positive emotions in positive psychology: The broaden-and-build theory of positive emotions. *American Psychologist*, 56(3): 218–26.

Fredrickson, B.L. and Joiner, T. (2002) Positive emotions trigger upward spirals toward emotional well-being. *Psychological Sciences*, 13(2): 172–5.

Kuhn, D.R. (1998) Caring for relatives with early stage Alzheimer's disease: An exploratory study. *American Journal of Alzheimer's Disease*, 13(4): 189–96.

Lazarus, R.S. and Folkman, S. (1984) *Stress, Appraisal, and Coping*. New York: Springer.

Levesque, L., Cossette, S. and Laurin, L. (1995) A multidimensional examination of the psychological and social well-being of caregivers of a demented relative. *Research on Aging*, 17(3): 332–60.

Malone Beach, E.E. and Zarit, S.H. (1995) Dimensions of social support and social conflict as predictors of caregiver depression. *International Psychogeriatrics*, 7(1): 25–38.

McCurry, S.M., Gibbons, L.E., Logsdon, R.G., Vitiello, M.V. and Teri, L. (2005) Nighttime insomnia treatment and education for Alzheimer's disease: A randomized controlled trial. *Journal of the American Geriatrics Society*, 53(5): 793–802.

Moniz-Cook, E., Agar, S., Gibson, G., Win, T. and Wang, M. (1998) A preliminary study of the effects of early intervention with people with dementia and their families in a memory clinic. *Aging and Mental Health*, 2(3): 199–211.

Pearlin, L. I., Mullan, J.T., Semple, S.J. and Skaff, M.M. (1990) Caregiving and the stress process: An overview of concepts and their measures. *The Gerontologist*, 30(5): 583–94.

Perrin, T. and May, H. (1999) *Well-being and Dementia: An Occupational Approach for Therapists and Carers*. Edinburgh: Churchill Livingstone.

Riedel, S.E., Fredman, L. and Langenberg, P. (1998) Associations among caregiving difficulties, burden, and rewards in caregivers to older post-rehabilitation patients. *Journal of Gerontology: Psychological Sciences*, 53B(3): 165–74.

Robertson, S.M., Zarit, S.H., Duncan, L.G., Rovine, M. and Femia, E.E. (In press) Family caregivers' patterns of positive and negative affect. *Family Relations*.

Schulz, R. and Beach, S.R. (1999) Caregiving as a risk factor for mortality: The caregiver health effects study. *Journal of the American Medical Association*, 282(3): 2215–19.

Schulz, R., O'Brien, A.T., Bookwala, T. and Fleissner, K. (1995) Psychiatric and physical morbidity effects of dementia caregiving: prevalence, correlates, and causes. *The Gerontologist*, 35(6): 771–91.

Son, J., Erno, A., Shea, D.G., Femia, E.E., Zarit, S.H. and Stephens, M.A.P. (2007) The caregiver stress process and health outcomes. *Aging and Health*, 19(6): 871–87.

Spillman, B.C. and Black, K. J. (2005) *Staying the Course: Trends in Family Caregiving*. Washington, DC: AARP Public Policy Institute.

Sundström, G., Johansson, L. and Hassing, L. (2002) The shifting balance of care in Sweden. *The Gerontologist*, 42(3): 350–5.

Teri, L., Logsdon, R.G., Uomoto, J. and McCurry, S.M. (1997) Behavioral treatment of depression in dementia patients: A controlled clinical trial. *Journals of Gerontology Series B-Psychological Sciences and Social Sciences*, 52B(4): 159–66.

Vitaliano, P.P., Zhang, J., and Scanlan, J.M. (2003) Is caregiving hazardous to one's physical health? A meta-analysis. *Psychological Bulletin*, 129(6): 946–72.

Whitlatch, C.J., Judge, K., Zarit, S.H., and Femia, E.E. (2006) A dyadic intervention for family caregivers and care receivers in early stage dementia. *The Gerontologist*, 46: 688–94.

Zarit, S.H., Femia, E.E., Watson, J., Rice-Oeschger, L. and Kakos, B. (2004) Memory Club: A group intervention for people with early-stage dementia and their care partners. *The Gerontologist*, 44(2): 262–9.

Zarit, S.H., Orr, N.K. and Zarit, J.M. (1985) *The Hidden Victims of Alzheimer's Disease: Families Under Stress*. New York: New York University Press.

Zarit, S.H. and Zarit, J.M. (1982) Families under stress: interventions for caregivers of senile dementia patients. *Psychotherapy: Theory, Research and Practice*, 19(4): 461–71.

Zarit, S.H. and Zarit, J.M. (2007) *Mental Disorders in Older Adults*, 2nd edn. New York: Guilford.

6

Toward a person-centred ethic in dementia care: doing right or being good?

Clive Baldwin

Learning objectives

By the end of this chapter you will:

- have a basic understanding of the basis of a person-centred ethic
- understand the relevance and applicability of a person-centred ethic to dementia care practice
- have practised applying a person-centred ethic in a case study

---

Introduction

Ethics is defined as both a set of principles of right conduct and a theory of moral values. In other words it covers both the principles we live by and the philosophical justification of those principles. Given that we all tend to see ourselves as people of goodwill, and given the pressures and concerns of caring for people with dementia, sometimes systematic reflection about the ethics of what one is doing may seem like another burden, a distraction, or worse, a hindrance to providing care.

Why then should we take the time and trouble to reflect? The answer to this question is multi-faceted:

- If ethics is about how we live with one another (right conduct) then ethical guidelines (the principles and values behind them) can act as a way of keeping society together.

- If there is a goal or purpose (telos) to human life, as Aristotle suggested, then living in a certain way may help us toward that goal. Ethics, in other words, helps us achieve the good life.

- Ethics provides practical support in guiding us when we face difficult situations, in protecting vulnerable people and in promoting good practice.

- Most importantly, acting ethically contributes to the well-being not only of those receiving our care but our own through establishing right relationships.

Much has, over the years, been written about person-centred dementia care. The pioneering work of Kitwood (see, for example, Kitwood 1997a) has had a major influence in the field and 'person-centred care' has, at least in name, become orthodoxy. As Innes *et al.* (2006) state:

> ... there is a general consensus that person-centred or quality care is care that: is focused on clients/users; promotes independence and autonomy rather than control; involves services that are reliable and flexible and chosen by users; and tends to be offered by those working in a collaborative/team philosophy.

(Innes *et al.* 2006: 9)

This way of understanding person-centred care, I suggest, takes as its working ethic a form of principlism – the ethical framework developed by Beauchamp and Childress (2001) – with autonomy as its key feature. This view of person-centred care – where care is reduced essentially to individual choice and flexible services (however necessary these may be), and its related ethic, is, I believe, a distorted version of the person-centred care envisaged by Kitwood – that is, care focused on upholding personhood.

It is my argument here that in relying on principlism for its ethical foundation, much that passes for person-centred care substitutes what is essentially a subset of decision-making theory for the deeper, more dynamic, dialogic and relational ethic that a person-centred approach requires.

In this chapter I will develop an outline of a person-centred ethic, based on upholding and developing personhood for people living with dementia. In brief my argument is thus: there are fundamental problems with principlism as an approach to ethics in the face of the onset and progression of dementia. These are laid out in the first two sections. I will then propose that personhood is, or should be, the central concept in a person-centred ethic. Following this I will suggest that personalism provides an alternative, more suitable, framework, though this approach requires some further development, focusing particularly on the concept of the narrative self and the uniqueness of persons. Finally, I will offer a brief case study for reflection.

The four principles of bioethics, or 'principlism'

Although there are many different ethical frameworks that we can draw on in dementia care practice, the framework that has become dominant is that developed by Beauchamp and Childress in their book *The Principles of Bioethics* (Beauchamp and Childress 2001). Beauchamp and Childress argue there are four *prima facie* principles to be upheld:

- autonomy: self-governance or being able to act freely in accordance with a self-chosen plan

- beneficence: an obligation to do good or contribute to the welfare of others

- non-maleficence: an obligation not to inflict harm on others

- justice: providing fair and equitable treatment.

According to Beauchamp and Childress these principles are prima facie in that each must be fulfilled unless it conflicts with an equal or stronger principle. For example, in certain circumstances we may think it necessary to act in a person's best interest even though that person does not agree with what is happening: a conflict between beneficence and autonomy.

Exercise 6.1   Thinking in a principlist way

Acquire a copy of your professional code of conduct. Read through the code identifying Beauchamp and Childress' four principles of bioethics as they are incorporated into the code.

The inadequacy of principlism

While principlism is the dominant framework in health care ethics, it is not without its critics (see, for example, Becker 2000; Campbell 1999; Clouser and Gert 1994; Harris 2003). My argument here, however, concerns the limits of principlism when we place personhood at the centre of our ethical reasoning: that is, principlism is simply not the approach best suited to the unique ethical challenges thrown up by the onset and progression of dementia and the requirements of person-centred care. I make this claim on the following basis:

- Principlism has nothing to say about personhood. While there is an implicit (modernist, Western, neo-liberal) anthropology within the principlist framework, personhood is not directly discussed as a salient feature in ethical reasoning and does not warrant even a passing notice in the index to *Principles of Biomedical Ethics*. This failure to address issues of personhood limits the usefulness and appropriateness of this approach in person-centred dementia care.

- By focusing on decision-making, principlism has little, if anything, to say about how such decisions emerge from and contribute to the trajectory of an individual's life in relationship with others nor how such decisions reflect and help construct the individuals who make those decisions. As is argued later, if personhood and its maintenance are a dialogical, relational process then the a-personal, abstract nature of principlism becomes less appropriate and useful as an ethical framework.

- Principlism is not located within any wider framework that provides guidance as to how we, as humans, should live. As such it is divorced from a sense of the Good (that is, any teleology, or purposeful development towards an ultimate end for life).

- Principlism has little, if anything, to say about the moral development of professionals (for a discussion of professional moral development see Kitwood 1997b). While it can provide a framework within which to act (and a framework to justify those actions) it is essentially a form of rule-following morality that contributes little to the moral development of its followers and, as Harris (2003) has pointed out, limits ethical creativity.

- The atomistic, individualistic nature of the principlist approach does not, and perhaps cannot, accommodate more communal approaches to decision-making, approaches more in keeping with a person-centred ethic that values relationships.

- That in establishing abstract principles that can make individuals replaceable, principlism fails to understand the uniqueness of the ethical encounter between two people (see Bauman 1993).

Exercise 6.2   The key features of personhood

What do you think are the key features personhood? Some would argue that rationality, self-awareness, self-interest, memory and psychological continuity are all essential to personhood. Others emphasize the relational qualities of personhood such as emotionality, the ability to give and receive love, creativity and relationships with others.

Make a list of those features that you think characterize personhood.

Then ask yourself whether these features apply to any or all of the following: a foetus; a chimpanzee; a human being in a coma; a child with severe autism; a very young baby; someone with very severe dementia; someone with mild dementia. Do you think it is possible to define personhood in this way?

Personhood as central to person-centred care

At the heart of Kitwood's conception of person-centred care was a sense of 'personhood', of what it means to be a person. Drawing on the work of Martin Buber, Kitwood argued that personhood depended not on ability or capacity but is a 'standing or status that is bestowed upon one human being, by others, in the context of relationship and social being. It implies recognition, respect and trust' (1997a: 8) and that personhood was the right of every human being regardless of capacity. Personhood is found – or rather realized – through the encounter with the Other (the 'Thou' in Buber's terminology) that was open to mystery and surprise.

In fashioning personhood in this way Kitwood drew attention to personhood as:

- an essentially relational concept – that is, one did not 'possess' personhood but personhood exists in the way one is treated

- essentially dynamic – that it could ebb and flow

- to some extent, situational – the social and physical environment could support and uphold or undermine personhood

- a unique encounter between two individuals that could not be legislated for without losing uniqueness.

Person-centred care, for Kitwood, thus flowed from a conception of personhood. Such care was to be aimed at upholding the personhood of the individual threatened by the onset and progression of dementia (the dementia itself not being the factor that undermined personhood, but the individual and social responses to the dementia).

Since Kitwood wrote, there has been much work done that has demonstrated that, contrary to the popular perception, for those people living with dementia, the Self remains. (See, for example, Sabat and Harré 1992; Klein *et al.* 2003; Surr 2006; see Chapter 7.) Such a Self may be vulnerable but is nevertheless retained in the face of the dementia and the response of others to the dementia.

Personalism as a basis for a person-centred ethic in dementia care

Having established the centrality of personhood I now turn to an ethical framework that offers the possibility of realizing that centrality – that of personalism. Unlike authors such as Brock (1993) and Harris (1985) who view personhood as distinct from being human, personalist authors start from the premise that personhood and being human are one and the same (see, for example, Bernardin 1980; McCarthy 1978; Palazzini 1994). Personhood is thus concerned with who we are rather than any particular features or capacities we might possess.

Personalism is an ethical framework that features a number of principles that are derived from its central tenet of the personhood of all human beings regardless of capacity. While this approach has been developed primarily with Catholic circles, there is nothing inherent within the approach that necessitates adherence to Catholicism, or indeed any faith.

For Palazzini, personalism has four fundamental principles:

- the fundamental value of human life – body, mind and soul

- the principle of totality or therapeutic principle – that the totality of life be considered in health-care actions

- the principle of freedom and responsibility – that 'to be free means to make responsible choices for ourselves and others'

- the principle of sociality and assistance – that life and health in society are promoted through promoting health and life of every individual and assistance is provided to whomsoever needs help and support (Palazzini 1994: 10).

Developing the personalist approach, Schotsmans (1999) draws on both Buber and Levinas and focuses on the uniqueness of persons, the relational and intersubjective nature of persons and the notion of participation in the wider society through communication and solidarity:

With these three fundamental value orientations in mind we can articulate a moral criterion, with a personalist meaning: we say that an act is morally good if it serves the humanum or human dignity, that is, if it in truth is beneficial to the human person adequately considered in these three basic value-orientations (dimensions and relationships): uniqueness, relational commitment and solidarity.

(Schotsmans 1999: 19)

Box 6.1   Case example

Consider the following account, taken from an interview with a family carer, Mrs Wellington:

> One time my husband was looking at a picture of a very young girl probably late teens, on the front page of a magazine and she was wearing very brief shorts and she had her thumb stuck in at quite a provocative attitude. I could hear him talking and when I came in here he had this book in his hand and he was saying, 'Go on, pull them down just a little bit, go on, go on' And it was really creepy; the voice, I'd never heard his voice like that before and so it really spooked me.

> Anyway, we were on holiday at the beach and he made some very inappropriate remarks to our eight-year-old grand-daughter, and I mean really inappropriate, the sort of things I'd only heard him saying to me when we were in bed together.

> Even after the incidents on holiday, which drew my attention to the fact that this was far more serious, I thought, 'No, if I tell professionals, am I going to get my husband into a court case or something?' Because I've been on courses about child abuse and I knew how serious it was. And even quite minor incidents have resulted in court cases and I was really, really very concerned that things would be taken out of my hands.

> But I didn't know how far I should go with the neighbours because before I had to keep my husband sort of locked in as it were because I knew that he would go out and stand and stare at children. I thought, 'How much do I tell people, how much do I warn them, how much can I let happen before I intervene?' I didn't want to go round painting this picture of some sort of sexual pervert but I felt it was important that people knew so that they could be aware.

While it would be possible to analyse the case example in Box 6.1 in terms of the four principles of bioethics, such an approach would seem not to do justice to the complexity of the situation. It is my contention that the issues raised in Box 6.1 do not revolve around 'what should be done?' (though that, of course, is part of it) but around how Mr and Mrs Wellington are together and how Mr Wellington is (and appears to be) in the world.

Mrs Wellington is obviously shocked by her husband's behaviour and realizes that it might be cause for concern because it could adversely affect other people. She experiences this behaviour as being out of character, a disruption to both the relationship she had with her husband and their history together (in personalist terms, a concern with the totality of the situation). At the same time she is aware of how others might perceive her husband (both if she informed them or if she did not) and how the workings of the system may adversely impact upon her husband should she seek professional advice.

Mrs Wellington is seemingly caught between her loyalty to (solidarity with) her husband and her desire to protect others (a concern for the wider community). In some ways, this reflects a conflict between her personal and professional selves. She is concerned to maintain her husband's dignity (not wanting him to be labelled a 'pervert'), yet also to be morally responsible to others in her actions.

The personalist approach would thus seem to be able to address some of the criticisms that I have levelled against principlism: the focus on personhood, looking at the totality of life, locating ethics in a wider framework of the Good and encompassing the relational aspects of what it means to be human. To develop this approach further I want to incorporate two features of narrative theory: the notion of the narrative self, and the intersection of character and narrativity. These two features, as I will outline below, help us to make concrete some of the above fundamental principles and address the issue of the moral development of those making decisions on behalf of others.

The narrative self and narrative ethics

It has become commonplace to refer to humans as narrative beings. The work of authors such as Macintyre (1984), Bruner (1987; 1996) and Taylor (1989) has had a great influence across disciplines, while recognizing that the notions of the narrative Self and life as narrative are not universally accepted (for example, see Strawson 2004). My starting point here is that human beings experience life, and their place in the flow of life, in narrative terms (broadly defined). In other words, our personhood is constructed and manifested in and through the narratives we tell about ourselves and the narratives that include us told by others. Personhood is thus personal and inter-personal, individual, social and institutional. And because narratives circulate in a world of other narratives (or as Taylor phrases it 'webs of interlocution') – sometimes competing for privilege with other narratives (for example, in two mutually exclusive narratives concerning the same events) – personhood can be both facilitated and vulnerable. For example, with the declining ability to construct narratives with the onset and progression of dementia, individuals may lose the discursive ability to perform their personhood through narrative for themselves but their personhood might be maintained by the narratives that surround them that are told by others. In this they are akin to Pirendello's *Six Characters in Search of an Author*, requiring another to complete their story. In this encounter we need, therefore, to be aware of the ethics of the narratives we construct and how they are constructed (see Baldwin 2005). The type of narrative and the process of narration are intimately bound up with the maintenance of personhood.

For example, it is possible to construct a narrative for/with/about a person living with dementia that focuses on deficit, 'challenging behaviour', loss of Self and difficulty:

The twenty-four houredness of it [caring], it is like having a baby. That, at stages you can't even go to the toilet without checking. So the twenty-four houredness of it and the, and the destruction of time because you are up and about in the night. ... The loss of the person, the loss of their contribution to your life and who they were and the shared memories. The loss of all that person and the gaining of another difficult person in their place.

(family carer)

Alternatively, the narrative could focus on retained abilities, expressions of Self, relationships and contribution:

Box 6.2

But it's interesting that despite the fact that she has a handicap in cognition and expression and all of these things, she can still form and make new relationships with other people in the home and she's very much assuming a role of trying to look after some of the elderly ladies and sort out. If they've lost something she'll take them round and look for it. And in some ways certainly I and some of the staff at the home feel that's an expression of the sort of things that she did when she was a schoolteacher. Sorting little lost little kids out and, and looking for things and helping them and being quite patient ...

(family carer)

Box 6.3

She's part of the home, she's part of the family and she enriches us in ways that are phenomenal sometimes. This is the lady who has never been particularly fond of babies but she met her two great nephews, one is 1 and one 4, she's met one of them before, they've come from Australia, and she was enthralled with the baby. She's never loved babies in her life but at this moment in time babies are what fits, she likes little babies and ... to have that amount of pleasure given you, it makes everything worthwhile.

(family carer)

The narrative in Box 6.1 marginalizes, excludes or distances the person from the company of the intact. The narratives in Box 6.2 and Box 6.3 acknowledge the personhood of the individual and bring her into communication, sociality and relationship. The narrative in Box 6.2 focuses on the sameness of people living with dementia (that is, their correspondence with the current meta-narrative of dementia). The narrative in Box 6.3 focuses on the uniqueness and the totality of the person.

The intersection of character and narrativity

The second aspect drawn from narrative theory that I want to introduce in support of a person-centred ethic focuses on how character and narrativity intersect. That is, how the narratives we live by give shape to our character which in turn shapes the narratives we construct.

The uniqueness of persons

For Kitwood, an essential part of person-centred care was a focus on the uniqueness of individuals. This follows from his position that personhood is relational, in that each of our relationships is unique. Focusing on uniqueness requires us to focus on the differences between us (for, by definition, similarity is not unique). A person-centred ethic, therefore, needs to focus on difference rather than similarity. In this, my argument is akin (though not as philosophical) as that of Emmanuel Levinas (1961).

According to Levinas ethics concerns the relationship between the Self and the Other. This relationship is presaged on the notion of radical difference – or alterity – that the Other is fundamentally and irreducibly different. However, we attempt to make others intelligible to ourselves by bringing them into conformity with our own perspective: for example, through attempts at normalization or the logico-scientificity of the medical model of dementia. From a person-centred approach this attempt is misguided because we can only understand the other person in all his/her own uniqueness by focusing on difference. Even Kitwood's reformulation of dementia as a dialectic between neurological impairment, personality, health, biography and social psychology simply extended the attempt to make the Other intelligible rather than challenging the attempt per se.

> **Exercise 6.3** Focusing on difference
>
> Think of a person living with dementia whom you know well. List all the ways in which that person is different from you. You may want to think of difference in terms of physical characteristics, genetics, history, social life, personality, family life, values, faith or spirituality, culture, tastes, activities, hopes, likes and dislikes, health, psychology, relationships, sense of humour, education, meaning-making behaviour, physiology.

The ethical relationship, however, is one that does not seek to reduce, negate or deny difference but one in which we respond out of our own sense of moral responsibility in relationship to the Other. The application of principlism is not an option as 'to reduce the Other who calls me as a unique self in the face-to-face to a set of a priori moral principles is a violence to her alterity' (Robbins 2000). One's response must be – as Kitwood (1997a) and Buber (2000) before him noted – a response of the I to the Thou, a spontaneous, open, surprising encounter – taking into account the uniqueness of the individual in his/her history and circumstances:

Box 6.4 Case example

Not only is every person with dementia an individual and the course of the illness is probably going to be very different for each person, depending upon, I think depending upon where the, which part of the brain is afflicted most, would bring a totally different pattern, so there are no easy answers. I think that is the first thing, that I feel there's no easy answers to looking after someone with dementia, there are no book pro forma if you like, you have to go with the individual.

So you've got the complete individuality not only of the person's illness, but the personality of the person who has the illness which may or may not have enormous changes to it.

So you've got loads of variables there, and then you mix in with that the skills and attitudes of a carer, of their primary carer, plus the kind of relationship they had with that person before the person became ill. And you can see how stuffing people into systems won't work because there are too many variables, too many thoughts and feelings and wishes which one should try to accommodate if the person is truly going to have what's, you know, a rather battered phrase now 'person-centred care' but that's what it needs to be.

(wife talking about caring for her husband)

Personalism revisited

Let us now return to personalism as an ethical framework. By introducing the notion of narrative personhood we do not have to rely on – but can also accommodate – a personhood dependent upon religious faith or metaphysics. Personhood so construed is inclusive and non-discriminatory. Furthermore, personhood, being constructed discursively, is also dynamic and dialogical, individual, social and institutional in a way that principlism is not, and could never be.

A case study in person-centred ethics

Box 6.5 Case example

Mr Gregory is a 76-year-old man, living at home with his wife of 52 years. He suffers from epilepsy which is currently controlled via medication and has been diagnosed as having Alzheimer's disease for which he has been prescribed an anti-dementia drug, gelantamine. His wife is keen to keep him at home with her for as long as is possible. They have some support from the social services: Mr Gregory goes to a day centre once a week; Mrs Gregory goes to a carers' support group once a month.

Mr Gregory is coping reasonably well though sometimes he becomes frustrated because he is no longer able to do things as well as he once could and expresses his frustration by shouting and occasionally throwing things.

Mr Gregory has recently started to refuse to take his medication because he thinks that the stomach upsets he experiences (the side effects of the medication) are due to his wife trying to make him ill. This has led to arguments, which Mrs Gregory finds particularly distressing as she says that she and her husband never argued before.

Mr Gregory recently went for his annual check-up with his GP. Mrs Gregory accompanied him, having already spoken to the doctor about her husband's anxiety and behaviour. The doctor prescribed a sedative, temazepam, and Mr Gregory agreed that this would probably be for the best. On returning home, however, Mr Gregory decided that he would not take the medication.

The following day, Mr and Mrs Gregory had an argument over the medication and Mr Gregory when leaving the room pushed his wife out of the way. She fell over and though shaken she was not badly hurt. She reported this to her daughter who was very concerned for her safety. That evening Mrs Gregory and her two children met to discuss the situation.

Mrs Gregory wants to believe that this was a one-off event. Her daughter thinks that the situation is more serious and is concerned for her mother's safety. Her son agrees but does not see any prospect of persuading his father to take the medication. He suggests that they think about possible residential care but his mother is not happy with that. They finally agree that the best course of action at this time is to get Mr Gregory to take his medication 'one way or another'.

Mr Gregory continued to refuse his medication and so Mrs Gregory has started to mix both the sedative and the anti-dementia drug in her husband's food, occasionally increasing the dosage of the sedative when her husband appears to be more anxious that usual. Since she has started doing this Mr Gregory is far less anxious and he and his wife have fewer arguments. Mr Gregory, however, sometimes complains of feeling very tired and has become less active.

Case study reflections

It is clear that the principlist framework could be applied easily to the case study in Box 6.5. Mr Gregory's autonomy in deciding whether or not to take his medication; the potential benefits of over-ruling Mr Gregory's choice (a conflict between the principles of beneficence and autonomy) in surreptitiously administering the medication in order that he be less agitated and able to remain at home with his wife longer; the potential harm of side effects and the damage to the relationship between Mr Gregory and his wife should he discover his wife's 'betrayal' and so on.

While such an analysis is reconcilable with a person-centred approach, it misses the central point – that of how Mr Gregory's personhood is to be maintained in the face of his dementia.

I want to suggest, heretically, that the issue of how the medication is administered is of secondary ethical concern here – there are much more important issues at stake. For the principlist approach the administration of medication is a 'problem' to be 'solved' through the application of prima facie principles.

For a person-centred ethic, the issue in the scenario in Box 6.5 is that Mr Gregory's personhood is under assault in a number of ways. First, his uniqueness is not being acknowledged or respected – the attempts to ensure he takes the medication are attempts by those around him (the cognitively and physically intact) to bring him into their way of seeing and doing things. Second, the shared narrative of Mr and Mrs Gregory that constructed their personhood together over many years is being disrupted. Mrs Gregory is thinking and acting differently than she had previously – 'acting out of character' – in the vain attempt that by doing so she can maintain what she and her husband had had before. In so doing the trajectory and dynamics of the narrative change – in effect constructing a different narrative – endangering Mr Gregory's personhood by cutting him adrift from the narratives that previously held his personhood in place. Third, the narratives that shaped Mr and Mrs Gregory's life together (in Taylor's words, the 'webs of interlocution') have shifted. The narratives that previously upheld Mr Gregory's personhood are in danger of being supplanted by the 'meta-narrative' of dementia that casts Mr Gregory's situation as a problem to be resolved (and Mr Gregory as someone whose behaviour has to be 'managed'). In so doing, relationships and solidarity are relegated to subsidiary features for ethical reflection and communication distorted or undermined. Fourth, Mr Gregory – in being excluded from the creation of the narrative in which he is a central character, in effect becoming narratively dispossessed (see Baldwin 2005) – is also being denied the opportunity to contribute to the personhood of other characters in the narrative. He is denied the possibility of giving to his wife – in the sense of easing her sense of burden, anxiety or uncertainty by cooperating in the construction of a jointly acceptable narrative that is respectful of all parties.

Finally, Mrs Gregory's moral development is linked to the stance she takes with regard to how to relate to her husband via the issue of medication: ... the kinds of decisions we confront, indeed the very way we describe a situation, is a function of the kind of character we have (Hauerwas 1977: 20).

Character, according to Hauerwas, is forged not through adherence to abstract principles or theories but by the stories of which we are a part and which form the milieu within which we live our lives. These stories tie together the contingencies that make up our lives and set the context for our moral judgement. In the example of Mrs Gregory, the stories that are at stake are not simply of how to get Mr Gregory to take his medication but long-term, shared narratives in which both Mr and Mrs Gregory have formed their characters and lives together. The intricate meanings bound up in those narratives go beyond the arguments raised by principlism to question the nature of the relationship and the character of Mrs Gregory within that relationship. By surreptitiously administering her husband's medication, Mrs Gregory – and her children – are changing the trajectory of the family narrative and thus their place within it. A previous narrative of a loving and faithful relationship slips into one of potential betrayal and deceit. And it is precisely because of this potential that it is vitally important to understand the underlying narratives and narrative dynamics so as to facilitate the best possible narrative in the circumstances.

A person-centred ethic would thus focus on seeking answers to questions such as the following:

- How do we enable Mr Gregory to participate in the co-construction of a meaningful narrative for him and his wife?

- Which narratives maintain Mr Gregory's personhood and which undermine it?

- How are these narratives institutionalized in policies and procedures?

- How do we acknowledge/celebrate Mr Gregory's uniqueness within those narratives?

- How do we express our solidarity with Mr Gregory in the face of dementia?

- How do we maintain (and even enhance) the relationship between Mr Gregory and his wife?

- In what ways can we maintain and enhance communication with Mr Gregory, now and in the future in terms of both process and technique?

- How do we support Mrs Gregory in maintaining narrative probity in changing (and possibly frightening) situations?

Exercise 6.4 Applying a person-centred ethic

Think again of the person living with dementia whom you thought of in Exercise 6.3. Try answering the questions above in relation to that person.

Debates and controversies

A person-centred ethic focuses on individuals and unique encounters. It is difficult, therefore, to legislate for those encounters. Such legislation – as found in professional codes of conduct, for example – attempt to remove the individual from that encounter and substitute a series of principles and guidelines (that any individual can follow). In so doing, such codes undermine the ethics of those encounters: my encounter with you is as unique as you and I and would not, and could not, be the same as my encounter with another. Such legislation substitutes the ethic of strangers for the ethic of intimacy demanded by person-centred care.

A person-centred ethic is challenging because it requires us to take personal responsibility for our actions; it is contentious because it removes the defence of 'following guidelines' when things go wrong. Professional codes of ethics, while ostensibly there to protect the vulnerable, also serve to protect professionals provided they follow the rules. Rules undermine the truly ethical encounter and hinder moral development.

Conclusion

In summary, a person-centred ethics has, at its heart, the maintenance of personhood as a relational, dynamic concept. Maintaining personhood – conceptualized in this way – involves:

- a respect for difference and uniqueness
- a respect for the totality of the situation
- the maintenance of narrative continuity
- solidarity with the vulnerable
- an awareness of how individuals are perceived and narratively constructed in the wider social sphere
- effective communication
- taking responsibility for our moral choices
- recognizing that our own moral personhood depends upon and is inextricable from that which we protect, maintain, construct or enhance for the person living with dementia.

Person-centred care necessitates a person-centred ethic which in turn necessitates that we become person-centred Selves. As unique individuals we are unsubstitutable in the ethical encounter. This is so because our engagement with Others is rooted in who we are, not simply what we do. A person-centred ethic, in essence, demands that we be good rather than simply do right, it requires of us a fundamental and unexceptionable orientation to Others. This orientation to Others, freed from rules, policies and procedures as the basis of ethical action, demands a discipline and awareness that other ethical frameworks do not. Why then should we bother? Why should we take this more difficult path? Because by focusing on the personhood of others, through solidarity, uniqueness, communication, narrative and character we all become better people.

Note

1. All quotes from family carers are taken from interviews for a research project on ethical issues facing family carers, funded by the Alzheimer's Society and undertaken at the Ethox Centre, University of Oxford.

Further information

The Kennedy Institute of Ethics is a resource for those who research and study ethics, as well as those who debate and make public policy.

The UK Clinical Ethics Network provides information and support to both developing and existing clinical ethics committees within the UK health service.

The Centre for Research on Personhood in Dementia in the University of British Columbia at Vancouver is an interdisciplinary research centre committed to addressing issues related to a personhood approach to dementia and dementia care.

DIPEx: Patient Experiences of Health and Illness is a website devoted to personal experiences of health and illness, including dementia.

Applied ethics resources on the web is a website devoted to ethics.

References

Baldwin, C. (2005) Narrative, ethics and severe mental illness. *Australian and New Zealand Journal of Psychiatry*, 39(11–12): 1022–9.

Bauman, Z. (1993) *Postmodern Ethics*. Oxford: Blackwell.

Beauchamp, T.L. and Childress, J.F. (2001) *Principles of Biomedical Ethics*, 5th edn. New York: Oxford University Press.

Becker, C.B. (2000) Problems of principlism in WASP bioethics (online). In: N. Norio Fujiki and D.R.J. Macer (eds) *Proceedings of the UNESCO Asian Bioethics Conference (ABC97) and the WHO-assisted Satellite Symposium on Medical Genetics Services, 3–8 Nov, 1997 in Kobe/Fukui, Japan*; 3rd MURS Japan International Symposium; 2nd Congress of the Asian Association of Bioethics; 6th International Bioethics Seminar in Fukui: 77–80. Available at: http://translate.google.com/translate?hl=en&sl=ja&u=http://eubios.info/ASIAE (accessed February 2008).

Bernardin, J.L. (1980) Personalist humanism: Value system for medicine. *Hospital Progress*, 61(3): 48–51.

Brock, D.W. (1993) *Life and Death: Philosophical Essays in Biomedical Ethics*. Cambridge: Cambridge University Press.

Bruner, J.S. (1987) Life as narrative. *Social Research*, 54(1): 11–32.

Bruner, J.S. (1996) A narrative model of self construction. *Psyke & Logos*, 17(1): 154–70.

Buber, M. (2000) *I and Thou*. Edinburgh: T and T Clark.

Campbell, A. (1999) Human dignity, human virtue – the lost dimensions of human bioethics. Keynote address: Christine Martin Lecture. In *proceedings of the 6th National Conference of the Australian Bioethics Association*, Hobart, October 1998, pp. 1–6.

Clouser, K.D. and Gert, B. (1994) Morality vs. principlism. In: R. Gillon (ed.) *Principles of Health Care Ethics*. Chichester: John Wiley and Sons, pp. 251–66.

Harris, J. (1985) *The Value of Life: An Introduction to Medical Ethics*. London: Routledge.

Harris, J. (2003) In praise of unprincipled ethics. *Journal of Medical Ethics*, 29(5): 303–6.

Hauerwas, S. (1977) *Truthfulness and Tragedy: Further Investigations. International Christian Ethics*. Notre Dame, In: University of Notre Dame Press.

Innes, A., Macpherson, S. and McCabe, L. (2006) *Promoting Person-centred Care at the Front Line*. York: Joseph Rowntree Foundation.

Kitwood, T. (1997a) *Dementia Reconsidered: The Person Comes First*. Buckingham: Open University Press.

Kitwood, T. (1997b) Professional and moral development for care work: Some observations on the process. *Journal of Moral Education*, 27(3): 401–11.

Klein, S.B., Cosmides, L. and Costabile, K.A. (2003) Preserved knowledge of self in a case of Alzheimer's dementia. *Social Cognition*, 21(2): 157–63.

Levinas, E. (1961) *Totality and Infinity*. Pittsburgh: Duquesne University Press.

Macintyre, A. (1984) *After Virtue: A Study in Moral Theory*. Notre Dame, Indiana: University of Notre Dame Press.

McCarthy, D.G. (1978) Personalism in health care. *Hospital Progress*, 59(5): 79–86.

Palazzini, L. (1994) Personalism and bioethics. *Ethics and Medicine: An International Christian Perspective on Bioethics*, 10(1): 7–11.

Robbins, B.D. (2000) *Emmanuel Levinas*. Available from: http://mythosandlogos.com/Levinas.html (accessed May 2007).

Sabat, S.R. and Harré, R. (1992) The construction and deconstruction of self in Alzheimer's disease. *Ageing and Society*, 12(4): 443–61.

Schotsmans, P. (1999) Personalism in medical ethics. *Ethical Perspectives*, 6(1): 10–20.

Strawson, G. (2004) Against narrativity. *Ratio (New series)*. XVII(4): 428–52.

Surr, C.A. (2006) Preservation of self in people with dementia living in residential care: A socio-biographical approach. *Social Science and Medicine*, 62(7): 1720–30.

Taylor, C. (1989) *Sources of the Self*. Cambridge: Cambridge University Press.

7

Being minded in dementia: persons and human beings

Julian C Hughes

Learning objectives

By the end of this chapter you will:

- have thought further about the breadth of skills and functions that go to make up our minds
- have learnt something about the externality of mind: the theory that our minds are not just in our heads
- have considered, therefore, how we should think of the person as being more than just what is or is not going on mentally, but rather have a broader view of personhood as reflecting our nature as situated, embodied agents
- have understood the importance of person-centred care, precisely because this is a way to recognize and enhance the standing of the individual with dementia as a human being-in-the-world worthy of respect

---

Introduction

Some years ago a person with dementia said to me, 'I'm one minded at the moment'. She meant that she could not think what she needed to say. She could not, as it were, get into the right groove. In this chapter I wish to consider some of the implications of this. And I wish to gesture in the direction of the link, which is too readily taken to be unbuckled, between being a person and being human.

To spell out my argument in more detail, the woman who said 'I'm one minded at the moment' meant that she had a problem to do with language as a result of her dementia. In the first section 'Being "one minded" in dementia' I shall point to the variety of ways in which a person with dementia might still be regarded as 'minded', even if there were a problem with language, or with other mental functions. This is a fairly basic point: to have a mind is to have all sorts of different mental skills; in dementia, some might be lost, but others are retained. But this basic point raises a more worrying possibility, what if *all* the skills were lost? What do I then become? Am I still a person or human being?

In the second section, 'Being "one minded" in public space', I present an argument that suggests the mind is not just in the head, it exists publicly, in the external world. This is trickier, but very important, because we tend to think our minds are inside us (they seem to be 'inner') and this leads to the possibility that our minds might be totally destroyed by a disease that destroys our brains. One important point to make is that dementia does *not* totally destroy our brains. But if it turns out that our minds are not just 'inner', as I shall argue, then what is going on (or not going on) in our brains is not the end of the story as far as we are concerned as minded individuals. We can still participate in the world by virtue of our interactions with other human beings.

The importance of this should be made clearer by the third section, 'Being a person'. Some people argue that to be a person is in some sense to have a mind. They argue, for instance, that to be a person is linked to having continuous memories (see section on Debates and Controversies). But since memory is affected by dementia, the suggestion is that the individual with dementia is not a person to the extent that his or her memory is affected. However, if we can argue that being minded and having memories is not just to do with what is going on in the head, then we can argue that neither is being a person. Hence, we are still persons even if we have severe dementia. At least, we can still retain our personhood if the external circumstances (the psychosocial environment or the ways in which we are treated) are right. Hence the importance of 'person-centred care', since this always implies a broad view of what it is to be a person.

Being 'one minded' in dementia

> **Exercise 7.1**   Awareness of our different minds
>
> Next time you forget something: (a) describe to yourself how you feel; (b) notice all the things you remember around the forgotten thing, including how you remember the words to describe your feelings.
>
> In this way you have demonstrated that we have huge numbers of memories, but also different types of memory. And, even if we had no memories, we would still have feelings and emotions. But can you imagine what it would be like to have no 'inner' goings-on at all, no feelings, understandings, desires and the like?

I wish to consider how people with dementia might think of themselves as problematically 'one minded'. According to cognitive neuropsychologists we have stores of knowledge, semantic stores, in which our knowledge of words and their meanings are kept. These semantic stores are quite distinct from our episodic memories (see Chapter 9). I might recall the *episode* when Auntie Bertha was stung by a bee in Bognor (i.e. episodic memory), but my recall of the *meaning* of the word 'bee' (or indeed 'Bognor') is not held in my episodic memory since it is a matter of semantic memory and is not tied to a particular episode.

The person who said 'I'm one minded at the moment' seemed, it might be argued, to be suggesting a failure of access to her semantic store. She was describing a transient frustration and, indeed, her general linguistic skills (despite some word-finding problems) were good. But what if it were no longer simply a case of awaiting access, waiting for the door to open, but what if the door (even when open) revealed only an increasingly empty space? Loss of semantic memory, loss of one's knowledge base, would entail a loss of one's knowledge of the world *perhaps*. To be stuck in a narrow linguistic groove would be a type of one mindedness; and the terror might be that the groove – one's knowable world – might inevitably become narrower still.

Of course we cannot be certain what it would be like not to have any semantic memory. Even if we could imagine a state in which a person had absolutely no knowledge, in the sense that he or she did not know any words or names, it is still not clear that the person would have no knowledge of the world, which is the reason for saying 'perhaps'. For, our knowledge of the world is not just based on knowing the names of things or knowing words. It might be that we could – even in severe dementia – retain an emotional understanding of the world, which would be another way of knowing it.

However, even if there is a certain sort of terror associated with dementia, does it have to be as bad as some people think it might be? In raising this question I am certainly not intending to suggest that dementia is a good thing: it can be very frustrating when only mild and a tragedy at the extreme. But it is still a way of being human and what I am suggesting is that, even in severe dementia (where semantic or episodic memory might be lost), there remain human possibilities.

The person who was 'one minded' was decidedly describing a problem associated with semantic memory. I have already pointed out that loss of semantic memory is one way in which a person might lose the world (or, at least, part of it). Of course we live in just one world. But there is a sense in which the one world can be understood in a variety of ways: intellectually, emotionally, aesthetically, and so on. It makes sense, therefore, to talk of the different worlds we can potentially inhabit. At one point I might exist in a world of loving family; at another, in the world of beautiful music. Some worlds might be closed off to me now (perhaps I cannot inhabit the world of mathematical theorems) and some worlds would be closed off to me if I were to develop dementia. But there is a sense in which, even if I were only 'one minded', I would at least have the potential of one world open to me. However, I am keen to make the more optimistic point in this chapter that even one mind is enough to open up for me, at least potentially, a whole lot of worlds.

The terror of dementia is partly associated with the fact that it is true that semantic memory can be lost. Note, however, that it is only *one* way in which the world is lost (and note, too, that when I implied this possibility previously I used the word 'perhaps'). I shall go on to argue that even if we were all 'one minded', we yet inhabit *many* worlds, despite dementia. But for now, partly to make this point, I wish to dwell on another way in which we might lose our world in dementia, which is to do with episodic memory.

Loss of memory has traditionally been regarded as the hallmark of dementia (albeit modern conceptions accept that alternative cognitive function might be affected early on) (National Collaborating Centre for Mental Health 2007). Typically it is recent memories for events or episodes that become problematic soonest, but gradually more remote memories are affected. For sure, this is another tragic way in which a world might be lost. Yet, a closer analysis reveals that memory is not just one thing. Perhaps my ability to recall events from a few minutes ago disappears, but I can still recollect things, even recent things, under other circumstances.

The psychologist Steven Sabat has hammered this point home in connection with standardized cognitive assessments. The mini-mental state examination (MMSE) (Folstein *et al.* 1975), for instance, is a good way to test recall, but it does not test much else (Sabat 2001). One of the lessons we learn from Sabat in this book (see Chapter 4), is that there are different ways to remember, for instance by recall and by recognition. His further point (see Sabat 2001) is a much harsher – but well-founded – criticism of the routine use of standardized cognitive tests such as the MMSE. If such a test so readily highlights defects but fails to highlight the person's remaining abilities then it cannot be regarded benignly. The use of objective cognitive tests might be warranted under specific circumstances, but might frequently fail when judged by the ethical principle of non-maleficence. (See Chapter 6 for a critique of the limitation of a principlist approach to resolving ethical dilemmas.) They can be regarded in this light as a form of defectology. In other words, tests like the MMSE can be regarded (especially when poorly used) as a good way to point out the person's defects rather than say anything positive. Indeed, carers of people with dementia complain that formal cognitive testing is one of the most upsetting things that can happen to the person with dementia (Hughes *et al.* 2002).

More striking, perhaps, are some of the stories in Professor Sabat's book *The Experience of Alzheimer's Disease* (Sabat 2001). Dr B was known to be in the moderate to severe stages of dementia as shown by formal assessments. When they were out walking Dr B would often suggest to Sabat that he should pick flowers for his daughter and towards the end of one of his meetings with Sabat, Dr B said: 'Um, but your daughter has a, um, you have to do with your daughter'. Sabat, because of their long association, knew that Dr B was concerned that Sabat might be late to pick up his daughter. Sabat comments:

> I find it fascinating that even when so many elements of cognitive ability are in some form of decline, there are still others remaining intact – others that, in their complexity, seem to require the presence of the very abilities which, when measured alone, are defective. In other words, expressing one's concern for the needs of another person ... would require that the person exhibiting that quality be able to pay attention, to retrieve from memory information about the cared-for person's needs, to be able to use language to communicate that concern, to understand the context of the situation, to name but a few abilities.

(Sabat 2001: 55–6)

Thus, in expressing concern about Sabat's daughter, Dr B was demonstrating a host of cognitive abilities that formal testing showed him to lack!

Now, to return to my theme, this incident shows strikingly how, although in a number of ways Dr B's world might have been considered constricted by his cognitive impairments, in this episode he was able to demonstrate a depth of human responses, which required intact cognitive, emotional and conative (i.e. volitional) abilities. In other words, Dr B was not only able to remember (a cognitive function) about Sabat's daughter, he conveyed an emotional concern about this and he demonstrated his wish that they should take action (conation) and leave so that she could be picked up. There is a sense, then, in which Dr B was also being 'one minded' and yet, in the real world (not the world of cognitive assessment) he was able to demonstrate a world of responses. Indeed, through Sabat's work we see how the increasingly 'one minded' Dr B can still occupy several different worlds – as patient, as caring friend, as research collaborator, as husband and father and so forth.

We were left with the feeling that being 'one minded' in dementia, if this means a loss of one's known world, would be terrifying. But in the case of remembering we have now seen how there are different ways of being minded that keep open several worlds; and being minded in these worlds is to be human, because the worlds of memory, concerned emotions and volitions (of the sort shown by Dr B), are human worlds.

In any case, loss of language (however devastating) does not inevitably involve a loss of meaning, which is why it can be so frustrating. The lady who said 'I'm one minded' knew at some level what she wanted to say (she knew what she meant), she just could not get to the words. This raises a question about whether meaning is ever lost completely. Still to have our understandings and meanings intact, but to be unable to demonstrate them by word or deed, would be a further way in which dementia might seem terrifying.

My inclination, as a clinician, is to doubt that it is really like this for people with severe dementia. I say this because the pathology of dementia is not the same as that of 'locked-in' syndrome. In this syndrome, the person, such as Jean-Dominique Bauby, has suffered a stroke that affects the brain stem, but the brain's cerebral cortex is intact. Bauby was able to communicate his meaning by blinking and thus dictated his immensely moving and instructive book *The Diving Bell and the Butterfly* (Bauby 1997). So, in locked-in syndrome the person's meanings and understandings of the world become completely inaccessible to others. In dementia, however, the pathology in and atrophy of the cortex would seem to make the persistence of this sort of linguistic meaning and understanding demonstrated by Bauby unlikely.

Nevertheless, we should exercise considerable caution here. First, dementia is not locked-in syndrome, where the cortex is intact, but nor is it persistent vegetative state, in which the cortex has essentially disappeared. In dementia, although there is pathology, the cortex remains (Esiri and Nagy 2002). Hence we might, at least, expect that there would be some sort of linguistic meaning and understanding, even if it might be difficult to interpret (see Chapter 12). Secondly, even where there are problems, a variety of abilities *do* persist and might yet be drawn upon by the person, like Dr B, as he or she interacts with the world. Thirdly, the existence of lucid episodes strongly suggests that certain understandings and meanings are retained, even in quite severe dementia (Normann *et al.* 1998). Lucid episodes occur when the person with dementia unexpectedly speaks or acts in such a way as to suggest a greater awareness of his or her situation than has been presumed. John Bayley suggested that his wife, the philosopher and author Iris Murdoch, had an inner world that survived, 'which Iris is determined to keep from me and shields me from' (Bayley 1998: 178); he spoke of utterances or activities that seemed to suggest a 'terrible lucidity' (Bayley 1998: 179).

We have also recounted the case of Mrs G who at one time, utterly dependent, seemed completely inaccessible, but after treatment with a cholinesterase inhibitor was able to talk to her doctor clearly and lucidly about things that had been said at an earlier appointment 'when she had been mute and unable to interact' (Aquilina and Hughes 2006: 149). In discussing this case we suggested that we should have a presupposition that the person has an inner life.

> The presupposition of the inner is grounded in a world in which it makes sense to regard even an incoherent utterance or an uncertain gesture as meaningful, if made by a human being, precisely because this is what we do all the time in our interactions with other human beings.

(Aquilina and Hughes 2006: 154)

We start to see, therefore, that while no one should be blamed for thinking that being 'one minded' in dementia might be terrifying, it is not inevitable that one's whole world will disappear, because we exist in a variety of ways, in a variety of human worlds. Not only do we exist through our retained abilities, as demonstrated by people like Dr B and Mrs G, but also we exist through our interactions with others. Our terror of dementia might in part be an understandable fear of the unknown; but it is also likely to reflect the fear that we shall be misunderstood, discounted, undermined, undervalued or disregarded. Yet it need not be like this: the point of person-centred care is precisely to guard against such possibilities (Brooker 2007; Kitwood 1997). The evidence is that, with the right care, the person's world – even if narrowed – can still remain humanly textured and retain its quality. Take, for example, in Box 7.1 this wife talking of her husband:

Box 7.1   Case example

... if you'd said to me ten years ago at the beginning of this illness, in ten years time my husband will become immobile, speechless, doubly incontinent, unable to do anything for himself ... And if somebody said to me, 'Does somebody in that state have any quality of life?' I think ten years ago I'd have said, 'No'. But working with him now, caring for him now, there is still quality of life there, there are still things that he appreciates. He likes the feel of the sun on his hands, he likes to see what he probably distinguishes as bright colours, ... He likes his music, he likes to be sung to, he likes to be played with in a way that you play with a small child and he loves human contact and cuddles and tickles and all these sorts of things. And yes, there is still a quality of life there.

(Hughes and Baldwin 2006: 100–1)

This takes us on to discuss the way in which being minded is not just a matter of something going on in our heads. It is also a matter of something happening externally in the public spaces of the world.

Being 'one minded' in public space

> **Exercise 7.2** How our minds reach out to the world
>
> Try to think of something, or remember something, that doesn't involve the world. A word such as 'cow' obviously links to the world. But even the number '2' does, because at root we come back to the idea of 2 somethings, such as cows. In doing this you are demonstrating to yourself the way in which your mind cannot be disconnected from the world.

Externalism stands over against those ways of thinking about the mind that always place it as something inner. Externalism states that 'the mental' cannot be characterized without reference to the world. In other words, a thought is always a thought about something or someone in the world; an intention is an intention to do something in the world; when we remember, we remember things that have happened to or been said by people in the world. The mind, on this view, is made up of, is peopled by, the world. This thesis has been encapsulated by the slogan: 'the mind just ain't in the head' (McCulloch 2003: 12).

Externalism is not the only way in which the mind can be understood, but I shall regard it as compelling without further argument (Hughes *et al.* 2006a). One of the main reasons for doing so is because of the fruitful ways in which externalism has implications for being 'one minded' in dementia. Having a mind, even if it has been adversely affected by dementia, entails as a constitutive feature (according to externalism) the potential to participate with the world.

Writing about externalism, McCulloch says, 'Doings and sayings are the primary bearers of content' (2003: 105). That is, meanings (the content of our minds) are conveyed by what we do and say. Hence, even if the person with dementia has lost speech, he or she might yet convey meaning by gesture and behaviour (see Chapters 11 and 14). Moreover, even when the person feels 'one minded', in the sense that she cannot access the right words, she still conveys meaning both by the things she *can* say as well as by her demeanour and tone. How might this be possible? Well, precisely because her human interlocutors can participate and engage with her in a space of meaning, which is the shared public world in which our minds interact. Furthermore, because we share this space (as Sabat did with Dr B) the possibility that we might facilitate her communication is always possible (Killick and Allan 2001; Sabat 2001; see Chapter 4 and Chapter 12).

The consequences of this approach to the mind are not unfamiliar: externalism supports many of the key tenets of person-centred care. If Mr Smith's mental life is world-involving, then others can help to sustain or to undermine Mr Smith's mindedness. In turn, this would be to enhance or detract from his personhood (Brooker 2004; Kitwood 1997). The tendency for someone's standing as a person to be undermined in dementia by 'malignant social psychology' was highlighted by Kitwood (1997). (Examples of how the person's 'social personae' can be undermined are given in Chapter 4.) On the view being encouraged here, it is always possible (in principle) to enter someone's mental world, to share with them meaning, even if this is unspoken, even if it is a matter of nuance and emotional tone.

So being 'one minded' is enough for any of us, because it inevitably entails the world. Indeed, one mind is enough to lead us to the many different worlds that we can inhabit together: worlds of thought and language, but also worlds of music, aesthetic enjoyment, touch and other sensations, worlds of meanings, drives, volitions and emotions. The multitude of worlds that we inhabit are open to *us* on account of our one mindedness. That is, the human mind (even just one of them!) opens us up to the world and is constituted (made up) by the world. Just as the mind has many aspects, so too we can enjoy, as human beings, many worlds. And the human mind situates us in the human world, where we share our mindedness, even in the midst of impairment. In the next section I shall flesh out what it means to be a person with dementia by considering the situated-embodied-agent view (Hughes 2001). This view of the person encourages and supports the ways in which externalism emphasizes our engagement with the world of variety, difference and change.

Being a person

> **Exercise 7.3** Developing awareness of the multilayered nature of our human existence
>
> Try to think of a personal friend without thinking of his or her life history, or culture, or values. Under what circumstances can we think of people in this way? Perhaps we can think administratively, or (in one rather cold sense) clinically, but can we think of people *personally* in this way?
>
> In engaging with this exercise you are demonstrating to yourself the extent to which we are inevitably *situated* as persons in a variety of human fields: cultural, social, historical, ethical, psychological, and so forth.

First, being a person entails *being situated*. This is a point of enormous consequence because we have the potential to be situated in so many different ways. We are situated within our own personal histories, which include our bodily, as well as our psychological, stories (see Chapter 10 on working with life history by Errollyn Bruce and Pam Schweitzer). We are embedded in familial, cultural, historical, societal, moral and legal contexts (see Chapter 27 on policies and politics by Jesse Ballenger). There is increasing recognition of the spiritual and religious aspects of our lives. All of this is of enormous consequence because it suggests the extent to which human lives cannot be circumscribed. Nor, therefore, should attempts be made to circumscribe the ways in which we might flourish or enjoy quality of life, even when we have a condition such as dementia (Hughes 2003).

To have dementia is in some sense or other to be different. The person who described herself as being 'one minded' was different because of her speech difficulty. But all human beings are unique. In some ways, being different makes one more human, because we are picked out by our differences. Difference, it seems, is the way to be an individual. Variety and difference, in short, are the spice of human life.

Secondly, being a person entails *being an agent*. In the modern Western world, being an autonomous agent seems almost quintessential (see Chapter 6). 'Being able to do things for myself because I want to', expresses much of the notion of liberty – uncritically formulated – that underpins modern democracies. 'Doings and sayings', remember are, according to McCulloch (2003: p. 105), the primary ways in which we pass on meaning or reveal our mindedness. To be unable *to do* would, at least to a marginal degree, start to challenge our sense of ourselves as minded. In many ways I am what I do. (See Chapter 3 for examples of how people with dementia express agency.)

Be all this as it may, it is important to recall that my standing as an agent, essential as it is with regards to personhood, is my standing as a *situated* agent. In other words my agentive possibilities are circumscribed by nature, by circumstance, by history and by my interdependence with others. Even if I can always be situated differently, I cannot act as an agent in just any way that I choose. In one sense this seems a trivial point: I cannot fly without considerable help; in the interest of my neighbours I cannot do whatever I want; and so on. But recall, my independence to act autonomously seemed to be quintessential to my standing as a person in Western society. There is something shocking about the realization that my autonomy can never be fully exercised. At the heart of my autonomy is my dependence, because I simply cannot live as an independent atom (as it were) isolated from the rest of humanity. Even real atoms interact! The interplay between autonomy and dependency in old age, especially in connection with long-term care, has been carefully detailed by Agich (2003).

If I were to become someone with dementia, things would change from how they are now, as they also would if I were to develop heart failure or lung disease. Perhaps finally I should only be able to demonstrate uncertain behaviour and make ambiguous gestures. There is, at least, the possibility that – inasmuch as agency persists – my actions, if not my language, might be understandable only to someone who knows me well. An interpretation might be required, but there is also the possibility of intuitive understanding, perhaps based on a form of tacit knowledge that draws from a common background of beliefs, values and reactions.

There are two important points to be drawn from this, first in connection with the background and, second, in connection with the notion of interpretation. Both points propel us into the third way of characterizing personhood, namely in terms of embodiment. Wittgenstein once wrote:

> We judge an action according to its background within human life ... Not what one person is doing now, but the whole hurly-burly, is the background against which we see an action, and it determines our judgement, our concepts, and our reactions.

(Wittgenstein 1980: 624, 629)

Hence, it can be argued, the gestures or behaviours of a person in the more severe stages of dementia will only make sense against the broad background that constitutes human life and *this* human life in particular. (A number of the other chapters in this book are relevant to this point; see Chapters 10, 14 and 12.) Our understanding of the person's actions, which might well in isolation seem meaningless, will require interpretation. The interpretation will be more successful if the person doing the interpreting (a) has considerable skill in this area and (b) has a deep knowledge of the person concerned. This knowledge is multilayered; it is biopsychosocial and spiritual at least. It requires an appreciation of all the ways in which we (and *this* person in particular) might be situated. The background is important because, for a human person, it is the human context without which and against which we make our judgements.

It is important to appreciate that part of the background to our interpretations stems from *our embodiment*. Being human beings of this kind entails being embodied thus. As Charles Taylor has suggested:

> Our body is not just the executant of the goals we frame. ... Our understanding itself is embodied. ... My sense of myself, of the footing I am on with others, is in large part also embodied.

> (Taylor 1995: 170–1)

Of course, on reflection, it should not be a surprise that the footing I am on with others is embodied; because this is the space of understanding we share: the human embodied world. But the idea that our understanding is itself embodied might seem surprising. A little thought should convince us that this is not too egregious. After all, communication generally involves bodily acts. The implications of the notion of bodily understanding run deeper still, however, because the idea goes against our ingrained tendency to regard the body and the spirit (or the inner, or simply the mind) as decidedly separate. On my view, our bodies should be regarded as ineluctably bound up with our inner, subjective natures. Interpretation of our bodily movements is the way to understand our inner meanings. Not only is this so as a matter of natural fact, but also it turns out to be true at a conceptual level: 'our understanding itself is embodied' (Taylor 1995: 170).

The philosopher Merleau-Ponty suggested this by the notion ascribed to him of the 'body-subject'. According to his way of thinking it is possible to argue that, 'Reflex or instinctual actions ... may be purposive but not consciously so ...' (Matthews 1996: 92). Wim Dekkers has expanded this understanding to elaborate his concept of 'bodily autonomy':

> The meaning of bodily autonomy that I am putting forward is a combination of the biomedical notion of bodily automatisms and the phenomenological idea of the lived body. Considered from this (combined) perspective, the human body lives its own life, to a high degree being independent of higher brain functions and conscious deliberations and intentions. The lived body demonstrates a 'tacit knowledge'. In a person with dementia, cognitive capabilities gradually disappear until the moment when the patient is no longer capable of exercising autonomy by making explicit decisions. This does not mean, however, that the patient's bodily knowledge, developed in the course of the patient's life, necessarily also disappears.

> (Dekkers 2004: 125)

A little later Dekkers states, 'Tacit bodily knowledge is based on the sedimentation of life narratives' (Dekkers 2004: 125). He uses this idea to argue that when people with severe dementia seem to resist artificial feeding, this should be taken as an expression of their bodily autonomy. Our gestures or resistances need to be understood in a broad human context and it is not unreasonable to presuppose the 'inner' life of a human being on the basis of actual human behaviour. As Wittgenstein famously remarked: 'The human body is the best picture of the human soul' (Wittgenstein 1958: 178).

Debates and controversies

Some philosophers have argued that personal identity is a matter of there being psychological continuity and connectedness. In other words, there should be some sort of link, provided by memory, between our psychological states over time (Parfit 1984; for a contrary view, see Hughes 2001).

If this were the case, it might be argued:

- that the person with dementia was not the same person he or she was before (Hope 1994)

- that the individual with dementia should not be considered a person at all and, therefore, any advance directives could be ignored (Buchanan 1988).

Some argue that, even if the self is eroded, the individual might still be worthy of moral concern (Luntley 2006); but the ethical implications of saying that someone with severe dementia is not a person need to be considered.

A number of philosophers and philosophical arguments have, however, been used to encourage the line that, even in severe dementia, there is still a person (see Hughes *et al.* 2006b).

Conclusion

The unbuckling of personhood from being human is possible inasmuch as it is possible to regard being a person as in some sense solely a matter of *inner* goings on. These inner processes might be thought of as the workings of a computer. They might be regarded more psychologically as consciousness. They might even be conceived in purely biological terms. In this chapter, however, I have focused on how being minded – having this sense of inner – is necessarily a potentially public, shared phenomenon. Therefore, being a person, which is characteristically to be minded, is typically to share potentially public spaces and to manifest the situated embodiment and agentive responses to the human world that constitute that world. Our interpretations of other human beings are instinctual and immediate because of our shared nature.

The arguments here suggest that people with dementia, because we all occupy the same human worldly groove, remain persons even in the severer stages of their disease. The requirement that we should be person-centred, therefore, stems from our being human. Indeed, the impetus behind the idea of person-centred care reflects and is supported by the sort of analysis offered in this chapter. Person-centredness, as a concept, was intended to move us away from a narrower, purely biomedical, view of dementia (Brooker 2007; Kitwood 1997). Not only does this seem to be a good thing from the perspective of people with dementia, but it also drops out of our philosophical discussion of what it might be to be minded in dementia. So there is conceptual backing to the ethical imperative to treat people with dementia as persons; that is, as human beings who are still capable of human interactions. The multifarious ways in which it is possible to be person-centred result from the variety of ways in which human beings can flourish. To occupy the human world – even with dementia – is to share a human significance through our mutual standing as inter-related and interdependent persons. For to be just 'one minded' as a human being is enough to allow the possibility of many personal worlds.

Further information

The **International Network for Philosophy and Psychiatry** (INPP) provides a collaborative research and education forum to support organizations and individuals involved in conceptual and ethical work in psychiatry and related disciplines.

References

Agich, G.J. (2003) *Dependence and Autonomy in Old Age: An Ethical Framework for Long-term Care*. Cambridge: Cambridge University Press.

Aquilina, C. and Hughes, J.C. (2006) The return of the living dead: agency lost and found? In: J.C. Hughes, S.J. Louw and S.R. Sabat (eds) *Dementia: Mind, Meaning, and the Person*. Oxford: Oxford University Press.

Bauby, J-D. (1997) *The Diving Bell and the Butterfly* (translated by J. Leggatt). London: Fourth Estate.

Bayley, J. (1998) *Iris: A Memoir of Iris Murdoch*. London: Abacus Books.

Brooker, D. (2004) What is person-centred care for people with dementia? *Reviews in Clinical Gerontology*, 13: 212–22.

Brooker, D. (2007) *Person-Centred Dementia Care: Making Services Better*. London: Jessica Kingsley.

Buchanan, A. (1988) Advance directives and the personal identity problem. *Philosophy and Public Affairs*, 17: 277–302.

Dekkers, W.J.M. (2004) Autonomy and the lived body in cases of severe dementia. In: R.B. Purtilo and H.A.M.J. ten Have (eds) *Ethical Foundations of Palliative Care for Alzheimer Disease*. Baltimore, MD: Johns Hopkins University Press.

Esiri, M. and Nagy, Z. (2002) Neuropathology. In: R. Jacoby and C. Oppenheimer (eds) *Psychiatry in the Elderly*, 3rd edn. Oxford: Oxford University Press.

Folstein, M.F., Folstein, S.E. and McHugh, P.R. (1975) Mini-mental state: a practical method for grading the cognitive state of patients for the clinician. *Journal of Psychiatric Research*, 12: 189–98.

Hope, T. (1994) Personal identity and psychiatric illness. In: A. Phillips Griffiths (ed.) *Philosophy, Psychology and Psychiatry*. Cambridge: Cambridge University Press.

Hughes, J.C. (2001) Views of the person with dementia. *Journal of Medical Ethics*, 27: 86–91.

Hughes, J.C. (2003) Quality of life in dementia: an ethical and philosophical perspective. *Expert Review of Pharmacoeconomics and Outcomes Research*, 3: 525–34.

Hughes, J.C. and Baldwin, C. (2006) *Ethical Issues in Dementia Care: Making Difficult Decisions*. London: Jessica Kingsley.

Hughes, J.C., Hope, T., Reader, S. and Rice, D. (2002) Dementia and ethics: a pilot study of the views of informal carers. *Journal of the Royal Society of Medicine*, 95: 242–6.

Hughes, J.C., Louw, S.J. and Sabat, S.R. (2006a) Seeing whole. In: J.C. Hughes, S.J. Louw and S.R. Sabat (eds) *Dementia: Mind, Meaning, and the Person*. Oxford: Oxford University Press.

Hughes, J.C., Louw, S.J. and Sabat, S.R. (eds) (2006b) *Dementia: Mind, Meaning, and the Person*. Oxford: Oxford University Press.

Killick, J. and Allan, K. (2001) *Communication and the Care of People with Dementia*. Buckingham: Open University Press.

Kitwood, T. (1997) *Dementia Reconsidered: The Person Comes First*. Buckingham: Open University Press.

Luntley, M. (2006) Keeping track, autobiography, and the conditions for self-erosion. In: J.C. Hughes, S.J. Louw and S.R. Sabat (eds) *Dementia: Mind, Meaning, and the Person*. Oxford: Oxford University Press.

Matthews, E. (1996) *Twentieth-Century French Philosophy*. Oxford: Oxford University Press.

McCulloch, G. (2003) *The Life of the Mind. An Essay on Phenomenological Externalism*. London: Routledge.

National Collaborating Centre for Mental Health (2007) *Dementia: The NICE-SCIE Guideline on Supporting People with Dementia and their Carers in Health and Social Care*. Leicester and London: The British Psychological Society and Gaskell.

Normann, H.K., Asplund, K. and Norberg, A. (1998) Episodes of lucidity in people with severe dementia as narrated by formal carers. *Journal of Advanced Nursing*, 28: 1295–300.

Parfit, D. (1984) *Reasons and Persons*. Oxford: Oxford University Press.

Sabat, S.R. (2001) *The Experience of Alzheimer's Disease: Life through a Tangled Veil*. Oxford and Malden MA: Blackwell.

Taylor, C. (1995) *Philosophical Arguments*. Cambridge, MA: Harvard University Press.

Wittgenstein, L. (1958) *Philosophical Investigations* (translated by G.E.M. Anscombe). Oxford: Blackwell.

Wittgenstein, L. (1980) *Remarks on the Philosophy of Psychology*. Vol II. (G.H. von Wright and H. Nyman (eds). translated by C.G. Luckhardt and M.A.E. Aue). Oxford: Blackwell.

PART TWO

Knowledge and skills for supporting people with dementia

8

Assessment and dementia

Gail Mountain

Learning objectives

By the end of this chapter you will be able to:

- outline the various purposes for which assessments are conducted with people with dementia and their family carers
- critically appraise the assessment process from the perspective of people with dementia and their family carers
- describe best practice of assessment with people with dementia and their family carers
- appreciate that on-going assessment is a feature of quality care for people with dementia and their family carers

Introduction

A changing view of the capacities of people with dementia, the push for early diagnosis and the potential of medication to allay symptoms are all pointing towards the need for a focus on person-centred assessment. Such assessment will complement the new forms of service provision which promote a person-centred approach including interventions to promote self-management and rehabilitation. New methods of assessment, which prioritize the views of the person with dementia and their family carer, are necessary in order to underpin service delivery.

Assessment is a systematic gathering of information. From a service perspective, the goal of assessment is to direct resources to where they are most needed (Meaney *et al.* 2005). For the person being assessed and their family carer, the results of assessment should indicate the services and interventions they need in order to maximize strengths and resources and achieve the best quality of life.

Assessment can serve a variety of different purposes and it is important that all who are involved in the process are clear about its purpose. Different purposes include:

- to assist the person with dementia or their carer to understand their needs and the services and interventions that can assist them

- to provide information which practitioners can use to make decisions about clients' eligibility for specific services

- to establish a baseline against which changes can be measured for clinical or research purposes.

This chapter describes the assessment process with people with dementia and their family carers, with a focus upon best practice to assist people to obtain the services they need in order to live a quality life with dementia. It includes attention to the need for clarity about the purpose for any assessment, best practice in the conduct of the assessment, and the importance of ensuring that information is shared between the assessor, the person with dementia and their family carer. A case study of a family coping with the impact of early dementia is used to illustrate various aspects of the process.

Reasons for assessment of people with dementia and their family carers

Until recently, a lack of treatment options and a prevailing view that management of person with dementia was largely palliative (even in the early stages of the condition) led to a limited repertoire of assessment options once the diagnosis was established. Assessment of the person with dementia tended to be undertaken to confirm failing capacities and needs for services due to increasing dependency rather than to identify active treatment and rehabilitative possibilities. The needs of the family carer predominated, with assessment concentrated upon services such as respite to support the caring role and to enable carers to continue caring (Levin *et al.* 1994).

Recently there has been a significant change in attitudes and understanding. Best practice in dementia care now includes a range of interventions to stimulate and support preserved abilities and self-management in the earlier stages of the condition. There is now an emphasis on promoting quality of life and maximizing the functioning of the person and their carer at all stages of the disease process (Graff *et al.* 2006; Mountain 2006; Vernooij-Dassen and Moniz-Cook 2005). Furthermore, it is increasingly recognized that interventions must take into account all aspects of the health and well-being of the person with dementia and their carer, mental, physical and spiritual. For appropriate interventions to be identified and delivered, they must be preceded by a relevant assessment of strengths and needs, with interventions to meet needs following on from assessment. The effectiveness of any intervention should then be examined through reassessment, and further interventions identified if required, as shown in Figure 8.1.

Thus assessment and provision of interventions should be a dynamic and interactive process, which fully engages the person and their carer and enables appropriate responses to be made to their needs over time (see Chapter 23). The complexity of what can be involved particularly when working with people who will have a range of needs resulting from older age and its consequences is described in the case study in Box 8.1.

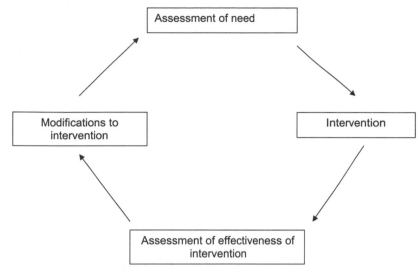

Figure 8.1 The assessment cycle

Box 8.1 Case example

Mrs Jones lives with husband of 40 years; they have no other family living nearby. She is newly diagnosed with Alzheimer's disease, even though she had been getting increasingly forgetful and anxious for the previous two years. Mr Jones is cognitively well but has limited mobility due to arthritis. He also has cardiovascular disease. He is the prime carer for his wife and has taken over responsibility for the majority of household tasks. They are both fearful for the future and Mr Jones feels isolated and unsupported at times. However, Mrs Jones has just been prescribed cognitive enhancing medication, which has led to improvements in her mental state. Health care staff plan to visit Mr and Mrs Jones in their own home to assess the effectiveness of Mrs Jones's memory enhancing medication, and also to assess the wider needs of both Mr and Mrs Jones within their own environment They are aware that Mrs Jones had a fall the previous year on the stairs at home and have also gathered that Mr Jones has recently slipped in the bath. At present the couple do not receive any social care services, so the visit will also explore these needs in preparation for a possible referral for social care.

The case study in Box 8.1 illustrates the extent of needs that might be uncovered when people first present with the symptoms of dementia. The age profile of people who are likely to develop the condition means that a whole range of unmet needs associated with the ageing process can co-exist (Xie *et al.* 2008), particularly if people have been coping with difficulties over a protracted period of time without any external help.

> **Exercise 8.1** Identifying and anticipating needs
>
> In the case example in Box 8.1, it appears that both Mrs Jones and her husband carer have some needs. Make a list of the needs you see for Mr Jones. In the past, many assessments would stop here. Now make a list of the needs you see, or might anticipate, for Mrs Jones. Can you think of any interventions that would meet the needs of both? What are some of Mrs Jones's needs that might be quite separate from what her husband needs?

Following initial assessment, the ongoing impact of dementia upon the individual combined with other factors like the changing family circumstances and the impact of the caring role upon family carers, will require a series of subsequent assessments in order to gauge the success of interventions as well as in response to changing needs over time. As such, assessment should be an on-going integral aspect of treatment and care. However, there are a number of well-established triggers, which can determine need for a specific type of assessment. These include the following:

Assessment for diagnostic reasons

The first, most important assessment is conducted for diagnostic purposes, usually in primary care or memory clinic settings (see Chapter 15). The outcome of this assessment should lead to a series of actions that assist the person and their carer to adjust to living with dementia and to receive the treatment, services and support that they require. There is a growing realization that people with dementia deserve to have an early diagnosis from an accurate, well-managed assessment so that treatment can commence as early as possible. This significant shift in philosophy of treatment care is described within guidelines for supporting people with dementia and their carers (NICE-SCIE 2006).

Assessment of the need for, and outcomes of, memory enhancing medication

Medical practitioners are required to determine the appropriateness of prescribing medication and following this, its effectiveness. The outcomes of the medication will then need to be monitored through reassessment over time.

Assessment of caregiver needs

As described in the case study, carers will frequently neglect their own needs. Additionally, changes in the person they care for due to the illness can be extremely distressing and the impact of the caring role can result in mental and physical problems for carers. Two types of assessment are often necessary; first, assessment of the health and well-being of the carer, which might be undertaken by health services staff, and, second, assessment to identify carer needs for services. In England, the Carers Equal Opportunities Act (2004) placed a duty upon social services departments to inform carers of their rights to an assessment which should include a discussion of carer involvement in education, work and leisure, with agencies being obliged to provide services in response to assessed needs if requested by the local authority.

Assessment for community-based services

This assessment will overlap with the previously described assessment of carer needs for services. The social care services that people with dementia and their carers may be eligible for include access to direct payments, assistive technologies for help and enablement, day care, help with meals and personal care in their home and respite care (for carers of people with moderate to severe dementia). The assessment for these and other community-based services usually incorporates identifying the level of functioning of the person with dementia, and the consequent needs of the carer as well as assessing financial eligibility for services.

Assessment following discharge from hospital

This form of assessment is concerned with determining the ability of the person to undertake activities of daily living safely prior to discharge from inpatient care, and is commonplace in acute medical care. They are part of a series of actions, which should start when the person is first admitted to hospital. There is a growing awareness that the common practice of setting aside the whole process in favour of one-off assessments does not accurately reflect ability to cope in the longer term and can be intimidating for the person and for their carer (Mountain and Pighills 2003). The aim is to identify the extent of risk (if any) the person poses to themselves and others if they are discharged to their former living arrangements and to ensure that the person and their caregiver are both properly prepared for return home. Therefore, shared decision-making between professionals, the person and their carer is promoted. These assessments can also inform whether a period of rehabilitation in an intermediate care setting might be beneficial, or alternatively whether need for residential care is indicated.

Assessment for admission to residential care

This will include assessment of need from the perspectives of the individual and their carer, as well as an assessment of financial means and therefore their contribution. Further details are addressed in Chapters 16, 18 and 19.

Assessment for research purposes

The focus on finding a cure for Alzheimer's disease and other dementias has led to people with dementia and their carers being involved in research as participants or informants. The introduction of memory enhancing medication has led to greater levels of research activity, both to assess the effectiveness of products and to determine further treatment possibilities. One of the unexpected benefits of the availability of medication for dementia has been a realization that people with dementia can benefit from psychosocial and rehabilitative interventions (see Chapter 14), with accompanying research activity also escalating as a result (Graff *et al.* 2006).

Assessment in response to specific needs

People with dementia tend to be older and are therefore likely to have needs as a result of physical health (Xie *et al.* 2008; see Chapter 13). Co-existing illnesses and impairments must also be identified and treated. Examples of assessments that may be relevant include those to identify depression and other mental health problems, to determine extent of physical impairment and dependency and to gauge the experience of pain.

Best practice in assessment

Assessments can be conducted in a variety of different ways, gathering different kinds of information. As discussed above, the starting point for any assessment is clarity as to its purpose. Once we are clear about the purpose of the assessment, we must ask ourselves:

- What is the information that is being sought through the assessment?
- Who should be assessed?
- What are the best ways of obtaining this information?
- How should the assessment be conducted?
- What happens to the information obtained through the assessment?

What information needs to be collected?

Each assessment is constructed to collect information in one or more domains. For the person with dementia, the global domains that might be assessed include:

- psychological functioning
- social functioning
- occupation and engagement
- physical health
- medication use.

Each domain will most likely be comprised of a number of different elements For example, assessment of occupation and engagement might include ability to undertake necessary tasks around the home, participation in chosen leisure activities and ability and opportunities to socialize outside the home.

For the caregiver, relevant assessment domains can include:

- physical health

- psychological well-being including experience of stress and burden
- social functioning
- participation outside the home
- available support
- medication use.

Who should be assessed?

As described in the case study, the assessment process with people with dementia frequently involves family such as spouses or partners and other relatives who are providing a caring role and, as a consequence, will have their own needs. It can also extend to neighbours and friends if they are involved in providing a substantial amount of assistance. The demands of caring for someone with dementia can be extensive and exhausting (Gilhooly 1984) and family and other informal carers will often have their own health and social care needs as a result of the demands stemming from the caring role (Wright 1986). For example, it can be difficult for a carer to attend the GP surgery if they do not feel able to leave the person for whom they are caring. Also, the carer's willingness to continue caring should not be taken for granted. Seddon and Robinson (2001) recommended that assessment of the needs of carers should be guided by a framework that includes full assessment of the carer's practical and emotional needs and the incorporation of a system for monitoring and review.

A further examination of the circumstances of Mr and Mrs Jones illustrated the range of difficulties and challenges they are living with, both as a couple and as individuals.

Box 8.2 Case example

Since diagnosis, Mrs Jones has received medication to enhance her memory. She is now able to think far more clearly but still has memory lapses. She wishes to consider how she can resume some responsibilities for the home, as well as some leisure interests. However, she is still fearful of falling. This fear has undermined her confidence, which can limit her activity and that of her husband, particularly outside the home. She is concerned about not being able to undertake household tasks to her previous standards and is also worried about Mr Jones's health.

Box 8.3 Case example

Mr Jones is committed to caring for his wife and wants them to stay together as a couple whatever the future may hold. His own health needs are concerning him though; he is not able to physically undertake certain tasks which he was previously responsible for in the home such as gardening. Also, getting to the supermarket is physically challenging due to the distance he has to walk while carrying shopping (he stopped driving several years ago). He needs to go to the GP for regular checks but over the last year has found it difficult to attend for appointments as Mrs Jones became anxious if he left her. Even though Mrs Jones is showing improvements he is finding it difficult to allow her to reassume tasks like cooking that she was previously responsible for, in case of accidents. He used to enjoy sport but now finds it impossible to attend local events and he also cannot concentrate on the TV.

In some circumstances, the needs of the person and their family carer should be addressed together and in others, it is more appropriate to see the person and their carer on separate occasions. In the case example in Box 8.3, both Mr and Mrs Jones may have difficulty expressing their true feelings about their situation as they might not want to appear disloyal to each other. This situation would need careful handling and possibly individual sessions.

What are the best methods for gathering this information?

The best methods for gathering information will depend upon the domains to be assessed. Methods of assessment can include the following:

- documentation of verbal information provided by the person and/or their carer often in response to key questions

- physiological tests and scans

- use of observation, with results of observation noted on check lists, providing a description of performance

- application of summed indices where the person is assessed on a number of items, but where the items to be summated will not have equal weight

- application of valid and reliable (standardized) instruments.

Complex assessment procedures such as those required to inform a complex plan of care will require a toolkit of measures, including standardized instruments and other forms of assessment (Department of Health 2001). Standardized instruments with proven psychometric properties provide an accurate measure, which is particularly valuable in providing a baseline measure, with further measurement providing an outcome. Important considerations in the choice of standardized instruments include their reliability, validity and sensitivity (Bowling 1997), whether training is required to use the instrument and the extent to which it enables the assessment process to be owned by the person being assessed. Even though standardized instruments are extremely valuable and their use is appropriate in many assessment situations, they cannot produce the quality and depth of information required for some purposes as they reduce actions, abilities and perceptions into concrete, easily understood statements so that there is no doubt as to their meaning. Such statements rarely take account of subtle difference in abilities of individuals or the complexity of the situations that might need to be assessed. Therefore, if assessment is being conducted for treatment and rehabilitative purposes, standardized measures will need to be supplemented by other forms of assessment such as interview and observation.

In the case of Mr and Mrs Jones, the initial assessment process is likely to take more than one visit and will require a combination of assessment through questioning and listening, observation and application of standardized measures.

Exercise 8.2   Conducting the most effective assessment

Looking again at the case example in Box 8.1 and your responses to Exercise 8.1, identify what specific information your assessment will include and about whom. Think about where, how and by whom the assessment should be carried out (see Chapter 12). Who will use the information? Who will be involved in deciding what support is necessary?

It is beyond the remit of this chapter to provide a comprehensive review of recommended assessment instruments for dementia, of which there are many. However, it is possible to consider the assessment methods and instruments that might be selected for use with Mr and Mrs Jones, taking account of the need to ensure that information is collected over time and not just as a result of one or two encounters.

To obtain the necessary information to plan treatment and services for Mr and Mrs Jones, assessment might incorporate the following:

Mrs Jones

Purpose of assessment	Assessment method	Appropriate instruments
Impact of memory enhancing medication and overall mental state	Measurement of cognitive function	Mini mental state examination (MMSE) (Folstein *et al.* 1975) General practitioner assessment of cognition (GPCOG) (Brodaty *et al.* 2002)
Needs for cognitive rehabilitation and assistance with enabling strategies to compensate for memory loss Ability to undertake functional tasks	Responses to key questions Structured observation with results leading to agreement between person being assessed and assessor regarding appropriate interventions or Measurement of IADL ability	Assessment of motor and process skills (AMPs) (Fisher 1999) Instrumental activities of daily living (IADL) (Lawton and Brody 1969)
Needs for leisure and socialization and experience of quality of life	Responses to key questions Measurement of life quality	Dementia quality of life (DEMQoL) (Smith *et al.* 2005)

Purpose of assessment	Assessment method	Appropriate instruments
Impact of fear of falling	Responses to key questions	
Worries and concerns		General health questionnaire (GHQ) (Goldberg and Williams 1988)

Mr Jones

Physical health needs

Ability to undertake necessary tasks	Assessment of medical and social needs Confidence in undertaking tasks	Easy-care (SISA) 1997 Short sense of competence questionnaire (Vernooji-Dassen *et al.* 1999)
Mental well-being	Assessment of experience of stress and burden	SF36 (Ware and Sherbourne 1992) General health questionnaire (Goldberg and Williams 1988)
Social care needs	Responses to key questions about daily routine and coping strategies	OPUS (Netten *et al.* 2002) Local authority carer needs assessment

Mr and Mrs Jones together

Appropriateness and safety of home environment

Shared worries and concerns	Responses to key questions about current concerns and concerns for the future	
Needs for community services	Community care assessment	Single Assessment Process (SAP) (Department of Health 2004)

How should the assessment be conducted?

The manner in which the assessment is conducted is very important. It is all too easy to forget the significance of the process for the user and their carer when it is part of everyday professional practice. The achievement of a quality assessment is demanding for all involved but its value cannot be underestimated (Godfrey 1998; Godfrey and Wistow 1997). Conversely, a poor assessment can leave the individual feeling disempowered and vulnerable, as well as failing to provide an accurate picture of the services required to meet their needs and those of their carer.

Conducting a quality assessment with people with dementia is a challenge for service providers, requiring a combination of knowledge and skills, which must be underpinned by an empathic approach and a willingness to listen. The encouragement of better assessment methods in practice settings demands new and improved assessment tools, which meet the needs of people with dementia and their carers, as well as of service providers. As previously mentioned, there is a growing awareness of the importance of partnering people with dementia and their carers in all encounters, including assessment.

Preparation and planning

As part of practicalities of undertaking any assessment, consideration should be given to who is most suited to conduct the process. Depending upon the reason for the assessment, it may for example be a person with a specific skill base, someone who the person being assessed knows and feels comfortable with or an individual with sufficient time available to ensure that the process is not rushed. The appropriateness of conducting hurried, one-off assessments, which do not allow the assessor to introduce themselves, listen to the person and invite questions is questionable with people with dementia, and those involved in their care, and is likely to cause anxiety and distress (Mountain and Pighills 2003).

Provision of information

Full information about the assessment process must be provided beforehand to the person being assessed (and to their carer if appropriate), ideally by the person who is to undertake the assessment so that any questions can be addressed beforehand. Pre-assessment, the person and their carer should be provided with information detailing where the assessment will take place, when and for how long, and what it will entail. Verbal information should be backed up with clear and readily comprehendible documentation, particularly if the process will involve potentially uncomfortable assessments, for example scans; or where the outcome will have particular significance such as assessments conducted for diagnostic purposes or those leading to decisions about provision of services. The extent of cognitive impairment that the person is experiencing is a further, important consideration and should lead to special considerations regarding how information is presented. When and how the person and their carer will be given the outcomes of the assessment should also be conveyed beforehand. Assessments undertaken for research purposes will necessitate obtaining ethical approval to undertake the assessment, followed by documented informed consent from the person and possibly from their carer before they can take place (National Research Ethics Services 2007).

Conduct during the assessment

The requirement for best practice during the assessment process is heightened when working with people with dementia and their carers. As previously described, the assessment location must be agreed with the person and their carer. The chosen venue should be quiet, comfortable and undisturbed. Through a review of assessment policy and implementation in health and social care, Nolan and Caldock (1996) identified a number of benchmarks for good assessment practice including undertaking the assessment in an appropriate setting, providing information, taking time to listen to the views of users and carers, providing constructive solutions and avoiding presenting the assessment as a hurdle which has to be overcome before services might be accessed. It is particularly important to allow the person with dementia plenty of time to talk freely as well as their carer. The challenge is to ensure that these benchmarks are met. Finally, the person and their carer should be provided with a written account of the outcomes of the assessment if possible.

Exercise 8.3   Recognizing individual needs in assessment

After reviewing Chapters 2, 3 and 4, think about where you might alter your assessment in response to cultural diversity, family differences or differences in the person with dementia.

Discuss how your assessment would be different, taking these things into consideration.

What happens to information obtained through the assessment?

The extent of assessment a person with dementia and their carers might experience can be excessive, as evidenced through the brief case example of Mr and Mrs Jones. Individuals can be subjected to several assessments of need, and if there is poor coordination across agencies, the same assessment might be repeated by different agencies within a short space of time. Also, a range of assessment methods may have to be applied to elicit the necessary information from the person with dementia, taking into account the impact of cognitive impairment (as demonstrated through the case study). In England, the need to avoid multiple assessments for community care has led to introduction of the Single Assessment Process which aims to recognize the full spectrum of health and social care needs, underpinned by a person-centred approach (Department of Health 2004). Outcomes of assessment are documented on the summary record. The requirement to update information over time, and the importance of information systems that facilitate sharing of assessment information across those involved are emphasized.

Implementation of the single assessment process is proving to be challenging, highlighting the need for enhanced staff training and for computerized systems, which enable information to be shared efficiently and confidentially across agencies, while at the same time allowing information to be shared with the person who has been assessed. The principles of information sharing promoted through the Single Assessment Process should pertain to all other forms of assessment.

Debates and controversies

We need to develop and test measures that can be used in rehabilitative and psychosocial practice. We must now seek to gain the person's perspective on their situation, rather than relying solely on the carer's viewpoint. The predominant practice to date has been to focus solely on carer views, reflecting the long-standing perceptions that a person with dementia is not able to give valid responses or views about their treatment and care. We now know that people can provide reliable and valid reports (Mozley *et al*. 1999; Whitlatch and Feinberg 2005). In England the implementation of the Mental Capacity Act 2005 is proving to be a further stimulus for change in assessment methods. This Act requires that the wishes of the vulnerable person are taken fully into account unless it can be proved that they definitely do not have the capacity to take decisions for themselves. Therefore assessments which lead to decisions which negate the views of the individual are no longer appropriate in the majority of cases.

In the past we have tended to focus on the measurement and management of carer burden. Now we are interested in providing education and other interventions to empower and enable carers to cope with the demands of their caring role. This in turn requires that we change existing assessment practice.

The content of some assessment instruments, and in particular those concerned with measuring activities of daily living, should take human functioning within an increasing technological world into account; for example ability to cope with commonly encountered technological devices within the home (Nygård and Starkhammer 2007).

Conclusion

Assessment is one of the most significant of care processes for people with dementia and their family carers. It is also very demanding for care providers and those seeking to undertake research. Good delivery requires a combination of good planning, skills and empathy. Prioritization of the needs of those being assessed together with careful listening can help to make it a positive experience despite the frequent and often palpable vulnerability of those being assessed.

Further information

The Royal College of Nursing produced a toolkit for *Nursing Assessment of Older People* in 2004. This is available for download from the Royal College of Nursing website.

The Social Care Institute for Excellence has a range of resources with respect to assessment available for download from their website. Of note on this website is a research review by Jo Moriarty on best practice in assessing the mental health needs of older people.

The New Zealand Guidelines Group has developed a best practice, evidence-based guideline providing recommendations for appropriate and effective processes for assessment of personal, social, functional and clinical needs in older people.

References

Bowling, A. (1997) *Research Methods in Health*. Milton Keynes: Open University Press.

Brodaty, H., Pond, D., Kemp, N., Luscombe, G., Harding, L., Berman, K. and Huppert, F.A. (2002) The GPCOG: a new screening instrument for dementia designed for General Practice. *Journal of the American Geriatrics Society*, 50: 530–4.

Department of Health (2001) *The National Service Framework for Older People*. London: Department of Health.

Department of Health (2004) HSC 2002/001; LAC (2002)1) *Guidance on the Single Assessment Process for Older People*. http://www.dh.gov.uk/en/PublicationsAndStatistics/LettersAndCirculars/HealthServiceCirculars/DH_4003995 (accessed 12 April 2008).

Fisher, A.G. (1999) *Assessment of Motor and Process Skills*, 3rd edn. Fort Collins Co: Three Star Press. http://colostate.edu/programs/AMPS (accessed 12 April 2008).

Folstein M.F., Folstein, S.E. and McHugh, P.R. (1975) 'Mini-mental state'. A practical method for grading the cognitive state of patients for the clinician. *Journal of Psychiatric Research*, 12(3): 189–98.

Gilhooly, M. (1984) The impact of caring on caregivers; factors associated with the psychological well-being of people supporting a demented relative in the community. *British Journal of Medical Psychology*, 57: 35–44.

Godfrey, M. (1988) *Older people with Mental Health Problems: A Literature Review*. University of Leeds: Nuffield Institute for Health.

Godfrey, M. and Wistow, G. (1997) The user perspective on managing for health and social care outcomes: the case of mental health. *Health and Social Care in the Community*, 5(5): 325–32.

Goldberg, D. and Williams, P. (1988) *General Health Questionnaire*. Windsor. NFER-Nelson.

Graff, M.J.L., Vernooij-Dassen, M.J.M., Thijssen, M., Dekker, J., Hoefnagels, W.H.L. and Olde Rikkert, M.G.M. (2006) Community based occupational therapy for patients with dementia and their caregivers: randomized controlled trial. *British Medical Journal*, 333: 1196.

Lawton, M.P. and Brody, E.M. (1969) Assessment of older people: self maintaining and instrumental activities of daily living. *The Gerontologist*, 9: 179–86.

Levin, E., Moriarty, J. and Gorbach, P. (1994) *Better for the Break*. London: NISW Research Unit, HMSO.

Meaney, A.M., Croke, M. and Kirby, M. (2005) Needs assessment in dementia. *International Journal of Geriatric Psychiatry*, 15: 86–9.

Mountain, G.A. (2006) Self management for people with dementia: An exploration of concepts and supporting evidence. *Dementia*, 5(3): 429–46.

Mountain, G.A. and Pighills, A. (2003) Pre-discharge home visits with older people: Time to review practice. *Health and Social Care in the Community*, 11(2): 146–54.

Mozley, C.G., Huxley, P., Sutcliffe, C., Bagley, H., Burns, A., Challis, D. and Cordingley, L. (1999) Not knowing where I am doesn't mean that I don't know what I like; cognitive impairment and quality of life responses in elderly people. *International Journal of Geriatric Psychiatry*, 14(9): 776–83.

National Institute for Health and Clinical Excellence and Social Care Institute for Excellence (2006) *Dementia: Supporting People with Dementia and their Carers in Health and Social Care.* NICE clinical guideline 42. London: NICE and SCIE.

Netten, A., Smith, P., Healey, A., Knapp, M., Ryan, M., Skatun, D. and Wykes, T. (2002) *OPUS: A Measure of Social Care Outcome for Older People.* PSSRU research summary 23. Personal Social Services Research Unit (PSSRU) University of Kent at Canterbury, Canterbury, Kent, CT2 7NF. http://www.pssru.ac.uk/pdf/rs023.pdf (accessed 12 April 2008).

Nolan, M. and Caldock, K. (1996) Assessment: identifying the barriers to good practice. *Health and Social Care in the Community*, 4(2): 77–85.

Nygård, L. and Starkhammer, S. (2007) The use of everyday technology by people with dementia living alone: mapping out the difficulties. *Aging and Mental Health*, 11(20): 144–55.

Seddon, D. and Robinson C.A. (2001) Carers of elderly people with dementia: assessment and the Carers Act. *Health and Social Care in the Community*, 9(3): 151–8.

Sheffield Institute for Studies on Ageing (SISA) (1997) *Easy-care: Elderly Assessment Instrument, UK Version.* University of Sheffield.

Smith, S.C., Lamping, D.L., Banerjee, S., Harwood, R., Foley, B.H., Smith, P., Cook, J.C., Murray, J., Prince, M., Levin, E., Mann, A. and Knapp, M. (2005) Measurement of health-related quality of life for people with dementia: development of a new instrument (DEMQOL) and an evaluation of current methodology. *Health Technology Assessment*, (9): 10.

Vernooji-Dassen, M.J., Felling, A.J., Brummelkamp, E., Dauzenberg, M.G., van den Bos, G.A. and Grol, R. (1999) Assessment of caregiver's competence in dealing with the burden of caregiving for a dementia patient: A short sense of competence questionnaire (SSCQ) suitable for clinical practice. *Journal of the American Geriatrics Society*, 47(2): 256–7.

Vernooij-Dassen, M.J. and Moniz-Cook, E. (2005) Editorial. Dementia. *International Journal of Social Research and Practice*, 4(2): 163–9.

Ware, J.E. and Sherbourne, C.D. (1992) The MOS 36-item short-form health survey (SF36). *Medical Care*, 30(6): 473–81.

Whitlatch, C.J. and Feinberg, L.F. (2005) Accuracy and consistency of responses from people with cognitive impairment. *Dementia*, 4: 171–83.

Wright, F.D. (1986) *Left to Care Alone*. Aldershot: Gower.

Xie, J., Brayne, C., Matthew, F.E. and MRC Cognitive Function and Ageing Study collaborators (2008) Survival times and people with dementia – analysis from a population based cohort study with 14 year follow up. *British Medical Journal*, 336: 258–65.

9

Supporting cognitive abilities

Jan Oyebode and Linda Clare

Learning objectives

By the end of this chapter you will:

- be aware of factors in the wider context that affect the choice of strategies for supporting cognitive functioning
- know about the major domains of cognitive functioning and how impairment in each might affect a person's day-to-day functioning
- be aware of the three major types of cognitive intervention: cognitive stimulation, cognitive training and cognitive rehabilitation, and the level of evidence for their effectiveness
- be able to plan cognitive stimulation sessions to suit people from a variety of backgrounds
- know about the steps included in developing a cognitive rehabilitation intervention
- know about the different strategies (internal and external) that can be used to enhance memory functioning

---

Introduction

Managing life with increasing cognitive impairment is at the centre of living with dementia. Damage to cognitive functions often starts with memory impairment, and progressively widens and worsens. As a consequence, over time a person with dementia will experience increasing problems in many aspects of everyday functioning, impairing independence and making social functioning difficult. Loss of memory means that self-identity is threatened. The person may have a lack of awareness and understanding of their situation and some of the internal resources they might formerly have used to enable them to cope are depleted by their dementia. Given this, it is evident that, as time goes by, those with dementia will require increasing assistance and support with aspects of life that depend on cognitive functioning.

This chapter considers how service providers can contribute to supporting the person with dementia, and those close to them, in managing this situation of increasing intellectual impairment, with the aim of reducing the degree of disability and handicap. The goal is to enable those with dementia to function to their maximum capacity, giving people more efficient and effective ways of using their remaining cognitive capacity, eroding any excess disability that has arisen through lack of opportunity or loss of confidence and enabling effective use of external environmental support.

There are a number of possible ways of intervening to address intellectual functioning. We outline here the drugs which aim to enhance cognitive functioning as well as the three main direct psychosocial approaches of cognitive rehabilitation, cognitive stimulation and cognitive training. Each of these approaches is supported at least to some extent by research evidence. Early in dementia interventions may be addressed directly with the person with dementia and their family whereas later, when it is more likely that the person is living in a residential setting, this may involve working with those staff who provide day-to-day care.

Although the subject of this chapter is supporting intellectual capacity, this does not mean we can focus solely on cognitive interventions. Any intervention needs to consider the person's awareness, ways of coping and living situation as well as their cognitive capacity, in order to achieve a positive outcome. Addressing factors such as these which are part of the wider context are essential to an effective response. This chapter does not address such interventions in depth but does situate work on cognitive functioning within a holistic framework, enabling interventions which directly target cognitive problems to be understood as part of wider person-centred and relationship-centred care.

Contextual factors which affect choice of strategies for supporting intellectual functioning

The degree of awareness, the person's coping style and the availability of social support will affect whether work to address difficulties can be carried out directly with the individual or whether it would be more effective to work with or through others. Each of these factors is briefly considered below.

Awareness

Awareness refers to the accuracy with which people judge aspects of their own situation and level of functioning, including their cognitive functioning and any associated difficulties. Where there is a specific issue that is causing concern which might become the focus of an intervention, then the professional needs to explore the person's awareness of that area in particular. People with dementia vary in the degree of awareness of their memory functioning from those who are vigilant to difficulties to those who appear unaware (Clare 2004a).

Box 9.1   Case example

A person who goes to their GP concerned about their tendency to be increasingly forgetful and who gives examples of forgetting appointments has a high level of awareness. Such a person might welcome the opportunity to develop strategies for addressing difficulties. This would contrast markedly with someone who repeatedly loses items and accuses her husband of hiding them or taking them. In this case, it may be her husband who goes to the doctor to express his concern. This situation would suggest a possible lack of awareness which would make it difficult to work directly with the person concerned.

As discussed in Chapter 4, in order to understand what it is like to live with dementia we need to consider the biological, psychological and social influences on that experience. In the same way, in order to explain the person's level of awareness we need to understand the relative contributions of biological, psychological and social factors to awareness (Clare 2004b). When a person is unaware, this may have as much to do with the social context or with their personal reactions as with cognitive impairment per se. Such an examination may provide us with suggestions for how to raise their awareness.

Box 9.2   Case example

When a person is making constant errors but is being protected from feedback by their spouse, it may be possible to discuss both the costs and benefits of providing more honest feedback with the carer. Where the person themselves seems to be using denial, it may be possible to work directly with them to address their fears and so on.

Coping

People with dementia have been described as using ways of coping that fall on a continuum from *self-maintaining* to *self-adjusting* (Clare 2002). Analysis of interviews with people with dementia found that those with a self-maintaining position aimed to find ways of continuing to live life in their usual way without necessarily absorbing the notion of having dementia into their identity, whereas those with self-adjusting ways of coping were more willing to accommodate their self-identity to having dementia. A person with a more self-adjusting style might be more willing to take part in open discussion of their difficulties whereas a person with a self-maintaining style might be more defensive, though possibly still willing to put effort into employing memory aids or trying memory strategies if this could help them maintain their usual way of life and avoid the risk of exposure of their difficulties to others.

Social context

A final contextual factor to consider is the social network of the individual. Care and intervention are provided through relationships, whether with relatives or with paid carers. The knowledge, resources and feelings of these carers need to be considered. We need to take their circumstances into account in designing interventions and pay attention to how much energy and time it is feasible for them to commit. Collaboratively designed interventions will have a better chance of success than those formulated by expert professionals alone, see Chapter 24.

If an intervention needs to rely on others then their understanding of the situation and their ways of coping will be important.

Box 9.3   Case example

A person with dementia might have memory loss which leads them to keep asking the same questions. The spouse may feel the person with dementia is asking the same thing repeatedly not because of cognitive impairment but in order to annoy them. In this situation, the carer could be given further information about the impact of memory loss that would help them to understand and have patience with their spouse. Such work would need to be undertaken before a suitable intervention to address the asking of repeated questions could be discussed.

In this section of the chapter we have outlined a number of aspects of the person's awareness, coping and social context that are important to consider when thinking about how to support cognitive functioning in someone with dementia. It is suggested that at this point you use the information from this section to consider the position of Mrs Margery Gubbins who is described in Exercise 9.1.

Exercise 9.1   Identifying the contextual influences

Mrs Margery Gubbins is a 76-year-old woman who lives at home with her husband, Roy. He has noticed that Margery has recently had difficulty with some everyday tasks. She seems to buy washing up liquid every time she goes shopping so that they now have about six unused bottles in their kitchen cupboard. He got quite cross about this but she said it would be useful if there was a shortage. More recently he even found a bottle hidden in their medicine cabinet. She seems to keep starting shopping lists but doesn't finish them or forgets to take them with her. She recently came home without her shopping and it turned out that she had forgotten to take her purse so could not pay when she got to the check-out. She said it was Roy's fault for taking it out of her handbag. Their grown-up son recently bought a new washing machine for them but Margery cannot seem to learn to use it. She says all these modern appliances have complicated instructions. He does not want his son to think he has bought something too hard for her to use and so he has not told him she is having any problems with it. He thinks his son means well. He appreciates that he has a busy job and needs his weekends to relax, though he would rather he came over and took them out from time to time rather than keep buying them things. Apart from these issues, Roy has noticed that Margery is not being as sociable as usual and seems to look for excuses not to go to the club where they would usually meet their friends. He has been trying to persuade Margery to go for a check up at the doctor's as he thinks this is a developing problem but Margery says it is only to be expected that someone her age will occasionally forget things and in any case, nothing could be done to improve her memory even if it is faulty.

Consider the above information and complete the following:

List three things that may indicate that Margery has some awareness of her memory problems.

List four ways of coping that Margery is using. Would you say these are predominantly self-maintaining or self-adjusting?

List three sources of actual or potential social support for Margery.

The nature of cognitive impairments in dementia

This section provides a brief overview of ways of understanding cognitive functioning in dementia.

Domains of cognitive functioning

Cognitive functioning can be divided into a number of domains, such as memory and attention, each of which contributes to effective cognitive functioning. The different cognitive functions vary in their importance in relation to different activities. The major domains are shown and defined in Table 9.1.

Table 9.1 Major domains of cognitive functioning and the impact of impairment on everyday life

Domain	Abilities subsumed	Everyday impact if impaired
Executive functions	Initiation of ideas and actions Switching of ideas and actions Planning and monitoring of ideas and actions	Apathy Perseveration Impulsive behaviour or actions not addressed in a logical sequence
Attention and concentration	Focusing on and sustaining attention to pertinent aspects of the environment Dividing attention as necessary between tasks	Distractibility Concentrating on one task to exclusion of another e.g. attending to doorbell and forgetting tap running in kitchen
Memory	Encoding new material Storing memories Recalling memories as necessary	No new memories formed Recent events forgotten Inability to recall events or names as needed
Language	Understanding what is said (i.e. receptive language) Being able to use words to express oneself (i.e. expressive language) Understanding written language Writing	Misunderstanding of conversations or instructions Lack of ability to express self verbally to others. 'Challenging behaviour' may occur as a form of communication Fails to understand labels, instructions, etc. Fails to fill out forms, write cards, etc

Domain	Abilities subsumed	Everyday impact if impaired
Visuo-spatial skills	Being able to identify objects Being able to recognize faces Being able to perceive orientation and positioning of objects in 3-dimensional space	Misidentifies objects e.g. unable to recognize a plate or a toilet seat Unable to find objects Lack of recognition of people Lack of recognition of things
Psycho-motor skills	Being able to manipulate objects singly or in relation to each other Being able to fit parts together to make a whole Being able to string together a series of actions	Problems with activities such as dressing, brushing teeth, using a knife and fork
Social and emotional intelligence	Understanding social cues Being able to put oneself in another's position Having empathy for others	Engages in socially unacceptable and uncharacteristic behaviour, causing offence or embarrassment to others

Of these domains, memory is usually the first function to be affected. People with dementia have difficulty developing new long-term memories. This is partly due to the difficulty they experience in encoding, or laying down, new memories (Germano and Kinsella 2005; Morris 2008; Morris and McKiernan 1994). This highlights the need to understand and support the process of encoding into memory and this is addressed below in the section on interventions.

In addition to memory, attention, executive function and word finding may also be affected. As dementia progresses, psychomotor functions become impaired and deficits in memory, attention, language and executive function become more widespread and more severe. Visuospatial perception and social cognition are usually affected only in the later stages.

Which domain to focus on when considering cognitive interventions

Interventions targeting coping with memory difficulties are likely to have particular importance in early dementia, since they are the most common early deficits and addressing them can have a major beneficial impact on the person's day-to-day life. However, other cognitive functions that are affected in early dementia such as impairment in attention and concentration may also be early targets for intervention.

As discussed in Chapter 4, key impairments differ according to the type of dementia a person has. Social cognition, for example, may be affected early in fronto-temporal dementia so may be a particular focus where this is the diagnosis.

As cognitive impairment spreads to affect a greater range of cognitive domains, new problems are likely to emerge and therefore the appropriate focus of intervention may change. In moderate dementia, the individual may have difficulty with lots of tasks and activities and may therefore withdraw and develop a layer of 'excess disability'. The focus may therefore be on providing an appropriately stimulating and enriching environment and maintaining practical skills and engagement in conversation. As dementia progresses it also becomes more likely that cognitive impairment, being more widespread and severe, will lead to behavioural difficulties, such as restless repeated attempts to leave the Home in which a person now lives to go to their former house. Finding ways to circumvent such behavioural difficulties may also then become an appropriate focus of cognitive interventions.

Identifying domains or areas of impairment can help to explain why a particular problem has arisen and can therefore also suggest possible ways of intervening.

Box 9.4　Case example

Mary is incontinent. Temporal disorientation, that is an inability to keep track of time, may mean she forgets that she needs to visit the toilet, whereas spatial disorientation may mean she cannot find her way there. Visuo-spatial impairment may cause problems her identifying the toilet and psycho-motor problems (known in this case as 'apraxia') may give her difficulty in manipulating her clothing. A timely prompt, a clearer sign on the toilet door combined with a cognitive rehabilitation programme using rehearsal (see below) and a change from trousers to a wrap-over skirt may all then help to avoid incidents of incontinence.

Interventions to support cognitive functioning

This section considers interventions that have been used to support cognitive functioning in people with dementia. The section defines some broad categories of cognitive intervention, reviews evidence for their effectiveness and looks at ways of applying them in dementia care.

Anti-dementia drugs

There are three drugs (donepezil, rivastigmine and galantamine) available at present that aim to improve or delay deterioration in cognitive functioning in dementia. They are collectively known as cholinesterase inhibitors (ChEIs) because they inhibit (i.e. delay) the breakdown of one of the brain chemicals (acetylcholine). This particular chemical is lost during Alzheimer's disease and the drug enables the small amounts that the brain does produce to work more effectively by enabling them to stay in the brain for longer. A recent Cochrane Review (Birks 2006) concluded that there was sufficient evidence to say that when used over a 6-month period the drugs produce small improvements in overall cognitive functioning (as measured by a general scale) as well as in activities of daily living and behaviour in people with mild to moderate Alzheimer's disease, with some evidence that improvements are similar in those with severe dementia.

In addition to drug treatments there are a range of psychosocial interventions which have been described as falling into three main types of cognitive training, cognitive stimulation and cognitive rehabilitation (Clare 2007; Clare and Woods 2008). See Table 9.2 where each is described alongside current research evidence for their effectiveness.

Table 9.2   Types of intervention to support cognitive functioning in people with dementia

Type	Definition	Aims
Cognitive training	Structured exercises that focus on defined cognitive functions such as memory, visuo-spatial reasoning or problem solving	To give sufficient practice to ensure that skills in particular cognitive domains are maintained or improved
Cognitive stimulation	Group activities centred on presentation and rehearsal of cognitive material in a social context.	To reduce excess disability and rebuild self-esteem
Cognitive rehabilitation	Bespoke intervention, based on knowledge of cognition and behaviour, that is applied directly in the real-life setting to address a particular difficulty	To improve quality of life and well-being through optimizing cognitive functioning in relation to everyday problems, and prevent or reduce excess disability

Cognitive training

Cognitive training typically involves practice of standardized tasks which focus on specific domains of cognition, such as memory, executive functions or attention. An appropriate domain can be selected to target areas which may be helpful for the person with dementia. The assumption is that exercising cognitive functions in the selected domain will strengthen performance either slowing deterioration or leading to a degree of improvement. The training may be offered through a number of modalities, for example using paper and pencil exercises, computerized programs or analogues of everyday tasks, and through a number of settings, for example in one-to-one interaction with carers or staff or in group settings. It may also be offered as part of a wider care programme.

Variability in the way cognitive training has been used makes its effectiveness hard to review. However, Clare (2007) provides a thorough discussion of studies evaluating individual and group cognitive training. The level of training that has been tested is fairly intense with typical studies involving 30–60-minute sessions delivered 3–7 times per week by staff or relatives. Some studies have reported significant improvements in the areas specifically targeted by the training, however, these benefits do not seem to generalize to wider aspects of daily life.

Cognitive stimulation

Cognitive stimulation has been defined as 'engagement in a range of group activities and discussions aimed at general enhancement of cognitive and social functioning'. In line with its broad aims, it has usually been evaluated in terms of its general impact on cognitive functioning using scales such as the Mini Mental State Examination (Folstein *et al.* 1975) rather than by measures in specific cognitive domains. Cognitive stimulation encompasses reality orientation, which focuses predominantly on current time and reminiscence therapy (RT) which focuses on past memories. These components will now be described in more detail.

Reality orientation (RO) operates through the presentation of information about orientation for time, person and place (Holden and Woods 1995). The assumption is that enabling someone to feel more orientated will increase well-being by providing anchors to the current environment and setting. The information is generally presented in a group setting and through various modalities, for example, participants may say the name of the day aloud, using prompting or cued recall if necessary; they may read it and write it and it may also be present on a reality orientation board in the general environment. RO has traditionally included other elements of orientation to the environment such as consideration of the weather, the season and topical associations with it, such as daffodils in spring and Christmas decorations in winter, and the news. Where orientation information can be tangibly provided, for example, through the group looking at seasonal items, members are encouraged to use all their senses to take in the information, for example, feeling, smelling and tasting an apple as well as looking at it. In the USA the early studies of RO were conducted in a classroom milieu to encourage pride in learning. In the UK they were conducted in an informal setting which included a cup of tea to encourage a relaxed atmosphere and social interaction. These differences indicate the need to adapt therapies in a culturally sensitive way that will encourage motivation and participation.

A systematic review of randomized controlled trials of RO (Spector *et al.* 2000a, 2000b) concluded from six controlled studies that there was some evidence that RO had benefits to both cognition and behaviour compared with control conditions. Since that review, additional studies have provided further evidence of significant impact of RO or cognitive stimulation on both cognitive functioning and quality of life (e.g. Orrell *et al.* 2005; Spector *et al.* 2003).

By contrast with RO, as discussed in Chapter 10, reminiscence therapy focuses on past memories. Topics might relate to particular periods of life, life events or daily activities. So, for example, discussion might take place on playground games, or rituals of courting the opposite sex. Memories are often prompted by materials such as photos, recordings or objects. An old skipping rope with wooden handles might provoke richer memories than an abstract conversation. Age Concern's Time Capsule (Age Concern 2007), which is described on their website as 'a fantastic opportunity for all generations to share their memories on a communal website' has a growing collection of personal accounts and photos covering the whole of the last century.

A systematic review of research on reminiscence (Woods *et al.* 2005) included five controlled trials, which found significant benefits on general behaviour, cognition and mood with improvement in the latter two areas being maintained at follow-up. There also appeared to be some advantages for staff who developed a better knowledge of the people with dementia with whom they were working. Where carers joined in reminiscence, they experienced a significant reduction in care-giver strain.

Overall, the research findings on cognitive stimulation suggest that sessions are worth providing in day and residential settings for those with mild to moderate dementia, possibly initially more intensively but then continuing on a weekly basis. The findings also suggest that people who are living at home might gain benefit from carers using the same approach.

Exercise 9.2   Cognitive stimulation

Outline a schedule for a cognitive stimulation session for each of the following groups:

- a group of Irish elders meeting in the spring

- a group of retired men in a rural area meeting in the summer

- a group of Afro-Caribbean women meeting in the autumn

- a group of women over 65 years of differing backgrounds meeting in the winter.

Each schedule should include:

- a symbol for group identity to suggest drawing on the RO board

- a non-cognitive warm-up exercise that will encourage group participation and be acceptable to the group members

- a reminiscence activity that will be enjoyable and relevant to the group as well as being cognitively stimulating for members, with a list of possible props to bring back memories

- an appropriate seasonal activity that will encourage multi-sensory stimulation.

Cognitive rehabilitation

Cognitive rehabilitation is the most recent type of direct cognitive intervention to be developed in work with people with dementia (Clare 2007). Although the term implies supporting recovery of function, the main focus is on optimizing remaining cognitive functioning, finding ways around difficulties, reducing their impact or helping someone to live more comfortably with their limitations. The approach aims to reduce disability by: identifying specific difficulties that have a cognitive basis; then applying strategies derived from knowledge of cognition and behaviour to address these difficulties. The focus is on understanding and intervening in relation to *specific* aspects of everyday functioning that are of importance to the person and those close to them.

Cognitive rehabilitation is not prescriptive or manualized. The basic ideas are drawn from knowledge of cognitive and behavioural psychology and are applied flexibly in individually tailored interventions appropriate to the priorities of the person and those closely involved with them. Examples of the principal techniques and their application are given below. Given that the approach is centred on the person's own unique needs and that the programme is designed especially for them, the approach fits well with the principles of person-centred dementia care.

There are a number of steps involved from setting appropriate feasible goals, through to assessment of outcome (see Table 9.3).

Table 9.3   Steps in cognitive rehabilitation (based on Clare 2007)

1   Determine whether the person is able or willing to indicate something that s/he would like to be different.

2   Identify the area to focus on – for example, memory problems, family relationships, or participation in activities.

3   Identify the specific issue to focus on – for example, remembering the names of people met during an activity.

4   Establish the baseline level of performance.

5   Identify the goal expressed in clear behavioural terms.

6   Identify the level of performance which will indicate that the goal is (a) wholly or (b) partially achieved.

7   Plan the intervention to address the goal, using appropriate methods and techniques.

8   Implement the intervention.

9   Monitor progress and adjust the intervention if necessary.

10 Evaluate the outcome of the intervention and decide on any further steps that may be needed.

The first step is to work with the person with dementia and other key individuals to decide on a meaningful, potentially achievable goal. In doing this it is important to bear in mind day-to-day difficulties that are important to the person and those close to them, the nature of their cognitive deficits and strengths, their awareness, ways of coping and their social context.

For example, goals selected by people with dementia and their families in recent work in our teams has included being able to take the correct number of tablets at the correct time, being able to work out what time of day it is without the person with dementia having to ring her son at his work, and being able to microwave meals.

Where the person has more severe dementia and cannot give consent, then it is important to consult others and to explicitly consider whether the proposed goal is in their best interest.

For example, a goal to find ways of stopping a person with dementia from shouting might make for a more peaceful environment for staff and fellow residents but might deprive the individual of their only means of gaining social contact. In this situation it would be important to have a modified goal such as 'to find a means for Mrs J to gain social contact without shouting'.

Once a clear and focused goal has been agreed, then the professional needs to decide what sort of strategies or techniques may enable this to be achieved. These may be *internal* or *external* to the person with dementia. internal strategies involve helping the person with dementia to optimize use of their cognitive resources. External strategies involve manipulation of the environment or the use of memory and cognitive aids and are used to reduce the load on cognitive resources that are already stretched.

There are a number of *internal learning strategies* that can be used to promote effective encoding and retrieval into episodic memory (Clare 2007):

- reducing the number of errors made during learning

- encouraging deep rather than superficial processing of the information to be learned

- encouraging encoding based on 'doing' rather than 'talking'

- encouraging encoding based on using several sorts of memory processes rather than one (e.g. visual, verbal and action memory; recognition and recall).

A focus on the external environment includes supporting memory and cognitive functioning through:

- the use of external memory aids and modern technologies

- the creative use of physical design

- life history books and memory wallets.

Use of external memory aids

The main functions of *external memory aids* are to prompt appropriate action, convey information that otherwise would not be remembered or trigger episodic memories that might be hard to access otherwise. Typical actions that may require prompting include taking tablets, preparing food or remembering an appointment. Typical prompts might include diaries or notebooks, signs, buzzers or phone calls. The prompt needs to be *timely*, it needs to be *specific* and it needs to be *accurate*.

For example, the buzzer which Dennis uses to remind him to take his tablets needs to occur at the moment the tablets need to be taken (timely); he needs to realize it is reminding him to take his tablets (specific) and it needs to be reset to buzz again at the correct time by his wife as it is of no use if it prompts him to take his next tablets too soon or not soon enough (accurate).

These aspects need to be carefully considered in planning use of external aids. Enlisting the help of others to ensure aids are up to date and timely make their use more efficient. Where possible, it is best to adapt aids the person already uses. For example, if a person uses a board to list their shopping requirements in their kitchen, then its use might be expanded to include key appointments.

Where new aids are introduced, a person is likely to need practice, using the internal strategies described above, to learn to use them.

For example, Clare *et al.* (2000) describe a woman with dementia who repetitively asked her husband about the date, causing friction in their relationship. An intervention was introduced using prompts to look at a calendar rather than ask her husband. This simple aid, combined with the practice in its use, led to a reduction in questioning and a reduction in tension in the relationship.

Modern technology has great potential to provide effective memory aids. Studies have looked at a range of devices that can support independent living, including the use of electronic, computer-based devices that can give specific reminders rather than conventional alarms that are non-specific (Baruch *et al.* 2004); devices to support sequences of activities (Orpwood *et al.* 2007); and those to decrease risk to safety due to forgetting, for example, cooker and tap monitors (Orpwood *et al.* 2004). This is likely to be an area that develops greatly in future.

Life history books and memory wallets

As we will see in Chapter 10, external reminders of past events can be helpful in reinforcing a sense of identity. Life story books can be constructed into which a person can paste reminders such as photos and postcards alongside diary entry-type script. These can be very useful to reinforce biographical memory. They may be particularly helpful at a point of disorientating transition such as when a person moves from home into residential care, and they serve a second purpose of enabling staff to have a feeling for the character and life of the person whose is in their care. On a less grand scale, memory wallets containing a sample of pictures and photographs of personally relevant events and people can easily be carried in a handbag or pocket and can enhance memories and interactions between a person with dementia and others (Bourgeois 1992).

Physical design

It is well accepted that buildings can be designed to allow those with physical disability to function independently. Similarly, physical aspects of buildings can be used to support cognitive functioning, helping to reduce cognitive errors and to promote independence and orientation. Features that can be taken into account range from the basic design through to the décor, furnishings and lighting. Although a detailed report on this area is outside the scope of this chapter, a good review is provided by Day *et al.* (2000).

In practice, a combination of internal strategies and external aids often works best. For example, Bird (2001) describes a woman living in a residential home who would become upset at not having her belongings and who would accuse staff of taking them. A relative and staff worked with her to establish a list of some of her favourite things indicating who she had given each to. She signed this list and it was made into a poster for the wall of her room (an external aid). An intervention was then undertaken to teach her to go and look at the poster when she became concerned about the whereabouts of her possessions (encoding based on doing rather than talking). This was done by asking her: 'What do you do when you worry about where your things have gone?' If she was unable to answer she would be given cues until she went to the poster (reducing the number of errors during learning). After regular practice this response became well established, leading to a point where the worry in itself would lead the woman to go and look at the poster in order to know where her belongings were and feel settled again.

Exercise 9.3   Designing a cognitive rehabilitation intervention

At the time of Exercise 9.1, Margery was having problems with her memory but was reluctant to openly acknowledge this or seek medical advice. Since that time, Margery has been persuaded by her husband to go the doctor's and has also had a memory clinic assessment which has established that she has dementia. She has become a little more willing to accept that she has difficulties and is pleased to hear there may be some assistance available. When you meet Margery and Roy to discuss areas that are stressful and where they might appreciate help, they say they wish she could still go shopping without making the sorts of errors noted earlier (buying the same item several times on successive trips, leaving her purse at home).

Develop a plan for steps 2–7 of a cognitive rehabilitation programme (see Table 9.3 for steps) to address this issue.

Debates and controversies

It could be said that focusing on improving and supporting cognitive functioning in people with dementia is putting effort into the wrong place. Progressive cognitive impairment is, after all, an inevitable consequence of having dementia. Trying to hold it back could be likened to King Canute trying to hold back the tide, which is why the gains in cognitive functioning achieved as a result of cognitive training are pretty modest. What is more, interventions that concentrate on cognitive functioning may be seen as forcing the person to face their deficits, putting them into embarrassing or shameful positions that expose their vulnerability. It might be seen as more comfortable and more constructive to put our resources into supporting emotional functioning and adaptation so as to ensure that those who have to suffer this condition can at least do so in a state of relative well-being.

We would argue, on the other hand, that working to find ways of enabling people with dementia to manage with the cognitive impairments that are core to the condition, can make a significant contribution to day-to-day functioning and hence self-esteem and well-being. Small gains in cognitive functioning, as illustrated by some of the examples above, may make a great difference to people's lives as long as the effort is carefully targeted towards personally tailored, meaningful goals. The mode of negotiation and delivery of cognitive interventions is crucial to their impact. An insensitive attempt to introduce cognitive interventions could increase distress and defensiveness. No-one wants to see people with dementia brutally corrected whenever they voice their confusion. However, a sensitive approach can be empowering and helpful and give an individual with dementia a sense of control and dignity. We hope this chapter has convinced you that individually designed, focused cognitive interventions have a key place in excellent dementia care.

Conclusion

This chapter has considered ways of supporting intellectual functioning in people with dementia. Drawing on research and practice we have attempted to demonstrate the place of cognitive training, cognitive stimulation and cognitive rehabilitation within holistic person-centred care for people with dementia.

There are four main types of intervention that directly address cognitive functioning in dementia. These are drug therapy, cognitive stimulation, cognitive training and cognitive rehabilitation. Cognitive stimulation involves engagement in a range of group activities and discussions aimed at generally enhancing cognitive and social functioning. Cognitive training involves systematic practice of standardized tasks designed to focus on particular domains of cognition. Cognitive rehabilitation comprises the personally tailored application of strategies derived from knowledge of cognition and behaviour to address specific difficulties. Strategies may be internal to the person and/or include external memory aids.

There is a growing body of evidence suggesting that all these approaches have a positive impact in enabling people with dementia to enhance their cognitive impairment and to minimize its consequences. Possibilities for cognitive interventions are influenced by a person's awareness, ways of coping and social supports. A holistic assessment is therefore needed to inform any intervention. People with dementia commonly have difficulty in encoding new long-term memories and memory may therefore be a particular focus of cognitive intervention in people with early dementia. People, however, vary in their cognitive strengths and weaknesses and a comprehensive assessment of cognitive functioning will help to identify preserved abilities to build on and impaired functions to address or circumvent. Later in the course of dementia, cognitive interventions may address wider domains of cognitive functioning.

Further information

Age Concern has a time capsule website which provides material on reminiscence and experience of past generations.

The Tangled Neuron is a website run by the daughter of Morris Friedell, a professor of sociology who wrote about his attempts at cognitive rehabilitation for his own dementia. His daughter states: 'This personal site chronicles my search for answers on my father's dementia. Although it's too late to help Dad, I hope any information I can find helps others.' The site includes discussion about cognitive rehabilitation.

Dementia Service Development Centre for Wales website includes information on current pertinent research on reminiscence, cognitive stimulation and cognitive rehabilitation.

References

Age Concern (2007) *The Time Capsule*. http://www.eurolinkage.org/AgeConcern/timecapsule.asp (accessed 31 January 2008).

Baruch, J., Downs, M., Baldwin, C. and Bruce, E. (2004) A case study in the use of technology to reassure and support a person with dementia. *Dementia,* 3: 372–7.

Bird, M. (2001) Behavioural difficulties and cued recall of adaptive behaviour in dementia: experimental and clinical evidence. *Neuropsychological Rehabilitation,* 11: 357–75.

Birks, J. (2006) Cholinesterase inhibitors for Alzheimer's disease. *Cochrane Database of Systematic Reviews.* Issue 1. http://www.mrw.interscience.wiley.com/cochrane/clsysrev/articles/CD005593 (accessed 9 August 2007).

Bourgeois, M. (1992) Evaluating memory wallets in conversations with persons with dementia. *Journal of Speech and Hearing Research,* 35: 1344–57.

Clare, L. (2002) We'll fight it as long as we can: coping with the onset of Alzheimer's disease. *Aging and Mental Health,* 6: 139–48.

Clare, L. (2004a) Awareness in early-stage Alzheimer's disease: a review of methods and evidence. *British Journal of Clinical Psychology,* 43: 177–96.

Clare, L. (2004b) The construction of awareness in early-stage Alzheimer's disease: a review of concepts and models. *British Journal of Clinical Psychology,* 43: 155–75.

Clare, L. (2007) *Neuropsychological Rehabilitation and People with Dementia.* Hove: Psychology Press.

Clare, L., Wilson, B.A., Carter, G., Breen, K., Gosses, A. and Hodges, J.R. (2000) Intervening with everyday memory problems in dementia of Alzheimer type: an errorless learning approach. *Journal of Clinical and Experimental Neuropsychology,* 22: 132–46.

Clare, L., Woods, B., Moniz-Cook, E.D., Spector, A. and Orrell, M. (2003) *Cognitive Rehabilitation and Cognitive Training for Early-stage Alzheimer's Disease and Vascular Dementia* (Cochrane Review). In *The Cochrane Library,* Issue 4, (2003) Chichester: John Wiley and Sons.

Day, K., Carreon D. and Stump, C. (2000) The therapeutic design of environments for people with dementia: a review of the empirical research. *The Gerontologist,* 40: 417–21.

Folstein, M., Folstein, S. and McHugh, P. (1975) Mini-mental state: a practical method for grading the cognitive state of patients for the clinician. *Journal of Psychiatric Research,* 12: 189–98.

Germano, C. and Kinsella G. (2005) Working memory and learning in early Alzheimer's disease. *Neuropsychology Review,* 15: 1–10.

Holden, U. and Woods, R.T. (1995) *Positive Approaches in Dementia Care* 3rd ed. Edinburgh: Churchill Livingstone.

Morris, R.G. (2008) The neuropsychology of dementia: Alzheimer's disease and other neurodegenerative disorders. In: R.T. Woods and L. Clare (eds) *Handbook of the Clinical Psychology of Ageing,* 2nd ed. Chichester: John Wiley and Sons, pp. 161–84.

Morris, R.G. and McKiernan, F. (1994) Neuropsychological investigations of dementia. In: A. Burns and R. Levy (eds) *Dementia.* London: Chapman and Hall.

Orpwood, R., Bjørneby, S., Hagen, I., Mäki, O, Faulkner, R. and Topo, P. (2004) User involvement in dementia product development. *Dementia,* 3: 263–79.

Orpwood, R., Sixsmith, A., Torrington, J., Chadd, J., Gibson, G. and Chalfont, G. (2007) Designing technology to support quality of life in people with dementia. *Technology and Disability,* 19: 103–12.

Orrell, M., Spector. A., Thorgrimsen., L. and Woods B. (2005) A pilot study examining the effectiveness of maintenance cognitive stimulation therapy (MCST) for people with dementia. *International Journal of Geriatric Psychiatry,* 20: 446–51.

Spector, A., Davies, S., Woods, B. and Orrell, M. (2000b) Reality orientation for dementia: a systematic review of the evidence of effectiveness from randomized controlled trials. *The Gerontologist,* 15: 404–7.

Spector, A., Orrell, M., Davies, S. and Woods, B. (2000a) Reality orientation for dementia. *Cochrane Database of Systematic Review,* (4): CD00(1119).

Spector, A., Thorgrimsen, L., Woods, B., Royan, L., Davies, S., Butterworth, M. and Orrell, M. (2003) Efficacy of an evidence-based cognitive stimulation therapy programme for people with dementia: randomised controlled trial. *British Journal of Psychiatry,* 183: 248–54.

Woods, B., Spector, A., Jones, C., Orrell, M. and Davies, S. (2005) Reminiscence therapy for dementia. *Cochrane Database of Systematic Reviews,* 18 (2): CD00(1120).

10

Working with life history

Errollyn Bruce and Pam Schweitzer

Learning objectives

By the end of this chapter you will:

- understand the key role of life history in providing person-centred care
- be familiar with ways to work with life history in dementia care
- understand the essentials of good practice in life history work

---

Introduction

Understanding a person's life history is necessary for person-centred care. We need to know where people have come from and what they have lived through in order to understand who they are now. Past experiences, especially if emotionally significant, influence how people perceive events in the present, and how they respond to them (Bell and Troxel 2001; Cheston and Bender 2000; Kitwood 1997). Knowledge of life history can provide caregivers with valuable clues about the meaning of words and actions that might at first sight appear meaningless or baffling.

In Chapter 4 Sabat explains what a biopsychosocial approach brings to our understanding of dementia. A key point is that the signs and symptoms of dementia are behavioural, but neurological impairment is not the only factor causing the behaviour we see. In his theory of dementia, Kitwood (1993) suggested that five factors influence behaviour, illustrating this with the equation:

$$SD = P + B + H + NI + SP$$

where SD = clinical presentation of dementia; P = personality; B = biography; H = health; NI = neurological impairment; and SP = social psychology.

From the equation we can see that biography (by which Kitwood meant life history) is identified as one the factors that interact to produce the clinical presentation of dementia in each individual. Kitwood (1997) stressed that we need knowledge and understanding of people's life histories to understand their experiences of dementia, their needs and their behaviour. Bell and Troxel (2001) have argued that life history is as important to holistic care as medical history is to medical care. They point out that both recent experiences and those from long past can be significant. While the effects of distressing parts of a person's life history can be very striking, it is clear that positive memories of the past can also shape the way that people experience the present.

The significance of life history is underlined if we see emotional care as a central element in dementia care, as it is widely recognized that an understanding of life history is important when working with emotional distress (Cheston and Bender 2000). Dementia is a very frightening condition, sometimes described as ongoing trauma (Miesen 2004). It puts people into an altered world (Perrin and May 2000), and the strangeness of the experience tends to activate the alarm system (Cheston and Bender 2000; Miesen 1992). The typical losses of late life mean that many people are coping with their dementia while destabilized by a series of unwelcome life changes (Kitwood 1997).

Profound insecurity, anxiety, depression and above all, loss, are features of the emotional experience of dementia (Cheston and Bender 2000; see Chapter 21). Loss of identity is a significant hazard. Loss of autobiographical memory weakens the narratives that contribute to identity (Cheston and Bender 2000), and appears to leave some people with dementia with a vague and shadowy sense of self (Bruce *et al.* 2002). Emotional care is needed to enable people to achieve tolerable levels of security, stability and confidence. This can be delivered in a more sensitive, appropriate and personalized way when the carer has, and reveals, a knowledge of the person's past.

Exercise 10.1   What would your carers need to know?

If you were to develop dementia and find yourself living in a care home, what do you think your carers would need to know about your life history in order to help them to:

- see you as a unique individual?

- support your identity?

- understand your feelings?

- provide a supportive social environment?

Terms and meanings

You will find a variety of terms used in this field, each with many definitions. Table 10.1 provides definitions of some of these terms.

Table 10.1   Definitions of terms

Term	Meaning
Life history	All that has happened in a person's life – their background, events in their life and how they felt about it all. We can gain a picture of this from records and stories told about a person's life, their social context and the times they lived through – as told by them and by others.

Term	Meaning
Biography	Usually refers to an account of a person's life compiled by another person, in contrast to autobiography where a person tells his or her own story. However, it is sometimes used to mean much the same as life history (e.g. in Kitwood's equation).
Life story	The story of a person's life, which like all stories, varies according to who is telling the story and the context in which it is told.
Reminiscence	The act or process of recalling the past (Butler 1963) – but there are a wide variety of definitions (Gibson 2004).
Reminiscence work	Making deliberate attempts to trigger memories of the past and use them as a vehicle for communication in the present. Reminiscence work provides opportunities for people to communicate about their memories in their own way, and is therefore important when using life history in dementia care.
Life review	Evaluating and coming to terms with the life one has lived. Some people engage in life review spontaneously, but more often life review refers to a planned one-to-one structured intervention (Haight and Haight 2007) leading to a personal history record. The worker needs counselling skills and the ability to act as a therapeutic listener (Gibson 2004).
Oral history	Collecting personal accounts of past experiences. The oral historian usually makes a selection of the most suitable material to include in a record or archive.
Autobiographical memory	Memory for one's own life story.
Narratives	The stories we construct to make sense of our experience.

The value of working with life history in dementia care

The evidence base

Life story work includes many different interventions with a variety of aims and objectives. Life story interventions are complex, and at their best when tailored to individual needs. This presents a challenge for research methods designed to investigate standard treatments that are expected to affect everyone in much the same way. Diversity in aims and approaches is reflected in diverse research methods (Moos and Bjorn 2006). Discussing life story work undertaken with a view to having an impact on care, McKeown *et al.* (2005) conclude that it has potential benefits, but high quality research is scarce. Discussing reminiscence, Woods (2002) suggests the need to use different outcome measures depending upon the aims and type of work done. He points out that we should not expect reminiscence to result in cognitive and behavioural improvement – more realistic aims might be to stimulate communication, foster identity, enhance mood and well-being, promote individualized care and improve autobiographical memory. Moos and Bjorn (2006) note a trend towards more rigorous quantitative studies but suggest that this is premature, since we still have a great deal to learn about how best to use life stories in the delivery of sensitive, individualized and effective support and care to people with dementia. Evidence from practice and qualitative studies suggests that working with life history can be very valuable to care workers, family members and people with dementia themselves (Bender *et al.* 1999).

The functions of reminiscence

Reminiscence was once thought to be an unhealthy preoccupation with the past, but over the past forty years there has been growing recognition that the natural habit of looking back and talking about the past can be positive and constructive. It is done by people of all ages, but can have various important functions for people as they grow older (Gibson 2004). Various authors have discussed the functions of reminiscence (Bender *et al.* 1999; Coleman 2004; Gibson 2004; Webster 2002) which can vary at different times and for different people. It has been suggested that reminiscence can be of value to people with dementia when it helps them to

- maintain a sense of coherence and continuity

- retain autobiographical memory

- retain a strong and positive sense of self

- re-experience the 'feel' of happier times in life

- communicate with others

- be sociable and build relationships

- engage in intimacy

- remember how past adversities were dealt with and use this experience with present difficulties

- engage in life review and preparation for death

- pass on family history and cultural heritage

- participate in enjoyable, stimulating and creative activities

- remember, share and use retained skills

- find an outlet for creativity.

Research on reminiscence has tended to focus on outcomes for clients but we also need to look at the impact of reminiscence on carers to fully appreciate its value (Gibson 2004). In a study by Pietrukowicz and Johnson (1991), care workers reported warmer feelings and better understanding of the people with dementia they cared for when they had knowledge of life histories. Warmth and understanding are clearly important for good relationships (Bender *et al.* 1999).

Family carers may also find that re-visiting the past improves their current relationship with the person they care for. For example, they may find that recalling happier times can help them to set current difficulties into the context of the relationship as a whole, and give meaning to their caring role (Schweitzer and Bruce 2008). Knowledge of life stories, whether gained from reminiscence work or elsewhere, has the potential to alter how people are perceived and understood by their carers, and thereby to influence relationships.

Ways in which life history is valuable in person-centred practice

Understanding the meaning behind what people say

Allan and Killick (see Chapter 12) discuss the impact of dementia on communication. Some of the changes that undermine easy communication are:

- cognitive changes, meaning that people with dementia perceive and understand the world differently

- difficulties with speech and language

- the tendency to avoid distressing topics, or speak about them indirectly or metaphorically.

To keep communication going, carers need to believe that there is meaning in what people with dementia say, and be prepared to make efforts to find meaning. Life history can often provide clues to meaning in metaphor, stories and speech that seems confused or irrelevant to the present (Barnet 2000; Cheston *et al.* 2004; Killick and Allan 2001).

Box 10.1   Case example

John started his working life in the Merchant Navy. As a member of a reminiscence group for people with dementia, he repeatedly talked about his experiences as a young sailor on trips to the West Indies. Life at sea was hard and dangerous, and more so if you joined a ship with a hostile crew. When this happened, he had to decide whether the captain was strong enough to protect him from these dangerous men. If he decided that he could not trust the captain, on reaching port he would jump ship and join another ship for the journey home. When he was in the reminiscence group, John had just started to attend a day centre and had not taken to it well. It seemed possible that it reminded him of his experiences in the merchant navy, and that he was trying to decide whether 'the crew' were dangerous and the 'captain' strong enough to protect him. This interpretation raised questions for workers supporting John and his wife – who desperately needed respite but did not want John to be unhappy. For example, would it be possible to reassure John that 'the crew' were not dangerous and that the 'captain' was strong and could be trusted to protect him? Or were there problems at the day centre (e.g. poorly managed conflicts between users,

> divided staff, weak management) meaning that John's feelings were grounded in reality, and it might be wise for him to 'jump ship'?
>
> (Rik Cheston, personal communication)

Understanding the messages in behaviour

Cohen-Mansfield (see Chapter 11) points out that behaviour can be seen as a form of communication. Understanding the language of behaviour requires us to work out the message or need conveyed by a person's actions. To do this we need an empathic understanding of the person's present experience, something that is often only possible if we have some knowledge about their past.

Box 10.2 Case example

Staff at Ivy Lodge were perplexed by Ida's behaviour. Every morning she would carry everything that she could move from her room down the corridor, and stack it in a quiet alcove that had been set up nicely for residents to sit in. She would become angry if anyone tried to prevent her from doing this, though she was happy to join other residents for tea breaks and lunch. Every afternoon she would move all the items back into her room. Some staff found her activities irritating, and suggested that there might be safety issues. Ida's daughter was contacted, and immediately explained her mother's behaviour in terms of her lifelong routines as a market trader. For nearly sixty years she had set up a stall each morning and packed it down in the afternoon. When staff understood what Ida was doing, they felt better about it.

The links between past and current experience are not always obvious, and it can sometimes take a considerable amount of detective work to find a plausible explanation. As the story of John illustrates, the links can be at an emotional level.

Providing individualized care

There is a risk that those receiving care feel like cogs in a large machine they do not control. In communal settings in particular, personal preferences are constrained by the needs of others, and for a number of reasons it tends to feel like public, rather than private, space. The impersonal feel can be reduced by small things that show that individuals are known, understood and valued.

Life history can often provide ideas about important details that can be used to make care personal rather than impersonal. In this context, recent life history may be as relevant as the deep past. For example, changes in routine have been identified as life events that have a clear impact on people with dementia (Orrell and Bebbington 1995). Allowing people to stick to habitual routines (e.g. getting up time, a sherry before lunch) is a relatively simple way to provide individualized care. In the example of Ida, understanding her old habits enabled staff to accept her need to continue with her activity, and also gave them ideas about ways to modify it to make it less exhausting for her, and safer.

Reinforcing a person's identity

Oyebode and Clare (see Chapter 9) remind us that memories of the past contribute to identity in the present. When dementia undermines autobiographical memory and disrupts the narratives that are important to identity, reminders of life history can be helpful. As Sabat (see Chapter 4) points out, recall is more severely impaired in people with dementia than recognition. People often retain the ability to recognize their own story when they can only recall fragments, or have difficulty communicating what they remember. If stories are collected and recorded well, carers can tell people their own stories (Naess 1998), which may help them maintain a stronger sense of self as dementia becomes more severe. However, Kitwood (1998: 106) stresses the 'great moral responsibility' of telling someone's story for them. Whereas it can be affirming and comforting to hear one's story told by someone who has understood it well, it can be confusing, irritating or insulting if misunderstood or told incorrectly. It is therefore very important to 'check back' with the person during the telling of their experience; this also helps the person to retain a sense of ownership of their story.

Tangible reminders of past times can be valuable in reinforcing identity. They include carefully chosen photographs, objects, work tools, souvenirs, school reports, prizes, everyday objects, songs (sung live or recorded by favourite stars of the past), local newspaper items from the past, and even familiar packaging from a previous era. Items like these can be used to make reminiscence products, such as life story books, collages, display boards, memory boxes, memory wallets and the life books made in structured life review (Haight and Haight 2007). These products need to be attractive and recognizable records capturing important elements in people's lives.

Reminiscence products can be a stimulus for communication and further reminiscence. They can be particularly helpful when identity is threatened by disorientating changes, such as hospitalization, bereavement or when moving into long-term care. By providing a reminder of the story so far, they can help people construct narratives which put difficult changes in context. They also provide staff with useful information and a valuable starting-point for conversation, enabling them to support the person's identity in a new environment.

Box 10.3 Case example

Noel made a memory box helped by an artist. Over a series of one-to-one sessions with the artist, Noel told stories, drew his memories and, with help from his wife, found photos and small objects relating to different aspects of his life in the Caribbean and in London. The artist worked with Noel to make a 3-D collage that featured his Caribbean background, his marriage to his wife in England and his love of camper van holidays with his wife in England with their sense of freedom and the open road.

Their wedding anniversary coincided with a reminiscence session, and they brought the memory box which led to a lively half hour of questions,

---

answers and story-telling which was pleasurable for all and extremely gratifying for them both. What began as a one-to-one reminiscence process became a product to be proud of, and this was a valuable stimulus for communication and further reminiscence.

Taking time to do reminiscence work with people with dementia can convey powerful messages to support a positive identity. Examples of these messages are 'We value you as person', 'We are interested in you as an individual', 'We respect you and your experience' (Woods 1998: 143–4). Tangible products of reminiscence can help to re-iterate these messages over a longer period of time.

Facilitating interaction

For many people, the loss of enjoyable conversation is a consequence of the biological and psychosocial changes associated with dementia. They may be psychologically isolated though surrounded by others. Knowing about people's lives makes it easier to communicate with them, and to find suitable memory triggers (e.g. pictures, objects, music) to stimulate interaction, whether based on verbal or non-verbal exchange. As well as being a convenient stimulus for interaction for staff and visitors, having objects that trigger memories to handle in the care environment can encourage conversation between users. The tangible reminders mentioned above can be particularly helpful in stimulating interaction, especially if they provide an attractive and accessible record of life stories (e.g. Bourgeois 1992). Computer-based systems using reminiscence to enhance communication are an interesting innovation (e.g. Alm *et al.* 2007).

Facilitating relationships between people with dementia

Shared experience is the basis of friendship. The experience of needing care is one that few people welcome, and is often not, on its own, a good basis for friendship among users of care services. Knowledge of life histories can help us to identify common ground between clients, and use this to foster relationships (Schweitzer and Bruce 2008). Bell and Troxel (2001) suggest introducing clients to each other repeatedly (saying, for example, 'Bill, this is Fred, he was a truck driver too, you know') while Bender *et al.* (1999) stress the value of reminiscence groups both for discovering common ground and for kindling interest in differences. Good use of life histories can help transform the experience of receiving care from feeling disconnected and misplaced among strangers, to finding some comfort from a sense of belonging and making meaningful connections with others.

Box 10.4 Case example

Lisbeth Prendegast, retired headmistress of a private school, and Maura O'Riley, a retired shop worker, both developed dementia in old age and were living in the same care home. They didn't get on. However, in a reminiscence session it emerged that they both had memories of church and family gatherings on Sundays in childhood, and shared the view that Sunday should be treated as a special day. This area of agreement helped to soften

> their feelings of animosity and staff were able to remind them of their shared opinions when they rubbed each other up the wrong way.

Providing ideas for occupation, engagement and activity

A person's life story can provide clues about the kind of occupation or activity that might suit them. Information has to be used thoughtfully, and ideas tested to see if they are appropriate. Tastes can change, and past passions may lose their appeal, but there can be some surprising threads of continuity. The skill often lies in seeing a way to evoke the 'feel' of an activity enjoyed in the past, without engendering any anxiety about performance.

Box 10.5 Case example

Betty was once a skilled dressmaker but no longer enjoyed sewing. It frustrated her, and was a distressing reminder of the skills she had lost. However, she still loved to handle fabrics, and enjoyed folding laundry. When given a basket of fabric samples, she enjoyed sorting through them and deciding what each could be used for. She enjoyed hearing and saying the names of the different fabrics and what they were used for.

Well-run reminiscence activities appeal to many people. For example, Brooker and Duce (2000) observed higher levels of well-being during a group reminiscence activity than during other group activities.

Exercise 10.2. Making use of what we know

Return to each of the vignettes in this section, and for each person with dementia:

● Consider how carers could make best use of life history information given in order to provide person-centred care.

● Comment on what more they might need to find out about the person's life to develop their work further.

Good practice when working with life history in dementia care

When doing life history work with people who have dementia, good practice is achieved by bringing together person-centred principles and the principles that underpin creative, communication-centred approaches to reminiscence. Whether we are gathering and recording information about life histories, running reminiscence sessions or responding to spontaneous reminiscence, it is important to value people and their stories, be sensitive to their emotional needs and careful to avoid malignant social psychology (Brooker 2007). This is not always easy, for example, it is very tempting to exchange looks that say 'there she goes again' when stories are repeated many times. However, it would be much more helpful to try to understand why a particular story is repeated, and to find out whether there is a connection – possibly at an emotional level – with the story told and a person's experiences in the present.

Ethical issues

Kenyon (1996) argues that frail elderly people have a right to have their stories known and understood, as this is often necessary for informed intervention. He argues that ignoring life history presents greater risks than working with it, though he points out that there is potential for harm and distress if life stories are not treated with respect. He stresses the need to see negotiated consent as an ongoing process, and to take steps to minimize negative consequences.

In the context of reminiscence work, Gibson (2004) talks in terms of contracting, that is, explaining what we are doing at each stage, and always offering people the chance to opt out. She points out that a heavy-handed approach to confidentiality may defeat the essential purpose of reminiscence – sharing, celebrating and communicating. Nevertheless, all involved with life history work need to take confidentiality seriously, and check out what can be recorded and made public, and what people would prefer to keep private.

Strong emotions may emerge during life history work, but in general this is unlikely to be harmful. Our lives include both happiness and distress, and many people prefer to remember both. Gibson (2004) stresses that workers must be able to accept and work with tears and anger, as well as smiles and laughter, and be prepared to refer appropriately in the unlikely event that recalling a traumatic memory leads to lasting disturbance.

Attitudes and skills

The attitudes and skills needed for reminiscence work are listed in Table 10.2. These are applicable to other ways of working with life history in dementia care. They are not tied to a particular background or training (Gibson 1998). They are closely related to the principles of person-centred care as described by Brooker (2007) – valuing people regardless of cognitive ability, approaching them as unique individuals, understanding the world from their perspective and creating a social environment that supports their psychological needs.

Table 10.2 Attitudes and skills for reminiscence work in dementia care

- Respecting and valuing people as unique individuals
- Genuine interest in the past and in people's life stories
- Willingness to listen to both painful and happy memories
- Not being frightened by strong emotions
- Giving good attention with active listening and a sense of being genuinely available to people
- Empathizing – sharing another's world without losing hold of your own
- Relating sensitively – not being a bull in a china shop or over-interpreting

- Being able to reflect critically on your own work

(Based on Gibson 1998: 18)

While there are undoubtedly some counselling skills and communication techniques that are helpful when doing reminiscence work with people who have dementia, skills and techniques are not everything. Believing that meaningful communication with people with dementia is possible, and having both the desire to communicate and the patience to keep trying are possibly the most important qualifications for reminiscence work (Gibson 1998).

Good practice in reminiscence work

There are different approaches to reminiscence work. Oyebode and Clare (see Chapter 9) characterize 'reminiscence therapy' as cognitive stimulation, and this may be appropriate in the case of 'recall and tell' approaches to reminiscence that are predominantly reliant on verbal communication, and delivered without particular attention to person-centred practice. However, the creative, communication-based approach, better suited to meet the needs of people with dementia (Schweitzer and Bruce 2008) shares many of the characteristics of cognitive rehabilitation.

The principles of good practice we set out here assume a creative communication-based approach to reminiscence interwoven with a person-centred approach to dementia. They apply whether reminiscence work is planned (e.g. as an activity; as part of gathering information about life history) or arises from a response to spontaneous reminiscence, but they need to be applied appropriately according to context and the needs of particular individuals.

Table 10.3   Good practice in reminiscence work

- Establishing rapport – e.g. making people feel that you are pleased to see them, and are happy to spend time in their company

- Being attentive to basic needs – e.g. check that people are comfortable and able to hear and see; reassure people if they are agitated or anxious, and do not expect them to concentrate on reminiscence if they are preoccupied by worries or distress

- Showing interest – e. g. being attentive, showing no signs of boredom or needing to be elsewhere

- Sensitivity – e.g. being receptive to the feelings people express, responding supportively; respecting people's interests and preferences

- Being non-judgmental – e.g. showing that you respect people's views and experiences, even if you disagree or feel shocked by what they are telling you

- Using cooperative conversational strategies – e.g. making sure that people with dementia take their turns in the conversation, leaving long pauses for them to come in; checking out your understanding by saying something like 'Have I got this right – you were saying that ....?'

- Having the ability to create an easy atmosphere – e.g. sharing the funny side of things, showing delight in what people are able to remember, appreciating the efforts they are making to participate

- Respecting the right to tell the story as they choose – e.g. recognizing that there may be an emotional truth in a story, even though 'the facts' are not accurate; avoiding showing people up by correcting mistakes or indicating that you don't believe what they are saying

- Approaching reminiscence with enthusiasm – e.g. modelling the activities by briefly relating an experience of your own, but not taking too much time over this

- Being prepared to let your hair down, thus licensing others to do the same (Schweitzer and Bruce 2008)

- Being person-centred – e.g. avoiding personal detractions, and making use of personal enhancers (Brooker 2007).

Good practice in creative communication-based reminiscence work requires us to be alert to ways to support each person, and careful to avoid anything that might undermine them. For example, we need to find ways round the fear of failure, and to play to the strengths of the people with whom we are working. If questioning seems to make a person's mind go blank, we need to avoid direct questions. If verbal communication has become difficult, we need to support it (for example, by allowing time for people to collect and express their thoughts) and explore other, non-verbal channels of communication (for example, asking people to show us, rather than tell us, how things were). We need to give people the best chance of receiving an idea and responding to it by stimulating all the senses (sight, hearing, touch, taste, smell and the body's sense of its own movements).

Group activities

When doing reminiscence work with a group, leaders need group skills. All members of the group need to feel secure and that their contributions are valued. Everyone needs to be given the opportunity to present something to the whole group, but no-one should feel under pressure to do so if they do not want to. People can gain a great deal by watching and listening to others' contributions and their incapacity or reluctance to join in should not be seen as a failure or met with disappointment. Group leaders need to build a sense of belonging, for example, by pointing out common ground and connections between people in the group. Leaders can 'amplify' people's contributions by repeating their story to the whole group, showing their appreciation of each individual and making connections with stories told by others in the group.

There need to be plenty of people available to listen to people with dementia, one-to-one wherever possible, because they often need to speak immediately to avoid forgetting what they want to say. If you are working alone, it is generally better to work with groups of three or four people (Heathcote 2007). In larger groups, it is a good idea to have a balance between small and large group activities, and there needs to be a leader or volunteer to work with each of the small groups (Schweitzer and Bruce 2008). Planning needs to take account of things such as deafness, and how long participants are able to concentrate when other people are speaking. There can be a great deal of humour and fun in reminiscence groups, but leaders should also be able to handle serious stories, and any feelings of anger or distress that arise from them (Bruce *et al.* 1999; Gibson 1998).

Spontaneous reminiscence and conversation

Recalling and talking about the past without being prompted by a question or a planned reminiscence activity is known as spontaneous reminiscence. Most carers are familiar with spontaneous reminiscence because many people with dementia enjoy talking about the past, describing how things used to be long ago or commenting on differences between then and now. Some have a story, or stories, which they tell repeatedly. Others may talk as though they are living in the past, for example, saying that they need to go out to fetch the children – who are now adults – from school.

Spontaneous reminiscence provides a springboard for conversation and understanding a person in the present, and best practice involves making the most of these opportunities. However, there are a number of reasons why family and paid carers do not encourage spontaneous reminiscence and the challenge for best practice is finding ways around these barriers.

Family carers often feel that chatting about the past is irrelevant when what they are missing and needing is talk about the present. However, some family members discover the power of the past to keep conversation going in the present, and are able to 'hold' a person's memories for them. In Box 10.6, an interview with the son of a man with dementia illustrates this phenomenon of 'holding' a person's memories.

Box 10.6   Case example

So I could get him to talk about these things from years and years and years ago and I can remember these things too ... And he liked that, so we always therefore managed to have quite a healthy little conversation going ... we had to talk about things he knew ... his old work colleagues and some of those fund of stories which came out of all that ... it's like pressing buttons ... immediately he'd be smiling and laughing and he'd remember ... And after a while he'd forget what the stories were but I could tell him them and then he'd remember ...

Not all family carers find this easy to do. For example, in Box 10.6, the wife of the man with dementia felt much less able to use the past as a way to connect with her husband than her son did. Deeply upset by her husband's decline, and resentful that he would chat to others, but not to her, she was unable to settle for conversation that did not meet her needs. The communication gap between them was widened by her stress, her deafness and her tendency to scold when he made mistakes. Family carers who are feeling overwhelmed by dementia and finding it hard to adjust their expectations need a lot of support and understanding. Given this, they may then be able to appreciate the importance of the past for those they are caring for, and change a little. Joint reminiscence sessions (Bruce *et al.* 1999) or other interventions that work with people with dementia and carers together may be helpful here.

Finding repeated stories boring, and feeling that 'living in the past' puts a person beyond their reach can be barriers for both family carers and paid staff. They may feel better about these things if they understand that listening to them and responding positively may be helping a person cope with very difficult present-day experiences. Remembering your own life story can be an important way to maintain identity, and repetition is a good way to remember. Believing that your mother is not far away is a reassuring thought when in a strange and threatening situation (Bruce 1999). These are examples of taking the perspective of a person with dementia – an important principle in both person-centred practice and reminiscence work.

For care workers, the culture of care can be a barrier. Findings from studies in long-term care settings suggest that people with dementia have very little conversation with care workers. Conversations tend to be brief and superficial; there is surprisingly little interaction during personal care (Cohen-Mansfield *et al.* 2007; Hallberg *et al.* 1990; Ward *et al.* 2005). However, in settings where communication and relationships are seen as a priority, there is evidence suggesting that staff can act very differently. There are reports of staff responding warmly to what people say, and using their knowledge of their clients' lives to facilitate further conversation (Bell and Troxel 2001; Vittoria 1998).

Ongoing support as well as education and training may be needed by both family and paid carers to facilitate best practice in this area. Carers need to know how to make the most of spontaneous reminiscence as an opportunity for conversation and communication, but to act on this knowledge they need to be in a supportive context.

Exercise 10.3 Learning from experience

After a smooth-running morning in the dementia unit, two care workers decided that there was time for an activity. They brought a box of reminiscence objects into the lounge and quickly helped a few people to move their chairs to make a group of nine people. Despite the moves, the chairs were not well placed and some people could not see or hear each other very well. The activity was run like a quiz game – residents who named an object correctly were praised. Those who didn't were asked to pass it on. Hilda held a pack of penny blue for quite a while, looking at it intently. She was asked to pass it on to the next person, and when she eventually spoke, no-one was listening. Lizzie was given the thimble and said quietly, 'A silver thimble. Mother had one. She made all our dresses – we had lovely clothes.' A worker said 'That's a lovely memory, Lizzie', and repeated what she had said so everyone could hear. Several other people chipped in with memories triggered by Lizzie's story. Sally began to cry when she was holding the darning mushroom. A worker said 'Are you crying about your brother?' and she nodded, continuing to cry. She was given no further attention. When she smelt the carbolic soap, Hetty began an animated story about her grandmother's chickens. When she paused one of the workers said, 'Hetty remembers a lot about her grandma's chickens but we're not talking about animals today, we're talking about household things.' Fred could not hear what was going on, and pointed out that it was raining outside. The activity ended abruptly without explanation when the staff were called away to help someone in the toilet.

What went well in the above example?

What areas of practice could be improved?

Good practice when gathering and using life history information

When collecting life histories, family members can be an invaluable source. They can provide an overview of a person's life, and may be able to supply the crucial details which make sense of mysterious fragments. However, it is good practice, if at all possible, to do some reminiscence work with the person concerned to get an understanding of how they remember and feel about the past.

In reminiscence work it is good practice to accept, and respect, different versions of a story. Every telling of a story is selective, and every story-teller will have their own particular bias, so we should not see one version as 'the facts' and others as erroneous. Making factual mistakes in recalling and recounting memories is a common consequence of cognitive decline. Fragments of memory from different times and places may be mixed; memories of films or books can be recalled as personal experiences; gaps in memory may be filled from imagination and what appear to be new stories with no basis in fact are sometimes created. It is not helpful to dismiss these phenomena as lies or manipulations. They illustrate the continued drive to make sense of experience and result from a person's particular profile of abilities and disabilities. There is often an emotional truth to be found in them, even if the details are confused. The importance given to a person's current and past views of their life relates to this issue. Perrin and May (2000) argued that our understanding should not be driven by a slavish commitment to the past and Murphy (1994) suggested that experiences right up to the present moment have a place in life histories. The challenge for good practice is to steer a person-centred course through the different versions of a life story.

There is value in considering how each person's life history is influencing their experience and behaviour in the present and what it can tell us about how they have dealt with past challenges (Bender *et al.* 1999). If this is to be done, life history information needs to be readily available, not buried in a filing cabinet. However, this raises issues of confidentiality, and it is important to check with client and family what they regard as private. Reminiscence products (life story books, etc.) raise awareness of life history, and it is worth making these and other non-confidential records easily accessible. To make links between life history and current needs, we often need to look behind life events and consider meanings and feelings. It can be helpful to share ideas and discuss possibilities with others, as this may help us to challenge our immediate assumptions and consider a wider range of alternative interpretations.

Debates and controversies

Family members and practitioners often express concern that working with life history may be harmful if it causes traumatic memories from the past to resurface. Many psychologists argue that recalling and speaking about unresolved distress is unlikely to lead to lasting harm, and may be necessary for resolution. However, the prospect of dealing with strong emotions can be alarming. In this debate it is important to consider what problems the recall of painful memories is likely to cause both for clients and for their caregivers – and how they can be handled in each case.

A very different area of debate concerns the place of psychosocial interventions (such as reminiscence work and life review) in dementia care. There is increasing evidence to support the view that psychosocial interventions compare well with current drug treatments in maintaining quality of life for people with dementia and their carers. They are free from adverse side effects, and not necessarily more expensive than drugs. Thus it can be argued psychosocial interventions should be available on the same basis as medication, given that the available drugs are unsuitable for many people and, where tolerated, may be less effective than psychosocial interventions. The opposing view is that while psychosocial interventions may be valuable as an adjunct to medication, they should take second place. More effective drug treatment will eventually become available and will be the best way to intervene in the long run. A question for this debate is whether the expectation that more effective medication will be found in future is good reason to limit the interventions offered to those who are living before this comes about.

Conclusion

While it is not easy to quantify and measure the benefits of life history work, ignoring the life stories of people with dementia is short-sighted and arguably irresponsible. Taking account of life history is essential for person-centred practice. The key question for practitioners is not whether to work with life history, but how best to do this work.

Further information

Age Exchange was established in 1983 to improve quality of life by valuing people's reminiscences.

The European Reminiscence Network aims to promote best practice in reminiscence work and to share experience across national frontiers.

Facilitated life story writing is a research project at the Sheridan Elder Research Center at McMaster University, Hamilton, Ontario, which aims to promote quality of life through the sharing of personal life stories.

The authors are collaborators on a research project evaluating the effectiveness of reminiscence groups for people with dementia and their family care-givers.

Further information about this pragmatic eight-centre trial of joint reminiscence and maintenance vs. usual treatment called RemCare is available from the **Bradford Dementia Group's** research web pages.

References

Alm, N., Dye, R., Gowans, G., Campbell, J., Astell, A. and Ellis, M. (2007) A communication support system for older people with dementia. *Computer,* 40 (5): 35–41.

Barnet, E. (2000) *Including the Person with Dementia in Designing and Delivering Care: 'I Need to be Me!'* London: Jessica Kingsley.

Bell, V. and Troxel, D. (2001) *The Best Friends Staff: Building a Culture of Care in Alzheimer's Programs.* Baltimore, MD: Health Professions Press.

Bender, M., Bauckham, P. and Norris, A. (1999) *The Therapeutic Purposes of Reminiscence.* London: Sage.

Bourgeois, M. (1992) Evaluating memory wallets in conversations with persons with dementia. *Journal of Speech and Hearing Research,* 35: 1344–57.

Brooker, D. (2007) *Person-centred Dementia Care: Making Services Better.* London: Jessica Kingsley.

Brooker, D.J.R. and Duce, L. (2000) Well-being and activity in dementia: a comparison of group reminiscence therapy, structured and goal-directed group activity and unstructured time. *Aging and Mental Health,* 4: 356–60.

Bruce, E. (1999) Holding onto the story: older people, narrative and dementia. In: G. Roberts and J. Holmes (eds) *Healing Stories: Narrative in Psychiatry and Psychotherapy.* Oxford: Oxford University Press, pp. 181–205.

Bruce, E., Hodgson, S. and Schweitzer, P. (1999) *Reminiscing with People with Dementia: A Handbook for Carers.* London: Age Exchange.

Bruce, E., Tibbs, M.A. and Surr, C. (2002) *A Special Kind of Care: Improving Well-being in People Living with Dementia.* Bradford Dementia Group, University of Bradford. http://www.brad.ac.uk/acad/health/dementia/research/methodist.php (accessed 12 April 2008).

Cheston, R. and Bender, M. (2000) *Understanding Dementia: The Man with the Worried Eyes.* London: Jessica Kingsley.

Cheston, R., Jones, K. and Gilliard, J. (2004) 'Falling into a hole': narrative and emotional change in a psychotherapy group for people with dementia. *Dementia,* 3(1): 95–103.

Cohen-Mansfield, J., Creedon, M.A., Malone, T., Parpura-Gill, A., Dakheel-Ali, M. and Heasly, C. (2007) Dressing of cognitively impaired nursing home residents: description and analysis. *The Gerontologist,* 46: 89–96.

Coleman, P.G. (2004) Uses of reminiscence: functions and benefits. *Aging and Mental Health,* 9(4): 291–4.

Gibson, F. (1998) *Reminiscence and Recall: A Guide to Good Practice*, 2nd ed. London: Age Concern.

Gibson, F. (2004) *The Past in the Present: Using Reminiscence in Health and Social Care.* Baltimore, MD: Health Professions Press.

Haight, B.K. and Haight, B.S. (2007) *The Handbook of Structured Life Review.* Baltimore, MD: Health Professions Press.

Hallberg, I.R., Norberg, A. and Eriksson, S. (1990) A comparison between the care of vocally disruptive patients and that of other residents at psychogeriatric wards. *Journal of Advanced Nursing,* 15: 267–75.

Heathcote, J. (2007) *Memories Are Made of This: Reminiscence Activities for Person-centred Care.* London: Alzheimer's Society.

Kenyon, G.M. (1996) Ethical issues in ageing and biography. *Ageing and Society,* 16(6): 659–76.

Killick, J. and Allan, S. (2001) *Communication and the Care of People with Dementia.* Buckingham: Open University Press.

Kitwood, T. (1993) Person and process in dementia. Reprinted in: C. Baldwin and A. Capstick (eds) (2007) *Tom Kitwood on Dementia: A Reader and Critical Commentary.* Maidenhead: Open University Press.

Kitwood, T. (1997) *Dementia Reconsidered.* Buckingham: Open University Press.

Kitwood, T. (1998) Life history and its vestiges: reminiscence work with people with dementia. In: P. Schweitzer (ed.) *Reminiscence in Dementia Care.* London: Age Exchange.

McKeown, J., Clarke, A. and Repper, J. (2005) Life story work in health and social care: systematic literature review. *Journal of Advanced Nursing,* 55(2): 237–47.

Miesen, B.M.L. (1992) Attachment theory and dementia. In: G.M.M. Jones and B.M.L. Miesen (eds) *Care-giving in Dementia: Research and Applications*, Vol. 1. London: Routledge, pp. 38–56.

Miesen, B.M.L. (2004) The psychology of dementia care: awareness and intangible loss. In: G.M.M. Jones and B.M.L. Miesen (eds) *Care-giving in Dementia: Research and Applications*, Vol. 4. London: Routledge, pp. 183–213.

Moos, I. and Bjorn, A. (2006) Use of the life story in the institutional care of people with dementia: review of intervention studies. *Ageing and Society*, 26: 431–54.

Murphy, C. (1994) *'It Started with a Sea-shell': Life Story Work and People with Dementia.* Stirling: Dementia Services Development Centre.

Naess, L. (1998) Reminiscence work with people with dementia. In: P. Schweitzer (ed.) *Reminiscence in Dementia Care.* London: Age Exchange.

Orrell, M. and Bebbington, P. (1995) Life events and senile dementia: admissions, deterioration and social environment change. *Psychological Medicine,* 25(2): 373–86.

Perrin, T. and May, H. (2000) *Well-being in Dementia: An Approach for Therapists and Carers.* Edinburgh: Churchill Livingstone.

Pietrukowicz, M.E. and Johnson, M.M.S. (1991) Using life histories to individualise nursing home staff attitudes towards residents. *The Gerontologist,* 31: 105–6.

Schweitzer, P. and Bruce, E. (2008) *Remembering Yesterday, Caring Today – Reminiscence in Dementia Care: A Guide to Good Practice.* London: Jessica Kingsley.

Vittoria, A.K. (1998) Preserving selves: identity work and dementia. *Research on Aging,* 20(1): 91–36.

Ward, R., Vass, A.A., Aggarwal, N., Garfield, C. and Cybyk, B. (2005) What is dementia care? 1. Dementia is communication. *Journal of Dementia Care,* 13(6): 16–19.

Webster, J.D. (2002) Reminiscence functions in adulthood: age, race and family dynamics correlates. In: J.D. Webster and B.K. Haight (eds) *Critical Advances in Reminiscence Work: From Theory to Applications.* New York: Springer Verlag.

Woods, R.T. (1998) Reminiscence as communication. In: P. Schweitzer (ed.) *Reminiscence in Dementia Care.* London: Age Exchange.

Woods, R.T. (2002) Non-pharmacological techniques. In: N. Qizilbash, L. Schneider, H. Chui *et al.* (eds) *Evidence-based Dementia Practice.* Oxford: Blackwell Science.

11

The language of behaviour

Jiska Cohen-Mansfield

Learning objectives

By the end of this chapter you will be able to:

- recognize that behaviour is a form of communication
- recognize that behaviour is often used to address unmet need
- identify a range of psychosocial approaches that can address needs
- appreciate the importance of knowing the individual person and their circumstance when seeking to understand the language of behaviour

---

Introduction

How we make sense of a person's behaviour, its cause and its purpose, is one of the most controversial issues in dementia care. This is an important area in dementia care because how we interpret a person's behaviour will influence how we respond. For example, if we consider a person's behaviour to result directly from brain dysfunction via disinhibition or via direct neurological activation of certain behaviours, such as screaming, we are more likely to propose drugs as a solution. If, on the other hand, we adopt a more bio-psychosocial approach to understanding dementia, we are more likely to seek explanations in the interaction between the person and their environment. As we have seen in Chapter 4, a bio-psychosocial approach argues that a person's behaviour is considered the result of interplay between neurobiology and the psychological and social environment. This chapter challenges the notion that behaviour is the direct result of neuropathology and argues instead that much behaviour is an attempt to address unmet needs – whether physical, psychological or social. According to this model, behaviour is a complex phenomenon affected by an interaction of cognitive impairment, physical health, mental health, past habits and personality, and environmental factors.

The chapter describes how a person with dementia experiences a decreased ability to meet their own needs. At the same time, people with dementia often find themselves in living or care situations which are either in direct opposition to, or in other ways fail to meet, their needs. Thus people with dementia rely on behaviour to fulfil and/or to communicate those needs. When this fails, they experience frustration and act in ways that others find challenging. The chapter presents a range of psychosocial interventions which can be employed to address the physical and psychosocial needs of people with dementia and argues for increased advocacy to support their research and use. Throughout the chapter evidence will be drawn from research with people with dementia in a range of care settings.

Needs and dementia

Maslow (1968) argued that humans are motivated by a group of hierarchically organized innate needs. The lowest layer involves mostly physiological needs (hunger, sleep, etc.), whereas the next layers include safety, belongingness and love, esteem and other higher-order needs. Once the lower need is satisfied, a person focuses on satisfying the higher needs. Results of observational studies of persons with severe cognitive impairment demonstrate that people with dementia, in common with all people, have higher order needs, such as those for social contact and sensory stimulation. While change has occurred in the person's ability to recognize, express and resolve these needs independently, and the environment often proves inadequate to address the needs, this does not mean the person no longer has such needs (see Table 11.1).

Table 11.1 Unmet needs: the effect of an interaction between human needs, cognitive impairment and an unfavourable environment

Human needs	Cognitive impairment	Unfavourable environment
Physiological – pain, health, physical discomfort	Unable to communicate needs	Environment does not comprehend the needs
Safety – uncomfortable environmental conditions	Unaware of needs of self	Environment does not provide for the needs
Love and belonging – need for social contacts	Unable to communicate the needs effectively	
Esteem- type of stimulation	Unable to use prior coping mechanisms	
Self-actualization – level of stimulation	Unable to obtain the means for meeting the need	

Based on Cohen-Mansfield (2000)

People with dementia express needs in common with all human beings (Cohen-Mansfield and Werner 1995), and as such these can be summarized under the hierarchy described by Maslow (1987).

Similar to Maslow's hierarchy of needs, Kitwood (1997) proposed a cluster of overlapping needs which, in his view, fall within one all-encompassing need, the need for love. These included the needs for comfort, attachment, inclusion, occupation and identity. By comfort he meant the need for tenderness and soothing of psychological pain; by attachment is meant the need for bonds with others; by inclusion, the need to be part of the group, part of the people club; by occupation, the need to be 'involved in the process of life'; by identity the need to 'know who one is' (Kitwood 1997: 83). He contended that many of these psychological needs go unmet in care environments. For Kitwood the key task of person-centred care was to meet these needs.

In our empirical research we have identified a range of physical, psychological and social needs. Physical needs include those related to pain, ill-health, and physical discomfort, including uncomfortable environmental conditions. Psychological and social needs include the need for social contacts and stimulation and those related to emotional discomfort (evident in affective states: depression, anxiety, frustration).

What makes the discussion of needs and dementia unique is that the dementia process results in a decreased ability to meet one's needs because of a decreased ability to communicate the needs, and a decreased ability to provide for oneself. As a result there is an imbalance in the interaction between lifelong habits and personality, current physical and mental states, and less than optimal environmental conditions. As such, most unmet needs arise because of the interaction between dementia-related impairments in both communication and a reduced ability to utilize the environment appropriately to fulfil the needs together with a social and physical environment which neither meets nor facilitates the meeting of these needs.

Understanding behaviour as an expression of unmet need

Exercise 11.1 Imagining unmet need

Think of the last time you felt hungry.

What led you to know that you were hungry? What did you do in response?

Were you able to meet your needs? What might you have done if you were unable to meet your needs?

How did your hunger affect your thinking? How did your hunger affect your behaviour?

Think of the last time you felt the need to talk to someone about something.

What happened in this circumstance? Were you able to meet your needs? How did your need to talk to someone affect your thinking? How did it affect your behaviour?

There has been a developing evidence base in support of the argument that behaviour is an expression of unmet needs (Algase *et al.* 1996; Cohen-Mansfield and Deutsch, 1996; Cohen-Mansfield and Werner, 1995). Thought of in this way, behaviour is a complex phenomenon affected by an interaction of cognitive impairment, physical health, mental health, past habits and personality, and environmental factors. Behaviour can be seen as an attempt to address unmet needs in one of several ways:

● The behaviour can aim to directly meet the need, e.g. when pacing may provide stimulation to alleviate the unmet needs for engagement, occupation and stimulation.

- The behaviour may aim to communicate the need, e.g. repetitious vocalizations which aim to draw attention to an unmet need

- The behaviour may represent the outcome of having an unmet need e.g. screaming as a result of frustration or pain.

From our research we have concluded that the main needs people with dementia seek to address through their behaviour include:

- unaddressed physical pain or discomfort

- lack of social contacts and loneliness

- boredom, inactivity, and sensory deprivation

- depression which may be the result of lack of positive experiences or lack of control.

Behaviour as an expression of physical pain and discomfort

Physical pain and ill health factors are associated with a range of verbal and vocal behaviours (Cohen-Mansfield *et al.* 1990). Hurley *et al.* (1992) reported an increase in vocalizations among patients experiencing fevers. The behaviour may be a direct manifestation of discomfort, a natural response to pain, and may be exacerbated in persons who are unable to communicate and therefore express their suffering through screaming. Alternatively, the vocally disruptive behaviour may be an attempt to communicate the discomfort under circumstances in which a cognitively impaired individual is no longer able to communicate more directly. While the relationship between health and physically aggressive behaviour is less clear, a positive association between aggressive behaviour and urinary tract infections has been reported (Ryden *et al.* 1991).

In contrast, people who engage in physically non-aggressive behaviour (e.g. pacing) have been reported to have fewer medical diagnoses than other nursing home residents, and have better appetites (Cohen-Mansfield *et al.* 1990). However, some people who pace suffer from akathaesia, an inner sense of restlessness, due to neurodegenerative disease or as an extrapyramidal reaction to antipsychotic or other drugs (Mutch 1992).

Sleep disturbance and fatigue are another aspect of health which has been linked to behaviour (Cohen-Mansfield and Marx 1990; Cohen-Mansfield *et al.* 1995). The impairment of circadian rhythms which is characteristic of Alzheimer's disease (e.g. Bliwise 1993) may also be related to behaviour. In particular, an increase in active behaviour in older individuals with dementia that occurs in the evening hours, beginning at a time near sunset, has been termed 'sundowning' (Bliwise 1994). It should be noted, however, that such behaviour is not related to the sunset or to the actual time of sunset. Many people experience restless behaviour more often in morning hours, while others manifest those at relatively uniform levels throughout the day (Cohen-Mansfield 2007).

Behaviour as an expression of uncomfortable environmental conditions

In an observational study of the nursing home environment, most behaviours that staff found difficult tended to increase when it was cold at night, and requests for attention increased when it was hot during the day (Cohen-Mansfield and Werner 1995). These findings suggest that discomfort may cause some behaviours.

Behaviour as an expression of need for social contact

Verbal/vocal behaviours, as well as some physically non-aggressive behaviours other than pacing and wandering, tended to increase in frequency when nursing home residents were alone, and to decrease when they were with others. Similarly, such behaviours decreased when staffing levels increased (Cohen-Mansfield and Werner 1995). These findings suggest that loneliness or the need for social contact may be at the root of verbal or vocal behaviours that distress others. This idea is supported by an intervention study (Cohen-Mansfield and Werner 1997) in which social interaction was more beneficial in decreasing verbal and vocal problem behaviours than the mere provision of pleasant stimuli, such as music.

Behaviour as an expression of need for stimulation

In the past, problem behaviours have been attributed to overstimulation or too much stimulation which cannot be processed because of the dementia. An observational study of the nursing home (Cohen-Mansfield *et al.* 1992a) did not support this hypothesis. In fact observations from this study found that the nursing home was a relatively monotonous place. Routine is the rule and activities and stimulation are infrequent (Cohen-Mansfield *et al.* 1992b). People often have nothing to do in long-term care settings. Most behaviours that others found difficult to manage increased when the older person was inactive, and decreased when structured activities were offered (Cohen-Mansfield and Werner 1995).

Therefore, the notion that problem behaviours result from understimulation and sensory deprivation has been proposed. According to this view, the person with dementia has a reduced ability to obtain stimulation and process it. Additionally, many of those living with dementia also have vision and hearing impairments which further decrease their ability to process stimuli. Finally, many of the nursing homes in which persons with dementia reside offer few activities or other positive stimuli. All of these factors result in a state of insufficient stimulation, which, at times, reaches a state of sensory deprivation to which the person responds with either self-stimulation or behaviours which manifest discontent because of this unmet need for stimulation. Studies on social deprivation in younger populations have shown that sensory deprivation can result in hallucinations and perceptual distortions, which may in turn lead to behaviours with which others have difficulty dealing. Even without hallucinations or perceptual changes, the sensory deprivation may evoke feelings of fear, loneliness and boredom, all resulting in the manifestation of problem behaviours. Several studies showed that providing sensory stimulation to nursing home residents decreased behavioural disturbances in general, and vocally disruptive behaviours in particular (Birchmore and Clague 1983; Mayers and Griffin 1990; Zachow 1984).

Behaviour in response to delusions and hallucinations

Delusions and hallucinations provide inappropriate internal stimuli, which may result in behaviour that others find difficult to understand. The relationship between behaviours and delusions or hallucinations has been documented repeatedly (Cohen-Mansfield *et al.* 1998; Deutsch *et al.* 1991; Lachs *et al.* 1992; Steiger *et al.* 1991). It is possible that, like other behaviours, those that are considered to be delusions and hallucinations also result from the interaction of the limited capabilities of the person with dementia and psycho-social and environmental situations that do not support the person (Cohen-Mansfield 2003).

Exercise 11.2　Needs-related behaviour

Think of the last time you saw someone with dementia behaving in a way you did not understand and which you found distressing. What was the person doing?

Thinking of this same person, do you think their needs for comfort, attachment, inclusion, occupation and identity were being met at the time? Which needs may not have been met? How might they have been?

Psychosocial interventions for meeting needs

Psychosocial interventions for meeting needs include those that address the need for social contact, engagement and relief from discomfort (see Table 11.2).

Table 11.2 Psychosocial interventions to address needs

Need	Social contacts			Engagement				Discomfort		
	Real human	Simulated significant others	Non-human	Provide		Accommodate behaviour		Pain/discomfort	Sleep	Discomfort during ADL
General treatment approach				Active	Passive	Decrease risk	Make behaviour more acceptable			
Interventions	One-on-one social interaction Small group interaction Massage	Simulated presence therapy Family videotapes	Pets Dolls	Walking Exercise Activity programmes Flower arranging	Provide hearing aids and glasses to allow persons to process ongoing stimulation Sensory stimulation Music Aromatherapy Massage	Environmental design, such as: tape on floor, covering doors or exits, relocating areas	Make behaviour more acceptable Activity apron Provide materials to handle Environmental design Changing the visual, auditory, and olfactory stimuli on corridors	Pain medication Repositioning Remove restrictions	Light therapy Melatonin Increase exercise and decrease awakening at night	Environmental redesign of bathing process (bird pictures and sounds in baths, offering food) Music during bath. Use of sponge bath rather than shower or bath Change location of meals

Based on Cohen-Mansfield (2000).

Many interventions address more than one of these, such as meaningful social contact alleviating both loneliness and boredom. A variety of psychosocial interventions have been described in the literature and summarized in reviews (Allen-Burge *et al.* 1999; Bates *et al.* 2004; Cohen-Mansfield 2001, 2003, 2004; Grasel *et al.* 2003; Kasl-Godley and Gatz 2000; Opie *et al.* 1999; Siders *et al.* 2004; Snowden *et al.* 2003).

Psychosocial approaches to the care of persons with dementia differ from pharmacological treatment in that they consider the interaction between the person, caregiver, environment and system of care. Such interventions generally provide more person-centred, individualized and personalized care, addressing their needs and considering their preferences.

Providing social support and contact

At the most basic level, providing social support and contact involves talking to persons with dementia, even if the caregiver conducts the majority of the conversation. One-on-one interaction is a potent intervention that can be provided by relatives, paid caregivers or volunteers. There are two major difficulties in providing positive social contact for persons with dementia: (1) these individuals may prefer socializing with loved ones rather than formal caregivers, and (2) providing one-on-one interaction with staff members can become costly. Two successful interventions that have addressed both of these issues are videotapes of family members addressing their relative with dementia (Cohen-Mansfield and Werner 1997; Werner *et al.* 2000) and simulated presence therapy (Camberg *et al.* 1999; Woods and Ashley 1995) in which a family member audiotapes his or her side of a telephone conversation, which is then played for the older person. Interventions addressing cost issues include training staff members to view all interactions with individuals in their care as opportunities for social contact (including during activities of daily living), and interaction videos for persons with dementia. These commercially produced videotapes often incorporate memories from the past and viewers are invited to sing along to familiar music. Pet therapy is another option (Churchill *et al.* 1997), and may include visits with dogs, cats, fish, or even plush stuffed animals or robotic pets (Libin and Cohen-Mansfield 2004). In addition to interaction with the animal, pet therapy provides a topic for interaction with other people. Dolls have also been used to simulate companions/babies, and massage may be an effective mechanism for social contact with persons with advanced dementia who lack verbal language.

Research results indicate that verbally disruptive behaviours often relate to social isolation; these behaviours decrease with the provision of appropriate ongoing social contact. In a study of verbally disruptive behaviours in the nursing home, both one-on-one social interaction and watching a videotape of a relative talking to the older person decreased verbal and vocal disruptive behaviours among residents who had manifested these behaviours at very high frequencies in comparison to a no-intervention condition (Cohen-Mansfield and Werner 1997). One-on-one interaction was more effective, though also more costly. There were also noticeable individual differences in response, with some persons benefiting more from one type of intervention. This suggests that additional factors, such as the person's prior relationship with relatives, must be taken into account when customizing the specific programme for each individual.

An individual with dementia's ability to communicate verbally declines in advanced dementia (see Chapter 12). As a result, communication skills on the part of the carer are crucial for maintaining quality of life and for understanding the perspective of the person with dementia. Caregivers must be educated in communication techniques, learning to observe, listen, speak, ask questions, and offer alternatives in ways that will maximize the individual's ability to receive and transmit information. Communication training for caregivers of persons with dementia focuses on environmental aspects of communication (e.g. approaching slowly, communicating at eye level), content, phrasing and interpreting nonverbal or confused verbal communication. Phrasing sentences in a short and clear way (Small *et al.* 2003), on a level compatible with the person's understanding (Hart and Wells 1997), and asking questions in a simple, yes/no format has been recommended as helpful. Others have advised using broad opening sentences, treating the person with dementia as an equal, sharing experiences and feelings, and finding topics that are meaningful (Tappen *et al.* 1997). Finally, caregivers must be aware that even when individuals with dementia do not speak in coherent sentences, their individual words may be meaningful, and their messages may be embedded in those words (see Chapter 12). Most essential is to not ignore, discount or negate the verbalizations of persons with dementia, but rather to view these as insights into their perspectives, and to use them to improve their situations whenever possible (Small and Gutman 2002; Ripich 1994; Ripich *et al.* 1995).

Providing relief from discomfort – medical and nursing care

Interventions addressing discomfort target pain, hearing and vision impairments, positioning problems, difficulties adjusting to ADLs, and unmet ADL-related needs. Interventions such as pain management, light therapy to improve sleep, reduction of discomfort by improved seating or positioning and removal of physical restraints have all been related to improvement in behaviour. Once needs have been identified, many of these interventions call for straightforward medical or nursing interventions, while others require more complex approaches, such as assessing pain.

Many articles have described the difficulties involved in assessing pain in this population (Cohen-Mansfield and Lipson 2002) and some recent findings suggest strategies for approaching these complexities (Cohen-Mansfield and Lipson 2008; Feldt 2000; Huffman and Kunik 2000). One small study found that pain medication reduced difficult behaviours and allowed discontinuation of psychotropic medication (Douzjian *et al.* 1998). Physical pain is frequently difficult to assess, but statements about not feeling well, or about being in pain, and unusual movements need to be examined. Looking at the person carefully for several minutes while sitting and during transfer may be beneficial for detecting signs of pain. Similarly, a change from the person's usual behaviour may be a sign of physical pain (Cohen-Mansfield *et al.* 1989). Caregivers' ratings for the assessment of pain together with a pain relief protocol may be especially useful for detection and treatment of pain in persons with dementia (Cohen-Mansfield and Lipson 2008).

Physical discomfort is very common in the nursing home and can range from thirst, to needing to go to the bathroom, to an uncomfortable sitting position. The reasons for such needs may be complex, such as insufficient staff to take persons to the bathroom, frequent urges to go to the bathroom, or the fear that the resident may choke if given regular liquids. Nevertheless, such issues need to be addressed.

One specific type of physical discomfort is the use of physical restraints, which have been shown to result in increased levels of agitation (Werner *et al.* 1989). The removal of physical restraints may eliminate those behaviours (Werner *et al.* 1994; Yeh *et al.* 2001).

A number of methods have been used to improve sleep and thereby decrease agitation, including the use of bright light therapy (Mishima *et al.* 1994; Okawa *et al.* 1991), use of melatonin (Cohen-Mansfield *et al.* 2000a), increased exercise (Zisselman *et al.* 1996), and a decrease in night-time interruptions (Alessi *et al.* 1999).

Improvement in eating or drinking, resulting from the use of enhanced light during meals, has been linked with a decrease in inappropriate behaviours (Koss and Gilmore 1998), as has the use of hearing aids (Leverett 1991; Palmer *et al.* 1999).

Changes in the methods and environment of providing activities of daily living have also been associated with reduction in inappropriate behaviours. For example, tape recordings and pictures of birds, flowing water and small animals in baths as well as offering food during bathing have been associated with a decrease of such behaviours during bathing (Whall *et al.* 1997). Person-centred showering and towel baths resulted in decreased agitation in comparison with usual bathing routines (Sloane *et al.* 2004). Similarly, changing location of meals from central dining to dining on the unit was effective in reducing patient-to-patient assaults on an Alzheimer's and related dementias unit (Negley and Manley 1990).

Providing engaging activities

Engaging persons with dementia can be accomplished by providing them with stimulation (passive engagement), providing activities (active engagement), and facilitating self-stimulation by accommodating inappropriate behaviours (see Table 11.2). Engaging persons may also involve the reduction of sensory barriers, as in the case of providing hearing aids. Providing stimulation includes the use of music, which should be tailored to the person's preferences (Gerdner 2000), and other sensory stimulation such as aromatherapy or touch therapy (Snyder *et al.* 1995). Music interventions take many forms, including listening to recorded music, playing musical games, dancing or moving to music, and singing. (Prior to initiating music therapy, hearing must be tested, and an amplifier, headphone, or hearing aid may be necessary.) One example of sensory stimulation is the 'Snoezelen' programme, which was developed in Holland and includes a variety of relaxing stimuli (Baillon *et al.* 2004).

More active engagement is usually offered in the form of structured activities, including group and individual activities. One such intervention, known as 'simple pleasures', includes a range of activities such as tetherball (Buettner 1999). Activity interventions may involve manipulation (e.g. ball throwing), nurturing (e.g. watering a plant), sorting, cooking, sewing, or sensory interventions as described above, such as music or tactile stimulation with a fabric book. Montessori-based activities are a set of activities based on Maria Montessori's principles (Camp *et al.* 2002), such as task breakdown, immediate feedback and use of everyday, real-world materials. Alternatively, the content of activities may be based on information regarding 'pleasant activities', that is, activities which were or are reinforcing to the individual (Teri and Logsdon 1991), or on information about the individual's role-identity in the past or in the present (Cohen-Mansfield *et al.* 2000b, 2006a, 2006b; Parpura-Gill and Cohen-Mansfield 2006). Activities can involve exercise (Zisselman *et al.* 1996), or they may incorporate an adaptation of activities of daily living, such as setting the table or cooking (Marsden *et al.*, 2001). Cognitive tasks are activities that stimulate cognitive and memory skills. Group examples include 'Question Asking Readings' in which a group reads a script accompanied by questions typed on cards that encourage participants to discuss related topics. Another group memory task is memory bingo, a game in which participants match beginnings and endings of popular sayings, which can also stimulate group discussion (Camp *et al.* 1996). Individual cognitive tasks include sorting cards or objects by category.

Interventions for accommodating pacing or wandering behaviour include outdoor walks (Cohen-Mansfield and Werner 1998a) and the use of wandering areas. Outdoor walks may take place in the company of a caregiver, in which case they also involve a social component, or they may occur in secure outdoor wandering areas (Cohen-Mansfield and Werner 1999; Namazi and Johnson 1992). Accommodating pacing and wandering often involves protection of others from trespassing while wandering. To prevent trespassing into another person's room or through emergency exit doors, doors and doorknobs can be camouflaged with cloth panels or murals, thereby disguising the doors. Additionally, providing alternative doors, which can be controlled by the person with dementia and permit movement into another secured area, can be useful in preventing people from getting into other persons' rooms (Namazi *et al.* 1989).

Inappropriate handling or the constant manipulation of objects can be accommodated by providing appropriate materials, such as books and pamphlets for handling (Cohen-Mansfield and Werner 1998a), and activity aprons (aprons that have buttons, zippers and other articles sewn on) providing appropriate and safe items for persons to handle. Similarly, rocking chairs and gliding swings have been used to accommodate restless behaviour and provide more acceptable stimulation.

Some verbally disruptive behaviour may serve self-stimulatory functions and may be associated with inactivity and boredom. Such behaviour is likely to be reduced when structured activities are offered. In the study described above (Cohen-Mansfield and Werner 1997), music chosen on the basis of the older person's past preferences significantly reduced verbally disruptive behaviours in comparison to a no treatment condition, although it was less effective than interventions aimed at social contact. The importance of individualizing the intervention to fit the participant was exemplified in a study by Gerdner (2000) who showed that music that was matched to the participant's past preferences was more effective than merely providing soothing music.

When the person's need calls for an activity, the specific type of activity offered needs to be matched to the person's level of cognitive functioning, sensory and physical abilities and deficits, as well as sense of identity and preferences (Parpura-Gill and Cohen-Mansfield 2006).

The specific choice of activity for the intervention would be determined by evaluating the older person on the following dimensions:

- current **sense of identity**, which usually includes some retained aspects of previously held identities, such as work role, family relationship, or preference for a certain type of leisure activity

- current **sensory abilities**, which include visual, auditory, smell and touch modalities. Mechanisms for augmentation of sensory abilities should be explored, including simple ones, such as better fitting eyeglasses, an auditory amplifier, better fitting hearing aids, etc.

- current **motor abilities**, including ability to walk, to wheel oneself, as well as dexterity

- an enhanced understanding of current **needs**, including social contact of any kind, longing for family, for daytime activity, for stimulation, for physical exercise, or for a specific meaningful activity, such as helping, or working

- an understanding of the person's past and present **habits and preferences** for daily life activities and the manner and environment in which they take place (Cohen-Mansfield and Jensen 2005a, 2005b; 2007a, 2007b).

The interactions of these factors will define the intervention that is most appropriate for the individual. A hypothetical-planning grid for matching activities to the needs of individuals is presented in Table 11.3.

Table 11.3 Choosing activities to suit needs and abilities

Abilities: primary modality	Needs/activity domains					
	Social contact	Family contact/home environment	Stimulation	Physical exercise/ self-stimulation	Meaningful activity/ increased sense of identity
Seeing	Home movies (H) Mirror (L) Video tape of someone talking to the person (E)	Video tape of family (E) Picture album of family (E) Increase family visits (E)	Show old movies (H) Place near a window with view to street or other activity (L) Display moving objects, such as bubbles and strands (L) Flower arranging, sorting shapes and colours, colouring (L)	Dancing (E)	Sheltered workshop (H)
Hearing	One-on-one social interaction (H) Group activities (H) Audiotape of someone talking to person (L)	Telephone calls with family (H) Audio tape of family member (L) Simulated presence therapy (L)	Books or tape (H) Trivia (H) Card games (H) Tapes of music the person used to like (E)	Moving to music (E)	Listening to religious services or music (E)
Moving	Arrange social visits (tea) (H) Go to religious services(H)		Rocking chair (E)	Walk in sheltered area (E) going outside (E)	Assembling materials (H) Cooking (H) Simulating work environment (H)
Touch-ing	Use of soft dolls (L) Massage therapy (E)	Use of object from home (E)	Massage therapy (E) Jacuzzi (E)	Handling different materials (L) Activity apron (L)	caring for or petting a dog or a cat (E)

H = Activities appropriate for higher cognitively functioning residents.
L = Activities appropriate for lower cognitively functioning residents.
E = Activities appropriate for both groups of residents.

Examples of the range of possible activities to use as stimulation can be found in research done by Bowlby (1993), Hellen (1998), Zgola (1987), Teri and Logsdon (1991) and Russen-Rondinone and DesRoberts (1996).

The actual utilization of psychosocial interventions in dementia falls far short of its potential. A number of systemic issues are responsible for this gap. Funding is lacking both for the practice of these interventions and for the acquisition of knowledge about them through systematic research. In the USA the commonly used alternative intervention of psychoactive medication is reimbursed, and the underlying structure for its delivery, such as physicians, medicine aids, pharmacy, monitoring and quality control systems, are largely in place. However, the provision of psychosocial interventions is generally not reimbursed, and a system for providing them is often absent. No one in the care system is currently responsible for assessing, observing, and analysing behaviour in order to determine its underlying cause and its impact on individuals' lives. The ability of paid carers to provide psychosocial interventions is further limited by lack of staff member knowledge, insufficient staffing levels, and stressful experiences within and outside the care situation (see Chapter 23).

Individualizing care for people with dementia: treatment routes for exploring agitation (TREA)

> **Exercise 11.3** Individualizing care
>
> Remember a time when you felt very sad. It is possible that several people tried to comfort you. You may have accepted some people's support while pushing others away.
>
> What might explain your willingness to accept help from one person while rejecting it from another?
>
> Might it have anything to do with how well understood you felt?

Addressing people's behavioural communication requires us to adopt a cyclical approach. This starts with assessment of the behaviour – describing the behaviour in detail and the circumstances in which it occurs. We then go on to hypothesize the cause of the behaviour, what need it is striving to meet. We propose an intervention, implement the intervention and then some time later reassess.

Once we have explored the possible causes for the person's behaviour – understood what the person is communicating through their behaviour – we then identify an intervention to match. The intervention may target a change in the environment, the behaviour of the staff member, the system of care, or the person with dementia. After the intervention is implemented, another evaluation is performed to determine whether the approach was helpful or whether it should be changed. A change may require a different intervention entirely, or may focus on a specific aspect of the intervention such as timing, dosage, or presentation style.

We need to have as the aim of our care improved quality of life and pleasure. To achieve this goal, we aim to either fulfil the person's need or to accommodate the behaviour that fulfils the need for the person. Therefore, the target of the intervention may be to reduce behaviour, or it may be to make it acceptable to the persons around. The job of care for people with dementia requires empathy, caring, or love for the person. This type of care has to be present throughout the different care activities. For example, 1:1 dressing is an opportunity for human contact, an opportunity for intimacy.

On the basis of our research we have proposed Treatment Routes for Exploring Agitation (TREA) as an approach for individualizing treatment plans in response to behaviours which others find distressing or that seem to indicate that the older person may be distressed. Such a plan involves several stages:

1   Hypothesize which need underlies behaviour.

2   Characterize the way in which the behaviour results from the need: does the behaviour attempt to accommodate the need? Does it express discomfort? Does it attempt to communicate the need?

3   Provide an intervention which either provides for the unmet need, or, alternatively, when the behaviour itself is alleviating the need, provide a method in which the behaviour can be accommodated.

When an intervention to provide for the unmet need is required, it needs to be matched to the person's sensory, mental, and physical abilities, as well as to the person's habits and preferences. The goal of the plan is to improve the quality of life for the patient, and to reduce the burden on caregivers.

The assumptions and principles underlying TREA

- A methodology for detecting the needs of the person with dementia is essential for proper care giving.

- The first step in developing a specific treatment plan for a specific person is to attempt to understand the cause of the behaviour, or the need it signals.

- Psychosocial approaches to behaviour should precede pharmacological approaches.

- Psychosocial approaches to behaviour need to be individualized.

Maximizing function and well-being necessitate a focus on the person–environment fit; both lifelong and current attributes must be considered in the development of methods to optimally address needs. Therefore, in developing a treatment plan, the remaining abilities, strengths, memories and needs should be utilized, as well as recognition of impairments, especially those in sensory perception and mobility. Unique characteristics of the individual such as past work, hobbies, important relationships, and sense of identity need to be explored to best match current activities to the person.

The TREA approach includes several key elements

Individualization of treatment as opposed to care for a group

Generally, persons with dementia are currently treated alike. In a typical nursing home, wake-up time and dining times are frequently guided by state regulations and by staffing issues more than by individual habits. Medication for dementia is guided more by market forces and by prescription habits than by individual differences. Group activities do not necessarily fit the participants' abilities and interests.

The detective rather than resigned approach

- Rather than assuming that the person suffering from dementia has lost all sense of self, our treatment of those persons should be a constant search for their personhood within the dementia.

- Commitment to understanding the person with dementia through communication with that individual and with appropriate informants.

- Formal caregivers' knowledge of their patients' past daily habits and identities are extremely limited (Cohen-Mansfield *et al.* 2000b) and need to be augmented by reports from other sources, most often family members (see Chapter 10). Communication with the older person also needs to be enhanced, so that the communicator listens to the underlying message rather than to the exact message conveyed.

Focus on prevention, accommodation, and flexibility as essential elements of intervention

- Prevention refers to structuring the environment in a manner that prevents the development of unmet needs. Examples include better control of temperature, facilitating activities, monitoring pain, and providing stimulation and social contact before any unmet needs are met.

- Accommodation involves ensuring that the design of the environment permits the person to express themselves through behaviours in a manner that fulfils the needs of the older person without imposing an undue burden on caregivers.

Box 11.1 Case example

Encouraging persons with dementia to walk in a sheltered garden allows them to manifest behaviour in an environment in which it is accepted as natural and which does not place them at risk or place a great burden on the caregiver (Cohen-Mansfield and Werner 1998b; Namazi and Johnson 1992). Gardens can include glasshouses and outdoor areas and need to be adapted to the weather conditions in order to allow yearlong use.

Similarly, in one study, pamphlets were provided for residents to take as their own (Cohen-Mansfield and Werner 1998b) as an acceptable way of accommodating behaviours which would otherwise be labelled 'inappropriate handling of things'.

Finally, even when the need is unclear, if the behaviour is not harmful, it is frequently best to accommodate it. Thus, simply accommodating the person's wish, even without understanding it, is frequently an appropriate route.

Box 11.2 Case example

An elderly woman was screaming next to the locked dining room door, obviously wanting to get in. It was not clear why she wanted to get in, as the room held no objects of interest or entertainment. Nevertheless, she should be let in as she would neither be hurt nor cause harm if let in.

Flexibility refers to the willingness and ability of caregivers to adjust elements of the older person's daily routine and environment to meet the resident's needs and/or wishes. This pertains to flexibility to accommodate biological needs (e.g. toileting times, feeding times) and psychosocial needs (e.g. social contacts, meaningful activities) which are tailored to the person's lifelong habits, identity, current physical disabilities (e.g. incontinence) and remaining abilities. Flexibility in mealtimes, type of food (e.g. finger food vs. regular cooked food), sleep times, and type of bathing (bath versus sponge bath) can all reduce the amount of conflict and ensuing disruptive behaviour by modifying the activities of daily living to accommodate the individual's needs, habits, moods, and tolerance.

The TREA approach utilizes a decision tree by which one arrives at the most likely cause of an agitated behaviour via assessment of the type of behaviour manifested, conditions surrounding the behaviour, and information about the individual's past preferences and needs. Once a cause has been hypothesized, a corresponding treatment is attempted. This effort is evaluated for effectiveness. If effective, the treatment is continued. If ineffective, or only partially effective, the next most likely cause is found and the corresponding treatment provided. The decision tree itself is a series of questions, beginning with the type of agitated behaviour (i.e., physically nonaggressive, physically aggressive, or verbally disruptive behaviours). Within each category, the decision tree guides the caregiver through the steps to be explored in order to ascertain the need most likely contributing to the manifested behaviour.

Debates and controversies

There is little consensus in either the literature or clinical practice about the definition of problem behaviours and theoretical frameworks used to understand and treat the problem behaviours of persons with dementia. Even the terminology used has been controversial. Some argue that terms such as problem behaviours, disruptive behaviours, challenging behaviours, disturbing behaviours, behavioural problems, and agitation are pejorative as they suggest the behaviour is intrinsically problematic rather than an indication of an environment which is failing to address people's needs.

Conclusion

As mentioned previously, there are several prerequisites to good psychosocial care of persons with dementia. In order to provide psychosocial interventions, the system of care must promote an atmosphere and practice of caring that goes beyond what is currently found in most care settings. A practice style that includes good communication skills, compassion and empathy by caregivers, as well as a high level of flexibility of direct care staff and the larger organization are needed, and are often lacking. In order to allow for alternative interventions, the system of care must promote autonomy and respect for the person with dementia and maximize flexibility in all procedures. Greater monetary resources must also be allocated for research to develop the knowledge necessary for optimizing such care. There is an urgent need to improve our ability to answer basic questions: Which interventions are efficacious for which individuals? Which aspects of an intervention are necessary for it to be efficacious? What are the active ingredients, or principles at work, in different interventions? Which personal characteristics (gender, culture, prior stress) should be considered in matching an intervention with an individual? What is the impact of the person delivering the intervention and the manner in which it is delivered? Only once these basic questions are answered can the issues of effectiveness and costs be properly addressed.

In order to increase the use of psychosocial interventions in dementia care, there is a need for public education and advocacy concerning the importance of such interventions and their support. Psychosocial interventions generally provide more personalized care for persons with dementia, addressing their needs, and thereby promoting quality of life.

Further information

The Dementia Behaviour Management Advisory Services in Australia were established to help people manage difficult behaviour and dementia. They support aged care workers and carers who are caring for people with dementia and related behaviours.

The National Dementia Behaviour Advisory Service (NDBAS) within Alzheimer's Australia provides advice on managing behaviours of concern to those who care for a person with dementia. This confidential assistance is available 24 hours a day to respite care staff, health professionals and carers.

References

Alessi, C.A., Yoon, E.J., Schnelle, J.F., Al-Samarrai, N.R. and Cruise P.A. (1999) A randomized trial of a combined physical acitivty and environmental intervention in nursing home residents: Do sleep and agitation improve? *Journal of the American Geriatrics Society,* 47(7): 784–91.

Algase, D., Beck, C., Kolanowski, A. *et al.* (1996) Need-driven dementia-compromised behavior: An alternative view of disruptive behavior. *American Journal of Alzheimer's Disease,* 11: 10–19.

Allen-Burge, R., Stevens, A.B. and Burgio, L.D. (1999) Effective behavioral interventions for decreasing dementia-related challenging behavior in nursing homes. *International Journal of Geriatric Psychiatry,* 14(3): 213–28.

Baillon, S., Van Diepen, E., Prettyman, R., Redman, J., Rooke, N. Campbell, R. (2004) A comparison of the effects of Snoezelen and reminiscence therapy on the agitated behaviour of patients with dementia. *International Journal of Geriatric Psychiatry,* 19: 1047–52.

Bates, J., Boote, J. and Beverley, C. (2004) Psychosocial interventions for people with a milder dementing illness: A systematic review. *Journal of Advanced Nursing,* 45(6): 644–58.

Birchmore, T. and Clague, S. (1983) A behavioural approach to reduce shouting. *Nursing Times,* 79: 37–9.

Bliwise, D.L. (1993) Sleep in normal aging and dementia. *Sleep,* 16(1): 40–81.

Bliwise, D.L. (1994) What is sundowning? *Journal of the American Geriatrics Society,* 42(9): 1009–11.

Bowlby, C. (1993) *Therapeutic Activities with Persons Disabled by Alzheimer's Disease and Related Disorders. Gaithersberg, MD: Aspen.*

Buettner, L.L. (1999) Simple pleasures: A multilevel sensorimotor intervention for nursing home residents with dementia. *American Journal of Alzheimer's Disease and Other Dementias,* 14(1): 41–52.

Camberg, L., Woods, P., Ooi, W.L. *et al.* (1999) Evaluation of simulated presence: A personalized approach to enhance well-being in persons with Alzheimer's disease [see comments]. *Journal of the American Geriatrics Society,* 47: 446–52.

Camp, C., Cohen-Mansfield, J. and Capezuti, E. (2002) Nonpharmacological interventions for dementia: Enhancing and maintaining mental health in long-term care residents. *Psychiatric Services,* 53(11): 1397–1404.

Camp, C.J., Foss, J.W., O'Hanlon A.M. and Stevens, A.B. (1996) Memory interventions for persons with dementia. *Applied Cognitive Psychology,* 10: 193–210.

Churchill, M., Safaoui, J., McCabe, B. and Baun, M. (1999) Using a therapy dog to alleviate the agitation and desocialization of people with Alzheimer's disease. *Journal of Psychosocial Nursing and Mental Health Services,* 37(4): 16–24.

Cohen-Mansfield, J. (2000) Nonpharmacological management of behavioural problems in persons with dementia: The TREA model. *Alzheimer's Care Quarterly,* 1(4): 22–34.

Cohen-Mansfield, J. (2001) Nonpharmacologic interventions for inappropriate behaviors in dementia: A review, summary, and critique. *American Journal of Geriatric Psychiatry*, 9(4): 361–81.

Cohen-Mansfield, J. (2003) Nonpharmacologic interventions for psychotic symptoms in dementia. *Journal of Geriatric Psychiatry and Neurology*, 16(4): 219–24.

Cohen-Mansfield, J. (2004) Cognitive and behavioral interventions for persons with dementia. In: *Encyclopedia of Applied Psychology*. Oxford: Elsevier Inc.

Cohen-Mansfield, J. (2007) Temporal patterns of agitation in dementia. *Journal of the American Geriatrics Society*, 15(5): 395–405.

Cohen-Mansfield, J., Billig, N., Lipson, S., Rosenthal, A. and Pawlson, L. (1990) Medical correlates of agitation in nursing home residents. *Gerontology*, 36(3): 150–8.

Cohen-Mansfield, J. and Deutsch, L. (1996) Agitation: Subtypes and their Mechanisms. *Seminars in Clinical Neuropsychiatry*, 1(4): 325–39.

Cohen-Mansfield, J., Garfinkel, D. and Lipson, S. (2000a) Melatonin for treatment of sundowning in elderly persons with dementia: A preliminary study. *Archives of Gerontology and Geriatrics*, 31: 65–76.

Cohen-Mansfield, J., Golander, H. and Arnheim, G. (2000) Self-identity in older persons suffering from dementia: Preliminary results. *Social Science and Medicine*, 51: 381–94.

Cohen-Mansfield, J. and Jensen, B. (2005a) Sleep-related habits and preferences in older adults: A pilot study of their range and self rated importance. *Behavioral Sleep Medicine*, 3(4): 209–26.

Cohen-Mansfield, J. and Jensen, B. (2005b) The preference and importance of bathing, toileting, and mouth care in older persons. *Gerontology*, 51(6): 375–85.

Cohen-Mansfield, J. and Jensen, B. (2007a) Self-maintenance habits and preferences in elderly (SHAPE): Reliability of reports of self-care preferences in older persons. *Aging: Clinical and Experimental Research*, 9(1): 61–8.

Cohen-Mansfield, J. and Jensen, B. (2007b) Dressing and grooming preferences of community-dwelling older adults. *Journal of Gerontological Nursing*, 33(2): 31–9.

Cohen-Mansfield, J. and Lipson, S. (2002) Pain in cognitively impaired nursing home residents: How well are physicians diagnosing it? *Journal of the American Geriatrics Society* 50(6): 1039–44.

Cohen-Mansfield, J. and Lipson, S. (2008) The utility of pain assessment for analgesic use in persons with dementia. *Pain,* 134(1–2): 16–23.

Cohen–Mansfield, J. and Marx, M.S. (1990) The relationship between sleep disturbances and agitation in a nursing home. *Journal of Aging and Health*, 2(1): 153–65. Also abstracted in *Abstracts in Social Gerontology*, 33(1): 114.

Cohen-Mansfield, J., Marx, M.S. and Rosenthal, A.S. (1989) A description of agitation in a nursing home. *Journal of Gerontology*, 44: 77–84.

Cohen-Mansfield, J., Marx, M.S. and Werner, P. (1992a) Observational data on time use and behavior problems in the nursing home. *Journal of Applied Gerontology*, 11(1): 111–21.

Cohen-Mansfield, J., Marx, M.S. and Werner, P. (1992b) Agitation in elderly persons: An integrative report of findings in a nursing home. *International Psychogeriatrics*, 4(Suppl. 2): 221–41.

Cohen-Mansfield, J., Parpura-Gill, A. and Golander, H. (2006a) Utilization of self identity roles for designing interventions for persons with dementia. *Journal of Gerontology: Psychological Sciences*, 61B(4): 202–12.

Cohen-Mansfield, J., Parpura-Gill., A. and Golander, H. (2006b) Salience of self-identity roles in persons with dementia: Differences in perceptions among patients themselves, family members and caregivers. *Social Science & Medicine*, 62(3): 745–57.

Cohen-Mansfield, J., Taylor, L. and Werner, P. (1998) Delusions and hallucinations in an adult day care population. *American Journal of Geriatric Psychiatry*, 6(2): 104–21.

Cohen-Mansfield, J. and Werner, P. (1995) Environmental influences on agitation: An integrative summary of an observational study. *American Journal of Alzheimer's Care and Related Disorders and Research*, 10(1): 32–7.

Cohen-Mansfield, J. and Werner, P. (1997) Management of verbally disruptive behaviors in nursing home residents. *Journal of Gerontology: Biological Sciences and Medical Sciences*, 52A(6): M369–M377.

Cohen-Mansfield, J. and Werner, P. (1998a) The effects of an enhanced environment on nursing home residents who pace. *The Gerontologist*, 38(2): 199–208.

Cohen-Mansfield, J. and Werner, P. (1998b) Visits to an outdoor garden: Impact on behavior and mood of nursing home residents who pace. In: B. Vellas, J. Fitten and G. Frisoni (eds) *Research and Practice in Alzheimer's Disease*. Paris: Serdi, pp. 419–36.

Cohen-Mansfield, J. and Werner, P. (1999) Outdoor wandering parks for persons with dementia: A survey of characteristics and use. *Alzheimer's Disease and Associated Disorders*, 13: 109–17.

Cohen-Mansfield, J., Werner, P. and Freedman, L. (1995) Sleep and agitation in agitated nursing home residents: An observational study. *Sleep*, 18(8): 674–80.

Deutsch, L.H., Bylsma, F.W., Rovner, B.W., Steele, C. and Folstein, M.F. (1991) Psychosis and physical aggression in probable Alzheimer's disease. *American Journal of Psychiatry*, 148(9): 1159–63.

Douzjian, M., Wilson, C., Shultz, M. *et al.* (1998) A program to use pain control medication to reduce psychotropic drug use in residents with difficult behavior. *Annals of Long Term Care*, 6(5): 174–9.

Feldt, K.S. (2000) Improving assessment and treatment of pain in cognitively impaired nursing home residents. *Annals of Long Term Care*, 8(9): 36–42.

Gerdner, L.A. (2000) Effects of individualized versus classical 'relaxation' music on the frequency of agitation in elderly persons with Alzheimer's disease and related disorders. *International Psychogeriatrics*, 12(1): 49–65.

Grasel, E., Wiltfang, J. and Kornhuber, J. (2003) Non-drug therapies for dementia: An overview of the current situation with regard to proof of effectiveness. *Dementia and Geriatric Cognitive Disorders*, 15(3): 115–25.

Hart, B. and Wells, D. (1997) The effects of language used by caregivers on agitation in residents with dementia. *Clinical Nurse Specialist*, 11(1): 20–3.

Hellen, C. (1999) *Alzheimer's Disease: Activity Focused Care*. Woburn, MA: Butterworth-Heinemann.

Huffman, J.C., Kunik, M.E. (2000) Assessment and understanding of pain in patients with dementia. *The Gerontologist*, 40(5): 574–81.

Hurley, A.C., Volicer, B.J., Hanrahan, P.A., Houde, S. and Volicer, L. (1992) Assessment of discomfort in advanced Alzheimer patients. *Research in Nursing and Health*, 15: 369–77.

Kasl-Godley, J. and Gatz, M. (2000) Psychosocial interventions for individuals with dementia: An integration of theory, therapy, and a clinical understanding of dementia. *Clinical Psychology Review*, 20(6): 755–82.

Kitwood, T. (1997) *Dementia Reconsidered: The Person Comes First*. Buckingham: Open University Press.

Lachs, M.S., Becker, M., Siegal, A.P. *et al.* (1992) Delusions and behavioral disturbances in cognitively impaired elderly persons. *Journal of the American Geriatrics Society*. 40(8): 768–73.

Leverett, M. (1991) Approaches to problem behaviors in dementia. *Physical and Occupational Therapy in Geriatrics*, 9(3–4): 93–105.

Libin, A. and Cohen-Mansfield, J. (2004) Therapeutic robocat for nursing home residents with dementia: Preliminary inquiry. *American Journal of Alzheimer's Disease and Other Dementias*, 19: 111–16.

Marsden, J.P., Meehan, R.A. and Calkins, M.P. (2001) Therapeutic kitchens for residents with dementia. *American Journal of Alzheimer's Disease and Other Dementias*. 16: 303–11.

Maslow, A.H. (1968) *Toward a Psychology of Being*. New York: D. Van Nostrand Co.

Maslow, A.H. (1987) *Motivation and Personality*, 3rd ed. New York: Harper and Row.

Mayers, K. and Griffin, M. (1990) The Play Project: Use of stimulus objects with demented patients. *Journal of Gerontological Nursing*, 16(1): 32–7.

Mishima, M.K., Okawa, M. and Hishikawa, Y. (1994) Morning bright light therapy for sleep and behavior disorders in elderly patients with dementia. *Acta Psychiatrica Scandanvica*, 89: 1–7.

Mutch, W.J. (1992) Parkinsonism and other movement disorders. In: J.C. Brocklehurst, R.C. Tallis and H.M. Fillit *Book of Geriatric Medicine and Gerontology*. Edinburgh: Churchill Livingstone, p. 423.

Namazi, K.H. and Johnson, B.D. (1992) Pertinent autonomy for residents with dementias: Modification of the physical environment to enhance independence. *American Journal of Alzheimer's Care and Related Disorders and Research*, 7(1): 16–21.

Namazi, K.H., Rosner, T.T. and Calkins, M.P. (1989) Visual barriers to prevent ambulatory Alzheimer's patients from exiting through an emergency door. *The Gerontologist*, 29(5): 699–702.

Negley, E.N. and Manley, J.T. (1990) Environmental interventions in assaultive behavior. *Journal of Gerontological Nursing*. 16: 29–33.

Okawa, M., Mishima, K., Hishikawa, Y., Hozumi, S., Hori, H. and Takashi, K. (1991) Circadian rhythm disorders in sleep – waking and body temperature in elderly patients with dementia and their treatment. *Sleep*, 14(6): 478–85.

Opie, J., Rosewarne, R. and O'Connor, D. (1999) The efficacy of psychosocial approaches to behaviour disorders in dementia: A systematic literature review. *Australia and New Zealand Journal of Psychiatry*, 33: 789–99.

Palmer, C.V., Adams, S.W., Bourgeois, M., Durrant, J. and Rossi, M. (1999) Reduction in caregiver-identified problem behavior in patients with Alzheimer Disease post hearing-aid fitting. *Journal of Speech, Language and Hearing Research*, 42: 312–28.

Parpura-Gill, A. and Cohen-Mansfield, J. (2006) Utilization of self-identity roles in individualized activities designed to enhance well-being in persons with dementia. In: L. Hyer and R.C. Intrieri (eds) *Geropsychological Interventions in Long-Term Care*. New York: Springer, pp. 157–84.

Ripich, D.N. (1994) Functional communication with AD patients: A caregiver training program. *Alzheimer's Disease and Associated Disorders*, 8(3): 95–109.

Ripich, D.N., Wykle, M. and Niles, S. (1995) Alzheimer's disease caregivers: the focused program. A communication skills training program helps nursing assistants to give better care to patients with disease. *Geriatric Nursing*, 16(1): 15–19.

Russen-Rondinone, T. and DesRoberts, A.M. (1996) Success through individual recreation: Working with the low-functioning resident with dementia or Alzheimer's disease. *American Journal of Alzheimer's Disease and Other Dementias*, 11(1): 32–5.

Ryden, M., Bossenmaier, M. and McLachlan, C. (1991) Aggressive behavior in cognitively impaired nursing home residents. *Research in Nursing and Health*, 4: 87–95.

Siders, C., Nelson, A., Brown, L.M. *et al.* (2004) Evidence for implementing nonpharmacological interventions for wandering. *Rehabilitative Nursing*, 29(6): 195–206.

Small, J.A. and Gutman, G. (2002) Recommended and reported use of communication strategies in Alzheimer caregiving. *Alzheimer's Disease and Associated Disorders*, 16: 270–8.

Small, J.A., Gutman, G., Makela, S. and Hillhouse, B. (2003) Effectiveness of communication strategies used by caregivers of persons with Alzheimer's disease during activities of daily living. *Journal of Speech, Language and Hearing Research*, 46: 353–67.

Sloane, P.D., Hoeffer, B., Mitchell, C.M. *et al.* (2004) Effect of person-centered showering and the towel bath on bathing-associated aggression, agitation, and discomfort in nursing home residents with dementia: A randomized, controlled trial. *Journal of the American Geriatrics Society*, 52: 1795–804.

Snowden, M., Sato, K. and Roy-Byrne, P. (2003) Assessment and treatment of nursing home residents with depression or behavioral symptoms associated with dementia: A review of the literature. *Journal of the American Geriatrics Society*, 51: 1305–17.

Snyder, M., Egan, E.C. and Burns, K.R. (1995) Interventions for decreasing agitation behaviors in persons with dementia. *Journal of Gerontology Nursing*, 21(7): 34–40.

Steiger, M., Quin, N., Toone, B. and Marsden, C. (1991) Off-period screaming accompanying motor fluctuations in Parkinson's disease. *Movement Disorders*, 6: 89–90.

Tappen, R.M., Williams-Burgess, C., Edelstein, J., Touhy, T. and Fishman, S. (1997) Communicating with individuals with Alzheimer's disease: Examination of recommended strategies. *Archives of Psychiatric Nursing*, 11(5): 249–56.

Teri, L. and Logsdon, R.G. (1991) Identifying pleasant activities for Alzheimer's disease patients: The pleasant events schedule–AD. *The Gerontologist*, 31(1): 124–7.

Werner, P., Cohen–Mansfield, J., Braun, J. and Marx, M.S. (1989) Physical restraints and agitation in nursing home residents. *Journal of the American Geriatrics Society*, 37(12): 1122–6.

Werner, P., Cohen-Mansfield, J., Fischer, J. and Segal, G. (2000) Characterization of family-generated videotapes for the management of verbally disruptive behaviors. *Journal of Applied Gerontology*, 19(1): 42–57.

Werner, P., Cohen-Mansfield, J., Koroknay, V. and Braun, J. (1994) Reducing restraints: Impact on staff attitudes. *Journal of Gerontology Nursing*. 20(12): 19–24.

Whall, A., Black, M., Groh, C., Yankou, D., Kupferschmid, B. and Foster, N. (1997) The effect of natural environments upon agitation and aggression in late stage dementia patients. *American Journal of Alzheimer's Disease and Other Dementias*, 12(5): 216–20.

Woods, P., Ashley, J., Snowden, M., Sato, K. and Roy-Byrne, P. (2003) Simulated presence therapy: Using selected memories to manage problem behaviors in Alzheimer's disease patients. *Geriatric Nursing* 16(1): 9–14.

Yeh, S.H., Lin, L.W., Wang, S.Y., Wu, S.Z., Lin, J.H. and Tsai, F.M. (2001) The outcomes of restraint reduction programme in nursing homes. Abstract (article in Chinese). *Hu Li Yan Jiu*; 9(2): 183–93.

Zachow, K.M. (1984) Helen, can you hear me? *Journal of Gerontological Nursing.* 18(8): 18–22.

Zgola, J.M.L. (1987) *Doing Things: A Guide to Programming Activities for Persons with Alzheimer's Disease and Related Disorders.* Baltimore, MD: Johns Hopkins University Press.

Zisselman, M.H,, Rovner, B.W., Shmuely, Y. and Ferrie, P. (1996) A pet therapy intervention with geriatric psychiatry inpatients. *American Journal of Occupational Therapy*, 50(1): 47–51.

12

Communication and relationships: an inclusive social world

Kate Allan and John Killick

Learning objectives

By the end of this chapter you will:

- understand the significance of communication in the lives of people with dementia, and those who support them
- have an appreciation of both the possibilities and challenges in terms of achieving genuine communication with people who have dementia in various contexts
- have considered a range of value-laden issues which are raised in the course of exploring this subject
- learn about two particular strands of communication work which show real promise in empowering people with dementia to share their views, experiences and needs, and in furthering the effort to understand the complexities of the condition

---

Introduction

As social animals, we conduct our lives in the context of relationships which rely on communication. Communicating with others – friends, relatives, colleagues, neighbours and fellow citizens – allows us to achieve the things we need to do to survive and flourish in all sorts of ways – physically, emotionally, in terms of activity and occupation, and at a spiritual level. Each of our individual relationships is unique and differs along a multitude of dimensions, for example, how the relationship formed, its purpose or core activities, its level of intimacy, style of communication involved. Our changing networks of relationships reflect the stage we are at in life and what is important to us.

Human communication is highly diverse. The use of language has been identified as one of the defining characteristics of the human species. Linguistic communication can take a variety of forms – spoken, written and signed. Alongside and interacting with language, we rely on many nonverbal channels of communication including facial expression, gesture, eye contact and touch. We also use a range of forms of creativity, for example, drama, painting, sculpture, photography, dance, film and literature. These may cross the boundary between language and nonverbal communication.

Communication plays a central part in our concept of identity, both as individuals and as members of groups. The particular ways in which each of us communicates form a large part of how others come to recognize us as unique individuals. However, the fact of our personal uniqueness exists within complex patterns of commonality which constitute another dimension of identity, that of culture.

As well as being very much a day-to-day, practical reality, the sphere of human communication and relationships is underpinned by many complex and value-laden issues:

- what counts as a valid relationship

- what is regarded as meaningful communication

- what happens to relationships when there are differences in power between people.

Work with people with dementia has a way of highlighting many of these issues, as we shall see in what follows.

The chapter begins by describing why communication is so fundamental to work with people with dementia. We then go on to chart the progress which brought about agreement that people continue to communicate no matter how cognitively disabled they are. Following this, we describe the state of current knowledge in the field, opening with a description of the changes typically associated with dementia which impact on communication and relationships, highlighting the role of psychological and social factors in such changes. This is followed by a discussion of the issues raised by communication and relationships within families, recognizing that most people with dementia live with family members, before going on to examine communication and relationships between care staff and people with dementia. Arguments for the usefulness of the concept of relationship-centred care in making explicit the centrality of relationship to good dementia care are discussed. Finally the chapter focuses on two overlapping areas within the field: communication using creative arts and communication with people with advanced dementia.

Dementia, communication and relationships

Twenty years ago it was generally believed that the development of dementia gradually destroyed the capacity of an individual to communicate and have meaningful relationships with others (Kitwood 1997). As discussed by Steve Sabat in Chapter 4, 'A bio-psycho-social approach', in the last 20 years there has been a move away from a purely medical understanding of dementia to a recognition of the psychological and social factors which influence its expression. As discussed by Julian Hughes in Chapter 7, 'Being minded in dementia', another significant change in the last 20 years has been the recognition that persons with dementia are still, first and foremost, persons, and with this comes the realization that just as communication plays a central role in all of our lives, the same applies to people with dementia.

The subject of communication can be seen as pertinent to work with people with dementia for a number of reasons. First of all Kitwood's argument about personhood (1997) asserts that all of us are only persons by virtue of being in relationship with others, meaning that communication is crucial to the reality of personhood. We signal our recognition of the personhood of other human beings by communicating with them. Whenever we stop attempting to communicate with those around us, we are withdrawing our regard for them as persons. And since we rely on others for the maintenance of our own personhood, we also damage ourselves.

Second, there can be no doubt that one of the major changes we see in persons with dementia is in the sphere of communication. More detailed discussion of the specific ways in which communication is commonly affected in dementia follows later.

A third reason why communication is a key issue to consider in understanding the needs of people with dementia arises out of the fact that although we have seen much progress in the past 20 years or so, we are still at an early stage of understanding the nature of dementia as a condition. Progress in this area must rely on genuine communication with people who live with dementia and those who support them (Cotrell and Schulz 1993).

Fourth, it is difficult to imagine any form of care or support which does not involve communication, and therefore quality care and effective support are dependent on achieving genuine communication. A large part of the rest of this chapter is concerned in various ways with this subject.

Our final reason for stressing the centrality of communication to the understanding of dementia draws on a more values-orientated perspective. The attempt to achieve genuine communication with persons who are experiencing such profound changes in their lives and relationships forces us to confront what are essentially moral issues about why and how we value persons. The bioethicist Stephen Post has drawn our attention to the 'hypercognitive' nature of much of Western culture, in which 'clarity of mind and economic productivity determine the value of a human life' (1995: 3). Within such a culture, our natural bias is to disregard or devalue the kinds of relationships and communication (with adults at least) which seem to lie outside the domain of full cognitive competence. Contact with people with dementia can invite us to value different aspects of being human, and to engage in different ways, for example at a physical, emotional or spiritual level.

In addressing some of these issues we will look not only at problems but also provide examples of situations in which the creativity and resourcefulness of those involved have resulted in new ways forward being found, and unhelpful assumptions being challenged. A favourite example of this comes from the writings of Laurel Rust (1986), who was working at the time in a care home, about her relationship with Amy:

> Amy and I have developed an intimacy that is hard to describe, an intimacy that makes me think of companionship differently because Amy does not know my name and has never asked. We sit and simply take up talking, wherever and whenever we are. Talking with Amy who 'exhibits no orientation to reality' is a wonderful experience in which we are always in the present, and the present could be anything we choose to create between us.

(Rust 1986: 140)

Changes in communication

We begin with a brief description of the changes in communication commonly seen in persons with dementia. The term aphasia is a general one used to refer to a range of difficulties with language, including those observed in dementia. Typical features in early to moderate dementia include difficulties with word finding which may result in the person 'talking around' the word that is causing difficulty, confusion with pronouns such as 'he' and 'she', reduced fluency overall, and difficulties with comprehension of more complex utterances. The later stages of the condition are frequently characterized by the emergence of features such as pronounced reduction of language use, difficulties producing sounds, the repetitive utterance of words or phrases, and the person becoming 'stuck' on repeating certain sounds. Whereas it is broadly true that individuals with dementia demonstrate a progressive picture as regards difficulties with language, research shows that considerable variability exists in patterns of change even between individuals diagnosed with the same form of dementia, and between different forms of the condition (Bryan and Maxim 2006).

It is important to note that the kinds of changes we see in the way individuals with dementia communicate do not necessarily arise directly from damage to the brain. Psychological factors such as loss of confidence, anxiety and depression can all have a profound effect on the way individuals communicate. Further to this, a major aspect of Kitwood's (1997) contribution to the reconceptualization of dementia was his illumination of the impact of a range of interpersonal processes which he termed 'malignant social psychology'. Examples of these are 'outpacing' when others consistently act or communicate at a pace which is too fast for the person with dementia, and 'objectification' which refers to the act of treating the person as if they were an inanimate object. Such processes, while not consciously intended to be damaging, have the effect of undermining the person's opportunities to communicate with others in a meaningful way and therefore to have their personhood enacted. Whatever their cause, however, changes in how people communicate often bring real distress to all parties, and can have a considerable impact on relationships. However, although such changes have traditionally been framed as evidence of an irreversible process of loss, the last decade or so has seen the emergence of alternative perspectives which question this kind of hopelessness.

Much less attention has been given to changes in the use of nonverbal forms of communication in persons with dementia. However, a study by Hubbard *et al.* (2002) has made an important contribution to this subject. Researchers spent time in a day centre identifying the incidence of nonverbal communication, both as an adjunct to speech and as a form of communication in its own right. They observed instances of people with dementia using nonverbal means to initiate interactions, to describe their own difficulties, and to signal needs such as visiting the toilet. Nonverbal humour was apparent, as was evidence that participants with dementia were active in interpreting others' nonverbal communication. The authors concluded that: 'recognizing and working with nonverbal communication may be one of the ways in which caregivers can contribute towards the preservation of self-identity and personae, and thus contribute towards improving quality of life and care' (Hubbard *et al.* 2002: 164).

The subject of nonverbal communication, and the strengths of people with dementia in this regard, needs much more exploration and development work.

The role of communication in well-being

> **Exercise 12.1** Using humour
>
> Cary Smith Henderson, a man with dementia, said: 'Laughing is absolutely wonderful. A sense of humour is probably the most important valuable thing you can have when you have Alzheimer's' (Henderson and Andrews 1998: 14).
>
> What roles do you think could humour play in helping people to live with dementia?
>
> Try to think of an example of the successful use of humour in a situation with someone with dementia.

We now move to considering the developments which have occurred in the dementia field following the positive impact of Kitwood's (1997) argument for a relationship-based concept of personhood, and attention to the social and psychological aspects of dementia. This has triggered a flourishing of many new and exciting ways of working, and many of these are concerned directly or indirectly with the subjects of communication and relationships. We now have a considerable body of findings from research, practice experience and accounts from people with dementia themselves, family members and friends which demonstrates that genuine communication is possible and vital to the well-being of all involved. This section of the chapter will present an overview of this learning.

Malcolm Goldsmith's book *Hearing the Voice of People with Dementia* (1996) represents a landmark in terms of thinking about communication. Based mainly on the views of those working in the field, Goldsmith's conclusion was unequivocal:

> It is possible to be involved in meaningful communication with the majority of people with dementia *but* we must be able to enter into their world, understand their sense of pace and time, recognize the problems of distraction and realize that there are many ways in which people express themselves and *it is our responsibility* to learn how to recognize these.

(Goldsmith 1996: 165, author's emphases)

Among many key messages of this work, including the importance of slowing the pace of communication, the effect of the environment on interaction, and the communicative function of so-called 'challenging behaviour', Goldsmith stressed the need to recognize the distinctiveness of the person's own subjective experience of dementia. As discussed by Alison Phinney in Chapter 3, we need to continue to find ways of learning more about the inner world of the person with dementia, and to understand the implications of this dimension for how we think about dementia as a condition and offer support to those who are living with it.

One very positive development of this need has come about through people with dementia themselves speaking out about their experiences, needs and views. This activity has taken a variety of forms including the publication of writings; the production of videos and DVDs featuring people talking about their perspectives; the appointment of people with dementia as voting members of organizations such as the Alzheimer's Society; their inclusion as speakers at conferences and other events, and the launch of organizations run by people with dementia which campaign for changes in attitudes and improvements in services. In the latter category there is the Scottish Dementia Working Group (which is now part of Alzheimer Scotland (www.alzscot.org/pages/sdwg/aboutus.htm), the Alzheimer's Forum (which is part of the Alzheimer's Society in England, Wales and Northern Ireland) and the Dementia Advocacy and Support Network International (www.dasninternational.org), which is a web-based organization enabling participation of people all over the world. The emergence of people with dementia themselves as a force for social change represents a significant step forward in addressing the problem of their long-standing social exclusion. This area of work is discussed more fully by Rachael Litherland in Chapter 22.

Communication in family contexts

In setting out to explore this subject, we are usefully reminded of the complexity of the terrain by Cary Smith Henderson, a man with young onset dementia who kept a journal about his experiences. He wrote:

> One of the things about this is – it's in the family and the family has not only me and my wife, but we have our children and the children have their spouses. In other words, this whole thing about Alzheimer's is not just about two people; it's about a whole mess of people. Not only our families but our extended families and their friends. It gets very very involved.
>
> (Henderson and Andrews 1998: 65)

As Henderson and Andrews (1998) so eloquently describe, the development of a condition such as dementia in one of its members is bound to affect the whole family. And, as we all know, families are complex! In addition to practical day-to-day routines and arrangements, financial matters and how decisions are made, there are all the intricate and involved emotional dimensions of relationships. Some of these relate to issues of power and deeply held values and beliefs. Most family relationships have a long history, and of course issues which go back many years can have an ongoing influence on the quality of our relationships with relatives. These multifaceted and personal issues are fundamental to our sense of who we are and how we fit into our social worlds. As each family is unique in its strengths and needs, the effect of dementia in one of its members will be unique. However, the changes which accompany dementia will represent a challenge to the established ways of most families' functioning in profound ways, and as relatives provide most of the care required by people with dementia, the challenges can be great (see Chapter 5).

Given the fundamental role of communication in enabling all those involved to live with dementia, there is a considerable body of work exploring ways for those who have known the person prior to the onset of their dementia to adjust their styles of communicating in order to support the continuation of relationships. An important contribution has been made by Steven Sabat (2001). His book largely consists of painstaking analyses of a series of interactions with a small number of individuals, and he describes some of the characteristics of successful conversations. He draws attention to the importance of turn-taking, of not interrupting and thus breaking the pattern, speaking clearly and slowly, and allowing the other person time to collect their thoughts. He has formulated the concept of 'indirect repair' which he defines as follows:

> Inquiring about the intention of the speaker, through the use of questions marked not by interrogatives but by intonation patterns, to the use of rephrasing what you think the speaker said and checking to see if you understood his or her meaning correctly.

> (Sabat 2001: 38–9)

By using such subtle 'cooperative strategies' one can help conversation to flow smoothly without outpacing the other person.

Using her knowledge and skills as a communication scientist and drawing on her experience of supporting her mother who had dementia, Jane Crisp (2000) has written about ways of 'keeping in touch' with a person with dementia. This includes advice about ways of making sense of apparently confused speech, and also responding in empathic and creative ways to the stories the person with dementia tells rather than dismissing a story as confused or simply untrue. There is also very good advice about understanding how nonverbal aspects of communication contribute to the whole picture.

While progress has been made in this area, we have a long way to go in developing the kinds of policies and practices which properly support the large number of people who provide care within a family context for people with dementia. However, despite the difficulties, we have begun to see the emergence of a kind of writing which demonstrates a balanced approach to both the possibility of gain and development, as well as the reality of loss. A notable example comes from a book written by Sunny Vogler called *Dementia: The Loss … The Love … The Laughter* (2003). The author had a very difficult relationship with her mother during her early life which was characterized by turmoil and estrangement. Having taken the decision to care for her mother when she developed dementia, she writes:

> Mother was different, and discovering who she was each day was a delight. The bitterness she had lived with was draining from her mind … and in its place was a new pleasant outlook that seemed to surprise and please us both. More than once she gave me a loving look and simply

whispered 'Thank you'. These were the rewards I had missed in my childhood and were so welcome now.

(Vogler 2003: 37)

Exercise 12.2   Dealing with a dilemma

You visit a service where you meet a number of people with dementia for the first time. One person seems especially drawn to you, and, on engaging in conversation, it becomes clear that the person is convinced that you are a much-missed relative, and is delighted that you have at last come to visit them.

How would you handle this situation?

What does this tell you about your values?

Communication and relationships with care staff

While most care for people with dementia is provided within a family, many experience care in an institutional setting. In this discussion we will consider two research projects which have closely examined the nature of communication and relationships in care homes. Prior to this, however, it seems important to remind ourselves that Kitwood's concept of personhood emphasizes that one can only be truly a person if we are recognized as such by others, and that this applies as much to staff as it does to the person with dementia. It follows, then, that the personhood of care staff is put at risk when communication is absent. This is demonstrated in the following quotation from a member of staff in a Swedish care setting:

> When you cannot get into contact with the patient you feel insufficient, without hope, dissatisfied or burnt out. Care seems meaningless. You lose your commitment.

(Ekman *et al.* 1991: 168)

The first of the studies we consider here was conducted by Anne Vittoria (1998) in an Alzheimer's special care unit in America. Vittoria observed that something special was occurring in the unit, and set out to investigate its nature. This resulted in her characterizing what she found as 'communicative care', and in an attempt to analyse the special characteristics of such care, Vittoria explores a range of concepts. These include 'felt meaning' which is 'non-cognitive understanding developed between residents and staff'; 'initiating' which is 'the process of entering into negotiation with a resident mindful of the possibilities'; and 'nurturing' which is 'building on achievements in a spirit of celebration', and involves 'recognizing a continuing *capacity for creating meaning* from those under one's care' (Vittoria 1998: 28, author's italics).

She concluded that successful care occurred when staff Certified Nurses' Aids (CNAs) were mindful of these aspects of interaction, and describes the caring situation generally in these terms:

> In this world, staff and residents are not positioned as benefactor–supplicant and caregiving is rooted in two things: the relationship between staff and residents ... and ... the relationship among the CNAs themselves as individuals and as a team ... Most important, the nature of care can *only* be understood within these relational connections between and among the staff and residents.

(Vittoria 1998: 129)

This study demonstrates that it is possible to provide high quality support for people with dementia where communication has its rightful central place. It also highlights the importance of high quality communication between members of staff supporting their sense of personhood.

However, the findings of a recent, large-scale UK study provides very different perspectives on the current situation of many people with dementia with regard to communication and relationships. The three-year study was carried out by Richard Ward and colleagues (Ward *et al.* 2005, 2006a, 2006b) and took place in various kinds of services. Its purpose was to investigate the skills required to provide good care for people with dementia. The findings summarized here concentrate on residential care. The field work involved direct observation and making video recordings of daily care work, together with interviews with persons with dementia, relatives and staff.

During the project the researchers formulated the view that 'dementia is communication' (Ward *et al.* 2005: 22), meaning that caring for people with dementia is essentially finding ways to communicate even when these may be unfamiliar or difficult to make sense of. Nevertheless, a major finding was that on average each individual person with dementia spent no more than 2% of the day in communication with care workers. Overall 78% of the encounters which did take place were concerned with specific care tasks, and much of this interaction proceeded in silence. When verbal interaction did occur, it was fairly impoverished and tended to conform to a routinized form of 'care speak' (Ward *et al.* 2005: 18). Encounters which were characterized by warmth were observed but these were infrequent. The authors comment that much of the behaviour of care staff seemed to serve to avoid rather than encourage communication.

On talking to staff about their experiences, a range of factors emerged which put these starkly negative findings in context. Staff participants described the tension they experience in being aware of opportunities to engage more fully with residents but being limited by the sheer amount of work to be done in a given time, and the way care tasks are organized. This highlights a crucial point: that although it may appear that an individual staff member has control over the way they respond to a resident on a given occasion, this encounter is actually part of a much larger, more complex and less visible system which exerts an influence on what takes place. Another implicit dimension is that of what the authors term the 'invisible workload' staff manage in terms of dealing with both their own emotional experiences regarding their work and in encountering emotion in residents (Ward *et al.* 2006a: 28). Those who look after people with dementia are described as an 'overlooked workforce' (Ward *et al.* 2006a: 28) who have little opportunity to share their experiences and reflect on their implications.

The authors describe many ways in which, despite the impoverishment of the general context, residents of care homes continue to communicate, and these bear a striking resemblance to the conclusions of Goldsmith (1996) 10 years previously. However, their overall conclusion is not an encouraging one:

> Evidence from our study suggests that the development of skills and of the potential for expertise in communication remains submerged and unsupported in dementia care settings. There is little opportunity for workers to share their insights or even to articulate what it is they do. The way care homes are organized fails to promote communication as a crucial dimension of care practice.

> (Ward *et al.* 2006b: 24)

This major study tells us that despite the advances in our understanding of the place of communication in supporting people with dementia, and the existence of examples of excellent practice, the general situation has not changed in fundamental ways. We clearly have a long way to go in putting what we know into action.

From person-centred to relationship-centred care

The impetus for much of the progress in this field has come from the emergence of the concept of person-centred care. The robustness and practical implications of this concept continue to be a focus of discussion and debate (Brooker 2006), and partly as a response to the problems of implementing such a model and a recognition that people exist within a network of relationships, the concept of 'relationship-centred care' has developed (Nolan *et al.* 2003).

In this vein, Adams and Gardiner (2005) explored different patterns of communication within dementia care triads, which typically comprise the person with the condition, a relative and a professional. They describe 'enabling dementia communication', which

> occurs when informal carers or health and social care professionals either help the person with dementia express their thoughts, feelings and wishes or represent the person with dementia as someone who is able to make decisions about their own care.

> (Adams and Gardiner 2005: 190)

Such communication arises through efforts to remove unwanted stimuli, get in the right position physically, promote equal participation, and be sensitive to nonverbal cues. 'Disabling' communication is characterized by practices such as interrupting, speaking on behalf of the person, using language which is too technical or complex, and talking out of earshot.

John Keady and Mike Nolan (2003) carried out a study exploring how couples, who were still at an early stage of coming to terms with the condition coped with this challenge. They interviewed both family members and persons with dementia. As a result of this, they identified four kinds of relationship. Three of these are variants on both partners working as single units, but one describes a situation where the partners are working together to make the best of the situation.

An example of what could be considered the latter type of relationship is described by Ingrid Hellström and colleagues (Hellström *et al.* 2005). They present a case study of a couple, Mr and Mrs Svensson, who are in their eighties and live in Sweden. Mrs Svensson developed dementia within four years of their getting married. This study provides both indications of what are successful approaches of communication, and also an example of how dementia is not always a burden which has damaging effects on relationships. They describe how 'whilst surprised by the diagnosis, for both partners this turn of events provided yet further meaning as to why they married late in life'. The researchers identified ways in which Mr Svensson included his wife in communication, and 'demonstrated both remarkable sensitivity to her needs and great ingenuity in providing assistance that actively reinforced, rather than undermined, his wife's sense of agency' (Hellström *et al.* 2005: 13). The authors' conclusions are that:

> rather than the person coming first in dementia … there is a case for considering that, for spouses at least, the 'couple' might be the primary focus. The concept of 'couplehood' therefore potentially provides a more nuanced understanding of the ways in which spouses 'do things together'.
>
> (Hellström *et al.* 2005: 19)

Mike Nolan and colleagues (Nolan *et al.* 2003) admit that the concept of relationship-centred care needs further clarification and development. Certainly whilst the model can be considered to correspond more closely to the reality of most people's lives, it does not seem likely that implementing such care on a widespread basis will prove any less of a challenge than that of delivering so-called person-centred care.

Communication through the arts

An exciting strand of work in the area of communication looks at the potential of creative activities as a means for people with dementia to express feelings, experiences and needs, and to maintain relationships and develop new ones. A seminal text in this field comes from Selly Jenny and Marilyn Oropeza in California (Jenny and Oropeza 1994). Their account of integrating painting into a day care programme in an Alzheimer's branch has inspired a great deal of subsequent work in this area. The authors comment:

> As we stand before their paintings, they call out to us in a way we cannot ignore. They tell us their stories in a language we all understand,

transmitted feelings and emotions trapped inside. Slipping beyond the language of words, their paintings show us glimpses of who they were and who they still are.

(Jenny and Oropeza 1994: back cover)

In the UK, appreciation of the capacity for meaningful communication through the arts began with John Killick's work in the field of poetry. On initially encountering people with dementia living in a nursing home, Killick (who is himself a writer and poet) found their speech and actions puzzling and even alienating. However, with a degree of immersion in the context he realized that while their language was not always easy to interpret in conventional terms, it had a metaphorical richness and used images which could, with the right kind of encouragement and attention, convey very powerful messages (Killick and Allan 2001). Killick's work has resulted in two books of poems exclusively from the words of people with dementia (Killick 1997; Killick and Cordonnier 2000).

One day a woman living in a nursing home and during a conversation with Killick demanded: 'The arts is all that's left. Give them us!' He took this as a cue for what the exploration of all the arts can contribute to communication. He mounted a series of pilot projects in different art forms throughout the UK, and this resulted in books, packs and videos demonstrating the role that creativity can play in supporting people with dementia. The publications also act as practice guides for those wishing to make use of these approaches (see www.dementia.stir.ac.uk). A more general volume about initiating, running and evaluating work in this area followed. This was a collaboration between Anne Davis Basting and Killick (2003); Basting had already developed a group storytelling method in the US called Timeslips (www.timeslips.org).

Occupational therapist Claire Craig is also a major contributor in this field. She considers the potential of participation in the arts to address issues of social exclusion by providing opportunities for gaining a sense of control, increasing self-esteem and challenging negative perceptions (Craig and Killick 2004). On the theme of supporting relationships she has discussed ways of involving family members in creative activities alongside their relatives with dementia (Craig 2004). The value of this kind of work to one person with dementia is expressed in her own words: 'We've been on a wonderful journey, you and I. What fun we've had laughing and singing. Holding a rainbow in our hands (Craig 2001: 38).

Communication with people with advanced dementia

Considerable progress has been made in exploring communication and relationships in the earlier years of dementia. A more testing challenge is that of making meaningful contact with persons with much more profound disabilities and those close to death.

Although there has been little such work undertaken in the UK, this field has been the focus of a stream of practice-orientated research in Scandinavia, including studies investigating the occurrence of 'episodes of lucidity' in persons with advanced dementia (e.g. Normann *et al.* 2006). These are short periods when the person is able to function at a much higher level or demonstrate a much greater degree of awareness than would be expected given the severity of their usual disabilities. Normann *et al.* report that over half of a sample of 97 persons with advanced dementia exhibited episodes of lucidity, and this reinforces the need to look beyond the usual negative perception of individuals' capacity for meaningful relationship and communication.

Within the last few years in the UK, and partly as a result of the growing recognition of the need for people with dementia to have access to palliative care services, there are signs that the challenges of communicating with people in the very extremes of dementia are receiving attention. One of the spurs for this development has come from outside of the dementia field. Over the past decade in the United States, Arnold and Amy Mindell have developed an approach to communicating with those in coma (mainly following acquired brain injury). The approach is called 'coma work' and its most basic elements involve attempting to establish communication with the person by matching breathing, and using voice and touch in time with breathing rhythm. It also involves observing evidence of sensory orientation, movement, posture and position, and a wide range of other nonverbal signals very closely, and feeding back observations to the person (Mindell 1997).

To our knowledge the originators of coma work have not undertaken work specifically with persons with dementia. However, in 2004 an article by Rosemary Clarke was published which described her experience of using this approach with her mother. She comments:

> My experience has been, at times, sublime and I believe for her empowering ... [It has] been infinitely precious and enriching for me, and I commend this approach to others who would like to both give and gain deep satisfaction in their contact with those with dementia who are, largely, beyond words.

(Clarke 2004: 23)

Exercise 12.3　Exploring silence

Think of some reasons why periods of silence during interactions with a person with dementia might be helpful.

Try out having some conversations with family, friends and persons with dementia where silence is a more prominent feature than usual.

Reflect on how these experiences felt, and any effects silence had on other aspects of communication.

The Mindells' work has not concentrated on people with dementia, but in North America two practitioners trained by the Mindells, Tom Richards and Stan Tomandl, have now published a book focusing on this area (Richards and Tomandl 2006). They call their adaptation of the method 'Process Work', and it takes account of the fact that people with dementia are not actually in a coma. The book has a strong narrative element as it follows Tomandl's father,

Stanley, on the final four-and-a-half years of his 18-year journey into Alzheimer's. During this period he was in a nursing home, and the co-authors visited him regularly and used the kinds of communicative strategies described above. Stanley's responses included hand squeezing, occasional clearly meaningful speech, eye contact, joining in with singing and expressive gestures. The book gets its title, *An Alzheimer's Surprise Party*, from the final celebration of Stanley's life, in which he took a very active part, only 24 hours before he died.

In a very small-scale exploration carried out in Australia by the authors of this chapter, only the most basic techniques of the coma work approach were used with a small number of persons and the initiative took place over a very short time. Nevertheless, clear evidence of communicative capacity was found in individuals who were considered extremely disabled. This demanded considerable investments of time, often characterized by uncertainty that the attention was welcomed, but efforts were rewarded with eye contact, hand pressure, facial expression and vocalizations, some of which were clearly discernible speech (Killick and Allan 2006). This work raised many questions about the remaining capacity for individuals with long-standing and severe disabilities to engage meaningfully, and also the ethical dimensions of such work.

These small-scale studies indicate the need for a much more extended exploration of the potential of individuals at such extremes to continue to communicate meaningfully. Apart from benefits to the individual, progress in this area stands to benefit both professional and family carers, who are often at a loss as to how to connect with a person who appears to be remote for much or all of the time. Learning gained from such work could also be used to confer advantages in communicating with people at an earlier point in their dementia journey.

We hope that this chapter has provided some sense of the progress and possibilities inherent in this area, as well as the challenges and complexities. We conclude with a quotation from Faith Gibson which is an answer to her own question: Can we risk person-centred communication?

> We must employ whatever power we have in the world of dementia care for this purpose. We must use our present knowledge, our skills and feelings, to communicate. We are morally obliged to continue working in extending our limited understanding, developing our embryonic skills, and taming our deep anxieties.

(Gibson 1999: 24)

Debates and controversies

We have already referred to how work with people with very advanced dementia raises ethical issues. This situation is the most extreme example of a power differential which has to be handled with great care. For example, how might we know if a person welcomes our attention or wishes to be left alone? How should we interpret very minimal or ambiguous signals which may or may not constitute an act of communication? In a world where resources are limited, how much time and energy should be devoted to attempts to connect with a person who may appear not to respond? And with increasing emphasis on evidence-based care, how should we value outcomes which are transient and difficult to record, such as the squeeze of one's hand or simply having a strong sense of the person being engaged and present?

Recently a lively debate has developed about whether it is ever justified to lie to a person with dementia. Research suggests that it is common practice for care staff when, for example, confronted with a person asking where their (long dead) spouse is, to tell them that their wife has gone out and will be back later. James *et al.* (2006) maintain that such an approach may be the most 'therapeutic' one if others such as attempting to meet needs or distract have failed. Walker (2007) argues that such situations call for a more nuanced and sophisticated approach with attention, for instance, to possible symbolic dimensions of what is happening. Another view is that lying almost always indicates a lack of respect for the person and that the desire to alleviate distress is not sufficient to justify using such a strategy (Müller-Hergl 2007).

Conclusion

This chapter has argued that communication is essential to being a person and to our relationships with others. While it is usual to see changes in ways of communicating in the person with dementia, the need to maintain contact with others, and do so in a range of ways, remains and is crucial to well-being. Those in a supporting role are equally reliant on authentic communication if they are not to experience a sense of alienation and perhaps burn-out.

Work in this field has investigated ways of enhancing communication in both professional care and family contexts, and we have seen the emergence of people with dementia themselves speaking out about their experiences and needs. Despite the development of greater understanding of what is needed and what works, however, research indicates that communication still does not have its rightful central place in how care is organized and provided.

The chapter introduced two areas of work within the field of communication, namely communication through creativity and approaches to communicating with people with very advanced dementia. While at an early stage of development, both of these avenues show real promise in enabling people with dementia to take a more active role in their own lives, and enhancing the well-being of all involved. They also stand to increase our understanding of what it means to live with dementia, and how we should respond to the many complex questions it raises.

Further information

The Scottish Dementia Working Group is a group run by people with dementia. It campaigns to improve services for people with dementia and to reduce prejudice and stigma.

The Timeslips Project encourages people with memory loss to exercise their imagination and creativity. It has generated hundreds of stories used to produce plays and art exhibits.

Dementia Positive is the authors' website which encourages communication, consultation and creativity in work with people who have dementia. Available at www.dementiapositive.co.uk

The Dementia Services Development Centre at Stirling University has hosted several arts-based projects.

References

Adams, T. and Gardiner, P. (2005) Communication and interaction within dementia care triads: Developing a theory for relationship-centred care. *Dementia,* 4(2): 185–205.

Basting, A.D. (2003) Looking back from loss: Views of the self in Alzheimer's disease. *Journal of Aging Studies,* 17: 87–99.

Basting, A.D. and Killick, J. (2003) *The Arts in Dementia Care: A Resource Guide.* New York: National Center for Creative Aging.

Brooker, D. (2006) *Person-centred Dementia Care; Making Services Better.* London: Jessica Kingsley.

Bryan, K. and Maxim, J. (2006) *Communication Disability in the Dementias.* London: Whurr.

Clarke, R. (2004) Precious experiences beyond words. *Journal of Dementia Care,* 12(3): 22–3.

Cotrell, V. and Schulz, R. (1993) The perspective of the patient with Alzheimer's Disease: A neglected dimension of dementia research. *The Gerontologist,* 33(2): 205–11.

Craig, C. (2001) *Celebrating the Person: A Practical Approach to Arts Activities.* Stirling: Dementia Services Development Centre.

Craig, C. (2004) Creativity for carers. *Signpost,* 8(3): 4–5.

Craig, C. and Killick, J. (2004) Reaching out with the arts: Meeting the person with dementia. In: A. Innes, C. Archibald and C. Murphy (eds) *Dementia and Social Inclusion: Marginalised Groups and Marginalised Areas of Dementia Research, Care and Practice.* London: Jessica Kingsley.

Crisp, J. (2000) *Keeping in Touch with Someone Who Has Alzheimer's.* Melbourne: Ausmed Publications.

Ekman, S.L., Norberg, A., Viitanen, M. and Winblad, B. (1991) Care of demented patients with severe communication problems. *Scandinavian Journal of Caring Sciences,* 5(3): 163–70.

Gibson, F. (1999) Can we risk person-centred communication? *Journal of Dementia Care,* 7(5): 20–4.

Goldsmith, M. (1996) *Hearing the Voice of People with Dementia: Opportunities and Obstacles.* London: Jessica Kingsley.

Hellström, I., Nolan, M. and Lundh, U. (2005) 'We do things together': A case study of 'couplehood' in dementia. *Dementia,* 4(1): 7–22.

Henderson, C.S. and Andrews, N. (1998) *Partial View: An Alzheimer's Journal.* Dallas, TX: Southern Methodist University Press.

Hubbard, G., Cook, A., Tester, S. and Downs, M. (2002) Beyond words: Older people with dementia using and interpreting nonverbal behaviour. *Journal of Aging Studies,* 16(2): 155–67.

James, I.A., Wood-Mitchell, A.J., Waterworth, A.M., Mackenzie, L.E. and Cunningham, J. (2006) Lying to people with dementia within care settings: Developing ethical guidelines for care settings. *International Journal of Geriatric Psychiatry,* 21(8): 800–1.

Jenny, S. and Oropeza, M. (1994) *Memories in the Making: A Program of Creative Art Expression for Alzheimer's Patients.* Orange Co, CA: Alzheimer's Association of Orange County.

Keady, J. and Nolan, M.R. (2003) The dynamics of dementia: Working together, working separately, or working alone? In: M.R. Nolan *et al.* (eds) *Partnerships in Family Care: Understanding the Caregiving Career.* Buckingham: Open University Press.

Killick, J. (1997) *You are Words: Dementia Poems.* London: Hawker Publications.

Killick, J. and Allan, K. (2001) *Communication and the Care of People with Dementia.* Buckingham: Open University Press.

Killick, J. and Allan, K. (2006) Good Sunset Project: making contact with those close to death. *Journal of Dementia Care,* 14(1): 22–4.

Killick, J. and Cordonnier, C. (2000) *Openings: Dementia Poems and Photographs.* London: Hawker.

Kitwood, T. (1997) *Dementia Reconsidered: The Person Comes First.* Buckingham: Open University Press.

Mindell, A. (1997) *Coma, a Healing Journey: A Guide for Families, Friends and Carers.* Portland, OR: Lao Tse Press.

Müller-Hergl, C. (2007) Distress does not justify lying. *Journal of Dementia Care,* 15(4): 10–11.

Nolan, M.R., Davies, S., Brown, J., Keady, J. and Nolan J. (2003) Beyond 'person-centred care': a new vision for gerontological nursing. *International Journal of Older People Nursing,* 13(3a): 45–53.

Normann, H.K., Asplund, K., Karlsson, S., Sandman, P.O. and Norberg, A. (2006) People with severe dementia exhibit episodes of lucidity: A population-based study. *Journal of Clinical Nursing,* 15(11): 1413–17.

Post, S.G. (1995) *The Moral Challenge of Alzheimer's Disease.* Baltimore, MD: Johns Hopkins University Press.

Richards, T. and Tomandl, S. (2006) *An Alzheimer's Surprise Party: New Sentient Communication Skills and Insights for Understanding and Relating to People with Dementia.* Interactive Media. http://www.tomrichards.com/publications.htm

Rust, L. (1986) Another part of the county. In: J. Alexander *et al.* (eds) *Women and Aging: An Anthology.* Corvallis, OR: Calyx, p. 140.

Sabat, S.R. (2001) *The Experience of Alzheimer's Disease: Life Through a Tangled Veil.* Oxford: Blackwell.

Vittoria, A.K. (1998) Preserving selves: Identity work and dementia. *Research on Aging,* 20(1): 91–136.

Vogler, S. (2003) *Dementia: The Loss … The Love … The Laughter.* Bloomington, IN: 1stBooks.

Walker, B. (2007) Communication: building up a toolkit of helpful responses. *Journal of Dementia Care,* 15(1): 28–31.

Ward, R., Vass, A.A., Aggarwal, N., Garfield, C. and Cybyk, B. (2005) What is dementia care? 1. Dementia is communication. *Journal of Dementia Care,* 13(6): 22–4.

Ward, R., Vass, A.A., Aggarwal, N., Garfield, C. and Cybyk, B. (2006a) What is dementia care? 2. An invisible workload. *Journal of Dementia Care,* 14(1): 28–30.

Ward, R., Vass, A.A., Aggarwal, N., Garfield, C. and Cybyk, B. (2006b) What is dementia care? 3. Seeing patterns, making sense. *Journal of Dementia Care,* 14(2): 22–4.

13

Supporting health and physical well-being

John Young

Learning objectives

By the end of this chapter you will:

- understand the important actions needed to promote health and well-being for people with early dementia
- understand the issues of delirium and falls, and how they might be prevented in people with moderate dementia
- understand the issue of swallowing difficulties that accompanies more advanced dementia
- understand the range of possible interventions to maintain the health and physical well-being during the 'career' of people living with dementia

---

Introduction

Evidence-based best practices for health promotion and disease prevention that constitute routine care for people in later life are *equally* applicable to people with dementia. Indeed, people with dementia may well accrue increased benefits by virtue of their additional vulnerability to some of the common ill-health situations that can arise in later life. Unfortunately, people with dementia are often excluded from routine best clinical practice due to pervading professional stigmatism, ignorance and misunderstandings (Iliffe and Manthorpe 2002). We will therefore present the arguments for a considered, proactive style of clinical care. Such an approach will ensure that people with dementia achieve sustained, optimum health and physical well-being. We will explore issues involved in providing advice and support to maintain health and physical well-being over the several years during the 'career' of someone living with dementia.

In the first part, we will look at health promotion for people in the early stages of dementia focusing on diet, primary and secondary prevention of vascular disease, promoting exercise and activity, and flu prevention. In the middle part we look at delirium, its definition, prevention and treatment, and the issue of falls prevention. In the last part of the chapter we discuss strategies for ameliorating the swallowing impairment that affects people at the end of their journey with dementia.

The beginning of the journey

> **Exercise 13.1**   Recently diagnosed with dementia
>
> Marjorie is a 75-year-old woman who has lived all her life in the same area. Since retiring as a teacher, she has written a weekly column in her local newspaper. Her husband died five years ago and, after a period of bereavement, she has re-formed her social life to include twice weekly luncheons with her daughter who lives nearby. Marjorie has had good health and rather dismisses her mini-stroke of two years ago and the high blood pressure that was diagnosed at that time. Recently, her memory has deteriorated and, on her daughter's insistence, she has attended the local memory clinic where a diagnosis of early Alzheimer's disease has been established and explained to Marjorie and her daughter. Her daughter now wants to know what should be done to keep her mother independent and living at home for as long as possible.
>
> What might you suggest?

We know that co-existing medical conditions in people with dementia are common. One prospective study identified 248 other medical problems in 124 of 200 older people with dementia attending an out-patient service (Larson *et al.* 1986). In order to promote health and physical well-being, the following areas could be highlighted for Marjorie:

- diet
- prevention of heart attacks and strokes
- promoting activity
- flu prevention.

We will discuss each of these in turn.

Dietary advice

We all know that we should eat a 'healthy and balanced' diet – but few of us do, and most of us are probably somewhat confused about the exact meaning of 'healthy and balanced'. To clarify this the UK government has developed a national dietary scheme called the '5 a Day' programme. It involves promotion of a deceptively simple message: 'to eat at least five portions (400g) of a variety of fruit and vegetables each day' (Department of Health 2003). It has been widely promoted in primary and secondary care. Should patients with early dementia like Marjorie be encouraged to adopt the '5 a Day' food habit?

Eating a diet that includes at least five portions of fruit and vegetables each day is known to be associated with a reduced risk for colorectal cancer, gastric cancer, possibly breast cancer, coronary heart disease, stroke, delayed cataract development and improved bowel function, quite an impressive list with an overall estimated 20% reduction in deaths from these conditions. Although the effects of diet on dementia progression are unclear (as discussed in Chapter 1), the potential for major disease avoidance by adopting the 5 a Day regime is equally valuable and applicable to people with or without early dementia. That is, it is ethically unjust to limit access to effective dietary advice on the basis of co-existing dementia. Moreover, one potential effect of the 5 a Day diet is that of stroke prevention with its attendant reduction in risk of further cognitive decline. This is a particularly well-evidenced outcome from the 5 a Day diet with eight studies involving over 250,000 subjects demonstrating a substantial 26% relative risk reduction in stroke associated with eating more than five portions of fruit and vegetables per day compared with less than three per day (He *et al.* 2006).

The '5 a Day' key messages are reproduced in Table 13.1.

Table 13.1   The '5 a day' programme

Eat a least five portions of a variety of fruit and vegetables each day.

Fresh, frozen, chilled, canned and dried fruit and vegetables and 100% juice all count.

One portion is 80g of fruit or vegetables: 1 medium apple **or** 1 medium banana **or** 3 tablespoonfuls of cooked vegetables **or** 1 cereal bowl of mixed salad **or** 1 glass (150 ml) **or** 100% orange juice.

The fruit and vegetables contained in convenience foods – such as ready meals, pasta sauces, soups and puddings – can contribute towards 5 a Day. But convenience foods can also be high in added salt, sugar or fat – which should only be eaten in moderation – so it's important always to check the nutrition information on food labels.

(Department of Health 2003: 15)

Fruit and vegetables are biologically highly active and contain a large variety of vitamins, minerals, and complex plant compounds called phyto-chemicals. Which of these many individual compounds is effective is unknown and, although it might be tempting to advise taking the various widely available vitamin and mineral tablet supplements, there is no evidence that these are effective. There is something intrinsically special about the natural food product and the complexity and interaction of the many biologically active ingredients.

In answer to the question posed in Exercise 13.1, Marjorie should be provided with information and advice about the '5 a Day' programme.

Treating vascular disease

Vascular disease is the leading cause of death in most regions of the world, mostly manifested by coronary heart disease and stroke. Over the past few decades, much progress has been made with effective prevention. As discussed by Stephan and Brayne (see Chapter 1), epidemiological evidence has demonstrated a link between grades of hypertension (high blood pressure) and both risk of future dementia and accelerated progress of existing dementia. Given Marjorie's history of hypertension and mini-strokes, she is at high risk of future vascular disease including strokes that would cause increased cognitive impairment. She would undoubtedly benefit from vascular disease prevention measures. What practical steps should be taken?

First, an assessment of vascular risk should be organized, usually by a member of the primary care team. Several lifestyle factors (smoking, poor diet, low activity), clinical factors (hypertension, diabetes, obesity, high cholesterol) and ageing predispose people to develop vascular disease. Estimating Marjorie's vascular risk will involve systematic questioning and testing to detect these factors. Thus, routine tests for Marjorie should include urine dip testing for blood and protein, and measurement of blood electrolytes and creatinine – all to detect possible kidney damage from high blood pressure. Blood glucose should be checked to test for diabetes. Measurement of total blood cholesterol and high-density lipoprotein (HDL: the 'good' cholesterol, higher levels in people who exercise regularly) should be done. Several blood pressure recordings should be taken to assess for high blood pressure and an electrocardiogram (ECG) arranged to detect possible associated heart damage. All this assessment information is then brought together and used to compute the cardiovascular risk, usually expressed as percentage risk for a vascular event over ten years, and to thereby determine if various vascular prevention treatments will be worthwhile.

We already know that Marjorie has the common condition of hypertension – present in about two-thirds of people of Marjorie's age. Should Marjorie's hypertension be treated, and, if so, what benefits might she get?

Treating hypertension

In Westernized societies, due to many factors – genetic, excess dietary salt, sedentary lifestyles – the blood pressure tends to gradually increase over the lifespan. This is not a disease in itself – high blood pressure rarely causes symptoms – but a high blood pressure increases the chance of several disease states including strokes, heart attacks, heart failure, kidney failure and poor circulation in the legs. High blood pressure has been subjected to intensive study. In a major review that incorporated 61 prospective observational studies involving over one million people, increased blood pressure was conclusively linked to vascular disease risk (Prospective Studies Collaboration 2002). These epidemiological findings have been confirmed in a substantial number of intervention randomized controlled trials (RCTs) – reducing blood pressure saves lives and improves quality of life by preventing heart disease and strokes. However, people with dementia were usually excluded from these research studies and it was unclear whether lowering blood pressure in people with both hypertension and dementia might be beneficial and reduce the rate of further cognitive decline by virtue of preventing future strokes, or, paradoxically, increase the rate of cognitive decline by the medication reducing overall brain blood flow. Fortunately recent research has helped clarify this clinical dilemma. This research has clearly demonstrated *reduced* cognitive decline in people with both dementia and hypertension receiving treatment to lower blood pressure. Important large-scale studies include: the Systolic Hypertension in Europe (Sys-Eur) study, the PROGRESS trial (investigating the benefits of blood pressure reduction after a minor stroke, just like Marjorie), the Heart Outcomes

Prevention Evaluation (HOPE) study (investigating the benefits of blood pressure reduction in patients with coronary artery disease) and the Study on Cognition and Prognosis in the Elderly (SCOPE) trial. In the UK, these studies have been incorporated into guidance by the National Institute for Health and Clinical Excellence (NICE) (2006a). It is therefore clear that Marjorie should be offered treatment for her hypertension.

Treatment of hypertension consists of lifestyle advice and drug therapy. Lifestyle advice is healthy diet (5 a Day); regular exercise (brisk walking, jogging, or cycling for 30–60 minutes three to five times each week); avoidance of excess alcohol (men: less than 21 units/week; women: less than 14 units/week); avoid excess caffeine (less than five cups per day); reduce dietary salt; provide advice and support to quit smoking. In most people, this advice will need to be supplemented by long-term medication using one or more of the several available effective blood pressure-lowering drugs. Risk of future vascular events can also be minimized by reducing blood cholesterol using one of the statin drugs and advising an anti-platelet drug, typically aspirin, to reduce the chance of blocked arteries (Joint British Societies Guidelines 2005).

In answer to the question posed in Exercise 13.1, Marjorie should be assessed for her future risk of vascular disease and the risk reduced by lifestyle advice and medication, particularly blood pressure-lowering treatment. This will reduce her risk of future strokes that will accelerate the rate of decline of her dementia.

Promoting activity

Most people in our society, including patients with dementia, have excessively sedentary lifestyles. Exercise and activity are associated with important health benefits at any age, including later life, and including people with dementia – it is never too late to commence regular exercise! Regular exercise can prevent or delay the onset of several diseases: osteoporosis, diabetes, hypertension, heart disease, stroke and possibly some cancers. Regular exercise can also reduce arthritis-related pain, improve sleep, prevent falls and fractures, and there are social benefits with amelioration of loneliness and depression.

The potential benefits of exercise have been specifically investigated and confirmed in people with dementia. A systematic review (30 RCTs; 2,020 subjects) has summarized the evidence and demonstrated that exercise training increases fitness, physical function, cognitive function and positive behaviour in people with dementia (Heyn *et al.* 2004). These findings suggest that regular physical activity represents an important, simple and safe protective factor for cognitive decline in people with dementia. People with dementia should be specifically counselled and encouraged to maintain, or if possible, increase their levels of activity.

In a review of the exercise literature in relation to older people, McMurdo (2000) concluded: 'Most of the health benefits (of exercise) can be gained by performing regular moderate intensity physical activity. [such as] ... walking, dancing, bowling or gardening.' These activities, rather than formalized exercise sessions such as gym classes, should be well within the grasp of the majority of older people, including most of those with early dementia. To this list we might also add cycling, step training, exercise to music and tai chi. Indeed, even frail older people in care homes (many of whom will have had dementia) obtained an improvement in health from appropriately constructed tasks such as chair exercises (McMurdo and Rennie 1993; Mulrow *et al.* 1993). The aim is to provide activities that are fun and will promote muscle strength, increase cardiovascular endurance and preserve joint mobility. The evidenced-based intensity requirement is for about 30 minutes activity on three to five occasions each week sufficient to cause slight but noticeable breathlessness.

In answer to the question posed in Exercise 13.1, Marjorie's lifestyle should be discussed in such a way as to explore opportunities for promoting and increasing physical activity.

Influenza prevention

Seasonal respiratory tract viral infections are a nuisance and affect everyone, including people with dementia. Influenza, or 'flu', is in a different league. Influenza is a highly infectious disease caused by the influenza viruses. Seasonal flu occurs every year, usually in the winter months. It spreads rapidly, person-to-person, mainly by airborne respiratory droplets (coughs and sneezes), particularly in highly populated environments such as care homes.

Most people will feel severely unwell with marked aches and pains, high fever, sore throat and runny nose. A few develop complications: viral pneumonia, secondary bacterial pneumonia, or sinusitis, or develop exacerbations of chronic medical conditions such as chronic heart failure or chronic bronchitis. These complications are more common in older people, particularly those older people with poor background health, hence the importance of influenza affecting people with dementia who are likely to develop increased confusion during an infection. Moreover, any carers are also likely to be affected, potentially becoming too unwell to continue their support, so precipitating a care crisis.

Influenza infections can be prevented in people with dementia and their carers by an annual vaccination each autumn. This provides 70–80% protection against infection during the winter months when influenza infection is commonest with the protection lasting about one year. UK government policy is to maximize cost effectiveness by offering the vaccination to the 'at risk' groups in our society (Department of Health 2007). The specific groups are all people over 65 years, and people who have chronic respiratory disease, chronic heart disease, chronic renal disease or diabetes. People with dementia are not a specified group but will be largely subsumed in the 'all people over 65 years' category. Additionally, influenza vaccination is recommended for residents of long-stay care home facilities, many of whom will have a dementia illness. Discretionary influenza vaccination can be provided to main 'carers of elderly and disabled' people (Department of Health 2007). It is also advised that health and social care staff directly involved with patient/client care should be immunized, partly to prevent staff contracting influenza and passing it on to the vulnerable people in their care, but also to minimize disruption caused by collective staff sickness (Department of Health 2007).

In answer to the question posed in Exercise 13.1, Marjorie and her daughter should be offered the flu vaccination each autumn.

The middle of the journey

Exercise 13.2 Delirium and dementia

Marjorie is now 81 years old. Her daughter phones to say that she is worried. She explains that her mother has been coping satisfactorily at home with home care and her own support but that two days ago she became incontinent of urine (unusual for her) and more confused in her conversation and that the home care team found her rather sleepy. She seems reluctant to get out of bed and doesn't seem interested in eating or drinking but appears rather uncomfortable and has been frequently rubbing her tummy. Sometimes her speech is slurred and it's hard to make out what she is trying to say.

What might be causing these changes in Marjorie?

What might have led to these changes?

What advice might you give?

Delirium

Marjorie has delirium and needs urgent medical attention. Delirium (also called acute or toxic confusion) is a common presentation of illness in people who have a dementia. The prevalence of delirium superimposed on dementia ranges from 22% to 89% of hospitalized and community populations aged over 65 years and older with dementia (Fick *et al.* 2002). Relatively little is known about the reasons for the strong association between delirium and dementia but a key factor is thought to be a deficiency in the neurotransmitter acetylcholine that is common to both conditions.

Delirium is characterized by recent onset of fluctuating inattention and confusion, linked to one or more triggering factors. Marjorie's presentation of new onset urinary incontinence suggests the triggering factor may be a urinary infection (but see below for other possible factors). Delirium is a serious illness. It is associated with mortality rates of 25–33%, functional decline, and symptoms persisting in some patients for up to 12 months (Young and Inouye 2007).

Detecting delirium

As is discussed by Thompson and colleagues (see Chapter 17), delirium is often poorly detected, being missed in about half of cases in hospital, and therefore poorly managed, resulting in sub-optimum outcomes. In our technologically driven health service, we are accustomed to reliable diagnostic tests (e.g. echocardiography for heart failure; blood sugar for diabetes). The diagnosis of delirium rests solely on clinical skills; there is no diagnostic test. This may be one reason why the condition is often unrecognized. However, several bedside diagnostic aids have been developed that provide a structured approach to assessing patients with suspected delirium. Table 13.2 describes the Confusion Assessment Method (CAM).

Table 13.2 The four items of the Confusion Assessment Method (CAM)

1.	Is there a history of recent onset confusion that has fluctuated? And:	0 or 1
2.	Attention impairment (count backwards from 20). And either:	0 or 1
3.	Is there disorganized thinking or incoherent speech? Or:	0 or 1
4.	Is the patient sleepy, lethargic or stuporose?	0 or 1
Score 3 or more = consider delirium		

The four items of the CAM provide prompts for the four cardinal features of delirium. Item 1, a history of recent onset, usually requires a history from a carer or relative. Spending time listening to carers, or supplementing the history by telephone enquiry, is time well spent. Impairment of attention can be simply observed as the patient loses the thread of their conversation or can be more formally detected by asking them to count backwards from 20. Disorganized thinking, or incoherent speech, and sleepiness can be detected during talking to the patient. This implies spending some time with the patient – and time is limited in hard-pressed medical assessment units or in casualty. This is one reason why delirium is not adequately detected. The confusion typically fluctuates with deceptively lucid moments. This once more underscores the critical importance of talking to carers such as Marjorie's daughter.

Causes of delirium: risk factors and precipitants

Delirium is a complex clinical syndrome that rarely has a single cause. A useful approach is to consider delirium as an interaction between underlying *risk factors* and *precipitants* (or triggering events). This allows for a simple two-stage assessment process. Moreover, the recognition of the risk factors for delirium opens up the important issue of delirium prevention, and the timely identification of delirium precipitants leads to early treatment, before the delirium syndrome has become fully established (Young and Inouye 2007). Risk factors for delirium are given in Table 13.3.

Table 13.3   Risk factors for delirium

- Old age
- Physical frailty
- Severe illness
- Dementia
- Infection
- Dehydration
- Visual impairment
- Deafness
- Polypharmacy (multiple medications being taken at the one time)
- Surgery (especially fractured neck of femur)
- Alcohol excess
- Renal (kidney) impairment
- Pain

Applying the risk factors in Table 13.3 to Marjorie, we find age and dementia as obvious risk factors but there are also clinical clues for pain (rubbing her tummy), constipation (abdominal discomfort, restlessness, reduced mobility and reluctant to eat or drink) and for dehydration (reluctant to drink). There may be others – drugs, malnutrition, visual or hearing impairment – as described below. Thus, delirium risk factors are not necessarily readily apparent but need to be actively sought by carefully applied observation. Tackling her constipation and dehydration at this early stage has the potential to minimize the impact of the delirium episode.

Precipitants for delirium

Precipitants are the factor or factors that can be identified as the responsible event that has triggered the episode of delirium. Common delirium precipitants are given in Table 13.4.

Table 13.4   Common precipitants for delirium

- Lower respiratory tract infection
- Urinary infection/urinary retention
- Faecal impaction/constipation
- Electrolyte disturbance (dehydration, renal failure, high or low sodium levels)
- Drugs (especially those affecting blood pressure or sedatives)

- Alcohol withdrawal
- Severe pain
- Neurological (stroke, epilepsy)

NB: Many patients have more than one cause.

The precipitants do not cause delirium in isolation but interact with the underlying predisposition at an individual person level. Thus, a major insult, such as a serious infection, is required to trigger delirium in a previously fit person, but only a minor change, for example, a change in medication, can result in delirium in a person at high risk such as someone like Marjorie with dementia. The probable delirium precipitants for Marjorie are a urinary infection (new onset incontinence), constipation, dehydration and pain.

The differentiation between risk factors and precipitants can appear confusing because some risk factors can also be precipitants! To understand the overlap better, it is helpful to separate two distinct clinical situations – people who are *at risk* of developing delirium (but have not yet done so), and people who *have developed* delirium. This explains why some risk factors can be reclassified as precipitants as the clinical situation changes. Thus, urinary retention/catheter (infection risk), medication, dehydration, constipation and pain are risk factors for delirium *and* can also be precipitants.

Preventing delirium

Perhaps the most important aspect of delirium is that there is good evidence it can be prevented in about one-third of patients (Young and Inouye 2007). As we have seen, many of the risk factors have been identified and many can be modified (e.g. hearing and visual impairment, medication, electrolyte disturbances, infections, environmental factors, urinary catheterization, nutrition, pain and constipation); and inappropriate medications may be the sole precipitant of delirium in 12–39% of cases (Young and Inouye 2007). To prevent episodes of delirium for Marjorie, the following steps should be taken.

Medication review

People with dementia are likely to be taking several medications for a range of age-associated conditions such as hypertension, chronic heart failure and arthritis. This is called polypharmacy. We have already seen that Marjorie might have been advised to take hypertension medication to reduce her risk of stroke. However, the balance between the benefits and side effects for any drug needs regular review. We know, for example, that in the middle part of the dementia journey blood pressure can fall due to dementia-related weight loss and changes in cardiovascular reflexes. Thus a treatment that was once highly appropriate may become potentially harmful and, particularly for drugs that are fat soluble and therefore capable of entering the brain, increase the risk of delirium.

The issue of polypharmacy in the UK was recognized in the National Service Framework for Older People with the recommendation for six-monthly medication reviews (Department of Health 2001). It is remarkable how many drugs can be safely discontinued. People with a moderate dementia frequently report they feel less 'muzzy', less sleepy or less dizzy a few weeks after stopping selected medication. It is therefore important for people with moderate dementia, with their carers, to obtain regular drug reviews. That is, to systematically review each medication in turn and to discuss if it is still necessary. These reviews can be added opportunistically to a visit to the general practitioner or specialist nurse, but is best achieved by a specific visit as careful deliberation and discussion are required to determine the best course of action.

The benefits of reducing the medication burden can be considerable in people with a moderate dementia. Taking more than six drugs is associated with a major risk of delirium development, and more than four medications are known to be a risk factor for falls (see below). In answer to the question posed in Exercise 13.2 Marjorie and her daughter should be encouraged to visit their primary care team for regular medication reviews.

Prevention of dehydration

Dehydration can develop insidiously in people with moderate dementia and will be an important risk factor for delirium for Marjorie. The causes are usually several – a dementia-associated loss of thirst sensation, lack of opportunity to drink, drinks placed out of easy reach, excessive diuretic medication, and sometimes excessive loss of body fluids through diarrhoea or vomiting. Early recognition of dehydration is difficult but a slow spring-back of the skin on the forehead after gently pinching it can be a useful indication. However, whenever there is doubt or concern about the presence of dehydration, it is important to take a blood sample and measure the electrolyte and urea concentrations.

Prevention of constipation

Prevention of constipation is important for people with dementia because it is a risk factor for delirium and a very common problem: about one-third of older people suffer from constipation (Petticrew *et al.* 1997).

There are many possible causes for constipation including serious disease such as colon cancer (alarm symptoms are rectal bleeding, alternating diarrhoea and constipation, weight loss, anaemia). But for Marjorie, the commonest reasons will be varying contributions from medications (many drugs cause constipation), diet low in fibre content, dehydration and lack of activity. A dementia-specific factor is impaired attention to the call-to-stool sensation. Constipation can progress to faecal impaction where the large bowel becomes loaded with hard faeces that irritate the colon lining and cause a paradoxical mucus-rich form of diarrhoea: a trap for the unwary – diarrhoea – but due to severe constipation.

Prevention involves withdrawal of constipative drugs (commonly codeine preparations, tricyclic antidepressants, and some hypertension medications), promotion of mobility, and increasing fluids and dietary fibre, with the option of using additional prescribed bulking agents such as Fybogel. In answer to the question posed in Exercise 13.2 Marjorie needs careful monitoring in order to detect and treat dehydration and constipation at an early stage.

Prevention of malnutrition

The adverse health consequences of over-eating and obesity have absorbed the attention of the media. But the main risk to people with dementia like Marjorie is under-eating and weight loss. 'Thousands of people are starving in the midst of plenty from want of attention to the ways which alone make it possible for them to take food.' So wrote Florence Nightingale in 1859 – it is sad that her observation is still applicable in the twenty-first century. The cause of under-eating is multifactorial. For Marjorie, her cognitive impairment and living alone will be two important risk factors but there may well be others as listed in Table 13.5.

Table 13.5 Common risk factors for malnutrition in older people

- Isolation/living alone
- Poverty
- Disability/chronic disease
- Lack of easy access to shops
- Depression/loss of interest in food
- Impaired taste, vision, smell, hearing
- Poor dentition/sore mouth
- Gastrointestinal diseases
- Loss of manual dexterity
- Cold house
- Bereavement
- Cognitive impairment

Marjorie may well be one of the 40% of older people who have features of malnutrition when admitted to hospital. The National Institute for Health and Clinical Excellence (NICE) (2006b) have recommended that all hospital inpatients and outpatients should be screened to identify malnutrition. There is no single diagnostic test for malnutrition but calculating the body mass index (BMI) is simple and reliable and is the preferred method recommended by NICE and should be included in health care assessments of people with dementia. Nutritional support should then be considered for people identified as at risk of malnutrition; or who are malnourished, typically with a BMI of less than 18.5 (see Table 13.6).

Table 13.6 Identifying people with malnutrition

Calculation of body mass index (BMI):

a) Weight measured in kilograms

b) Height measured in metres

BMI = $\dfrac{\text{Weight}}{(\text{Height})^2}$

BMI < 18.5 is indicative of under nutrition

People at risk of malnutrition:

- Have eaten little or nothing for 5 days
- Are unable to take in food properly
- Have conditions causing increase nutritional needs.

People who are malnourished:

- Have BMI of < 18.5
- Have unintentional weight loss of > 10% over 3–6 months
- Have BMI < 20 and unintentional weight loss of > 5% over 3–6 months.

If Marjorie has a BMI of less than 18.5, further enquiry is necessary to identify causes and remedies. Commonly, it is due to contributions from ill-fitting or absent dentures, loss of interest in food (ensure depression is not overlooked), forgetfulness about meals, difficulty with planning meals, or difficulty preparing and cooking meals. Providing meals at home or increasing the social opportunities for meals may be required but individualized care plans need to be negotiated that fully respect the wishes of Marjorie and her family. Marjorie is more likely to eat foods she is familiar with, she may require longer mealtimes with gentle encouragement, and finger foods can be enjoyable and increase intake (Biernacki and Barratt 2001). In answer to the question posed in Exercise 13.2, Marjorie should be monitored for under-nutrition by being weighed regularly.

Exercise 13.3 Falls at home

Marjorie has been finding it increasingly difficult to get up from her chair and often needs a little help. Also, she has started walking in the house more slowly and tends to place her hands on items of furniture for balance as she walks. She is found one morning lying on the floor by the home care staff. Marjorie is upset and cannot recall what exactly happened but it seems she fell while going to the toilet during the night.

What would you suggest?

Reducing falls risk

Falls are a common occurrence in people like Marjorie who have dementia and are aged over 75 years because age and cognitive impairment are important risk factors for falls. The risk of falls associated with dementia is partly caused by impaired balance reactions due to slower brain processing as a consequence of the dementia, partly because dementia is associated with impairment of cardiovascular reflexes that help maintain blood pressure when standing, and partly due to risk factors common to many older people (e.g. multiple drugs, environmental hazards, poor eyesight, inappropriate footwear, painful feet). Difficulty getting out of a chair, and slow walking, are early warning signs for an impending fall event. Marjorie might be expected to have an annual falls incidence of around 60% (twice that of people without dementia), and to have an increased risk of a head injury or a major injury such as a fracture (Tinetti *et al.* 1988). Head injury is a particular concern to people with dementia because observational studies have repeatedly identified head injury as an exacerbating factor associated with a step change in cognitive decline. Why this is so is unclear: In some ways the neuropathology of dementia is exacerbated by the response to a head injury. Preventing falls in people with dementia is therefore an important aspect of their care.

NICE has produced guidance on the steps required to prevent falls. The recommendation is for people like Marjorie who have a high risk of falls to be assessed by 'health care professionals with appropriate skills and experience, normally in the setting of the specialist falls service' (NICE 2004: 6). Specialist falls prevention services are widely, but not yet universally, available and can be accessed through primary care. The prevention assessment is designed to identify the falls risk factors and to construct an individual treatment plan to address them. These multifactorial prevention interventions have been successful in preventing falls in at-risk people, including people with cognitive impairment (Close *et al.* 1999; Tinetti *et al.* 1994). The interventions required include improving balance and walking through physiotherapist-led exercises, medication reviews to discontinue drugs that can impair balance, assessment of vision, advice on footwear, attention to foot problems by a chiropodist, and detailed medical assessment if there is any concern that the falls are due to blackouts (NICE 2004).

Assessment of the home environment is also essential. Common situations that can be improved are attention to loose mats and carpets; provision of non-slip bathmats; provision of additional rails in showers, around baths and toilets and to stairs and steps; removing trailing electric cords; and improved lighting, especially in critical areas such as stair wells. Equally important is to check footwear. There have been several 'sloppy slipper' campaigns to replace inadequate and dangerous slippers and thereby reduce the risk of falls. Simple, cheap home modifications, provided after assessment by an experienced occupational therapist, have been associated with a reduction in falls (Cumming *et al.* 1999). In answer to the question posed in Exercise 13.3, Marjorie should be offered a falls prevention assessment that includes a home environment assessment by the local falls prevention service.

Towards the end of the journey

> **Exercise 13.4** Difficulty swallowing
>
> Marjorie is now 85 years old, still living at home but has become much more dependent; she spends much of the day lying in bed with only brief periods sitting in a chair. Her daughter visits several times each day but Marjorie doesn't always recognize her. She now needs assistance to eat her food and the home care staff are worried because there have been some choking episodes.
>
> What would you advise?

Impairment of swallowing (dysphagia)

Marjorie now has advanced dementia. Optimizing her health and well-being requires continuing attention to the issues discussed above: medication reviews to reduce her risk of delirium, prevention/early detection of dehydration and constipation, and prevention of malnutrition. But Marjorie is now developing a further problem – impairment of swallowing. This is a common, probably inevitable, feature in people with more advanced dementia (Ratnaike 2002).

Difficulty in swallowing liquids or solids is referred to as *dysphagia*. The act of swallowing is complex and involves a highly coordinated sequence of muscle contractions that move mouth contents safely over the upper airway and into the oesophagus. Initiation and control are by a swallowing centre located in one cerebral hemisphere. This centre can become damaged by the neuropathology of dementia (or by a stroke lesion). A further issue is that the muscles involved with swallowing are composed of skeletal muscle and therefore subject to the generalized wasting and weakness that affect all muscles in people who adopt a sedentary, chairfast lifestyle. This disuse atrophy is progressive and a critical stage is reached when there is just sufficient swallowing function capacity for usual health but with a loss of functional reserve such that a stressor event (commonly an infection) unmasks the loss of reserve and manifests as acute dysphagia. With hindsight, it is usually possible with careful enquiry to obtain a history of recent occasional choking, particularly with liquids, as minor episodes of aspiration have occurred. This can be used as an early warning symptom of impending dysphagia providing a window of opportunity to consider selected special feeding techniques described below. The principal complications of dysphagia are aspiration pneumonia, malnutrition and dehydration – all of which are unpleasant and distressing and have a high mortality.

Timely identification of the early features of dysphagia is important as it can prevent an episode of aspiration pneumonia. The early features include a moist sounding voice or a moist cough (both features of liquid pooling in the various pouches around the back of the throat), or coughing immediately after sipping a drink (implies some abnormal penetration of fluid into the larynx). If any of these features are present, it is imperative that drinks and food are withheld ('nil by mouth') and a specialist swallowing assessment is requested –

usually from a speech and language therapist. Often one or more compensatory measures will be recommended – careful head and body positioning, attention to consistency of food (no runny liquids or lumps), smaller, more frequent meals and using a slow, spoon-by-spoon presentation, including a double swallow if cooperation is possible, frequent checking of mouth contents to ensure no accumulation is occurring and careful watching for fatigue. Meals should be flexible and timed with periods of greatest wakefulness. Marjorie's concentration will be impaired and it is important that disturbances and distractions are minimized. 'Feeders', cups with spouts, popular in elderly care settings, must be banned. They create a fast jet of liquid liable to overwhelm the deficient swallow mechanism landing the fluid at the back of the mouth and straight into the airway. When in doubt, always present fluids a spoon at a time, and use a commercial thickening agent (such as 'Thick and Easy'). Thickened fluids are much less likely to penetrate into the larynx.

If the dysphagia is more severe and persistent, tube feeding may need to be considered. Nasogastric tubes with liquid feeds can be useful in the short term if swallowing deteriorates during an acute illness such as a urinary infection. This can buy time for a few days while it is hoped the swallowing will improve. However, nasogastric tubes are poorly tolerated and are often quickly removed by the patient, particularly in people like Marjorie with advanced dementia who have difficulty retaining the information about the purpose of the tube.

Persistent dysphagia prompts consideration for a percutaneous endoscopic gastrostomy (PEG) feeding tube system. Here a feeding tube is located in the stomach via the overlying skin under local anaesthetic using an upper gastrointestinal endoscope procedure. As the patient is sedated, the procedure is usually well tolerated by people with dementia so that the immediate complication rate (haemorrhage, infection and perforation) is very low. The main issue, however, is not the technical aspects of the procedure, but in determining whether it is the right course of action, considering the long-term complications, particularly the high rate of aspiration pneumonia due to aspiration of saliva or aspiration/reflux of gastric contents. A review by Gillick (2000) suggests that such artificial feeding neither prolongs life nor prevents aspiration pneumonia but is associated with discomfort and distress. The overriding ethical principle is to consider how the supported feeding will impact on quality of life and to what extent the life of the person is meaningful. In the UK, in clinical practice a pragmatic approach is usually adopted so that when the dementia (or any other condition) has severely impacted on awareness to an extent that, for example, the person no longer appears able to appreciate the presence and contact of people close to him/her, then prolonged PEG feeding has little to offer.

Debates and controversies

There are a variety of debates and controversies in the area of promoting health and well-being for people with dementia. One key area which attracts controversy is the extent to which the involvement of a multidisciplinary team improves outcomes for people with dementia, and within this argument what the composition of the multi-disciplinary team should be.

Another area of controversy is regarding admission to acute care for people with moderate dementia who become acutely unwell. There are discrepant views of the benefits for people with dementia of being treated in hospital or in their own homes. It is still unclear which system offers best cost effectiveness, and therefore how resources should be deployed.

With respect to delirium there is no consensus regarding whether our current crisis management response is the most cost-effective approach, or whether we should develop care systems based on prevention.

Finally, with respect to patients with advanced dementia, it is unclear whether we should struggle to maintain sufficient food intake, or whether this apparently humane approach simply prolongs the period of decline and its associated poor quality of life.

Conclusion

There are a range of interventions to promote and sustain optimal health and physical well-being for people with various stages of dementia. We have an established evidence base of their effectiveness. As the dementia progresses, different priorities emerge. This implies that regular reviews need be organized if health care crises are to be minimized and physical well-being promoted. The aim should be to identify early indications of changing health to ensure there is the best opportunity to implement a process of proactive management. Involving family members is key to the success of this process.

There is much that can and should be done to promote and sustain optimal health and physical well-being for people with dementia. We can think of prevention and intervention as focusing on various points along a person's journey with dementia. For people with mild dementia, as for all people, it is important to provide advice about health promotion including exercise, diet and flu prevention, and to ensure they are assessed for vascular disease prevention. An increasing risk of delirium becomes a major issue for people with moderate dementia and this can be reduced by regular drug reviews and prevention of malnutrition, dehydration and constipation. Also, the risk of falls and injury becomes an important threat to health. Action is needed to optimize the safety of the home, give advice on footwear, and improve walking balance to reduce this risk. In advanced dementia, a deterioration of swallowing with its attendant risk of aspiration pneumonia is an important and distressing issue and some simple preventative measures can be helpful.

Further information

National Institute for Health and Clinical Excellence (2006) *Dementia: Supporting People with Dementia and their Carers in Health and Social Care.* Clinical Guideline No. 42. London: NICE.

Royal College of Physicians (2006) *The Prevention, Diagnosis and Management of Delirium in Older People.* London: Royal College of Physicians.

Age Concern (2006) *Hungry to Be Heard: The Scandal of Malnourished Older People in Hospital.* London: Age Concern.

Royal College of Psychiatrists. *Delirious about Dementia: Towards Better Services for Patients with Cognitive Impairment.* London Royal College of Psychiatrists.

The State Government of Victoria, Australia, Department of Human Services has produced guidance on best practice in acute care, including prevention, assessment and management of delirium.

References

Biernacki, C. and Barratt, J. (2001) Improving the nutritional status of people with dementia. *British Journal of Nursing,* 10: 1104–14.

Close, J., Ellis, M., Hooper, R., Glucksman, E., Jackson, S. and Swift, C. (1999) Prevention of falls in the elderly trial: the PROFET study. *Lancet,* 353: 93–7.

Cumming, R.G., Thomas, M., Szongi, G., Salkeld, G., O'Neil, E., Westbury, C. and Frampton, G. (1999) Home visits by an occupational therapist for assessment and modification of environmental hazards: a randomised trial of falls prevention. *Journal of the American Geriatrics Society,* 47: 1397–402.

Department of Health (2001) *National Service Framework for Older People.* London: Department of Health.

Department of Health (2003) *A Local 5 A DAY Initiative: A Handbook for Delivery. Booklet 2.* Available from: http://www.dh.gov.uk/en/Publichcalth/Healthimprovement/FiveADay/indcx.htm (accessed 12 April 2008).

Department of Health (2007) *Flu Prevention.* Available from: http://www.dh.gov.uk/en/Publichealth/Flu/Flugeneralinformation/indcx.htm (accessed 12 April 2008).

Fick, D.M., Agostini, J.V. and Inouye, S.K. (2002) Delirium superimposed on dementia: a systematic review. *Journal of the American Geriatrics Association,* 50: 1723–32.

Gillick, M.R. (2000) Rethinking the role of tube feeding in patients with advanced dementia. *New England Journal of Medicine,* 342: 206–10.

He, F.J., Nowson, C.A., and MacGregor, G.A. (2006) Fruit and vegetable consumption and stroke: meta-analysis of cohort studies. *Lancet,* 367: 320–6.

Heyn, P., Abreu, B.C. and Ottenbacher, K.J. (2004) The effects of exercise training on elderly persons with cognitive impairment and dementia: a meta-analysis. *Archives of Physical Medicine and Rehabilitation,* 85: 1694–704.

Iliffe, S. and Manthorpe, J. (2002) Dementia in the community: challenges for primary care development. *Reviews in Clinical Gerontology,* 12: 243–52.

Joint British Societies (2005) Guidelines on Prevention of Cardiovascular Disease in Clinical Practice. *Heart,* 91: suppl V. Available from: http://heart.bmj.com/cgi/content/extract/91/suppl_5/v1 (accessed 12 April 2008).

Larson, E.B., Reifler, B.V., Summi, S.M. *et al.* (1986) Diagnostic tests in the evaluation of dementia: a prospective study of 200 elderly out-patients. *Archives of Internal Medicine,* 146: 1917–22.

McMurdo, M.E.T. (2000) A healthy old age: realistic or futile goal? *British Medical Journal,* 321: 1149–51.

McMurdo, M.E.T. and Rennie, L.A. (1993) A controlled trial of exercise by residents of old people's homes. *Age and Ageing,* 22: 11–15.

Mulrow, C.D., Gerety, M.B., Kanteen, D., DeNino, L.A. and Cornell, J.E. (1993) Effects of physical therapy on functional status of nursing home residents. *Journal of the American Geriatrics Society,* 41: 326–8.

National Institute for Health and Clinical Excellence (2004) *Falls: The Assessment and Prevention of Falls in Older People.* Clinical Guidance No. 21. London: NICE. Available from: http://guidance.nice.org.uk/CG21/guidance/pdf/English (accessed 12 April 2008).

National Institute for Health and Clinical Excellence (2006a) *Hypertension: Management of Hypertension in Adults in Primary Care.* Clinical Guideline No. 34. London: NICE. Available from: http://guidance.nice.org.uk/CG34/?c=91497 (accessed 12 April 2008).

National Institute for Health and Clinical Excellence. (2006b) *Nutrition Support in Adults: Oral Nutrition Support, Enteral Tube Feeding and Parenteral Nutrition.* Clinical Guideline No. 32. London: NICE. Available from: http://guidance.nice.org.uk/CG32/?c=91500 (accessed 12 April 2008).

Petticrew, M., Watt, I. and Sheldon, T. (1997) Systematic review of the effectiveness of laxatives in the elderly. *Health Technology Assessment,* 1(13). Available from: http://www.hta.ac.uk/execsumm/summ113.shtml (accessed 12 April 2008).

Prospective Studies Collaboration (2002) Age specific relevance of usual blood pressure to vascular mortality: a meta-analysis of individual data for one million adults in 61 prospective studies. *Lancet,* 360: 1903–13.

Ratnaike, R.N. (2002) Dysphagia: implications for older people. *Review of Clinical Gerontology,* 12: 283–94.

Tinetti, M.F., Baker, D.I., McAvay, G., Claus, E.B., Garrett, P., Gottschalk, M. *et al.* (1994) A multifactorial intervention to reduce falls risk among elderly people living in the community. *New England Journal of Medicine,* 331: 821–7.

Tinetti, M.F., Speechley, M., and Ginter, S.F. (1988) Risk factors for falls among elderly persons living in the community. *New England Journal of Medicine,* 319: 1701–7.

Young, J. and Inouye, S.K. (2007) Clinical review: delirium in older people. *British Medical Journal,* 334: 842–6.

14

Understanding and alleviating emotional distress

Chris Rewston and Esme Moniz-Cook

Learning objectives

By the end of this chapter you will:

- understand that emotional distress is a normal part of the human experience
- appreciate that emotional distress is caused by an interaction between internal states and the external environment
- understand the importance of the social and interpersonal environment in alleviating emotional distress for people with dementia
- recognize that understanding psychological approaches to alleviating emotional distress is important to providing quality dementia care

---

Introduction

People with dementia, families and care staff may all at some time experience distressing emotions. These can be expressed both verbally and behaviourally. For some, these emotions can develop into states of anxiety and depression. In this chapter we will present a psychological understanding of anxiety and depression, using predominantly cognitive-behavioural concepts. We demonstrate how prolonged emotional distress can lead to anxiety and depression. We argue that emotional distress is not an inevitable symptom of living with dementia, but is a reasonable human reaction to the perceived threats associated with dementia. Finally, we discuss circumstances which may lead to emotional distress in people living with dementia including adjusting to living with a diagnosis of dementia; misinterpretations and difficulty processing information; personality and coping style; and the emotional distress of those around them – families and care staff.

A psychological understanding of emotional distress

Emotional distress is a broad concept that includes a range of feelings including hostility, fear, panic, anger, embarrassment and shame. Psychological theories have much to offer us in terms of our understanding and response to people experiencing emotional distress. The focus of this chapter will be on cognitive-behavioural approaches which have an established evidence-base for alleviating emotional distress, particularly anxiety and depression. These approaches focus on the relationships among a person's thoughts, feelings and behaviours (Roth and Pilling 2008).

Cognitive-behavioural understandings of emotional distress suggest that this to alert the person to a perceived threat within their external (i.e. physical or social) or internal (i.e. physiological or mental state) environment (Eysenck 1992). For example, a person may hear an unexpected noise and become fearful of a burglar, or may experience chest pain and fear a heart attack. If s/he takes action to ensure that the house is secure, or realizes that the chest pain was due to exercise at the gym, the fear is short-lived. In these cases the individual's 'remedial action' i.e. ensuring that the house is secured or attributing chest pain to exercise, is sufficient to reduce distress. When the chosen remedial actions are ineffective in addressing the perceived threat – such as hiding under the bedding due to fear of a burglar or avoiding exertion to prevent a heart attack, prolonged distress can develop into anxiety and depression. Anxiety is associated with heightened physiological and psychological arousal in response to a perceived threat. When the response to threat is apprehension or avoidance, a state of anxiety is maintained.

Depression, on the other hand, is characterized by lowered mood that is manifested as sadness, passivity or low energy. Thus, at the extreme ends of the continuum of emotional distress, the behaviours associated with anxiety and depression are often distinct. For example, restlessness and agitation are commonly associated with anxiety while acts of omission such as passivity and reduced arousal characterize depression (Clark and Watson 1991).

Cognitive-behavioural perspectives on anxiety and depression

From a cognitive-behavioural perspective, addressing the experience of anxiety requires an understanding of what happens when someone is over-aroused. Most people have at some point felt anxious about a situation, which is often short-lived or limited to specific events, such as taking an examination or public speaking. Not surprisingly, anxiety is 'preparatory', activating both psychological and physical systems to prepare for a 'threat' that has yet to occur. This 'anticipated anxiety' is associated with the 'fight or flight' system that is often related to fear about a forthcoming or 'looming' event which alerts the person to a perceived threat in order to activate the required remedial action.

Cognitive-behavioural models of anxiety suggest that people who tend to interpret bodily sensations in a catastrophic way are more likely to experience panic. In turn, panic can lead to a response style of either hyper-vigilance and over-monitoring of bodily functioning or to avoidance. The consequences of these types of responses is to increase both over-arousal and anxiety (Laidlaw *et al.* 2003). Cognitive theories of anxiety are supported by research which demonstrates that people who are prone to anxiety are more sensitive and vigilant to possible threat from their environments, particularly when in stressful conditions. They are also likely to show biases in what information they attend to in their environment and this in turn influences thinking styles that they are more likely to perceive a potential threat (Rewston *et al.* 2007).

Thus they might react with exaggerated apprehension when faced with uncertainty or may present with chronic worry when environmental circumstances are perceived as uncontrollable. Coping strategies to address or reduce the fear will only be effective if, as noted previously, these do not maintain over-arousal. For example, avoidant coping behaviours such as closing the eyes or pacing (i.e. escaping from the fear or the 'flight' response) may initially reduce arousal but will eventually fail, as they do not address the cause of the initial concern. In contrast, direct problem-solving or action to address the feared situation is likely to result in a longer term solution and less anxiety.

Box 14.1   Case example

Mr Green felt anxious whenever he had to speak at his local church committee. As each monthly meeting approached he would start to worry about how others viewed him. He could picture himself making mistakes in front of his colleagues, sweating and being ridiculed. To prevent his fears becoming reality he believed it was better to remain very quiet at the meetings. He would also spend much of his attention focused on worry about how others perceived him. Such avoidance and hyper-vigilance had the paradoxical effect of reducing his concentration on important information and increasing his anxiety-related perspiration. Mr Green addressed these problems by altering his behaviour in the meetings. He made deliberate efforts to increase his contribution and involvement. From this he learnt that his predictions about making mistakes and excessive sweating were incorrect and his confidence returned.

As with anxiety, mild forms of depression are a common experience for many, where feelings of sadness can be a reaction to a specific event and which usually disperses in a few days. In contrast with anxiety where cognitions are focused on anticipation of a future threat, depressive thinking is characterized by cognitions related to the past (Rewston *et al.* 2007). Depressive mood is thought to bias thinking styles towards introversive rumination of personal losses, failures and short-comings. Ruminative thinking styles often result in selective recall of negative personal memories and events, thus reinforcing the existing sense of hopelessness and low self-esteem in depressive states. This in turn impacts on the efficacy of potential remedial action and exacerbates the sense of despair and associated withdrawal.

Psychological understanding of emotional distress experienced by people with dementia

We will now apply this cognitive-behavioural understanding of emotional distress to the care and support of people with dementia. In common with all human beings people with dementia will experience fear, despair and other symptoms of emotional distress. Some emotions, if prolonged, may lead to anxiety and depression. Our interest in this section is to understand what we can do to alleviate the intensity and duration of these distressing emotions for people with dementia to prevent their escalation to anxiety and depression.

This begins with recognition that these emotions are part of everyday life and not an inevitable consequence of dementia. Viewing emotional distress as a symptom of dementia, rather than as a normal response experienced by all people, places us at risk of dismissing the distress as something related to the illness, which we can do nothing about. On the other hand, seeing distress as a human response to internal or external threats, or to learned ways of responding, provides an opening for remediation by reducing distress.

There is an increasing body of literature on applying cognitive and behavioural theories to understanding emotional distress in people with dementia (James 1999a, b). For example, Cheston Jones and Gilliard (2006) describe how behavioural strategies of avoidance, concealment and denial sometimes used by people with dementia are used to avoid shame.

As noted previously, when depression and anxiety are seen as normal human responses for all people, including those with dementia, this can open the way for the use of multiple therapies to address their distress. Examples of such therapies can be found in Woods' (2001) overview of psychotherapeutic approaches for people with dementia. Updates on the talking therapies (Heason 2005), cognitive-behavioural therapy (Laidlaw *et al.* 2003) and supportive psychotherapy (Junaid and Hedge 2007) are now emerging. There are particular examples of psychotherapy for people with dementia, such as cognitive-behavioural therapy and relaxation strategies offered individually (Scholey and Woods 2003; Suhr *et al.* 1999; Walker, 2004) or in groups (Kipling and Bailey 1999), interpersonal therapy (James *et al.* 2003) and group psychotherapy (Cheston *et al.* 2003; Mills and Bartlett 2006). These have all demonstrated some success in alleviating anxiety and depression in people with dementia (Teri *et al.* 1997). Texts on cognitive analytic (Hepple and Sutton 2004) and psychoanalytic approaches (Balfour 2007) for the treatment of anxiety and depression in dementia are also emerging as are supportive group service interventions conceptualized as 'Alzheimer's cafés' (Thompson 2006). One memory clinic randomized trial of brief psychodynamic interpersonal therapy reported no evidence to support the widespread introduction of brief psychotherapy in early dementia (Burns *et al.* 2005). Such a finding highlights the view that providing psychological care for people with dementia requires concept-driven, person-specific formulations that are set within an adequate knowledge base, to guide the clinician on the choice of psychotherapy that will best suit the person's need (Bird and Moniz-Cook 2008; Moniz-Cook 2008).

Reasons people with dementia experience emotional distress

We will now examine four common reasons for emotional distress in people with dementia:

- adjusting to having a diagnosis of dementia
- cognitive changes in perception and information processing
- personality and coping style
- emotional distress of others

Adjusting to having a diagnosis of dementia

Living with dementia is an emotional as well as a cognitive experience (Woods 2001) and therefore it requires an emotional as well as cognitive adjustment. Many people with dementia experience anxiety and depression, although this is by no means inevitable and, significantly, where people are adequately supported, less distress is observed. Clare *et al.* (2002) reported that 40% of people recently diagnosed experience anxiety while 17% experience depression. Lower levels of anxiety heave been reported for those attending a memory clinic where individually tailored post-diagnostic support was in place. Lower levels of anxiety and depression have been noted for those attending a memory clinic where Moniz-Cook *et al.* (2001a) reported levels as low as 14% for anxiety and 2% for depression, while Harrison (2005) reported that 22% of attendees experienced anxiety and 9% depression. This may reflect the wide range of human responses to life events that exist, a difference in what was provided at the clinics, a difference in population, or methodological differences in the studies described.

A study of 50 older people who were attending a memory clinic for a diagnostic work-up found that their prevailing emotions were fear and anticipated shame. These included negative images of family experiences and socially stigmatizing images of 'vegetating elders' in care facilities (Moniz-Cook *et al.* 2006). People with dementia anticipated feeling shame in relation to 'incontinence', 'immobility' and relationships damaged by 'incoherence'. A better understanding of these negative emotions will hopefully lead to greater use of services, such as counselling for the person with dementia as well as their carers (Cheston and Bender 2003).

Reduction of anxiety can also be achieved by families using, 'emotion-orientated communication' where carers learn to use both verbal and nonverbal communication as a means of empathizing with and validating their disorientated relatives in a nonjudgmental way that allows the person with dementia to freely express their distress (Finnema *et al.* 2000). People with dementia will experience understandable emotional distress associated with their experiences of cognitive decline and this may become acute at times as illustrated in Box 14.2.

Box 14.2   Case example

Mr Howe, aged 78, has a vascular dementia. First seen at the memory clinic, where few day-to-day problems were noted by either him or his wife, their only concern was that when he awoke to use the toilet at night, he would occasionally pace about the house anxiously looking for his 'mother'. Sometimes he also addressed his wife as 'mother' and, according to her, became 'incoherent and upset', when she attempted to correct his mistake. Both Mr and Mrs Howe feared that he was becoming like his now deceased mother, who 'did not know them' when they used to visit her at a care home, some twenty years previously. Mr Howe described the 'strange feelings' of disorientation' he felt at these and other times as a significant concern for him. Mrs Howe learned to assist in alleviating Mr Howe's distress with soothing reassurance at such times and later she demonstrated to hospital staff during an admission to a surgical ward, how they too might reassure her husband, when he became agitated and attempted to leave the ward, while 'looking for his mother'.

As demonstrated in Box 14.2, emotional support alleviated Mr Howe's emotional distress by preventing sustained over-arousal. In this case, early in his experience of living with dementia, Mr Howe's distress was understood as his response to what he understood about dementia (Moniz-Cook *et al.* 2006) and his reduced cognitive capacity. The source of his anxieties was his ability to remember while not being able to exercise control over his own cognition – a psychological process known as 'meta-cognition'. His anxieties were not alleviated with his pacing, itself an avoidant coping strategy, which failed to reduce over-arousal. Cognitive theories describe this type of coping with the stress of dementia as 'safety-seeking behaviours' (James and Sabin 2002). Safety-seeking behaviours are behaviours employed in threatening situations. They are either mental or physical actions (e.g. counting to ten, holding on to things) that the person believes are necessary to reduce the likelihood of the threat occurring. These behaviours may not actually resolve the distress and instead can increase over-arousal and anxiety states.

As seen in Box 14.2 Mr Howe's wife's initial unsuccessful attempts to communicate by correcting her husband's mistake, acted to maintain his over-arousal. When she learned to direct communication to his emotional experience, he was able to use these messages to address the source of his distress. In Mr Howe's case the source of his distress was the strange feelings associated with reduced cognition. Thus 'here and now' emotion-orientated communication (Finnema *et al.* 2000) allowed Mr Howe to cope with his concerns. This in turn enhanced his sense of competence and his capacity to solve problems (Teasdale and Barnard 1993; Williams 1994).

Misinterpretations and difficulties with processing information

Cortical changes associated with dementia can lead to misunderstanding of the interpersonal and physical environments (Stokes 2000). Changes in perception may alter the person's interpretation and evaluation of what constitutes a threat. The resulting 'misidentification' of objects and people within the environment can lead to events being processed as potentially threatening, such as seeing oneself in a mirror as an intruder, thus causing anxiety. This anxiety, in turn, may be expressed verbally and through behaviour. For example, loud noises may be interpreted as threatening or signalling immediate danger, or impairments in attention and information processing could impact on the person's ability to distract themselves from unpleasant thoughts and memories.

Emotional distress due to 'misidentification' of what is said or what is seen in conjunction with reduced information processing capacity, is common in dementia (Stokes 2000). Therefore, reducing ambiguity in the environment and within interpersonal encounters can reduce distress, as is illustrated below in the case of Mr Dee. When impaired communication ability or misperceptions (Holden and Stokes 2002) are addressed alongside a thorough investigation of the person's physical environment (lighting conditions, noise levels) and the person's beliefs, past fears or dislikes, distress in people with dementia can be resolved (Moniz-Cook 2003; Moniz-Cook *et al.* 2001b; 2003).

Box 14.3   Case example

Mr Dee is a retired fireman living in residential care. Staff reported that he was occasionally distressed and shouted out at night when alone in his bedroom. When staff appeared, he pointed at the door and began screaming. When staff tried to calm him, he responded with verbal aggression and if approached, he shoved and hit out. Their view was that he was protesting about having to retire to his room at night. However, the explanation for his distress was found in the way he processed visual information and his autobiographically-based belief system. It appeared that Mr Dee had always believed it was his duty to use his strong physique to protect others from harm. His misinterpretation of his dressing gown (hanging on the back of his bedroom door) as an unknown intruder, reflected a serious threat. His initial misperception of the dressing gown as an intruder had generalized into a vicious circle of expectation, which influenced his future perception of the robe at night. His associated hostility towards staff was seen as an understandable response to this 'threatening' situation i.e. being returned to an unsafe situation which he could not make safe. Remedial action was taken by removing the robe from its location. The associated reductions in night-time distress were sustained by improving the lighting and by staff 'checking' doors and windows in a calm, reassuring way (i.e. emotion-orientated communication) on the now much reduced occasions when he shouted out at night.

Personality and coping style

The standard neuropsychiatric model contends that a developing dementia heralds a change in personality and that this is reflected in behaviour. However, Stokes (2000) argues that these behavioural changes reflect a reasonable attempt by the person with dementia to use adaptive defences in response to fears of cognitive decline. Thus, to avoid fear, a person might attempt to cope with their experience of cognitive failure by denying errors, blaming others for lost items, or covering up for mistakes they may have made (see Chapter 9). If such compensatory coping strategies do not reduce anxiety, this can result in continued stress. Studies of emotional responses to a diagnosis of dementia suggest that different types of coping strategies exist such as minimizing the difficulty, remaining optimistic or taking actions to maximize life quality and that each style can be associated with some risk such as increased fear, anxiety or emotional dependency (Moniz-Cook 2008). Even in the later stages of dementia, people are thought to retain their personal preferences and purposes (Cheston and Bender 2003) with a strong continuity of prior behaviour patterns, such as purposeful activity, personal appearance and hygiene (Moniz-Cook 2001) (see Chapter 11). Expression of purposefulness or defensive coping, if perceived to be 'unreasonable' because it challenges the norms and rules of the context within which it occurs, is often construed by others as 'challenging behaviour' and considered to be inevitable 'symptoms' of dementia.

Theories of personality have been used to understand individual differences in responses to dementia. For example, Kitwood *et al.* (1995: 29–31) describe six response profiles in a group of 112 people with dementia in care homes;

Hilton and Moniz-Cook (2004) note two profiles differing on personality, coping and thinking styles. These differences were associated with vulnerability to distress in 63 people with dementia in care homes. Harrison (2005) describes similar profile-dependent vulnerability to anxiety and depression in memory clinic attendees, noting that a person who habitually overestimates a potential threat is likely to become fearful and anxious following a subtle change in circumstances, as was seen in the case of Mr Howe above. These emotional reactions are in themselves not a consequence of pathological changes in personality, but instead are understandable, albeit not always conscious, human response to cognitive loss and the associated continual task of having to interpret a complex and potentially threatening environment.

Empirical support for stability in aspects of personality can have important implications for the philosophy that underpins person-centred dementia care. Here we have outlined how knowledge and theories from the psychology of personality and individual differences can be used to understand the normal but unique lived experiences, attitudes and beliefs that influence coping with dementia. Predictions based on conceptualizations of personal-vulnerability profiles (Harrison 2005; Hilton and Moniz-Cook 2004) can allow the clinician to target psychological support. This has the potential to minimize sustained distress and progression to anxiety or depression in people with dementia. Understanding the sources of distress in dementia (James 1999a, b; James 2002; James and Sabin 2002) also open avenues by which the stress of living with dementia can be reduced, preventing anxiety and depression (Moniz-Cook 2008).

Exercise 14.1 Distress within the context of personal identity

Read the following vignette and then consider the questions that follow:

Mrs Willis, a 75-year-old ex-bank manager, had retired early through stress-related illness and was diagnosed with vascular dementia some three years ago. Overall she and her husband were managing well at home. However, at times during the day, Mr Willis was upset by his wife's apparently changed behaviour towards him. He reported that she was argumentative and verbally aggressive, which was unusual for her. Mrs Willis, a gentle person who placed high value on important relationships such as that of her husband, now spent long periods in front of the television, with her word-finding problems sometimes limiting conversations. Occasionally she would anxiously pace about looking for things to do. Mr and Mrs Willis had no children and Mrs Willis reported that she and her husband had always depended on each other. All their married life he had apparently reassured her that she was appreciated, needed and had supported her in her productive work life. When she retired, she maintained her need to be productive by focusing her efforts on her husband and their home.

Mr Willis, a reserved man, had also appreciated his wife's efforts and now found it hard when she became frustrated, for example, when they were in the kitchen. Her attempts to join in meal preparations were often unsuccessful, particularly when using the cooker or locating food from the refrigerator. When her husband tried to help her she became angry with him. Mr Willis had gradually taken charge of cooking – a task his wife had previously enjoyed sharing with him. Now it appeared she would anxiously look for him when she heard him preparing their meals in the kitchen. Mr Willis would then attempt to distract his wife from her frustration directing her away from meal preparation and encouraging her to sit in the lounge and converse with him. Mrs Willis complied by sitting down, although at these times her word-finding difficulties were more marked and her conversation less fluent. She often became tearful when alone in the lounge, including when her husband returned to the kitchen.

1   What in Mrs Willis's history might offer suggestions about her psychological needs?

2   What is the effect of the consequence of dementia (i.e. in this case not preparing meals) on Mrs Willis's current thinking?

3   What interpersonal information might be exacerbating her distress at these times?

4   What aspect(s) of the above factors might be maintaining her distress? For example, were there any 'safety-seeking behaviours' being used by Mr Willis to reduce any potential threat to himself or his wife?

Emotional distress of others

A family or staff carer's emotional reactions to the subtle changes in their care-recipients' behaviour can exacerbate distress, thus increasing the risks of anxiety and depressive states in the person with dementia (see Bird and Moniz-Cook 2008, for an overview). In family settings this may hamper the person's opportunities to continue living in their own home (de Vugt *et al.* 2004), whereas in care homes associations with perceived challenging behaviour (Moniz-Cook *et al.* 2000) can lead to overuse of sedatives and sometimes make things worse for the person with dementia. Furthermore the family care-giving literature suggests that carers are themselves vulnerable to distress (Harrison 2005) and psychological support offered to them can be of benefit (Jang *et al.* 2004). (See Chapter 5.) Thus the causes of carer distress can be reduced in both carers and their relative with dementia by taking a psychological approach (Marriott *et al.* 2000).

The care home literature also suggests that some staff may protect themselves from distress by distancing themselves from the care recipient (Moniz-Cook 2001). This type of carer coping response runs the risk of negative impacts on their empathy with residents. Supportive interventions to reduce staff disengagement can improve staff coping and empathy, resulting in a positive impact on resident anxiety and depression, which in turn improves both resident and staff well-being (Bird and Moniz-Cook 2008).

Exercise 14.2   The impact of carer stress

Read the following vignette and consider the questions that follow:

Mrs Sale, the primary carer for her husband with dementia, was highly anxious. She felt unable to feel comfortable if she did not know his whereabouts. She received some respite from her worries when he attended day care twice weekly, but her significant sense of pressure remained for the rest of the time. Central to her distress was her concern about her husband's safety because of his dementia. Mrs Sale admitted that much of her time was occupied with worrying about her husband's well-being and that that she was now continuously 'on edge' about him. She was significantly worried about the growing sense of responsibility that she now felt – this was new for her as in the past she had depended on him. She was also frustrated that their once pleasurable lifestyle was apparently diminishing. Her high anxiety resulted in her feeling that she had to check out that he was safe. Thus she would check that he was not near the cooker, shut doors to prevent him entering 'unsafe' places or repeatedly look out for him in the home.

Mr Sale, a calm, dependable and autonomous man, perceived his wife's new and unusual behaviour towards him as belittling and became angry when she interfered with the simple things he did, such as making a drink. This resulted in significant friction between them. The consequences were that Mrs Sale's beliefs that dementia was associated with personality change were reinforced, since in the past Mr Sale had been her mainstay and support and very rarely was he cross with her; and Mr Sale became sensitive and guarded about any attempts by his wife to assist him, whether he needed her practical help or not.

1   What might be the source of threat that has contributed to Mrs Sale's heightened arousal and anxiety?

2   What might be maintaining her arousal and associated anxiety state?

3   What are Mrs Sale's assumptions about her husband's dementia (i.e. her understanding of the meaning of dementia)?

4   What is the effect of her beliefs on (a) herself; and (b) her husband?

5   What might be the focus of psychological intervention in the case of Mr and Mrs Sale?

The case of Mr and Mrs Sale in Exercise 14.2 describes a spouse carer who was herself vulnerable to distress (Harrison 2005). Her husband who had cognitive impairments due to a dementia tried to support her, as he had always done. However, her beliefs about dementia combined with her growing sense of responsibility for him and her sustained over-arousal, served to maintain her distress and also undermined her husband's sense of efficacy.

Debates and controversies

We are in danger of assuming that because we have an emerging evidence base for the effectiveness of psychological approaches, such as those informed by cognitive-behavioural theories, that we should apply this approach to all people with dementia. However, such approaches should be individualized and tailored to address each person's unique concerns and circumstances. There is no theoretical or empirical basis for using cognitive-behaviour therapy, cognitive-analytic therapy, or any other psycho-therapy with all people with dementia. We might ask ourselves then why we consider randomized controlled trials to be the gold standard for demonstrating outcomes of psychological approaches to distress in dementia. Is this really consistent with an individualized and person-centred approach to care?

Conclusion

In this chapter we suggest that emotional distress in people with dementia is not inevitable. We have focused on cognitive-behavioural approaches to understanding and alleviating emotional distress in people with dementia. Central to the cognitive-behavioural approach is the notion that emotional distress can be influenced by a person's internal state, including their personal thinking styles. Equally important is the idea that this thinking occurs in the context of interactions with others and with the physical environment. Therefore, social and interpersonal environments are important moderating influences to the potentially distressing experience of cognitive decline in dementia.

Success in preventing and alleviating distress in people with dementia is often dependent on families and staff carers, who require training and support. Service providers need to ensure the availability of specialists who are skilled in using psychological knowledge of what leads to and maintains emotional distress in dementia. Such knowledge allows for the development of individualized, person-centred 'theories' about what that person might experience as a threat. This in turn will guide the choice of person-centred, psychological intervention required to prevent or alleviate distress in a person with dementia.

Further information

PSIGE provides a forum for psychologists with an interest in work with older people.

The British Association for Behavioural and Cognitive Psychotherapies (BA-BCP) is an interest group for people involved in the practice and theory of behavioural and cognitive psychotherapy./

References

Balfour, A. (2007) Facts, phenomenology and psychoanalytic contributions to dementia care. In: R. Davenhill (ed.) *Looking into Later Life: A Psychoanalytic Approach to Depression and Dementia in Old Age.* London: Karnac Books, pp. 222–47.

Bird, M. and Moniz-Cook, E.D. (2008) Challenging behaviour in dementia: a psychosocial approach to intervention. In: R.T. Woods and L. Clare (eds) *Handbook of the Clinical Psychology of Ageing.* Chichester: Wiley, pp. 571–94.

Burns, A., Gutherie, E., Marino-Francis, F. *et al.* (2005) Brief psychotherapy in Alzheimer's disease: randomised controlled trial. *British Journal of Psychiatry,* 187: 143–7.

Cheston, R. and Bender, M. (2003) *Understanding Dementia: The Man with the Worried Eyes.* London: Jessica Kingsley.

Cheston, R., Jones, K. and Gilliard, J. (2003) Group psychotherapy and people with dementia. *Aging and Mental Health,* 7: 452–61.

Cheston, R., Jones, K. and Gilliard, J. (2006) Psychotherapeutic groups for people with dementia: the Dementia Voice Group Psychotherapy Project. In: B.M.L. Miesen and G.M.M. Jones (eds) *Caregiving in Dementia: Research and Applications,* Vol 4. Hove: Routledge, pp. 251–70.

Clare, L., Wilson, B. A., Carter, G., Breen, K., Berrios, G. E. and Hodges, J. R. (2002) Depression and anxiety in memory clinic attenders and their carers: implications for evaluating the effectiveness of cognitive rehabilitation interventions. *International Journal of Geriatric Psychiatry,* 17: 962–7.

Clark, L. A. and Watson, D. (1991) Tripartite model of anxiety and depression: Psychometric evidence and taxonomic implications. *Journal of Abnormal Psychology,* 100: 316–36.

de Vugt, M.E., Stevens, F., Aalten, P., Lousberg, R., Jaspers, N., Winkens, I., Jolles, J. and Verhey, F.R. (2004) Do caregiver management strategies influence patient behaviour in dementia? *International Journal of Geriatric Psychiatry,* 19: 85–92.

Eysenck, M.W. (1992) *Anxiety: The Cognitive Perspective.* Hove: Psychology Press.

Finnema, E., Dröes, R.M., Ribble, M. and Van Tillberg, W. (2000) The effects of emotion-orientated approaches in the care of persons suffering from dementia: a review of the literature. *International Journal of Geriatric Psychiatry,* 15: 141–61.

Harrison, J. (2005) The relationship between personality and psychological distress in older people with dementia and their family caregivers. ClinPsyD thesis, University of Hull, UK.

Heason, S. (2005) Talking therapy as a psychological intervention for people with dementia: a literature review. *Psychology Specialists Working with Older People Newsletter,* 89: 24–31.

Hepple, J. and Sutton, L. (2004) *Cognitive Analytic Therapy and Later Life: A New Perspective on Old Age.* Hove: Routledge.

Hilton, C. and Moniz-Cook, E. (2004) Examining the personality dimensions of sociotropy and autonomy in older people with dementia: their relevance to person centred care. *Behavioural and Cognitive Psychotherapy,* 32: 457–65.

Holden, U. and Stokes, G. (2002) Neuropsychological impairments and rehabilitation approaches. In: G. Stokes and F. Goudie (eds) *The Essential Dementia Care Handbook: A Good Practice Guide.* Bicester: Speechmark Publishing, pp. 92–101.

James, I. (1999a) Using a cognitive rationale to conceptualize anxiety in people with dementia. *Behavioural and Cognitive Psychotherapy,* 27: 345–51.

James, I. (1999b) A cognitive conceptualization of distress in people with dementia. *Clinical Psychology Forum,* 133: 21–5.

James, I. (2002) Treatment of distress in people with severe dementia using cognitive-behavioural concepts. In: S. Benson (ed.) *Dementia Topics for the Millennium and Beyond.* London: Hawker Publications, pp. 145–9.

James, I., Postma, K. and Mackenzie, L. (2003) Using an IPT conceptualization to treat a depressed person with dementia. *Behavioural and Cognitive Psychotherapy,* 31: 451–6.

James, I. and Sabin, N. (2002) Safety seeking behaviours. *Dementia: International Journal of Social Practice,* 1: 37–45.

Jang, Y., Clay, O.J., Roth, D.L., Haley, W.E. and Mittelman, M.S. (2004) Neuroticism and longitudinal change in caregiver depression: impact of a spouse-caregiver intervention program. *The Gerontologist,* 44: 311–17.

Junaid, O. and Hedge, S. (2007) Supportive psychotherapy in dementia. *Advances in Psychiatric Treatment,* 13: 17–23.

Kipling, T. and Bailey, M. (1999) The feasibility of a cognitive behavioural therapy group for men with mild/moderate cognitive impairment. *Behavioural and Cognitive Psychotherapy,* 27: 189–93.

Kitwood, T., Buckland, S. and Petre, T. (1995) *Brighter Futures: A Report on Research into Provision for Persons with Dementia in Residential Homes, Nursing Homes and Sheltered Housing.* Anchor Housing Association, Oxon. Available at: http://www.anchor.org.uk/publications_pdfs/brighter-futures.pdf (accessed 12 April 2008).

Laidlaw, K., Thompson, L.W., Dick-Siskin, L. and Gallagher-Thompson, D. (2003) *Cognitive Behaviour Therapy with Older People.* Chichester: John Wiley and Sons.

Marriott, A., Donaldson, C., Tarrier, N. *et al.* (2000) Effectiveness of cognitive-behavioural family intervention in reducing the burden of care in carers of patients with Alzheimer's disease. *British Journal of Psychiatry,* 176: 557–62.

Mills, M. and Bartlett, E. (2006) Experiential support groups for people in the early to moderate stages of dementia. In: B.M.L. Miesen and G.M.M. Jones (eds) *Caregiving in Dementia: Research and Applications,* Vol. 4. Hove: Routledge, pp. 271–90.

Moniz-Cook, E.D. (2001) Behavioural disturbance in care homes. PhD thesis, University of Wales, Bangor.

Moniz-Cook, E.D. (2003) Mealtime challenges for people with dementia and staff in care homes – a psychological perspective. In: M. Marshall (ed.) *The Food Book*. London: Hawker Publications, pp. 109–13.

Moniz-Cook, E.D. (2008) Assessment and psychosocial intervention for older people with suspected dementia: a memory clinic perspective. In: K. Laidlaw and B. Knight (eds) *Handbook of Emotional Disorders in Late Life: Assessment and Treatment*. New York: Oxford University Press, pp. 421–51.

Moniz-Cook, E.D., Gardiner, E. and Woods, R.T. (2000) Staff factors associated with the perception of behaviour as challenging in residential and nursing homes. *Aging and Mental Health*, 4: 48–55.

Moniz-Cook, E.D., Manthorpe, J., Carr, I., Gibson, G. and Vernooij-Dassen, M. (2006) Facing the future: a qualitative study of older people referred to a memory clinic prior to assessment and diagnosis. *Dementia: The International Journal of Social Research and Practice*, 5: 375–95.

Moniz-Cook, E.D., Stokes, G. and Agar, S. (2003) Difficult behaviour and dementia in nursing homes: five cases of psychosocial intervention. *International Journal of Clinical Psychology and Psychotherapy*, 10: 197–208.

Moniz-Cook, E.D., Wang, M., Campion, P., Gardiner, E., Carr, I., Gibson, G. and Duggan, P. (2001a) Early psychosocial intervention through a memory clinic – a randomised controlled trial. *Gerontology*, 47: 526.

Moniz-Cook, E.D., Woods, R.T. and Richards, K. (2001b) Functional analysis of challenging behaviour in dementia: the role of superstition. *International Journal of Geriatric Psychiatry*, 16: 45–56.

Rewston, C., Clarke, C., Moniz-Cook, E. and Waddington, R. (2007) Distinguishing worry from rumination in older people: A preliminary investigation. *Aging and Mental Health*, 11: 604–61.

Roth, A.D. and Pilling, S. (2008) Using an evidence-based methodology to identify the competences required to deliver effective cognitive and behavioural therapy for depression and anxiety disorders. *Behavioural and Cognitive Psychotherapy*, 36(2): 129–47.

Scholey, K.A. and Woods, B.T. (2003) A series of brief cognitive therapy interventions of people experiencing both dementia and depression: a description of techniques and common themes. *Clinical Psychology and Psychotherapy*, 10: 175–85.

Stokes, G. (2000) *Challenging Behaviour in Dementia: A Person Centred Approach*. Bicester: Winslow Press.

Suhr, J., Anderson, S. and Tranel, D. (1999) Progressive muscle relaxation in the management of behavioural disturbance in alzheimer's disease. *Neuropsychological Rehabilitation*, 9: 31–44.

Teasdale, J. and Barnard, P. (1993) *A Review of Affect, Cognition and Change*. Hove: Lawrence Erlbaum Associates.

Teri, L., Logsdon, R. G., Uomoto, J., and McCurry, S. (1997) Behavioral treatment of depression in dementia patients: A controlled clinical trial. *Journals of Gerontology B: Psychological Sciences and Social Sciences,* 52B 159–66.

Thompson, A. (2006) Qualitative evaluation of an Alzheimer café as an ongoing supportive group intervention. In: B.M.L. Miesen and G.M.M. Jones (eds) *Caregiving in Dementia: Research and Applications,* Vol. 4. Hove: Routledge, pp. 291–312.

Walker, D.A. (2004) Cognitive behavioural therapy for depression in a person with Alzheimer's dementia. *Behavioural and Cognitive Psychotherapy,* 32: 495–500.

Williams, M.J. (1994) Interacting cognitive subsystems and unvoiced murmurs. *Cognition and Emotion,* 8: 571–9.

Woods, R.T. (2001) Discovering the person with Alzheimer's disease: cognitive, emotional and behavioural aspects. *Aging & Mental Health,* 5(Suppl 1): S7–S16.

PART THREE

Journeys through dementia care

15

Diagnosis and early support

Richard H Fortinsky

Learning objectives

By the end of this chapter you will:

- be able to discuss the importance and application of the principles of uncertainty and partnership from the first symptoms of dementia to diagnosis
- be able to explain how different ethnic and cultural groups view the symptoms of dementia and seek information
- be able to explain the implications of results from clinical trials intended to improve diagnosis and early support of people with dementia in the primary care setting
- understand the types of early support services for people with dementia and their families

---

Introduction

Dementia has become a global health issue in the twenty-first century, owing largely to the ageing of populations in all developed countries and many developing countries throughout the world. Symptoms characteristic of dementia, regardless of the cause, include: progressive loss of memory; increasingly impaired judgement, decision-making and verbal communication; mood changes; and increased inability to conduct activities of living ranging from driving to grocery shopping to personal care (Alzheimer's Association 2007; Alzheimer's Society 2007; NICE-SCIE 2006). Because the trajectory and accumulation of these symptoms vary widely among individuals in terms of time intervals and intensity, there is a tremendous amount of uncertainty among people affected by these symptoms and their family members regarding when to seek help from health care professionals to determine a diagnosis and answer questions they have about prognosis and treatment options. Once a diagnosis of Alzheimer's disease or vascular dementia is made, persons with dementia and their families face questions about what support services are available in the community to help them plan for the future and manage symptoms as they worsen. For most families living with the daily challenges of dementia, the goal is to enable the person with dementia to live in the comfort of her or his home with as much dignity as possible, as long as support services in the local community can be identified and marshalled to help enable them to achieve this goal.

This chapter focuses on the phase of the dementia journey beginning with the initial recognition of symptoms, proceeding through the acquisition of a diagnosis and ending when the person diagnosed with dementia is still living at home but with symptoms progressed to the point where they and their family carers receive some degree of health and social care assistance. For purposes of this chapter, then, 'early support' refers to health and social care services in the statutory (public) and voluntary (private) sectors provided during the time that a person with dementia resides in a home setting and any involved family carers are actively engaged in helping the person remain at home.

The chapter is divided into four interrelated sections — time before the diagnosis, making the diagnosis, disclosing the diagnosis, and early support after the diagnosis. Each section highlights the degree to which uncertainty remains a key problem throughout the dementia journey among persons with dementia, family carers, and health and social care practitioners.

Before the diagnosis

The time between symptom development and diagnosis is characterized by increasing uncertainty for most people with dementia and their families. A recent large-scale survey of more than 600 family carers from six European countries found that the average length of time between symptom recognition and a diagnosis of symptoms was 20 months, with an average range from 10 months in Germany to 32 months in the UK (Bond *et al.* 2005). Research on the pre-diagnosis phase of the dementia journey, between memory symptom recognition and diagnosis by a health care practitioner, is quite limited. Although there is growing research about the self-described experience of living with dementia, we are just beginning to understand the ways in which persons with dementia symptoms feel about and respond to their symptoms before a diagnosis is made (see Chapter 3). The challenge in this type of research is locating and interviewing persons living with dementia during the time period between recognition of symptoms and receiving a diagnosis from a physician or memory clinic practitioners.

To date, the only known study to capture this pre-diagnosis window was conducted in England. The study included 48 people attending a memory clinic for assessment of their symptoms who were later diagnosed with Alzheimer's disease and/or vascular dementia as a result of this clinic assessment (Moniz-Cook *et al.* 2006). Separate interviews were conducted with these subjects (age range 66–87 years) and with their accompanying family members (nearly all spouses or adult children). Subjects were exclusively British Caucasians residing in urban or suburban settings at the time of the study. Results from this study illustrated the principle of uncertainty at this pre-diagnosis stage of the dementia journey from the perspective of persons with dementia symptoms. Uncertainty arose primarily from not knowing whether the course of their symptoms would mirror those experienced previously by loved ones who had been affected by dementia. Findings also revealed uncertainty among persons with dementia and their family members in the form of a lack of awareness about support that might enable the person with dementia to live at home as long as possible.

There is a growing literature about how family members become aware and react to dementia symptoms prior to diagnosis. Although most published studies are based on fairly small sample sizes, insights can be gained from this literature about the views of ethnically diverse family carers. Wilson (1989) developed an elegant model of co-resident family carer experiences over time based on retrospective reports, including stages occurring prior to diagnosis. Initially, these carers noticed behaviours that were out of the ordinary (stage one), but did not become concerned until such behaviours began to accumulate. At this point the person with dementia could no longer rationalize, normalize or discount the behaviours (stage two). Their greatest period of uncertainty was during the third stage in which they realized that explanations must be sought. Often a sentinel event actually triggered the move to seek a diagnosis, such as a driving-related incident. Wilson's work and subsequent research by Keady and Nolan (2003) helped clarify that family members most often internalize their roles as 'carers' only after seeking and receiving a diagnosis from a physician or other health care professional.

Research conducted with family members in the United States revealed that they often waited considerable periods of time after first noticing symptoms before seeking a diagnosis. Reasons for this waiting period included those echoed in the study by Wilson (1989): attributing memory lapses and other symptoms to normal ageing and not having proper information to distinguish symptoms as problematic, but also including perceived barriers such as lack of physician confirmation of a problem, the cost of diagnostic services, and lack of access to medical specialists (Boise *et al.* 1999; Wackerbarth *et al.* 2002).

Ethnic and cultural diversity before the diagnosis

Studies in the United States have also tapped ethnic diversity in searching for how family carers interpret dementia symptoms before seeking a diagnosis. Mahoney and colleagues (2005) conducted retrospective interviews in either focus group or personal interview format with small samples of African American, Chinese and Latino family carers. The Latino group included individuals from six different countries of origin including Puerto Rico and five Central or South American countries, providing clear evidence of the wide cultural heritage represented by Latinos in the United States (Gallagher-Thompson *et al.* 2003; Weineck *et al.* 2004). Across the three groups, initial impressions of their relatives' memory loss were attributed to normal ageing, although cultural explanations for this attribution varied: for African Americans, 'old timer's disease'; for Chinese, 'hu tu', signifying forgetfulness in old age, as well as bad 'feng shui' or negative environmental energies; and for Latinos, 'el loco' or 'craziness'. All family carer groups reported normalizing their response to early symptoms but tactics varied: among African Americans, the ethic of strong respect for elders supported quiet tolerance of symptoms while marshalling extended family support; among Latinos, normalization was prompted mainly by not wishing to upset the person with symptoms; and among Chinese, normalization was couched in terms of keeping mental health problems hidden to avoid community awareness and social stigmatization. Triggering events to seek help outside the family were common across all three groups as well, leading to advice from community confidantes and subsequently medical sources to establish a diagnosis. Chinese carers mentioned the most hostility upon seeking informal advice due to the stigma attached to dementia in that community (Mahoney *et al.* 2005).

These results strongly suggest that remarkable cross-cultural similarities are found in the reaction of carers to symptoms in the pre-diagnosis phase of the dementia journey. Cultural differences tended to emerge, however, in the wider social world of these families as they sought information and support when symptoms persisted. Another study of carers from diverse ethnic backgrounds, including African Americans, Chinese, Latinos and European Americans (whites) found subtle group differences in reasons that symptoms were attributed to old age rather than to a disease process, but more striking differences were seen in how cultural meanings were reinforced through immediate family members' interactions with other family and community members (Dilworth-Anderson and Gibson 2002). This study and another study comparing white American carers with African Americans, Asian Americans and Latinos (Hinton *et al.* 2005) also found that whites were more likely to attribute biomedical, or disease, explanations to symptoms, while carers from other ethnic groups subscribed more often to folk or mixed folk/biomedical explanations. For additional literature on ethnic and cultural diversity in the context of dementia, see Chapter 3.

Exercise 15.1   Seeking help before the diagnosis

Talk with a family carer about how he/she went about seeking information and help when their relative's memory problems became apparent

Draw a diagram depicting the people with whom he/she attempted to form a partnership to reduce his/her uncertainty.

Making the diagnosis

More than two decades of scientific work has yielded only modest knowledge about the underlying causes of changes that occur in the brain in persons with various types of dementia. The most current American update on Alzheimer's disease and related dementia concludes that:

> different types of dementia are historically associated with distinct symptom patterns and distinguishing microscopic brain abnormalities. Increasing evidence from long-term epidemiological observation and autopsy studies suggests these distinctions are somewhat artificial. Symptoms and pathologies frequently overlap, and can be further complicated by coexisting health conditions.

(Alzheimer's Association 2007)

This is the level of scientific uncertainty that a physician walks into whenever a patient presents in the office with persistent memory loss complaints, often in tandem with a concerned spouse or adult child.

The pursuit of a diagnosis confronting physicians occurs against a back-drop of broader uncertainty that begins during medical training. Fifty years ago, medical sociologist Renee Fox published the first results of her intensive observational studies of medical education; many of her conclusions resonate loudly today. She recognized that medical uncertainty arises from a combination of the sheer volume of material that physicians-in-training are expected to digest and the gaps in scientific knowledge underlying the educational material imparted during training (Fox 1957). Because uncertainty borders the edges of knowledge, rapid advances in technology enabling exploration of previously uncharted terrain within the human body lead to yet more medical uncertainty (Gerrity *et al.* 1992). Examples of recent technological advances that relate directly to dementia diagnosis include the rise of genetic mapping (Fox 2002), brain imaging techniques, and drug discoveries (Post and Whitehouse 1998). The importance of medical prognosis is another source of uncertainty (Fox 2002), with direct relevance to questions that persons with diagnosed dementia and their family carers ask regarding 'what will happen next?'

From a strictly clinical standpoint, the degree of uncertainty in making a diagnosis of dementia should be considerably minimized by the publication and wide dissemination of clinical practice guidelines for primary care physicians and specialists. Very briefly, most guidelines recommend taking a careful history of memory and other cognitive impairment symptoms; conducting laboratory tests to rule out potentially treatable or reversible metabolic causes of dementia such as thyroid dysfunction and infections; conducting neuropsychological batteries of performance and interview-based tests to determine the types of and severity of cognitive impairments; and brain imaging techniques such as non-contrast computed tomography (CT scans) or magnetic resonance imaging (MRI scans).

In the UK, evidence-based practice guidelines for dementia diagnosis and management were released in 2006 by the National Institute for Health and Clinical Excellence and Social Care Institute for Excellence (NICE-SCIE) under the sponsorship of the National Health Service. These guidelines are quite explicit regarding laboratory and other diagnostic testing procedures that should be performed, and provide clear guidance for primary care practitioners about how to obtain specialist assistance when implementing diagnostic procedures. Within the past decade a number of similarly explicit evidence-based clinical practice guidelines have been published in the United States but, unlike in the UK, these guidelines do not carry the sponsorship or sanction of the federal government. Instead, they have been sanctioned by physician specialty organizations and advocacy organizations in the voluntary sector (American Geriatrics Society (AGS) 2003; Small *et al.* 1997). In Canada, the College of Family Physicians published a management guide for primary care of people with dementia (Pimlott *et al.* 2006). Other Canadian guidelines for evaluating people suspected of having dementia have also been published (Patterson *et al.* 1999). The AGS guidelines are abstracted from practice parameters published in 2001 by Quality Standard Subcommittees of the American Neurological Association. It is noteworthy that both the AGS guidelines and the NICE-SCIE guidelines refer to the same diagnostic formulations – the National Institute of Neurologic, Communicative Disorders and

Stroke-Alzheimer's Disease and Related Disorders Association Work Group – to help physicians arrive at a differential diagnosis (i.e., to distinguish vascular dementia from Alzheimer's disease).

Despite this widely available clinical guidance to help physicians make a diagnosis, research based on medical record reviews and surveys of primary care physicians has consistently found sub-optimal levels of diagnostic performance in the United Kingdom (Audit Commission 2002), the United States (Callahan *et al.* 1995; Fortinsky and Wasson 1997; Valcour *et al.* 2000), Canada (Pimlott *et al.* 2006) and Australia (Brodaty *et al.* 1994). These poor diagnostic performance results are explained in large part by primary care physician reports of reservations about their capacity to confidently arrive at a diagnosis of dementia symptoms (Boise *et al.* 1999). Unfortunately, physician reluctance to make the diagnosis in the face of their uncertainty has the added effect of prolonging uncertainty for the patient and family. Another reaction in the face of uncertainty is to make a diagnosis that is possibly premature in order to placate the patient and family and to begin a regimen of medications to address cognitive symptoms, an approach that carries its own risks (Iliffe and Manthorpe 2004).

Exercise 15.2   Finding support and reducing uncertainty: What is available?

Go online to search for support in your community for persons with dementia.

Think about the uncertainties faced by persons with dementia and their carers and how the services available might reduce, or add to their uncertainty.

Make a list of support available in your community and the support that seems to be missing.

Clinical trials to improve diagnosis

Several recently published studies with practising primary care physicians and other practitioners provide partial evidence of the value of educational interventions to improve their dementia diagnosis practices. In the United Kingdom, 35 primary care practices in London and central Scotland were randomly assigned to one of four trial arms: an electronic tutorial carried on a CD-ROM; decision support software built into the electronic medical record; in-person workshops convened at the practice site; or no intervention (Downs *et al.* 2006). The primary outcome measures were dementia detection rates and concordance with the clinical practice guidelines in the UK that preceded the 2006 NICE-SCIE guidelines. Results indicated that dementia detection rates were statistically significantly higher than control group practices in the intervention groups that received decision support software and in-person educational workshops (both $p<0.05$). No group differences were found, however, in concordance with clinical practice guidelines for dementia diagnosis or management after the trial compared to before; concordance scores remained low in all study arms after the trial. This study lends support for specific types of educational interventions in improving detection of dementia in primary care, but provides little guidance for ways to improve concordance with clinical practice guidelines for dementia diagnosis or management.

In primary care interventions in the United States, two studies employed nurses and social workers in primary care clinics to determine their effects on dementia diagnosis and dementia management practices in the practice sites. The first study involved 18 primary care practices in Southern California that were randomly assigned to either receive or not receive dementia guideline-based disease management led by non-physician primary care providers. Results indicated that practices with care coordinators in place did follow clinical practice guidelines in a greater proportion of patients than in practices without care coordinators (Vickrey *et al.* 2006). However, this same study did not produce improved provider self-reported knowledge about or attitudes favourable to dementia care (Chodosh *et al.* 2006).

A similar primary care enhancement intervention in a different part of the United States also found significantly improved dementia diagnosis practices concordant with clinical guidelines, but this study did not explore provider knowledge or attitudes about dementia care (Callahan *et al.* 2006).

Taken together, these studies demonstrate that it is possible to introduce educational programmes directly into primary care settings and achieve modest impacts on dementia detection rates, and that enhanced primary care settings involving nurses or social workers can achieve improved dementia diagnosis practices. One important limitation of the latter types of studies is that in the United States the primary care enhancement models tested are quite resource-intensive and it is not clear that they could be replicated in most primary care settings with more constrained resources unless public policy changes are made to help finance these initiatives (Covinsky and Johnston 2006).

Numerous reasons have been cited for the lack of adherence to dementia diagnosis clinical guidelines among primary care physicians. Reported barriers to adequate dementia diagnosis by primary care physicians include: attitudes of futility toward making a diagnosis in the absence of effective drug therapies; concerns about consequences of making an incorrect diagnosis due to the stigma of dementia; limited professional training in mental health disorders of later life; the complexity of dementia as a psychological and biological disorder with variable signs and symptoms; and the lack of specialists to confirm primary care physician suspicions, especially in rural areas (Boise *et al.* 1999; Cody *et al.* 2002; Iliffe and Manthorpe 2002; Teel 2004).

Disclosing the diagnosis

Numerous studies, using a variety of methodologies, have examined attitudes to disclosing the diagnosis of dementia, current practice regarding disclosure, factors influencing disclosure, the impacts of disclosure on people with dementia, and carers' views on disclosure. At first glance, it is surprising that there would be any difference in opinion or practice regarding practitioners disclosing a dementia diagnosis to persons and family carers; preference for disclosure would appear to be universal among all participants in the dementia care triad in order to relieve uncertainty about the cause of dementia symptoms and to initiate post-diagnosis treatment and early support service strategies. Empirical results, however, suggest a much more complex reality.

Bamford and colleagues published the most comprehensive review of dementia disclosure research to date, systematically summarizing methods and results of 59 studies completed through September 2003 (Bamford *et al.* 2004). In the same year, Carpenter and Dave (2004) published a review of opinion and practice regarding dementia diagnostic disclosure, and also proposed a research agenda based on identified gaps in the published literature. Both reviews combined results regardless if respondents were physicians, carers, or persons with dementia. Both studies found wide variation in physicians' disclosure practices, preferences among carers to inform their relatives about the diagnosis, and preferences among persons with dementia to learn the diagnosis.

The most common reasons in favour of diagnostic disclosure revealed by the studies reviewed by Bamford and colleagues (2004) were: to facilitate planning (10 studies); psychological benefit to the person with dementia and/or carers (9); the person's right to know the diagnosis (6); and to maximize treatment possibilities (6). Conversely, most common reasons against diagnostic disclosure included: risk of causing emotional distress (12 studies); inability of the person with dementia to understand and/or retain diagnosis (10); no benefits, costs outweigh benefits (8); lack of a cure or effective treatments (6); and stigma associated with dementia (6). Based on their review, it is clear that existing studies demonstrate wide variability in all dimensions of disclosure and thus indicate a significant discrepancy between current practice and the guidance about disclosure in policy documents (e.g. Department of Health 2001) and professional journals (Drickamer and Lachs 1992). It is noteworthy that some of the reasons expressed by physicians for withholding the diagnosis in these studies are similar to reasons why physicians are reluctant to pursue diagnostic assessments, particularly due to the lack of effective therapies and perceived stigma of labelling patients with the diagnosis.

Both reviews concluded that the perspectives of people with dementia, in comparison to carers and professionals, appear relatively neglected in the disclosure literature, although this imbalance is slowly being rectified in more recent years. From an ethical perspective, Carpenter and Dave (2004) noted that a dementia diagnosis is the 'property' of the person to whom it applies, and that individual has the right to share or withhold that information with others. Indeed, a more recent study of a small sample of persons with dementia found that although they were comfortable sharing their diagnosis with family members and other loved ones, they were reluctant to do so with people beyond their immediate circle of family and close friends (Langdon *et al.* 2007).

Exercise 15.3 Training professional carers: What they learn and what is missing

Visit a local medical school and talk with a faculty member or administrator responsible for the curriculum about how medical students are exposed to older adults with memory problems during their training years.

Consider how this curriculum addresses the challenges of medical uncertainty as discussed in this chapter.

Early support after the diagnosis

The final section of the chapter describes research concerning the needs of patients and their carers immediately following diagnosis and summarizes the rapidly expanding range of support services available in the community from the public or statutory sector, and from the voluntary or private sector, for people with diagnosed dementia and their families in order to supplement family care. Examples of such programmes are drawn primarily from the UK and the United States. Programmes at this phase of the dementia journey are intended mainly to address the uncertainties facing people with newly diagnosed dementia and/or their family carers in the areas of adjustment to the diagnosis itself, legal and financial planning, and anticipatory feelings of isolation.

Many of the concerns voiced by subjects in the study conducted with pre-diagnosed persons by Moniz-Cook and colleagues (2006), mentioned earlier in this chapter, are highly relevant to the development of early support services. This study found that the most prominent worries among pre-diagnosed persons were their loss of bodily function (especially incontinence), and the impact on family members of the anticipated diagnosis and their anticipated further cognitive and functional decline. This study identified another important concern that is highly salient to the development of early support services – subjects' desires to maintain social activities and physical activities such as gardening, exercise, and sustaining their valued personal relationships with loved ones as long as possible. If a diagnosis were made, most subjects in this study reported wanting 'reassurance about what to do' in the future almost exclusively as a function of taking medications to forestall symptom progression, highlighting the lack of awareness about support services available to them (Moniz-Cook *et al.* 2006).

However, this study did not address how persons with dementia went about seeking information from lay sources prior to visiting their GP, nor about what prompted them to actually visit their GP about their memory-related concerns. Clues about these issues could inform efforts in many countries to develop 'social messages' about how persons and families concerned about memory loss could seek assistance to obtain a diagnostic work-up and initiate early support services.

Partnerships

Many studies summarized in this chapter suggest the potential value to people with dementia and their family carers of forming partnerships from the earliest phases of the dementia journey. The principle of partnership in the context of dementia can be viewed broadly as any effort to help minimize uncertainty in dementia care, at any phase along the dementia journey. The goal in forming dementia care partnerships is to integrate the views and knowledge of numerous stakeholders to help resolve the numerous uncertainties in dementia care. Partnerships can be formed between people with dementia and their family members; among people with dementia, family carers, and one health care professional such as physicians (Fortinsky 2001) or community mental health nurses (Nolan *et al.* 2003); and among health and social care practitioners and voluntary sector organizations on behalf of persons with dementia and family carers (Abendstern *et al.* 2006; Kumpers *et al.* 2006).

In the UK, the Department of Health (2001), in its landmark *National Service Framework for Older People*, introduced the term 'partnership' into the health policy lexicon. This policy document called for the rapid development of 'knowledge-based practice and partnership working between those who use and those who provide services; between different clinicians and practitioners; across different parts of the NHS; between the NHS and local government; between the public, voluntary and private sectors and reaching out to individuals, groups and organizations within the community'.

This policy principle has led to the gradual evolution during the first decade of the twenty-first century of statutory relationships among primary care trusts, mental health trusts, and local social services councils throughout the UK to improve dementia care. The language of 'partnership working' has become a staple in policy pronouncements in the UK about how to resolve deficiencies in care coordination and effectiveness regarding older adults with dementia and other mental health problems.

A series of public policy directives in the UK during this decade (Care Services Improvement Partnership 2005; Department of Health 2001; NICE-SCIE 2006) have provided considerable guidance about how early support services for older adults with mental health problems (as dementia is classified) should evolve through partnerships among primary care trusts, mental health trusts, local social services councils, and local voluntary sector organizations. These policy directives have led to careful considerations about how multi-professional teamwork can develop most successfully to meet the needs and maximize outcomes among persons with dementia and family carers (Manthorpe *et al.* 2003).

In the USA, the Program for all Inclusive Care for the Elderly (PACE) and the Wisconsin Partnership Program were both designed and developed specifically to integrate services and providers from across settings and organizations, creating ongoing partnerships among providers (Kane *et al.* 2006; Mukamel *et al.* 2007). In the Wisconsin Partnership Program, the consumer was afforded a more central position in decision-making, creating a working partnership between consumers and the network of providers. However, both of these programmes are quite limited, serving a small overall number of people with dementia.

In the UK, nurses with community mental health training are assuming increasingly central roles in early support service environment. These nurses are receiving special training in dementia care, and are working in partnership with family carers and persons with dementia during the stage immediately following diagnosis (Nolan *et al.* 2003; Woods *et al.* 2003).

Also in the UK, the Partnerships for Older People Projects (POPPS) have been established in 29 locales with funding from the Department of Health. The overall goal of POPPS is to provide earlier and preventive services for older people with or at risk for mental health problems. Partnerships have been forged between statutory and voluntary sector organizations in most POPPS communities. Embedded within many POPPS projects are creative early support services for people with early stage dementia and their carers, including 'well-being cafés' where people can meet in a relaxed atmosphere to discuss their challenges and accomplishments in the face of living with dementia. The aim of these cafés is to improve the mood of users by reduce anxiety and depressive feelings.

In many countries, support groups for those recently diagnosed have been established to allow frank exchanges of emotions and information among individuals facing the common future of life with dementia. In essence, these groups represent informal partnerships in response to the uncertainties that lie ahead after a dementia diagnosis is made. These support groups were pioneered by the work of Yale (1999). More recently a class-based programme designed for persons in early stages of dementia and their family carers was implemented in the United States and evaluated by Zarit and colleagues (2004). Known as the Memory Club, this programme allows for interaction time among dyads as well as within the groups of diagnosed individuals and family carers. Many positive features of this programme were voiced by participants in a preliminary evaluation, including the ability to plan for the future in a nurturing setting and joint problem solving to strengthen the couple's relationship (Zarit *et al.* 2004).

An important early support programme that has not yet developed to its full potential is counselling immediately around the time of a diagnosis. One example of this type of service was a brief individualized intervention at the time of diagnosis at a memory clinic, and individuals participating were found to experience positive benefits (Moniz-Cook *et al.* 1998).

An excellent monograph summarizing the current scope of early support services for persons with dementia and family carers in the UK is *Getting on With Living: A Guide to Developing Early Dementia Support Services* (Cantley and Smith 2007). This report provides a comprehensive overview of the background and evolution of a wide range of early support services throughout the country. For example, several localities initiated new early support services in response to an initiative by a voluntary sector organization, the Mental Health Foundation. Known as dementia advice and support (DASS) projects, five of the DASS pilot services were based in the voluntary sector and one in an NHS trust. All offered the provision of information to people with early dementia and their families; one-to-one, or group, support and advice, and befriending, an in-home companion service for people living alone with dementia. Other types of early support services developed through the DASS projects included tutoring about memory management through the use of prompts and memoire aids; helping the person with dementia with personal care by monitoring and prompting personal hygiene and domestic activities such as laundry; and conflict resolution programmes between different members of a family concerning the person with dementia.

In the United States, early support services for persons and families living with dementia have developed through a more modest public policy directive from the national Administration on Aging, which provides funding to states for Family Caregiver Support Programs. States have a wide degree of flexibility in how to develop dementia care services for families under this directive. Other early support service initiatives have been developed primarily as randomized trials of interventions to assist family carers with funding from the National Institutes of Health. Two rounds of projects known as the Resources for Enhancing Alzheimer's Caregiver Health (REACH and REACH 2) have been completed and evaluated, with results showing promising effects on carer outcomes (Belle *et al.* 2006; Gitlin *et al.* 2003) (see Chapter 16).

Recommendations

Before the diagnosis:

- Conduct research with larger samples of ethnically diverse subjects to illuminate how people with dementia and family carers form partnerships with family, friends, and other informal members of their local communities in order to address their uncertainties from the time troubling memory loss symptoms are identified.

- Conduct research with larger samples of persons with memory loss to refine how their awareness of changes in cognition and capacities develop over time.

- Disseminate results of this research to advocacy groups, physicians and other practitioners to sensitize them to the concerns they should address with patients and families at the time of diagnosis.

- Using patients' personal stories, train health and social care practitioners about how to incorporate unique ethnic and cultural issues into professional advice and guidance once the diagnosis is made.

After diagnosis:

- Develop and test the value of brief counselling interventions for people and their family carers at the time of diagnosis.

- Develop and test partnership models in community settings away from academic health centres, where primary care is practised most commonly, particularly involving the use of nurses with specialized training in mental health problems of older adults.

- Conduct cross-national policy and best practice comparisons to determine how the most promising initiatives to improve dementia care through creative partnerships can be adapted to the realities of other countries where such policies and practices do not currently exist.

- Conduct cross-national intervention research in medical schools and post-graduate medical training settings to reduce uncertainty that presently presents barriers to improved dementia diagnosis and diagnostic disclosure practices.

Debates and controversies

One ongoing debate in diagnosis of dementia is how soon after memory loss symptoms are noticed by family members and friends should they discuss their concerns with the person showing symptoms. We do not have sufficient knowledge about whether it is better to diagnose dementia earlier, and if so, for whom and under what circumstances is an earlier diagnosis better.

Another debate concerns who 'owns' the diagnosis. Opinions differ on whether the individual with dementia owns the diagnosis and should be told, allowing the person with symptoms to decide whether and when to share the diagnosis with family members. Others believe that family members should be told, allowing them to determine whether, when and how the individual with dementia will be told of the diagnosis. Clearly, many providers and family members continue to keep this information from people who are showing symptoms of dementia, believing this is the right thing to do. We need to better understand the implications of telling, as well as the timing and method of telling.

There has been discussion about whether services should be tailored to specific ethnic groups, as separate from other care recipients. While opinions differ on this, at this point we simply have insufficient knowledge about the implications of either separate or integrated service delivery systems. Nor do we know how to best tailor services within a programme to respond to different ethnic.

Finally, we are lacking agreement on the best methods of training physicians and other health care professionals to recognize, diagnose and manage memory problems in middle-aged and older adults. Creating effective providers will require more effective training programmes, especially those in primary care. At this point, we have insufficient guidance on these topics.

Conclusion

The journey from initial symptom recognition to diagnosis is characterized by uncertainty for both persons with dementia and family carers. Uncertainty about the trajectory of symptoms and impact of symptoms on loved ones and future care needs are commonly experienced. While the meanings of symptoms in early dementia are culturally determined to some extent, carers from many ethnic and cultural groups seek information from other family members and community confidantes before seeking medical counsel. Physicians also report considerable uncertainty regarding dementia diagnosis and diagnostic disclosure, and suboptimal clinical performance revealed in research supports their reported uncertainty. Clinical trials to date have yielded modest results in improving physicians' diagnostic behaviour, and enhanced primary care trials have led to improved outcomes among persons with dementia and family carers. The degree to which these limited promising results can be widely disseminated and replicated remains unclear. Policy initiatives in England have led to the development of dementia care partnerships across primary care, mental health and social services sectors. Community mental health nurses with dementia care training represent potential links between persons with dementia, family carers and physicians to improve partnerships and reduce uncertainties before and immediately following dementia diagnosis. Further research is needed to determine how professional educational programmes can be improved to produce future physicians and other practitioners with greater knowledge about memory loss and related cognitive problems to help reduce uncertainty and improve health-related outcomes in earlier stages of the dementia journey.

Further information

The Health and Social Care Change Agent Team (CAT) was established in January 2002 to tackle delayed transfers of care (or delayed hospital discharges) and associated arrangements.

The U.S. Administration on Aging Alzheimer's Resource Room is a website where families, caregivers, and professionals can find information about the Alzheimer's Demonstration Program, including information on support and assistance, and providing services to caregivers.

References

Abendstern, M., Reilly, S., Hughes, J., Venables, D. and Challis, D. (2006) Levels of integration and specialisation within professional community teams for people with dementia. *International Journal of Geriatric Psychiatry*, 21: 77–85.

Alzheimer's Association (2007) *Alzheimer's Disease Facts and Figures*. Chicago, IL: Alzheimer's Association.

Alzheimer's Society (2007) *Dementia UK*. London: Alzheimer's Society.

American Geriatrics Society Clinical Practice Committee (2003) Guidelines abstracted from the American Academy of Neurology's dementia guidelines for early detection, diagnosis, and management of dementia. *Journal of the American Geriatrics Society*, 51: 869–73.

Audit Commission (2002) *Forget Me Not 2002: Developing Mental Health Services for Older People in England*. London: Audit Commission.

Bamford, C., Lamont, S., Eccles, M., Robinson, L., May, C. and Bond, J. (2004) Disclosing a diagnosis of dementia: A systematic review. *International Journal of Geriatric Psychiatry*, 19: 151–69.

Belle, S.H., Burgio, L., Burns, R., Coon, D., Czaja, S.J., Gallagher-Thompson, D. *et al.* (2006) Enhancing the quality of life of dementia caregivers from different ethnic or racial groups. *Annals of Internal Medicine*, 145: 727–38.

Boise, L., Camicioli, R., Morgan, D., Rose, J.H. and Congleton, L. (1999) Diagnosing dementia: Perspectives of primary care physicians. *The Gerontologist*, 39: 457–64.

Bond, J., Stave, C., Sganga, A., Vincenzino, O., O'Connell, B. and Stanley, R.L. (2005) Inequalities in dementia care across Europe: Key findings of the Facing Dementia survey. *International Journal of Clinical Practice*, 59 (Suppl. 146): 8–14.

Brodaty, H., Howarth, G.C., Mant, A. and Kurrle, S.E. (1994) General practice and dementia: A national survey of Australian GPs. *Medical Journal of Australia*, 160: 10–44.

Callahan, C.M., Boustani, M.A., Unverzagt, F.W., Austrom, M.G., Damush, T.M., Perkins, A.J. *et al.* (2006) Effectiveness of collaborative care for older adults with Alzheimer's disease in primary care: A randomized controlled trial. *Journal of the American Medical Association*, 295: 2148–57.

Callahan, C.M., Hendrie, H.C. and Tierney, W.M. (1995) Documentation and evaluation of cognitive impairment in elderly primary care patients. *Annals of Internal Medicine*, 122: 422–9.

Cantley, C. and Smith, M. (2007) *Getting on with Living: A Guide to Developing Early Dementia Support Services*. London: Mental Health Foundation.

Care Services Improvement Partnership (2005) *Everybody's Business. Integrated Mental Health Services for Older Adults: A Service Development Guide*. London: Department of Health.

Carpenter, B. and Dave, J. (2004) Disclosing a dementia diagnosis: A review of opinion and practice, and a proposed research agenda. *The Gerontologist*, 44: 149–58.

Chodosh, J., Berry, E., Lee, M., Connor, K., DeMonte, R., Ganiats, T. *et al.* (2006) Effect of a dementia care management intervention on primary care provider knowledge, attitudes, and perceptions of quality of care. *Journal of the American Geriatrics Society*, 54: 311–17.

Cody, M., Beck, C., Shue, V.M. and Pope, S. (2002) Reported practices of primary care physicians in the diagnosis and management of dementia. *Aging & Mental Health*, 6: 72–6.

Covinsky, K.E. and Johnston, C.B. (2006) Envisioning better approaches for dementia care. Editorial. *Annals of Internal Medicine*, 145: 780–1.

Department of Health (2001) *National Service Framework for Older People: Modern Standards and Service Models*. London: Department of Health.

Dilworth-Anderson, P. and Gibson, B.E. (2002) The cultural influence of values, norms, meanings, and perceptions in understanding dementia in ethnic minorities. *Alzheimer's Disease and Associated Disorders*, 16 (Suppl 2): S56–S63.

Downs, M., Turner, S., Bryans, M., Wilcock, J., Keady, J., Levin, E. *et al.* (2006) Effectiveness of educational interventions in improving detection and management of dementia in primary care: Cluster randomised controlled study. *British Medical Journal*, 332: 692–6.

Drickamer, M.A. and Lachs, M.S. (1992) Should patients with Alzheimer's disease be told their diagnosis? *New England Journal of Medicine*, 326: 947–51.

Fortinsky, R.H. (2001) Health care triads and dementia care: integrative framework and future directions. *Aging & Mental Health*, 5 (Suppl 1): S35–S48.

Fortinsky, R.H. and Wasson, J. (1997) How do physicians diagnose dementia? Evidence from clinical vignette responses. *American Journal of Alzheimer's Disease*, 12: 51–61.

Fox, R.C. (1957) Training for uncertainty. In: R.K. Merton, G. Reader and P.L. Kendall (eds) *The Student Physician: Introductory Studies in the Sociology of Medical Education*. Cambridge, MA: Harvard University Press, pp. 207–41.

Fox, R.C. (2002) Medical uncertainty revisited. In: G. Bendelow, M. Carpenter, C. Vautier and S. Williams (eds) *Gender, Health, and Healing: The Public/Private Divide*. London: Routledge, pp. 236–53.

Gallagher-Thompson, D., Solano, N., Coon, D. and Arean, P. (2003) Recruitment and retention of Latino dementia family caregivers in intervention research: Issues to face, lessons to learn. *The Gerontologist*, 43: 45–51.

Gerrity, M.S., Earp, J.L., DeVellis, R.F. and Light, D.W. (1992) Uncertainty and professional work: Perceptions of physicians in clinical practice. *American Journal of Sociology*, 97: 1022–51.

Gitlin, L.N., Belle, S.H., Burgio, L.D., Czaja, S.J., Mahoney, D., Gallagher-Thompson, D. *et al.* (2003) Effect of multicomponent interventions on caregiver burden and depression: the REACH multisite initiative at 6-month follow-up. *Psychology and Aging,* 18: 361–74.

Hinton, L., Franz, C.E., Yeo, G. and Levkoff, S.E. (2005) Conceptions of dementia in a multiethnic sample of family caregivers. *Journal of the American Geriatrics Society*, 53: 1405–10.

Iliffe, S. and Manthorpe, J. (2002) Dementia in the community: Challenges for primary care development. *Reviews in Clinical Gerontology*, 12: 243–52.

Iliffe, S. and Manthorpe, J. (2004) The hazards of early recognition of dementia: A risk assessment. *Aging & Mental Health*, 8: 99–105.

Kane, R., Homyak, P., Bershadsky, B. and Flood, S. (2006) Variations on a theme called PACE. *Journal of Gerontology: Biological and Medical Sciences*, 61(7): 698–3.

Keady, J. and Nolan, M. (2003) The dynamics of dementia: Working together, working separately, or working alone? In: M. Nolan, U. Lundh, G. Grant and J. Keady (eds) *Partnerships in Family Care: Understanding the Caregiving Career*. Maidenhead: Open University Press, pp. 15–32.

Kumpers, S., Mur, I., Hardy, B., van Raak, A. and Maarse, H. (2006) Integrating dementia care in England and The Netherlands: Four comparative local case studies. *Health & Place*, 12: 404–20.

Langdon, S.A., Eagle, A. and Warner, J. (2007) Making sense of dementia in the social world: A qualitative study. *Social Science & Medicine*, 64: 989–1000.

Mahoney, D.F., Cloutterbuck, J., Neary, S. and Zhan, L. (2005) African-American, Chinese, and Latino family caregivers' impressions of the onset and diagnosis of dementia: Cross-cultural similarities and differences. *The Gerontologist*, 45: 783–92.

Manthorpe, J., Iliffe, S. and Eden, A. (2003) The implications of the early recognition of dementia for multiprofessional teamworking: Conflicts and contradictions in practitioner perspectives. *Dementia*, 2: 163–79.

Moniz-Cook, E., Agar, S., Gibson, G., Win, T. and Wang, M. (1998) A preliminary study of the effects of early intervention with people with dementia and their families in a memory clinic. *Aging & Mental Health*, 2: 199–211.

Moniz-Cook, E., Manthorpe, J., Carr, I., Gibson, G. and Vernooij-Dassen, M. (2006) Facing the future: A qualitative study of older people referred to a memory clinic prior to assessment and diagnosis. *Dementia*, 5: 375–95.

Mukamel, D., Peterson, D., Temkin-Greener, H., Delavan, R., Gross, D., Kunitz, S.J. and Williams, T.F. (2007) Program characteristics and enrollees' outcomes in the Program of All-Inclusive Care for the Elderly (PACE). *Milbank Quarterly*, 85(3): 499–531.

National Institute for Health and Clinical Excellence and Social Care Institute for Excellence (2006) *Dementia: Supporting People with Dementia and Their Carers in Health and Social Care*. London: NICE-SCIE.

Nolan, M., Lundh, U., Grant, G. and Keady, J. (eds) *Partnerships in Family Care: Understanding the Caregiving Career*. Maidenhead: Open University Press.

Patterson, C.J., Gautheir, S., Bergman, H., Cohen, C.A., Feightner, J.W., Feldman, H. *et al.* (1999) The recognition, assessment, and management of dementing disorders: Conclusions from the Canadian Consensus Conference on Dementia. *Canadian Medical Association Journal*, 12 (suppl): S1–S15.

Pimlott, N.J.G., Siegal, K., Persaud, M., Slaughter, S., Cohen, C., Hollingworth, G. *et al.* (2006) Management of dementia by family physicians in academic settings. *Canadian Family Physician*, 52: 1108–15.

Post, S.G. and Whitehouse, P.J. (1998) Emerging anti-dementia drugs: A preliminary ethical view. *Journal of the American Geriatrics Society*, 46: 784–7.

Small, G.W., Rabins, P.V., Barry, P.P. *et al.* (1997) Diagnosis and treatment of Alzheimer's disease and related disorders: Consensus statement of the American Association for Geriatric Psychiatry, the Alzheimer's Association, and the American Geriatrics Society. *Journal of the American Medical Association*, 278: 1363–71.

Teel, C.S. (2004) Rural practitioners' experience in dementia diagnosis and treatment. *Aging & Mental Health*, 8: 422–9.

Valcour, V., Masaki, K., Curb, J. and Blanchette, P. (2000) The detection of dementia in the primary care setting. *Archives of Internal Medicine*, 160: 2964–8.

Vickrey, B.G., Mittman, B.S., Connor, K.I., Pearson, M.L., Della Penna, R.D., Ganiats, T.G. *et al.* (2006) The effect of a disease management intervention on quality and outcomes of dementia care. *Annals of Internal Medicine*, 145: 713–26.

Wackerbarth, S., Streams, M. and Smith, M. (2002) Capturing the insights of family caregivers: Survey item generation with a coupled interview/focus group process. *Qualitative Health Research*, 12: 1141–54.

Weineck, R.M., Jacobs, E.A., Stone, L.C., Ortega, A.N. and Burstin, H. (2004) Hispanic health care disparities: Challenging the myth of a monolithic Hispanic population. *Medical Care*, 42: 313–20.

Wilson, H.S. (1989) Family caregivers: The experience of Alzheimer's disease. *Applied Nursing Research*, 2: 40–5.

Woods, R.T., Wills, W., Higginson, I.J., Hobbins, J. and Whitby, M. (2003) Support in the community for people with dementia and their carers: A comparative outcome study of specialist mental health service interventions. *International Journal of Geriatric Psychiatry*, 18: 298–307.

Yale, R. (1999) Support groups and other services for individuals with early stage Alzheimer's disease. *Generations*, 23: 57–61.

Zarit, S., Femia, E.E., Watson, J., Rice-Oeschger, L. and Kakos, B. (2004) Memory club: A group intervention for people with early-stage dementia and their care partners. *The Gerontologist*, 44: 262–9.

16

Living at home

Georgina Charlesworth

Learning objectives

By the end of this chapter you will be able to:

- discuss 'living with dementia' from the perspectives of the person with dementia and the family carer

- understand the tensions between safety and personhood

- identify the social networks associated with different types of service use

---

Introduction

> Most people with dementia are able to live in their own homes for most of their lives, and most care is given by families.

> (NCCMH 2007: 98)

Nearly two-thirds of people with dementia live at home (PSSRU 2007). The time between diagnosis of dementia and the need for nursing care is up to seven years, depending on the type of dementia and the physical health of the person, although with improved diagnostic processes the post-diagnosis duration may be increasing. During this post-diagnosis time, the person with dementia will need emotional support and increasing levels of assistance with activities of daily living. The increased care needs of the person with dementia affect family carers' lives whether cohabiting with the person with dementia, living within the same locality or 'at a distance'. The consequences of caring have been extensively studied, identifying carers as being at risk of physical exhaustion, emotional burnout, financial hardship and social isolation. Carers of people with dementia have higher levels of stress and distress than other caring populations (Ory *et al.* 1999). Stressed and distressed carers have higher mortality and morbidity than non-carers, and carer distress is one of the predictors of institutionalization of the person with dementia. Governments around the world have begun recognizing the needs of carers, while in the UK, the needs of family carers have been specifically recognized in successive policies over the past two decades (for a review, see Stevenson 2003).

In many countries, an overriding objective for social care is to maintain people with dementia in their own home for as long as possible (Department of Health 2001; Department of Health/Care Services Improvement Partnership

2005). To achieve this, both health and social care interventions will be necessary. In 2007, in the UK, the National Institute for Health and Clinical Excellence (NICE) in conjunction with the Social Care Institute for Excellence (SCIE) published a joint guideline on the care of people with dementia and their carers (NCCMH 2007). It was the first time the two organizations had come together to produce a joint guideline, highlighting the importance of joint health and social care working in the field of dementia. The NICE-SCIE recommendations for interventions for the person with dementia in the mild to moderate stages included cognitive stimulation, support groups and 'environmental modifications to aid independent functioning, including assistive technology' (NCCMH 2007). Psychological therapies such as cognitive-behavioural therapy (CBT) were also recommended for people with dementia with co-morbid anxiety and/or depression.

The NICE-SCIE recommendations for carers (NCCMH 2007) were:

- individual or group psycho-education

- peer-support groups with other carers, tailored to the needs of individuals depending on the stage of dementia of the person being cared for and other characteristics

- support and information by telephone and through the internet

- training courses about dementia, services and benefits, and communication and problem solving in the care of people with dementia

- involvement of other family members as well as the primary carer in family meetings.

Not all interventions for the person with dementia or their families will be appropriate or necessary in all circumstances, but the complexity of many situations will demand that multiple interventions should be considered. Care planning should be 'needs led', and should be specifically developed for both the person with dementia and their carer. Support needs for both carers and people with dementia can be summarized as falling within three categories: informational, instrumental and emotional. Informational support refers to advice and knowledge, instrumental support is that which assists with daily living needs such as housework, shopping, transportation and personal care, and emotional support includes having an available confidante (Wills 1985). Both carers and people with dementia are likely to demonstrate needs in each category, although there may be discrepancies in perception of need between assessors and the assessed.

Even when needs have been identified and services are available, accessing and using support are not entirely straightforward. Both carers and people with dementia may deny their need for support or choose not to use services from which they may benefit. For the person with dementia, an apparent denial of need may be a strategy to protect their sense of self, or may be related to a lack of awareness of their own cognitive difficulties. A denial of cognitive deficits, or lack of awareness as to the extent of difficulties with cognition and activities of daily living, is not uncommon in dementia, although there is a range of conceptual and methodological issues that needs to be addressed in research into awareness and deficits in awareness (Clare *et al.* 2004). For the carer, personal needs may be denied due to the carer's focus on the care recipient.

Exercise 16.1 presents an opportunity to consider the informational, instrumental and emotional needs of Mrs James (a person with dementia living alone), and the needs of her daughter, Kay (an 'extra-resident' carer), who visits on a daily basis. Were Kay a co-resident carer, she could provide prompts that ensure safety but visiting family, friends or service providers cannot offer such a high level of monitoring and support. Mrs James' needs and willingness to accept services will depend on her level of awareness of the incidents described, and on her perception of risk.

Exercise 16.1   Identifying needs

Mrs James is a 78-year-old widow who lives alone in the house she shared with her husband for 50 years. She has been experiencing increasing memory problems that started before her husband died, but which seemed to worsen after his death. Her daughter, Kay, insisted that her mother visit her GP, and Mrs James was referred to a Memory Clinic where she received the diagnosis of an Alzheimer's type dementia. Kay, who visits every day, has become concerned for her mother's safety following a number of incidents: Mrs James left the front door open when she went to the local shop; she left the bath tap running when she went to answer the phone; and she forgot to turn off the gas after she had been warming some soup. Fortunately there had been no great damage done on any occasion, but Kay is worried about what may happen next.

What are Mrs James' needs (informational, instrumental, emotional)?

What may Kay's needs be (informational, instrumental, emotional)?

What might some reasons be for either Mrs James or Kay refusing services to meet these needs?

Needs for those 'home alone'

People with dementia living at home alone are 20 times more likely to move into residential or nursing care than those living with a family member (Banerjee *et al.* 2003). This suggests that needs of people with dementia living alone are not being met, and indeed a study of community dwelling people with dementia in Ireland showed that people living alone with dementia were more likely to have unmet needs than their counterparts with a co-resident carer (Mcaney *et al.* 2005).

Some guidance for assessing the needs of people with dementia can be gained from using the Care Needs Assessment Pack for Dementia (CareNap-D; McWalter *et al.* 1998) that includes seven domains of need for the community dwelling person with dementia:

- health and mobility
- self-care and toileting

- social interaction
- thinking and memory
- behaviour and mental state
- housecare
- community living.

Comparing the needs of people with dementia living alone with the needs of those with a co-resident carer, the domains of thinking/memory, housecare and community living are more likely to be unmet (Meaney *et al.* 2005). The thinking/memory domain includes the specific items 'recognizing strangers' and 'remembering routines'; the housecare domain includes 'using the cooker', 'securing the home', 'appliance safety' and 'safety with gas'; and the community living domain includes 'taking medication', 'using the phone' and 'managing finances'. If a person with dementia has unmet needs in any of these areas, they are in a vulnerable situation in terms of their own safety and the safety of the home.

Maintaining the person in their own home requires a balance between minimizing risk and maximizing independence. A range of gadgets and devices has been developed to supplement carer-provided prompts and safeguards for aspects of daily living, and are collectively known as 'assistive technologies'. They include 'low technology' solutions such as day/night indicators, bath and cooker monitoring and shut off devices, medicine reminders, lost item locators, automatic lights, door alarms and programmable telephones. Evaluations of assistive technologies indicate that they can be of benefit where devices are reliable, aesthetically pleasing, meet an acknowledged need and are easy to install and use (Cash 2004; Gilliard *et al.* 2004). Where devices are 'user operated' it is also necessary that the person with dementia is both motivated and capable of operating them. Training techniques may be of benefit, such as those used within cognitive rehabilitation (see Chapter 9), but the level of awareness of the person with dementia will be an important factor in its success or otherwise.

For people in early stages of dementia, technological advances are also helping to meet informational needs. The internet has become a resource for both informational and emotional support, and in the UK both the Alzheimer's Society and Alzheimer's Scotland have web-pages for those with a diagnosis of dementia. Not only can written information and advice be downloaded but also problems can be shared through online discussion groups. For example, the Dementia Advocacy and Support Network is a worldwide organization for mutual self-help for people with a diagnosis of dementia (DASNI; www.dasn-international.org).

Caring for a person with dementia at home

Family carers who live with the person with dementia ('co-resident') often describe greater difficulty than those who live elsewhere ('extra-resident'), although there may be a confound with other characteristics such as age and kinship, given co-resident carers are often spouses whereas extra-resident carers are more commonly adult offspring. The pattern of associations between care-related stressors and outcomes are different for spouses and adult children. For example, physical impairments and behaviour problems of the care-recipient and a longer duration of care provision show stronger associations with carer 'burden' in spousal carers than in adult children (Pinquart and Sörensen 2003). This may be due to spouses also living with age-associated chronic illness, and to adult children being more likely to have alternative roles and social activities that may buffer against long-lasting stress. In other words, the available resources differ between the co-resident spouses and extra-resident adult offspring and lead to differing needs for both the carer and the person with dementia.

Models such as the 'Stress Process Model of Caring' (Pearlin *et al.* 1990) help us understand some of the individual differences between carers. (See Chapter 5.) Their model suggests that carer outcomes such as physical and psychological well-being are influenced by contextual factors (e.g. kinship, age, ethnicity, socioeconomic status), stressors (e.g. behavioural and psychological problems of the person with dementia; need for activities of daily living assistance), intrapsychic and interpersonal strains (e.g. divided loyalties between work and caring, or caring for parents or own children) and resources (e.g. coping, social support). The model would predict that carers have a better outcome where stressors and strains are minimized and resources are maximized.

The Stress Process Model formed the basis for Aneshensel and colleagues' (1995) 3-year longitudinal study of 555 carers for persons with dementia in the USA. The resulting book, *Profiles in Caregiving: The Unexpected Career*, emphasized the importance of changing needs over time when determining support.

> The form, content, and timing of intervention should depend to a considerable extent on where caregivers are in their careers, and involve an understanding of what has passed before and what is likely to lie ahead. That is, the problems encountered today should be viewed against the backdrop of yesterday and with an eye towards tomorrow.
>
> (Aneshensel *et al.* 1995: 306)

Aneshensel and colleagues subdivide the 'caregiving career' into the stages of role acquisition, role enactment and role disengagement, with role enactment covering both in-home care and involvement with the person with dementia post-admission to residential, nursing or continuing care. They referred to the stage of in-home caring as the 'long haul' for carers, and highlight the development of the carer from being illness-naïve to being experientially knowledgeable, and from having pre-caring levels of resources to being socially, personally and economically depleted. Their recommended interventions would be stress management and resource enhancement. More specifically, interventions to enhance psychosocial resources would include:

- carer education

- behaviour management techniques
- problem solving training
- personal counselling for emotional distress.

Similar to the NICE-SCIE guidelines, Aneshensel and colleagues suggest that a multifaceted approach is likely to be required. Extensive work has been undertaken in the United States to develop and evaluate a structured multi-component intervention for family carers of people with Alzheimer's Disease or related disorders. The Resources for Enhancing Alzheimer's Caregiver Health (REACH; http://www.edc.pitt.edu/reach) initiative started in 1995 funded by the National Institutes of Health. Its primary purpose was to develop and test new ways to help families manage the daily activities and the stresses of caring for people with Alzheimer's Disease or a related disorder. Building upon the findings of REACH I, REACH II was funded in 2001 to design and test an intervention targeting depression, burden, self-care and healthy behaviours, social support and problem behaviours in the person with dementia. Intervention strategies included education, stress and mood management techniques, communication skills and problem solving delivered in 12 sessions over six months. Carers in the intervention group from the three different ethnic or racial groups studied (Hispanic or Latino, white or Caucasian, and black or African American) all improved in quality of life compared to those in the control group (Belle *et al.* 2006).

In the UK, a multifaceted approach entails contact with a 'mixed economy' of care in which statutory, private and voluntary sectors provide community services in addition to the support given by family and friends. Britain has a long tradition of voluntary action, and the emphasis on partnership in recent government policies has given voluntary, community and user organizations a more central role in the delivery of services (Taylor 1997). At the same time, social service departments have been encouraged to develop local markets in care by providing fewer direct care services themselves and commissioning independent service providers (Ware *et al.* 2001).

Taking Mrs James and her daughter Kay (see Exercise 16.1) to illustrate the potential 'mixed economy' of care provision, informational need on 'safety in the home' may be met through information leaflets downloaded from a national voluntary sector organization such as the Alzheimer's Society by an occupational therapist employed through health or social services. Instrumental support may be provided through the private purchase and fitting of assistive technology by Kay's husband, and emotional needs met through local support groups and befriending services provided by a local voluntary sector organization funded by the local authority. If Mrs James were to attend a day centre, possibly run by the local authority or a voluntary organization, she might also receive transport from either the day centre provider or an alternative third party.

Understanding the inter-relationships of care-providers within the mixed economy is vital as introducing a new service to a family, or to a locality, may impact existing services. As state provision of welfare services increased in some countries, concern was expressed that the introduction of services would lead to a withdrawal, or 'crowding out' of family support. This concern has not been borne out. Indeed international comparisons have found evidence for accumulation of help from statutory and family supporters, that is a 'crowding in' of support (Künemund and Rein 1999; Motel-Klingebiel *et al.* 2005). Family care is often seen as 'saving' the state from the need to provide formal care, that is family care substituting for formal care for the person with dementia (Nelson *et al.* 2002; Nordberg *et al.* 2005). Schneider *et al.* (2003) viewed services as supplementing family support in the early stages of dementia care, followed by formal services substituting for family care as the person with dementia entered residential care. They also reported that service inputs for the person with dementia predicted higher family care inputs. In practice, this means that care planners can realistically hope that by introducing new services to meet needs they will reduce the number of unmet needs and enable families to continue caring.

Part of the role of the carer can be to 'case manage' the service provision for the person with dementia. This can be a challenging task when multiple services have been put in place. Exercise 16.2 describes provision of multiple services for Mr O'Keefe who has dementia and for his disabled wife. The services are provided by a range of organizations and involve day care, home care sitting services and a lunch club. Mrs O'Keefe experiences difficulties with these, but does not know who to contact.

Exercise 16.2 Carers' experience of the 'mixed economy' of care

Mrs O'Keefe, who has disabling arthritis, cares for her husband who has a diagnosis of vascular dementia and has marked difficulties in self-care. A care assessor visited, and arranged: a daily home care service to help with washing/bathing and dressing (private sector provider); two days per week day care (local authority); one day per week jointly at a lunch club (voluntary sector); and two hours per fortnight sitting service (voluntary sector). A few weeks after the various services were introduced, Mrs O'Keefe asked the lunch club coordinator if she could cancel everything as she was feeling more exhausted than she had before all the services started. On further enquiry, the lunch club coordinator identified Mrs O'Keefe's particular concerns as:

- feeling uncomfortable that someone else is doing 'her work'

- feeling frustrated at the unreliability of arrival time for homecare workers, day hospital transport and sitters

- feeling nervous and unsettled that a 'stream of strangers' was passing through the house

- that the home carers dressed Mr O'Keefe differently to the carer, and did not put his tie on even when she laid it out with his other clothes

- finding it difficult to tidy round in preparation for the care worker's arrival

- not being able to keep up with the laundry given the amount of towels used.

Mrs O'Keefe had no concerns about the lunch club, and indeed rather enjoyed her time there.

> As a voluntary sector worker with no responsibility for, or knowledge of, the other providers, what would you say to Mrs O'Keefe? Is it your role to make suggestions or offer advice? Can you relay messages on her behalf?

Had services been running smoothly, Mrs O'Keefe in Exercise 16.2 might not even have become aware that the services were provided by multiple organizations. Similarly, if the care assessor is able to review services and offers to act as advocate, then Mrs O'Keefe will not need to learn about any differing organizational policies and procedures. Otherwise, before she can begin to address any of the issues raised, she will need to build up a picture of which provider is responsible for each service, who the key contacts are for each service, and the best way of triggering review procedures within each service. Perhaps counter-intuitively, non-resident carers may find it easier to build up a picture of services as their contacts are predominantly with managers by phone, post or e-mail. 'Case managing' services requires a level of communication skills and assertiveness that carers may not have needed to develop through other phases in their lives, and thereby can be an additional burden.

The focus of many services for family carers is instrumental support or respite. However, Aneshensel and colleagues (1995) suggest that emotional support may have a greater influence on the course of stressors than instrumental support. Social relationships influence the physical and mental well-being of older people, but carers report less social interaction and fewer friendships with carers of people with dementia at risk of experiencing a reduction in their social network due to a lack of opportunities to socialize and/or the stigma associated with a dementing illness.

Social networks have been shown to effect access to resources and capacities to cope with life events (Wenger 1996). Constituent features of support networks include proximity to kin, proportions of involved family, friends and neighbours and levels of interaction with family, friends and community groups. The patterning of these features has been used to distinguish five network types (Wenger 1991):

- family dependent – small network and high dependency on local family

- locally integrated – extends beyond tighter family or household groups to include local family, friends, neighbours; good community involvement maintained

- locally self-contained – rely mostly on neighbours, although there may be contact with a family member; community involvement low

- wider community-focused – absence of local family and high levels of community involvement

- private restricted – no local family or other contacts and no community involvement.

These network types demonstrate some predictive power as to the demands made on health and social services. Locally integrated support networks appear more open to gaining new information and more able to adapt to a greater range of changes and pressures. People with dementia are most likely to remain in the community where their support networks are 'locally integrated', or 'family dependent'. Carers are thought most likely to require face-to-face support in 'locally self-contained' and 'private restricted' support networks.

How can emotional support for carers be enhanced if their social resources are being depleted? Although formal cognitive-behavioural therapies are recommended for psychologically distressed carers (NCCMH 2007), formal therapy may neither be available nor desirable for other carers. Only a fraction of psychological support is provided by psychological therapists, and there is much in common between informal and formal helping, such as empathy, positive regard and genuineness (Barker and Pistrang 2002). Indeed, Faust and Zlotnick (1995) found that, for mild to moderate mental health problems, the benefits of informal helping by mental health paraprofessionals, such as clergy and family doctors, are roughly the same as that of professional, formal helping, carried out by psychiatrists and psychologists. Most psychological support is provided through an individual's social network and there are examples of interventions designed to mobilize support networks.

The New York University Silberstein Aging and Dementia Research Center has a long-standing research programme into a psychosocial intervention for spouse-carers of people with dementia, designed to provide counselling and provide social support over the entire course of caring. A particular emphasis was on the mobilization of local family support through family counselling sessions, with the aim of enhancing the social resources of the carer. Higher levels of emotional support, more visits and having more network members to whom carers felt close predicted carers' satisfaction with their social support network (Drentea *et al.* 2006) and in turn satisfaction with social support predicted better mental health outcomes (Roth *et al.* 2005).

Not all carers have locally available family, and an alternative approach to enhancing social networks is through befriending. The Health Technology Assessment programme in the UK recently supported research into befriending of family carers by trained lay volunteers. The Befriending and Costs of Caring (BECCA) trial was a randomized controlled cost-effectiveness trial of access to a 'befriender facilitator' for family carers of people with dementia (Charlesworth *et al.* 2008). The study involved 236 family carers of people with dementia randomized to either intervention ('access to a befriender facilitator') or control (usual care). The level of support provided by families was related to the network type with carers in family dependent and locally integrated network types being more likely to receive regular support from family and friends, and carers in private restricted network types being most likely to have no support from family or friends (Charlesworth *et al.* 2007). Intervention group carers were put in contact with a local voluntary sector-based befriender facilitator and given the opportunity to be matched with a trained lay befriender who could provide 'a listening ear, companionship and conversation'. Only 1 in 3 of those offered befriending engaged with a befriender for the target six months and there was no evidence for either effectiveness or cost effectiveness of 'access to a befriender facilitator'. However, carers in the private restricted network were most likely to engage with the befriending intervention and least likely to see the care-recipient move into residential, nursing or continuing care (Charlesworth *et al.* 2007).

Lack of service uptake by carers is well known for both standard services and research interventions. Although awareness is a vital precursor to service use (Brodaty *et al.* 2005), awareness alone does not lead to increased uptake of services. Other factors include work status, socioeconomic status and level of burden (Bass and Noelker 1987; Miller and McFall 1991). Lack of time is associated with non-uptake although increased burden, depression or distress may increase uptake (Monahan *et al.* 1992). It is apparent that no single service is appropriate for all carers, and that carers needs may change over the years spent supporting the care recipient.

Over time, carer mental health and well-being may be steady, decline or show a period of decline followed by improvement. These different trajectories have been described respectively as the 'trait', 'wear and tear' and 'adaptation' models (see Haley and Pardo 1989; Townsend *et al.* 1989). Pinquart and Sörensen (2003) concluded that the relationship between duration of care and carer outcome is best explained by either the trait or adaptation model.

Although the predominant literature on carer well-being has focused on the stresses and burdens of caring, there is an emerging body of evidence on the Positive Aspects of Caring (PAC). Positive aspects include satisfactions with caring, enjoyable aspects of caregiving, feeling fulfilled or important; finding a sense of companionship and meaning within the relationship, feeling pride in one's own abilities to handle crisis. Cohen and colleagues (2002) found that 73% carers are able to generate 1 or more PAC, and Andren *et al.* (2005) found 51% of spouse carers and 66% adult-offspring carers reported either 'great deal' or 'quite a lot' of satisfaction. Individuals reporting higher PAC report less depression and burden and greater subjective health than those who did not endorse PAC (Cohen *et al.* 2002). Perceived uplifts are associated with lower levels of carer burden and depression. The ability to identify PAC seems to be influenced by racial or cultural factors, with African American carers scoring more highly on PAC than white Americans, and the relationship between PAC and race seems to be partially mediated by religiosity (Roff *et al.* 2004).

The mechanism of the relationship between positive and negative aspects of caring is not yet known. Hypotheses for the relationship are that uplifts reduce the negative effects of caring on outcome, or that distressed carers are less likely to perceive PACs. The finding that perceived uplifts are largely independent of objective stressors suggests that uplifts are rooted in other aspects of the carer – care-recipient relationship, or related to carer's personality or motivation (Pinquart and Sörensen 2003).

The care dyad

The most successful interventions appear to be those that involve both the carer and the care recipient (Brodaty *et al.* 2003). This is in the context of documented 'concordance' between the mental and physical health states of partners (Meyler *et al.* 2007). The well-being of one partner influences the well-being of the other, and the coping strategies of one partner influence the adjustment of the other. For example, Marriott and colleagues (2000) demonstrated that a cognitive-behavioural intervention not only reduced carer stress, but also led to a smaller increase in behavioural disturbance in the person with dementia.

The importance of supporting both the person with dementia and their carer was acknowledged by the launch of the Alzheimer's Society's magazine *Living with Dementia* which aims to help people with dementia and carers cope together (www.alzheimers.org.uk/News_and_campaigns/Newsletters).

A systematic review of evidence for effects of combined interventions for both the family carer and the person with dementia demonstrated a beneficial impact on the general health of carers, the mental health of people with dementia and a delay in admittance to long-stay care (Smits *et al.* 2007).

Transition to and from home care to care home

The proportion of people with dementia living in care homes rises with age, from 27% for those aged between 65 and 74, to 61% for those aged over 90. This demographic is most likely due to spouses being less willing to use care homes for their partners than are adult children for their parents. Differences in views on the desirability of institutionalization result in family role conflicts. This is illustrated in Exercise 16.3, where a carer is faced not only with the difficulty of making decisions on behalf of her husband, but also needs to navigate the associated conflicts within her family.

Exercise 16.3   Decision to institutionalize

Mrs Roberts's husband, Michael, has had increasing difficulties with memory and activities of daily living over the past five years. They have been married for 58 years, and have rarely been apart during that time. Their four children have all married and have grown-up children of their own. Various children and grandchildren were helping out with household tasks, but as Michael's condition worsened a number of conflicts arose, with some family members accusing others of not 'pulling their weight'. To try to reduce arguments, Mrs Roberts contacted social services and a package of care was arranged for Michael including both day care and daily personal care. Mrs Roberts hoped that if her family saw that she and her husband were not reliant on them for help, then the disagreements would stop. As time went by, Michael's abilities further declined and the topic of residential care was raised. Arguments within the family restarted, with strongly voiced views being aired both for and against. Mrs Roberts was concerned that whatever decision she made would leave her alienated from one part of her family.

What are the consequences for a carer of feeling isolated and unsupported within the family?

What should the role of involved workers be in supporting a carer in such circumstances?

When is the 'right time' to consider moving a person with dementia from home into care?

Exercise 16.3 illustrates the way in which family conflict can reduce the amount of emotional support available to a carer. A carer's family and friends may 'distance' themselves physically and/or psychologically from the carer and care recipient (Jones and Peters 1992; Clyburn *et al.* 2000; Upton and Reed 2006). The carer's burden may be increased through being faced with the family conflict in addition to a decision on institutionalization.

Debates and controversies

For many years most services were directed at family carers. For example, respite services were designed to give the carer a break with relatively little attention paid to its psychotherapeutic potential for people with dementia. Today we still lack clarity as to whether such services are for persons with dementia or for carers.

While we know the importance of social networks and social support, we have yet to agree on the most effective methods of assessing families and social networks.

There is considerable debate over whether services prevent or facilitate institutional care. Some argue that once carers experience some support they realize how much they need, while others argue that were services provided in a more proactive versus reactive fashion, carers would continue caring for longer.

Conclusion

The purpose of this chapter was to explore the experience of people living at home with dementia and the people who care for them at home. Reviews of research and of public policy suggest that support of both carers and people with dementia contributes to personal well-being and the ability to continue care, and that the most effective interventions take both into consideration. Research also documents that, while sometimes causing extreme distress, caring can be rewarding and despite the challenges of living with dementia, there is an increasing literature on the positive aspects. Carers of people with dementia have benefited less from interventions than other carer populations (Sörenson *et al.* 2002) highlighting the need for development work.

Acknowledgements

The Befriending and Costs of Caring (BECCA) trial was funded through a Health Technology Assessment (HTA project no 99/34/07; ISRCTN08130075) Primary Research grant to Charlesworth (UCL) Mugford, Poland, Harvey, Price, Reynolds and Shepstone (University of East Anglia) with additional funding from Norfolk and Suffolk Social Service, the King's Lynn and West Norfolk Branch of the Alzheimer's Society and an ad hoc grant from the Department of Health; the Mixed Economy in the Care of Dementia (MECADA) project is a secondary analysis of the BECCA data funded through an ESRC small grant to Charlesworth, Higgs and Poland (RES-000–22–2020 co-investigators Higgs and Poland). The views and opinions expressed in this chapter are those of the author and do not necessarily reflect those of funders.

Further information

There are websites designed for people with dementia on the **Alzheimer Scotland Action on Dementia** website. The **Alzheimer's Society** web pages provide direct information to both people with dementia and their carers.

The **UK government** has created a website for carers. It includes a range of topics from crime and education to living environment to tax questions and travel. The site is not exclusive to dementia, but more generally addresses disability.

Many countries have **non-government dementia care organizations** that serve as resources and advocates for people with dementia and their carers.

There are also organizations established primarily to support informal carers, such as the **National Family Caregivers Association** (NFCA) USA and **Carers UK**.

References

Andren, S. and Elmstahl, S. (2005) Family caregivers' subjective experiences of satisfaction in dementia care: aspects of burden, subjective health and sense of coherence. *Scandinavian Journal of Caring Sciences*, 19: 157–68.

Aneshensel, C.S., Pearlin, L.I., Mullan, J.T., Zarit, S.H. and Whitlatch, C.J. (1995) *Profiles in Caregiving: The Unexpected Career*. London: Academic Press.

Banerjee, S., Murray, J., Foley, B., Atkins, L., Schneider, J. and Mann, A. (2003) Predictors of institutionalization in people with dementia. *Journal of Neurology, Neurosurgery and Psychiatry*, 74(9): 1315–16.

Barker, C. and Pistrang, N. (2002) Psychotherapy and social support. *Clinical Psychology Review*, 22(3): 361–79.

Bass, D.M. and Noelker, L.S. (1987) The influence of family caregivers on elders' use of in-home services. *Journal of Health and Social Behaviour*, 28: 184–96.

Belle, S.H., Burgio, L., Burns, R., Coon, D., Czaja, S.J., Gallagher-Thompson, D. *et al.* (2006) Enhancing the quality of life of dementia caregivers from different ethnic or racial groups. *Annals of Internal Medicine*, 145: 727–38.

Brodaty, H., Green, A. and Koschera, A. (2003) Meta-analysis of psychosocial interventions for caregivers of people with dementia. *Journal of the American Geriatrics Society*, 51: 657–64.

Brodaty, H., Thompson, C. and Thompson, M.F. (2005) Why caregivers of people with dementia and memory loss don't use services. *International Journal of Geriatric Psychiatry*, 20: 537–46.

Cash, M. (2004) At home with AT (assistive technology): An evaluation of the practical and ethical implications of assistive technology and devices to support people with dementia and their carers. *Dementia Voice* www.dementia-voice.org.uk (accessed 31 March 2008).

Charlesworth, G., Shepstone, L., Wilson, E., Thalanany, M., Mugford, M. and Poland, F. (2008) Does befriending by trained lay workers improve psychological well-being and quality of life for carers of people with dementia and at what cost? A randomised controlled trial. *HTA Journals Series*, 12(4). Available at: www.hta.ac.uk/1233 (accessed 31 March 2008).

Charlesworth, G., Tzimoula, X., Higgs, P. and Poland, F. (2007) Social networks, befriending and support for family carers of people with dementia. *Quality in Ageing: Policy, Practice and Research*, 8(2): 37–44.

Clare, L., Wilson, B.A., Carter, G., Roth, I. and Hodges, J. (2004) Awareness in early-stage Alzheimer's disease: relationship to outcome of cognitive rehabilitation. *Journal of Clinical and Experimental Neuropsychology*, 26: 215–26.

Clyburn, L.D., Stones, M.J., Hadjistavropoulos, T. and Tuokko, H. (2000) Predicting caregiver burden and depression in Alzheimer's disease. *Journals of Gerontology. Series B: Psychological Sciences and Social Sciences*, 55: S2–S13.

Cohen, C.A., Colantonio, A. and Vernich, L. (2002) Positive aspects of caregiving: rounding out the caregiver experience. *International Journal of Geriatric Psychiatry*, 17: 184–8.

Department of Health (2001) *National Service Framework for Older People*. London: Department of Health.

Department of Health/Care Services Improvement Partnership (2005) *Everybody's Business – Integrated Mental Health Services for Older Adults: A Service Development Guide*. London: Department of Health.

Drentea, P., Clay, O.J., Roth, D.L. and Mittelman, M.S. (2006) Predictors of improvement in social support: five-year effects of a structured intervention for caregivers of spouses with Alzheimer's disease. *Social Science and Medicine*, 63: 957–67.

Faust, D. and Zlotnick, C. (1995) Another dodo bird verdict? Revisiting the comparative effectiveness of professional and paraprofessional therapists. *Clinical Psychology and Psychotherapy*, 2(3): 157.

Gilliard, J., Dementia Voice and Hagen, I. (2004) *Enabling Technologies for People with Dementia*. Cross-national analysis report, available from: www.dementia-voice.org.uk. Project website: www.enableproject.org (accessed 24 March 2008).

Haley, W.E. and Pardo, K.M. (1989) Relationship of severity of dementia to caregiving stressors. *Psychology and Aging*, 4: 389–92.

Jones, D.A. and Peters, T.J. (1992). Caring for elderly dependants: effects on the carers' quality of life. *Age and Ageing*, 21: 421–8.

Künemund, H. and Rein, M. (1999) There is more to receiving than needing: theoretical arguments and empirical explorations of crowding in and crowding out. *Ageing and Society*, 19: 93–121.

Marriott, A., Donaldson, C., Tarrier, N. and Burns, A. (2000) Effectiveness of cognitive behavoural family intervention in reducing the burden of care in carers of patients with Alzheimer's Disease. *British Journal of Psychiatry*, 176: 557–62.

McWalter, G., Toner, H., McWalter, A., Eastwood, J., Marshall, M. and Turvey, T. (1998) A community needs assessment: the Care Needs Assessment pack for dementia (CareNap-D), its development, reliability and validity. *International Journal of Geriatric Psychiatry*, 13: 16.

Meaney, A.M., Croke, M. and Kirby, M. (2005) Needs assessment in dementia. *International Journal of Geriatric Psychiatry*, 20: 322–9.

Meyler, D., Stimpson, J.P. and Peek, M.K. (2007) Health concordance within couples: a systematic review. *Social Science and Medicine*, 64(11): 2297–310.

Miller, B. and McFall, S. (1991) The effect of caregivers' burden on change in frail older person's use of formal helpers. *Journal of Health and Social Behaviour*, 32: 165–79.

Monahan, D.J., Green, V.L. and Coleman, P. (1992) Caregiver support groups: factors affecting use of services. *Social Work*, 37: 254–60.

Motel-Klingebiel, A., Tesch-Roemer, C. and von Kondratowitz, H-J. (2005) Welfare states do not crowd out the family: evidence for mixed responsibility from comparative analysis. *Ageing and Society*, 25: 863–82.

National Collaborating Centre for Mental Health (2007) *Dementia: The NICE-SCIE Guideline on Supporting People with Dementia and Their Carers in Health and Social Care*. National Clinical Practice Guideline 42. London: British Psychological Society and Royal College of Psychiatrists.

Nelson, T., Livingston, G., Knapp, M., Manela, M., Kitchen, G. and Katona, C. (2002) Slicing the health service cake: the Islington study. *Age and Ageing*, 31: 445–50.

Nordberg, G., von Strauss, E., Kareholt, I., Johansson, L. and Wimo, A. (2005) The amount of informal and formal care among non-demented and demented elderly persons – results from a Swedish population-based study. *International Journal of Geriatric Psychiatry*, 20: 862–71.

Ory, M.G., Hoffman, R.R., Yee, J.L., Tennstedt, S. and Schulz, R. (1999) Prevalence and impact of caregiving: a detailed comparison between dementia and nondementia caregivers. *The Gerontologist*, 39(2): 177–85.

Pearlin, L.I., Mullan, J.T., Semple, S.J. and Skaff, M.M. (1990) Caregiving and the stress process: an overview of the concepts and their measures. *The Gerontologist*, 30: 583–94.

Personal Social Services Research Unit (PSSRU) at the London School of Economics and the Institute of Psychiatry at King's College London (2007) *Dementia UK: The Full Report: A Report into the Prevalence and Cost of Dementia*. London: Alzheimer's Society.

Pinquart, M. and Sörensen, S. (2003) Associations of stressors and uplifts of caregiving with caregiver burden and depressive mood: a meta-analysis. *Journal of Gerontology: Psychological Sciences*, 58B(2): 112–28.

Roff, L.L., Burgio, L.D., Gitlin, L., Nichols, L., Chaplin, W. and Hardin, J.M. (2004) Positive aspects of Alzheimer's caregiving: the role of race. *Journal of Gerontology: Psychological Sciences*, 59B(4): 185–90.

Roth, D.L., Mittelman, M.S., Clay, O.J., Madan, A. and Haley, W.E. (2005) Changes in social support as mediators of the impact of a psychosocial intervention for spouse caregivers of persons with Alzheimer's disease. *Psychology and Aging*, 20(4): 634–44.

Schneider, J., Hallam, J., Islam, M., Murray, J., Foley, B., Atkins, L., Banerjee, S. and Mann, A. (2003) Formal and informal care for people with dementia: variations in costs over time. *Ageing and Society*, 23: 303–26.

Smits, C.H.M., de Lange, J., Droes, R-M., Meiland, F., Vernooij-Dassen, M. and Pot, A.M. (2007) Effects of combined intervention programmes for people with dementia living at home and their caregivers: a systematic review. *International Journal of Geriatric Psychiatry*, 22: 1181–93.

Sörensen, S., Pinquart, M. and Duberstein, P. (2002) How effective are interventions with caregivers? An updated meta-analysis. *The Gerontologist*, 42: 356–72.

Stevenson, F. (2003) Community care and informal caring. In: G. Scambler (ed.) *Sociology as Applied to Medicine*. London: Elsevier.

Taylor, M. (1997) *The Best of Both Worlds: Partnership between Government and Voluntary Organisations: York: YPS for Joseph Rowntree Foundation*.

Townsend, A., Noelker, L., Deimling, G. and Bass, D. (1989) Longitudinal impact of interhouse caregiving on adult children's mental health. *Psychology and Ageing*, 4: 393–401.

Upton, N. and Reed, V. (2006) The influence of social support on caregiver coping. *International Journal of Psychiatric Nursing Research*, 11: 1256–67.

Ware P., Matosevic T., Forder J. *et al.* (2001) Movement and change: independent sector domiciliary care providers between 1995 and 1999. *Health and Social Care in the Community*, 9(6): 334–40.

Wenger, G.C. (1991) A network typology: from theory to practice. *Journal of Aging Studies*, 5(2): 147–62.

Wenger, G.C. (1996) Social networks and gerontology. *Reviews in Clinical Gerontology*, 6: 285–93.

Wills, T.A. (1985) Supportive functions of interpersonal relationships. In: S. Cohen and S.L. Syme (eds) *Social Support and Health*. Orlando, FL: Academic Press.

17

Care of people with dementia in the general hospital

Fiona Thompson, Deborah Girling, Susan Green and Clare Wai

Learning objectives

By the end of this chapter you will:

- be aware of the prevalence of dementia in the general hospital
- understand why it is important that dementia is identified early in the hospital admission
- know how to take steps to prevent deterioration in health for persons with dementia who are admitted to hospital
- be familiar with steps to reduce length of stay and optimize the chance of returning home

---

Introduction

Older persons with dementia are admitted to hospital and remain in hospital for a variety of reasons. Maintaining a high quality of care for patients during their hospital stay and a high quality of life post-discharge requires a comprehensive and sensitive approach to assessment and care while in hospital. An optimal stay balances thorough clinical management of the medical condition with maintenance of cognitive and functional ability while also attending to quality of life. For patients with dementia, this careful and sensitive management requires specialized knowledge, an understanding of how to communicate with people who have dementia (see Chapter 12) and inclusion of patients in decisions about their care (see Chapter 22). Since care of people with dementia requires specialized expertise, failure to recognize dementia decreases the likelihood that they will receive the care they need.

While patients with dementia face many risks as a consequence of hospitalization, hospital admission can also provide an important opportunity to establish a diagnosis for previously undiagnosed symptoms (see Chapter 15), to discuss treatment and to establish a support structure for the patient and family. If the admission reflects a breakdown in care or carer strain, a hospital stay presents an opportunity to review the situation and find alternative or additional sources of support for patients and caregivers (see Chapter 16).

This chapter describes the prevalence of dementia in the general hospital, the reasons people with dementia are admitted to hospital, particular risks of hospitalization for people with dementia, strategies for optimizing outcomes, suggestions for keeping patients involved in decision-making, and models of hospital care that are designed to improve care of people with dementia.

Prevalence of dementia in hospitalized patients

Estimates from the United Kingdom and the USA suggest older patients with dementia comprise between 20% and 25% of people in a typical general hospital (Department of Health 2001; Silverstein and Maslow 2006) and that a quarter of older patients presenting to the accident and emergency department after a fall had cognitive impairment (Shaw *et al.* 2003).

Research has shown that the diagnosis of dementia in the general hospital is often missed (Ardern *et al.* 1993; Harwood *et al.* 1997). One study documented that it is unrecognized as often as 50% of the time. In some cases, it is unrecognized because the diagnosis has not been made, while in other cases it is known but not recorded on admission (Silverstein and Maslow 2006).

Given the prevalence of hospitalization-related factors that affect the patient's quality of life, it is important that anyone caring for patients in the general hospital is familiar with good patient care and an understanding of dementia.

Reasons for admission to hospital

Patients with dementia are admitted to hospital for all the same reasons that people without dementia are admitted, most of which are unrelated to the dementia. This includes a range of medical and/or social reasons such as heart disease, cancer or accidents. Lyketsos *et al.* (2000) also found that psychotic symptoms related to alcohol use were relatively common reasons for hospital admission of patients with dementia.

While many hospitalizations are unavoidable, the quality of primary care is an important determinant of hospital admissions for older people with dementia (Hutt *et al.* 2004). Improving primary care for dementia patients by means of increasing the knowledge of primary care providers about dementia care would certainly decrease the need for at least some hospital admissions for these individuals. In particular, enhancing the ability of primary care providers to communicate with people who have dementia (see Chapters 4, 9, 11, 12) and creating more effective community partnerships with other services (see Chapter 15) might delay or prevent hospital admissions. Finally, effective management of chronic illnesses in the community has been shown to decrease the need for hospitalization of older people. This is particularly important for people with dementia.

Risks to people with dementia in hospitals

The general hospital presents a hostile and disorienting environment for the person with dementia. People with dementia are particularly vulnerable to changes in their environment. They may behave in ways that are difficult to manage in a busy 'acute' ward setting, requiring more nursing staff time than other patients (Erkinjuntti *et al.* 1988; Fulmer *et al.* 2001).

While complications from hospital stays are common among all older adults, people with dementia are more likely than people without dementia to be hospitalized and are at particular risk of developing complications related to their hospital stay (Silverstein and Maslow 2006). Complications are related to deterioration in both cognitive and physical functioning, the distress related to change in environment or unmet needs and to the failure of staff to recognize and address their needs (see Chapter 14). These complications can lead to prolonged hospital stays, increasing likelihood of further complications, increasing the likelihood of requiring institutional care on discharge and greatly diminishing their quality of life.

While the evidence is mixed concerning the mortality rate of people with dementia, there is evidence suggesting a higher post-discharge mortality rate (Lyketsos *et al.* 2000). One study documented a two-fold increase in death following hospitalization for hip fracture in patients with dementia as compared to similar patients without dementia (Holmes and House 2000).

A thorough history on admission increases recognition of dementia in persons previously undiagnosed and ensures an understanding of their needs early in the admission. Listening to the concerns of carers may reveal cognitive problems preceding the admission that can be used to clarify the diagnosis. However, people with cognitive impairment who were functioning well in a familiar home environment often become profoundly disorientated within a general hospital setting.

Care planning can then consider the probable increase in need for help and supervision while in hospital. In particular, the likelihood of patients becoming confused, distressed and agitated should be considered and strategies to prevent these outcomes should be considered. A range of factors is known to cause distress and agitation in people with dementia. These are presented in Table 17.1.

Table 17.1 Factors which cause distress and agitation

Physical environment

- lack of familiarity

- changes in bed or ward

- noise, bright lights, and other disturbances

Physical health

- pain

- poor food or fluid intake

- constipation

- medications

Social environment

- inconsistency of staff
- infrequent interaction with staff or family

Mental health

- cognitive deterioration
- depression and anxiety

Delirium

Another major risk for people with dementia who are admitted to hospital is the development of delirium. Delirium is characterized by a disturbance of consciousness and change in cognition that develops over a short period of time. It may be associated with perceptual disturbance, typically visual hallucinations or other psychiatric symptoms such as disturbance of mood and paranoia. Other patients with delirium may be quiet and lethargic. There is a tendency for the disturbance to fluctuate during the course of the day.

Patients who are admitted to hospital with symptoms of dementia may indeed have dementia or may have delirium with a reversible underlying cause of their cognitive symptoms such as urine infections and dehydration.

Differentiating between delirium and dementia is difficult and often both are present. As well as the patient's presentation, the chronology of the deterioration is significant for distinguishing the two. History from a carer or others familiar with the patient is helpful in establishing the time course of the symptoms of confusion and the patient's level of function at home. A wealth of other background information can be useful in determining whether the patient has dementia, delirium, or both. Underlying causal factors such as alcohol misuse and medication history should be carefully explored.

Distinguishing between the two conditions is important, as management primarily depends on the underlying cause. Caution should be used in determining the patient's baseline as cognitive status on admission might reflect delirium, rather than the patient's capacity prior to becoming ill.

Table 17.2   Diagnostic guidelines for delirium (World Health Organization 1992)

- Impaired, fluctuating consciousness and attention
- Global disturbance of cognition
- Psychomotor agitation/retardation
- Disturbance of sleep–wake cycle
- Emotional disturbance
- Usually rapid onset
- Hallucinations in any modality

Delirium is a direct consequence of a physical cause such as a medical condition, drug withdrawal or intoxication and may be evident on or arise during admission. Dementia is the biggest single risk factor for delirium, a condition that significantly increases morbidity and mortality (Elie *et al.* 1998; Francis *et al.* 1990; Inouye *et al.* 1999; Pompei *et al.* 1994). Non-detection of delirium in the emergency department has also been associated with an increased six months mortality rate (Kakuma *et al.* 2003). Overall, delirium complicates one quarter of admissions to the acute hospital in patients over the age of 70 (Francis *et al.* 1990). A review of studies identifying risk factors for delirium found that advanced age, medical illness, sensory impairment, psychotropic medication use, abnormal biochemistry results and alcohol misuse were consistently associated with delirium (Elie *et al.* 1998; Francis *et al.* 1990).

Delirium carries the risk of a permanent decline in cognitive function (Francis and Kapoor 1992), making these patients less likely to manage independently when discharged from hospital. Given the potential for poor prognosis if not treated, it is important that signs of delirium are identified early and appropriate care is provided.

Length of stay

Patients with dementia represent a large proportion of patients who remain in hospital for prolonged periods of time. One study showed that almost 30% of patients with dementia remained in hospital for over three months in comparison to 6% of patients without dementia (Erkinjuntti *et al.* 1988). One reason for this was inadequate social support and lack of placement options. Another reason is the higher incidence of complications (Silverstein and Maslow 2006).

Numerous studies have shown that dementia is an independent risk factor for increased length of stay in hospital (Erkinjuntti *et al.* 1988; Holmes and House 2000; King *et al.* 2006). Other factors that are often associated with dementia such as co-morbid psychiatric illness, medical illness and reduced ability with 'activities of daily living' also contribute to longer periods of stay. Patients with dementia living independently prior to admission are less likely than people without dementia to return to independent living on discharge from hospital (MacNeill and Lichtenberg 1997). Unfortunately, a longer stay in hospital may result in deskilling and reduce further their ability to return home.

Intensive rehabilitation may reduce the length of stay as shown in patients with mild to moderate dementia following a hip fracture and promote a successful return to independent living (Huusko *et al.* 2000). Applying a 'social model' of care that consists of an intensive effort to identify dementia and to begin working on discharge soon after admission, may also help in reducing complications and length of admission (Lyketsos *et al.* 2000).

Optimizing patient outcomes

The need for proactive management highlights the importance of being aware of an established diagnosis or making a new diagnosis early in the admission. Some patients may be overtly agitated or causing a disturbance on the ward. However, others may be suffering from similar levels of distress without being noticed. Therefore, it is important that staff proactively monitor all patients with dementia and implement preventive processes, taking care not to interpret a lack of visible distress as an absence of distress.

Essentially, good hospital care mirrors good dementia care. This includes recognizing dementia, timely diagnosis and treatment of reversible aetiology, education and support for relatives, initiating treatment, having an awareness of potentially complicating factors, preventing agitation and thorough discharge planning.

Nursing patients with delirium

Given that the risk of developing delirium increases in the presence of the multiple risk factors, it would follow that good clinical practice will seek to identify and modify these risk factors wherever possible. Preventing delirium will decrease the need for reactive approaches to managing delirium, for example, the use of sedative medications, which often result in adverse events such as falls and further deterioration of cognitive function (Inouye *et al.* 1999, 2003).

Patients with delirium may be distressed, agitated and difficult to manage on an acute medical ward. Once the underlying cause is identified and addressed, distress and agitation should be managed with environmental intervention including frequent contact with staff and placement in a well-lit room, possibly with other patients and with cues to help orientation. A one:one nurse/patient ratio provides reassurance and increases monitoring and safety. Low stimulus environments and minimizing the impact of sensory impairment (i.e. use of hearing aids or glasses) will minimize disorientation. Family presence can also be quite comforting, reducing the level of distress. These measures will improve outcome regardless of whether the condition is dementia, delirium or both.

Other helpful interventions include:

- continuity of location and staff (avoidance of unnecessary move)
- patient orientation to their environment
- explanation of interventions
- glasses and hearing aids used (switched on)
- quick identification and remedy of pain, thirst or the need for the toilet
- family may be able to reassure a disorientated relative but may themselves need explanation and reassurance
- careful attention to diet and fluid intake
- mobility encouraged
- monitoring of bowel and bladder function.

Medication with psychotropic drugs may be necessary to address agitation but should never be the first line of intervention. Medications should only be used when non-pharmacological efforts are ineffective and should not be used as a substitute for good nursing care as they can actually make the situation worse and have other problematic side effects. The British Geriatric Society and the American Psychiatric Association offers guidance on environmental and pharmacological management of delirium (American Psychiatric Association 1999; British Geriatric Society 2006).

Early discharge planning

Ideally, discharge planning starts on admission. This allows time to identify difficulties the patient may have been having at home prior to admission and provide important information about the patient's current level of functioning. History should be gathered from the patient, relatives, carers, GP or other professionals involved in the community. It is especially important to ask if the patient is known to mental health services. Careful assessment of the needs of the person with dementia and their carers, and liaison with professional community staff can facilitate early discharge.

Admission to hospital, especially with prolonged stay, causes disruption to social networks in the community and functional decline which reduces the likelihood of a successful return home. Hospital staff with limited community experience can be risk averse and in the presence of dementia consider institutional care the only option.

Table 17.3 Information required for effective discharge planning

- Patients' attitudes and wishes
- Family input concerning attitudes and wishes
- Current level/types of care
- Current accommodation
- Personal care needs
- Mobility
- Food provision and preparation
- Medications-organization and compliance
- Finances
- Sleep habits
- Wandering or getting lost
- Weekly structure and social outlets
- Vulnerability and risk of exploitation

Obstacles may be overcome with the implementation of simple strategies including rationalization of medication to simpler regimes, increased home care, day-centre attendance and meals-on-wheels. Multidisciplinary teams are the most effective way to achieve this.

Exercise 17.1 Preventing hospital-related decline

Mr A is an 83-year-old man who lives alone and has no known history of cognitive impairment. He rarely attends his GP surgery. He comes to the emergency department of his local hospital following a fall. He is admitted because he is unsteady on his feet and is found to have a urinary tract infection. On the first night in hospital he becomes very restless and confused repeatedly leaving his bed area and protesting that he is being held a prisoner. When staff try to guide him back to his bed he becomes agitated, shouting for help and hitting out.

What possible factors may be contributing to Mr A's confusion? Consider factors relevant both to the individual and to the environment.

What might be done to remedy underlying causes and relieve the distress Mr A is experiencing?

Differential diagnoses include dementia, delirium, psychosis and depression. Mr A has been exposed to at least two unfamiliar environments and a series of unfamiliar people in his first 24 hours in hospital. The ward activity and noise may be confusing and frightening. Where is the toilet, where can he get a drink? These may often be highly relevant factors for elderly patients in hospital described as 'restless' or 'wandering'. Attention to these environmental issues may reduce distress and disorientation The possibility of an acute confusional state or delirium should be considered. In Mr A's case the urinary tract infection for which he is commencing treatment may be one underlying factor for his acute confusion.

Involving patients in decision-making

The patient should be central to decision-making. In a busy ward environment, decisions may be made without taking the time to involve the patient. Conflicts between patient and hospital staff may arise in the context of admission, treatment or in planning discharge. Research in the general medical population has shown that cognitive impairment and increasing age are both associated with a lack of capacity to consent to treatment (Raymont *et al.* 2004). However, while one should be mindful that someone with dementia might lack the capacity to make certain decisions, the diagnosis of dementia does not necessarily render someone incapable of making decisions. A study in the USA demonstrated that persons with moderate dementia made decisions that were consistent over time, suggesting that they understood what was being asked and that their responses reflected true preferences (Feinberg and Whitlatch 2001). There is a common misconception among clinicians that patients with dementia cannot understand or participate in treatment decisions.

The UK and many other countries including the USA, Canada and Australia have adopted a functional approach to testing capacity for decision-making. This tests the process of decision-making rather than either the person's condition (status) or someone else's perception of the wisdom of their decision (Wong *et al.* 1999). The process by which a person is judged to be able to make a decision is their understanding of and ability to weigh up the information required to come to a decision.

This process works by providing information about the nature and purpose of the decision and likely outcomes. When presented in a way that optimizes the person's understanding, their capacity can be enhanced, allowing them to participate in decisions about their care. For example, the use of visual aids and choosing the best time of day to assess the patient or treating an underlying condition that is causing increased confusion can enhance the person's capacity to participate in decisions.

If a person is determined to lack capacity, collateral information from family and carers may help to guide in determining best interest. See Wilkinson (2002) for an extensive discussion of using proxies for people with dementia.

Determining the patient's best interest

- Is the person likely to regain capacity, e.g. is it likely that their mental state will improve during the admission, and if so, can the decision be made at that time?

- Can participation in decision-making be improved? Would involvement of the occupational therapist or speech therapist help to improve your ability to understand the patient?

- Could the medical staff explain proposed interventions in lay terms?

- What are the person's wishes (current or past)? Maybe collateral information from the family would shed some light on the person's wishes.

- Does the person have beliefs or values that may affect this decision?

- Has the person named someone else to make decisions on their behalf?

It is important to remember that the person's best interests may not equate to the professional's ideal management plan or to the least risky option.

Exercise 17.2 Thinking about options for the future

Mr A has been treated with antibiotics, has recovered from his urinary tract infection and is more settled on the ward. He remains disoriented to time and place, and history from his daughter suggests a gradual decline in memory over the last two years. She is concerned that he is unable to look after himself at home and needs to be discharged to a residential home or supportive accommodation. He has not been eating properly and gets muddled with the days of the week. He has a social life that is unstructured and he sometimes forgets what he was supposed to be doing that day. He has on one occasion wandered out of the house at 3 a.m. as he thought that it was afternoon.

On cognitive testing he scores 20/30 on mini mental state examination (MMSE). Computerized tomography confirms vascular dementia and he is on appropriate medication to minimize risk factors for further vascular change. Mr A is adamant that he wants to return home because he loves his garden and his friends who live locally.

What factors should be considered in assessing his ability to cope at home?

Should Mr A make his own decisions about where he lives?

In the event of him being incapable of making these decisions, how would you determine what to do next?

How might you enable him to be discharged home?

A thorough history should be taken and further exploration of his daughter's concerns should be made. Objective assessment by nursing staff, occupational therapists and physiotherapists offers further clarification of his level of function. Some hospitals allow a trial of self-medication to assess patients' ability to manage their own treatment routine. Ascertain what level of support he has had in his own home prior to admission. This enables you to paint a picture of how he was coping and to test his level of understanding when you assess him.

People are presumed to be able to make decisions about their own welfare. Sometimes, this ability to make a decision may be in doubt if, for example, the person appears to be making a decision without fully appraising the situation or if the person has a condition that may impair decision-making. Mr A's capacity to make a decision about where he should be discharged to should be assessed. If he retains capacity, then the choice is his. If he lacks capacity, any decision about placement should be in his best interest. His wishes remain important and should be central to determining best interest.

In determining capacity, one should assess whether or not Mr A understands the information required to make a decision. This involves understanding the specific difficulties he has in functioning at home, including any associated risk. He should be able to retain this information in order to weigh up the factors important in coming to a decision. He then needs to communicate this information to the assessor. All efforts should be made to enhance his capacity – this may involve writing things down or assessment by occupational therapy to demonstrate difficulties.

If Mr A lacks capacity to make a decision about discharge, then any decision made for him should be in his best interest. Mr A has clearly stated that he wants to go home. Although this may carry some risk, factors influencing his quality of life are important and offer weight in determining best interest. Sometimes compromise between the two has to be made.

Services may be put in place to enable Mr A to be discharged home. These may include home-care to assist with activities of daily living and to provide structure to his week. He may require help with shopping and cooking or need meals delivered. Medicines support agencies, rationalization of medication or dosette boxes may help with medication compliance. If he is unable to manage his financial affairs, legal advice should be sought.

Models of care

People with dementia may be admitted to various wards in the general hospital, depending on presenting illness or bed management. With this in mind, all staff should be able to recognize dementia and its impact on patient care and be able to identify a need for specialist input. UK guidelines state that hospitals should ensure that all patients with known or suspected dementia have access to specialist dementia services and that staff have appropriate training in dementia care (Department of Health 2001; NICE 2006).

Over the last decade, various innovative models of care have been created to improve hospital care for older people. Three main (and similar) types of specialist geriatric services for the acute care of older people can be found in several countries: specialist geriatric wards on the basis of age, integrated care in which specialists in old age medicine work with physicians on several wards in an integrated team and admission to specialist wards for older people based on clinical needs such as complexity or frailty (Metz and Labrooy 2005). In the UK, these approaches are fundamentally derived from the multidisciplinary models of assessment and rehabilitation first described in the 1940s (Parker 2005).

In the USA, nurses have been more extensively used as specialists in acute care for geriatric patients. Clinical nurse specialists (CNS), geriatric resource nurses (GRN) and gerontological nurse specialists (GNS) have advanced skills and knowledge in the care of older people. Their activities include promoting best practices, initiating clinical protocols and following patients throughout the hospital stay and post-discharge. Their roles are often interfaced with specialized units similar to those in the UK, such as the acute care of the elderly unit (ACE) and geriatric evaluation and management unit (GEM). Founded in the 1990s, the Nurses Improving Care for Health System Elders (NICHE) offers a range of resources for both individual nurses and hospitals to develop, use and evaluate best-practice care. Specialist geriatric assessment can have an impact on functional status, well-being and the likelihood of entry to nursing home care; however, some services actually exclude older people with dementia.

In Australia, dementia clinical nurse consultants were created to provide expert advice, education and support to families of patients with dementia and to staff working on acute care wards of hospitals.

In the UK, service models such as proactive care of older people undergoing surgery (POPS) and older persons' assessment and liaison team (OPAL), created by geriatricians, use the comprehensive geriatric assessment (CGA) approach to screen older people admitted under the care of acute surgical and medical teams, respectively.

The OPAL team, consisting of a nurse, a senior physiotherapist and a geriatrician, screen all acute medical patients over 70 years of age within 24 hours of admission in a preadmission unit and facilitate the best discharge or admission options for these patients. Early assessment by the OPAL team identifies those patients who require intensive geriatric care leading to improved care and decreased length of stay (Harari *et al.* 2007). Clinical issues including detection and management of delirium, end of life issues of care home residents, rapid discharge and investigation of patients with falls and management of potential readmissions may be addressed (Martin 2005).

The 'Discharge from Hospital Good Practice Checklist', specifically for patients with dementia, was produced by the Change Agent Team (Department of Health 2003) and has been widely used by councils and their NHS partners to assess their discharge arrangements and identify changes required.

Models of specialist psychiatric care

Psychiatry plays an important part in providing mental health care for people with dementia, assisting with diagnosis or management of dementia and related mental health problems, offering advice on placement options, or a combination of these. Many referrals to psychiatry services request advice on placement or request an assessment of the patient's ability to make decisions about their care. Brindle and Holmes (2005) described the roles that psychiatric services play in assessing capacity: education of other professionals; provision of specialist input in more complex cases; provision of information on the range of services available to support older people with dementia so that options may be fully understood.

There are a variety of models of psychiatric care for patients with dementia in the general hospital (Royal College of Psychiatrists 2005). These involve varying degrees of integration between acute hospital and mental health staff. The most suitable model for a given hospital will depend on hospital size, prevalence of dementia and available resources.

In a standard sector model, mental health staff are based outside the general hospital and provide consultation with an individual patient at the request of general hospital staff. This model aids continuity if the patient requires specialist follow-up on discharge from hospital. However, as staff are not specifically appointed to or present in the general hospital, delays to consultation are inevitable and intensive follow-up less practical. This model does not generally provide for regular contact with hospital staff. An enhanced sector model has increased resources within the sector team to enable a rapid response to referrals.

The liaison mental health nurse is a nurse specialist whose role is dedicated to the general hospital enabling a rapid response and ongoing input in cases where the patient is remaining in hospital and needs follow-up of their mental health problems during this admission. This follow-up may be intensive requiring reviews on a daily basis, similar to that provided if a patient is being offered intensive input from mental health services either at home or in a psychiatry in-patient setting. The role of a liaison mental health nurse covers four domains: expert practice, professional leadership; education, training and development, and practice and service development. In the clinical settings, the liaison nurse focuses on practical and care-oriented interventions.

In Australia, the impact of the consultation-liaison nursing role has been studied and has often demonstrated improved access of general hospital patients to specialist mental health care and valued expert assistance to staff (Sharrock *et al.* 2006). Liaison psychiatric nurses for older people are also effective in improving nursing care for older patients on medical wards and facilitating appropriate discharge options. Sometimes a liaison psychiatrist has dedicated sessions in the general hospital. Similarly, this provides for rapid response to referrals, follow-up and education. The psychiatrist is medically trained and has a broad understanding of medical problems and provides diagnosis and treatment.

This liaison multidisciplinary team brings a much wider range of expertise and includes occupational therapy, social work and support work along with the above medical and nursing input. This allows all aspects of a patient's care related to their dementia to be addressed within one team. When comparing this liaison model to a consultation or reactive model, the liaison model is found to promote greater numbers of referrals and improved diagnostic accuracy among those making referrals in the longer term (Swanwick *et al.* 1993).

A shared ward enables physicians and psychiatrists to have joint responsibility for patient care. This enables both medical and psychiatric care at inpatient intensity to be provided at the same time, avoiding compromise of psychiatric care in a medical ward and medical care in a psychiatric ward.

Exercise 17.3 A turn for the worse

Mr A developed a chest infection which prolonged his stay in hospital. He has become withdrawn and has reduced his food and fluid intake. He has told staff that he does not feel like eating. While previously, he watched TV to pass time, he is no longer doing this.

What diagnoses would you consider?

How would you proceed?

Possible diagnoses include delirium, further deterioration in cognitive function secondary to prolonged admission or recent infection. He also presents with reduced appetite and has stopped doing an activity that he previously enjoyed. This may be due to a loss of interest, an inability to concentrate or sensory impairment. Some of these symptoms are indicative of a depressive episode. Depression is prevalent among older hospital inpatients and, in combination with cognitive impairment, further increases the length of stay.

The patient should be urgently assessed by the medical team looking after the patient to identify and treat the underlying cause of a delirium if present. Poor food and fluid intake should be highlighted and monitored by nursing staff as he is at risk of dehydration and electrolyte disturbance.

Assessment by a team skilled in differentiating between these possibilities should be made. He may require treatment for depression and need regular follow-up by the mental health team. A liaison team can offer ongoing psychological support and monitoring of mental state during the admission. They will also provide guidance to the ward staff in monitoring depressive symptoms longitudinally. At the point of discharge the team will advise or arrange follow-up with the appropriate mental health team or the patient's GP.

International comparisons

It is difficult to compare the effectiveness of various specialist nurses and care models across the world, as there are marked differences in training curricula of nurses and doctors, health care costs, provision and systems, resources, culture and practices; however, it is a common global theme that general hospital staff require enhanced skills and knowledge to look after the complex needs of older people with dementia.

Globally, there is an abundance of guidelines on best practice and government frameworks to inform staff and service providers in ways to improve the care of older people with dementia in a general hospital setting and the common themes are comprehensive assessment, appropriate skills, training and attitudes, person-centred care. Young *et al.* (2003) stressed that these principles were never intended to be implemented in isolation, as an end to itself and education and training should be for staff across the whole of the hospital system.

In the UK, the Royal College of Psychiatrists' document *Who Cares Wins* (2005) and the *National Service Framework for Older People* (Department of Health 2001) highlighted the importance of a skill mix necessary to meet the complex needs of older people. In Australia, the government initiative advocated care in the right place at the right time for people with dementia and has published the *National Framework for Action on Dementia 2006–2010* (NSW Department of Health 2006) which highlighted workforce training as one of its five key priorities. The development of the liaison mental health nurse in the 1960s in the USA and in the 1980s in the UK and Australia has improved access to this training by virtue of the dedicated sessions in the general hospital.

Nurses working in non-psychiatric settings often feel that they are not adequately prepared to meet the mental health needs of patients. It is a challenge for general nurses in acute general hospitals to provide person-centred care due to numerous constraints, for example, lack of knowledge and skills, staff mix ratios, turnover rates of regular staff and use of temporary staff, lack of resources and space, and complex medical and surgical needs of patients. This clearly has implications for patient care as psychological difficulties often go undetected when working under pressure and clinical workload has to be prioritized.

Table 17.4   Knowledge and skills needed to work with patients who have dementia

Identifying symptoms and signs of dementia

Identifying delirium

Identifying depressive or psychotic symptoms

Course of the illness

Cognitive and person-centred stimulation

Understanding how to optimize care in older people

Understanding how to maintain fluid balance and prevent infection

Understanding how to communicate with someone who has dementia (see Chapters 4, 11, 12)

Understanding how to manage the environment to prevent agitation

Understanding the judicious use of psychotropic medication

Being comfortable working in an interdisciplinary team

Participating in early discharge planning

Understanding how to assess risks of hospitalization for someone with dementia

Debates and controversies

Although much is known about the impact of hospitalization on people with dementia, there is still considerable debate and controversy over who is best placed and experienced to lead the care, what specialists should be involved in hospital care of people with dementia, and how carers should respond to the person with dementia. In addition to the controversy over this question, there is much we simply do not understand about how best to care for people with dementia who are acutely ill.

Other important debates involve the role of mental health professionals in the care of acutely ill people with dementia, the best methods of involving mental health expertise and the type of liaisons that will most effectively meet their needs.

In most developed countries the funding for mental health services is separate from funding for acute care. Continuing this division will likely continue to create gaps in services for people with dementia who develop acute illnesses.

Conclusion

Dementia is common among hospitalized older adults but is often missed or is misdiagnosed. Accurate diagnosis early in hospital admission is important as it sets the course for appropriate intervention and discharge planning. People with dementia are at increased risk of developing complications and experiencing a prolonged hospital stay, often leading to long-term disability. In particular, failure to detect and manage delirium appropriately can lead to serious negative outcomes. Much is known about ways to decrease hospital risks for people with dementia, although widespread implementation of these risk reduction processes has not yet been achieved.

Further information

The National Institute for Health and Clinical Excellence in the UK provides guidelines for management of dementia. Their website is designed primarily for professionals.

The British Geriatrics Society, a professional organization of doctors practising geriatric medicine in the UK, has a website for professionals. Among the reports is 'Delirious about Dementia', a document from a consensus group formed by BGS and Faculty of Old Age Psychiatry.

The UK National Audit Office has established a website that outlines the services and supports recommended for people with dementia. The site includes several reports on dementia services available and recommended.

The **American Psychiatric Association** provides guidance and identifies published research for psychiatrists on diagnosing and treating dementia.

The **Mental Capacity Act UK 2005** includes discussion of dementia. It addresses decision-making capacity in people with dementia, including decisions made in acute care settings.

References

American Psychiatric Association (1999) Practice Guideline for the Treatment of Patients with Delirium. *American Journal of Psychiatry*, 156(Suppl 5): 1–20. http://www.psychiatryonline.com/content.aspx?aid=42494 (accessed 10 April 2008).

Ardern, M., Mayou, R., Feldman, E and Hawton, K. (1993) Cognitive impairment in the elderly medically ill: how often is it missed? *International Journal of Geriatric Psychiatry*, 8: 929–37.

Brindle, N. and Holmes, J. (2005) Capacity and coercion: dilemmas in the discharge of older people with dementia from general hospital settings. *Age and Ageing*, 34: 16–20.

British Geriatric Society (2006) *Guidelines for the Prevention, Diagnosis and Management of Delirium in Older People in Hospital*. London: BGS.

Department of Health (2001) *National Service Framework for Older People*. London: The Stationery Office.

Department of Health (2003) Discharge from hospital. Getting it right for people with dementia. A supplementary checklist to help with planning the discharge from acute general hospital settings of people with dementia. Available at http://www.dh.gov.uk (accessed 10 April 2008).

Elie, M., Cole, M.G., Primeau, F.J. and Bellavance, F. (1998) Delirium risk factors in elderly hospitalised patients. *Journal of General Internal Medicine*, 13: 204–12.

Erkinjuntti, T., Autio, L. and Wistrom, J. (1988) Dementia in medical wards. *Journal of Clinical Epidemiology*, 41: 123–6.

Feinberg, L. and Whitlatch, C. (2001) Are persons with cognitive impairment able to state consistent choices? *The Gerontologist*, 41(3): 374–82.

Francis, J. and Kapoor, W. (1992) Prognosis after hospital discharge of older medical patients with delirium. *Journal of the American Geriatrics Society*, 40: 601–6.

Francis, J., Martin, D., Kapoor, W.N. (1990) A prospective study of delirium in hospitalised elderly. *Journal of the American Medical Association*, 263: 1097–101.

Fulmer, T., Foreman, M., Walker, M. and Montgomery, K. (2001) *Critical Care Nursing of the Elderly*. New York: Springer Publishing Co.

Harari, D., Martin, F., Buttery, A., O'Neill, S., Hopper, A. (2007) The Older Persons' Assessment and Liaison Team: Evaluation of comprehensive geriatric assessment in acute medical inpatients. *Age and Ageing. Advance Access.* Available at: http://ageing.oxfordjournals.org/papbyrecent.dtl (accessed 6 January 2008).

Harwood, D.M.J., Hope, T. and Jacoby, R. (1997) Cognitive impairment in medical inpatients. II: Do physicians miss cognitive impairment? *Age and Aging*, 26: 37–9.

Holmes, J. and House, A. (2000) Psychiatric illness predicts poor outcome after hip fracture: a prospective cohort study. *Psychological Medicine*, 30: 921–9.

Hutt, R., Rosen, R., and McCauley, J. (2004) *Case-managing long-term conditions: what impact does it have in the treatment of older people?* London: King's Fund. Available at http://www.kingsfund.org.uk/pdf/casemanagment.pdf (accessed 10 April 2008).

Huusko, T. *et al.* (2000) Randomised, clinically controlled trial of intensive geriatric rehabilitation in patients with hip fracture: subgroup analysis of patients with dementia. *British Medical Journal*, 321: 1107–11.

Inouye, S.K., Bogardus, S.T., Charpentier, P.A., Leo-Summers, L., Acampora, D., Holford, T.R. and Cooney, L.M. Jr. (1999) A multicomponent intervention to prevent delirium in hospitalised older adults. *New England Journal of Medicine*, 340: 669–76.

Inouye, S., Bogardus, S., Vitagliano, G., Desai, M., Williams, C. and Grady, J. (2003) Burden of Illness Score for Elderly Persons: risk adjustment incorporating the cumulative impact of diseases, physiologic abnormalities, and functional impairments. *Medical Care* 41(1): 70–83.

Kakuma, R., Galbaud du Fort, G., Arsenault, L., Perrault, A., Platt, R., Monnette, J., Moride, Y. and Wolfson, C. (2003) Delirium in older emergency department patients discharged home: effect on survival. *Journal of the American Geriatrics Society*, 51(4): 443–50.

King, B., Jones, C. and Brand, C. (2006) Relationship between dementia and length of stay of general medical patients admitted to acute care. *Australasian Journal on Ageing*, 25: 20–3.

Lyketsos, C.G., Sheppard, J-M.E. and Rabins, P.V. (2000) Dementia in elderly persons in a general hospital. *American Journal of Psychiatry*, 157: 704–7.

MacNeill, S. and Lichtenberg, P. (1997) Home alone: the role of cognition in return to independent living. *Archives of Physical Medicine and Rehabilitation*, 78: 755–8.

Martin, F.C. (2005) POPS and OPAL – progress is possible. *BGS Newsletter*, March. Available at: http://www.bgsnet.org.uk/July106NL/8_pops_opal.htm (accessed 6 January 2008).

Metz, D.H. and Labrooy, S.J. (2005) The future of geriatric medicine in an era of patient choice. *Age and Ageing*, 34: 553–5.

National Institute for Health and Clinical Excellence (NICE) (2006) *Supporting People with Dementia and their Carers in Health and Social Care*. Clinical Guideline 42. London: NICE.

NSW Department of Health (2006) *National Framework for Action on Dementia 2006–2010*. North Sydney: NSW Department of Health. Available at: http://www.health.gov.au/internet/wcms/publishing.nsf/Content/D64BD892C 6FDD167CA2572180007E717/$File/nfad.pdf (accessed 10 April 2008).

Parker, S.G. (2005) *Do Current Discharge Arrangements from Inpatient Hospital Care for the Elderly Reduce Admission Rates, the Length of Inpatient Stay or Mortality, or Improve Health Status?* Copenhagen: WHO Regional Office for Europe (Health Evidence Network report). Available at: http://www.euro.who.int/Document/E87542.pdf (accessed 10 April 2008).

Pompei, P., Foreman, M., Rudberg, M.A., Inouye, S.K., Braund, V., and Cassel, C.K. (1994) Delirium in hospitalized older persons: outcomes and predictors. *Journal of the American Geriatrics Society*, 42: 809–15.

Raymont, V., Bingley, W., Buchanan, A., David, A., Hayward, P., Wesseley, S. and Hotopf, M. (2004) Prevalence of mental incapacity in medical inpatients and associated risk factors: a cross-sectional study. *Lancet*, 364: 1421–7.

Royal College of Psychiatrists (2005) *Who Cares Wins: Improving the Outcome for Older People Admitted to the General Hospital*. Report of a Working Group for the Faculty of Old Age Psychiatry. London: RCP.

Sharrock, J., Grigg, M., Happell, B., Keeble-Devlin, B. and Jennings, S. (2006) The mental health nurse: a valuable addition to the consultation-liaison team. *International Journal of Mental Health Nursing*, 15: 35–43.

Shaw, F.E., Bond, J., Richardson, D.A. *et al.* (2003) Multifactorial intervention after a fall in older people with cognitive impairment and dementia presenting to the accident and emergency department: randomised controlled trial. *British Medical Journal*, 326: 73–9.

Silverstein, N. and Maslow, K. (eds) (2006) *Improving Hospital Care for Persons with Dementia*. New York: Springer Publishing.

Swanwick, G.R.J., Lee, H., Clare, A.W. and Lawlor, B.A. (1993) Consultation--liaison psychiatry: A comparison of two service models for geriatric patients. *International Journal of Geriatric Psychiatry*, 9: 495–9.

Wilkinson, H. (ed.) (2002) *The Perspectives of People with Dementia: Research Methods and Motivations*. London: Jessica Kingsley.

Wong, J., Clare, I., Gunn, M. and Holland, A. (1999) Capacity to make healthcare decisions: its importance in clinical practice. *Psychological Medicine*, 29: 437–46.

World Health Organization (1992) *The ICD-10 Classification of Mental and Behavioural Disorders*. Geneva: WHO.

Young, J., Sturdy, D. and Bhattacharjee, G. (2003) *Approaches to Improving General Hospital Care of Older People*. Available at: http://www.dh.gov.uk (accessed 10 April 2008).

18

The role of specialist housing in supporting older people with dementia

Simon Evans, Sarah Vallelly and Karen Croucher

Learning objectives

By the end of this chapter, you will be able to:

- discuss the changing social policy discourse which has underpinned the development of specialist housing settings for older people

- understand the key differences between the main models of specialist housing for older people

- identify the key challenges involved in providing specialist housing for people with dementia and their family carers

---

Introduction

Housing is increasingly recognized as an important resource for achieving health and social care policy goals. The latter half of the twentieth century and the early years of the twenty-first have been marked by a number of key socio-demographic trends that have profound implications for housing. In particular, the increase in life expectancy, decrease in household size and growth in owner occupation are having a considerable impact. Over this same period the emphasis of public policy has shifted from caring for frail older people in institutional settings to providing care and support for them in their own homes or other environments that are as 'domestic' or 'homely' as possible. This shift towards 'care in the community' (Means 1997) has led to rapid growth in the provision of housing with care.

There has often been a lack of understanding of dementia among housing and social care professionals and an over-emphasis on the potential levels of risk associated with supporting people in the community. Together these can lead to the exclusion of people with dementia from community-based care and housing services and pressures to moving to institutional care settings instead, particularly as their condition progresses (Cox 1998). Housing is about more than bricks and mortar and the notion of 'home' is an important framing concept in cultural theory about identity. Home is the repository of memories, the place where we literally represent our private selves through photographs, ornaments and possessions (Darke 1994). The concept of home is therefore key to the concept of identify when the processes of memory are impaired and the self is fragmented, as is often the case when people have dementia.

In many nations, dementia has become an increasingly important issue for government and a priority area for national policy development. In the UK, this was acknowledged by the Department of Health in their National Dementia Strategy (2008). The strategy has been developed with three main goals in mind: to improve awareness of dementia; to improve early diagnosis and intervention; and to improve the quality of care for people with dementia, their carers and families. The success of the strategy is contingent on a whole systems approach which has a broader focus than health and social care. The dementia strategy recognizes the value of the housing sector to promoting the well-being of people with dementia. In the USA, government recognition and support of appropriate housing for people with dementia have been less substantial and varies widely by state (see Chapter 22).

This chapter provides an overview of housing with care, including who it is for, the identifying features of different models and their key aims and objectives. It also explores how well specialist housing settings can meet these broad aims for people with dementia, particularly in terms of supporting independence, choice and well-being. The chapter begins by describing the most common forms of housing with care and comparing their key features. It then goes on to consider the social and policy context in which housing with care has become increasingly popular in recent years and the importance of the concept of 'home' for people with dementia. A third section considers how appropriate and achievable these aims are for people with dementia by reviewing the existing evidence and identifying gaps in the knowledge base. Finally, the reader is offered a summary of the key issues and some further debating points.

Models of housing with care

Specialist housing for older people has been around in one form or another for many years. More recently there has been increasing recognition of the role that housing can play in promoting quality of life, health, independence and well-being for older people. However, the terminology associated with older people's housing often lacks clarity and can be confusing for the public and professionals.

In sheltered housing there are typically 30 or 40 flats and/or bungalows with an emergency alarm system and basic communal facilities such as a lounge and a laundry. On-site support is usually provided by a manager (sometimes called a scheme, housing or court manager or 'warden'). Sheltered housing does not normally provide care, but residents are able to get care and support from social services like anyone else in the community who is eligible. Sheltered housing was initially designed with active older people (55+) in mind. Most of it was developed by councils and housing associations in the 1960s and 1970s. The majority of sheltered housing stock was initially developed for rental. Over the last fifteen years, some older developments show signs of being 'difficult to let', particularly in unpopular locations or with a high proportion of bed-sit (studio) flats (Tinker *et al.* 1995). Other sheltered housing has struggled to meet the increasing care and support needs of residents as they become older and frailer. In the USA, a similar phenomenon has occurred with residents in many independent apartment buildings being mostly older, and becoming frailer. These have come to be known as 'naturally occurring retirement communities' (Masotti *et al.* 2006). They are mostly found near a particular cluster of services including: transportation, pharmacy, grocery, post office. With no formal services on site, housing managers have done their best to respond to changing needs. This has frequently led to tension over whether increasing frailty is sufficient reason for asking a resident to leave (Masotti *et al.* 2006).

In the mid-1990s in the UK, 'extra care' or 'very sheltered' housing began to emerge as a model, largely due to a growing focus on the needs of an ageing and increasingly frail population and the search for alternatives to institutional settings for care. Extra care housing is now firmly established as a popular form of housing with care provision for older people. In the UK, extra care housing is a key plank of government policy in terms of its aims to promote choice, independence and well-being for older people. Many different models of extra care have been developed and the flexibility of this form of provision is one of its key strengths. However, this flexibility also makes extra care hard to define. Put simply, extra care offers housing that has the full legal rights associated with being a tenant or home owner, along with 24-hour on-site care that can be delivered flexibly according to a person's changing needs. In the USA, this type of housing (referred to as 'assisted living') has also experienced an explosion in growth. In some cases they stand alone while in others they are formally linked to either retirement communities, residential aged care (nursing homes), or both, providing a continuum of care and support (Sikorska-Simmons and Wright 2007). Many states are now developing guidelines for developers and care providers in these settings. Many of these settings are dementia-specific. One of the most pressing challenges for assisted living is how to provide a safe environment for people with dementia (Bellantonio *et al.* 2008; Rasin and Kautz 2007; Zimmerman *et al.* 2007).

Extra care housing and assisted living are designed to promote independence and well-being, ideally to provide a 'home for life' by supporting 'ageing in place'. Different provider organizations have placed varying emphasis on the housing or care element of their provision, depending on whether they position their schemes as alternatives to residential care or as a replacement for traditional sheltered housing. A key feature of extra care housing is that it is less institutional than residential care and each resident has their own front door. It is fundamentally about 'quality of life' not just 'quality of care'. This type of housing can be for rent, outright sale or part ownership, and some developments are mixed tenure, offering homes for sale and for rent. Extra care housing and assisted living are designed to wheelchair-accessible standards and with many flats designed or adapted for wheelchair users.

Retirement villages are another increasingly popular housing option for older people, driven by a range of factors including the ageing population, the development of new lifestyles in older life, improved health into old age, and a general recognition of the need for greater choice and flexibility in housing options for older people (Heywood *et al.* 2002). One feature that distinguishes retirement villages from other forms of housing with care is the diversity of residents and their needs. They are also usually bigger than other forms of housing with care. In the UK they tend to accommodate 200–300 residents, while in the USA there is a wide range from less than 100 residents to several thousand in retirement communities or cities. Such economies of scale allow a wide range of facilities and social and recreational activities. Flexible care is typically available, including home help, personal care, health care, home maintenance, eating facilities and transport.

Table 18.1 summarizes the key features of each of these models of housing with care.

Exercise 18.1   The benefits of housing with care

List the key aims of extra care housing/assisted living in the left-hand column of a table like the one below. Now, think about the specific challenges that this represents and, against each aim, list the key issues or barriers in terms of achieving these goals for people with dementia. How realistic are they? Label the third column 'successful outcomes' and think about what type of evidence would be necessary to demonstrate this. The following example may help:

Key aim	Dementia-specific challenges	Evidence required to demonstrate successful outcome
To provide a 'home for life'	Balancing risk, security and independence Complex care needs Challenging behaviours	Quantitative data on length of residence and reasons for tenancies ending

---

Role of housing with care for people with dementia

This section explores what we currently know about housing with care for people with dementia. It draws largely on the research evidence but is also based on the experiences of people with dementia and their carers.

A review of the literature relating to housing and dementia care (O'Malley and Croucher 2005) found very few studies that had attempted to investigate the role and capacity of different models of 'specialist' housing for later life with regard to the needs and preferences of people with dementia. Only one study to date has focused exclusively on extra care housing for people with dementia. This study, called 'Opening doors to independence' (Vallelly *et al.* 2006), found that the benefits of extra care housing were recognized by people with dementia, particularly in terms of the care and support provided, relationships with other residents, feeling safe and being able to choose how they spent their time. The relatives of residents with dementia felt that extra care housing offered them reassurance that help was readily available when needed, particularly in a crisis. In some instances family relationships were said to improve when people with dementia moved to extra care housing. Nearly all the residents with dementia were frequently visited by family members who provided much informal support. Other studies (e.g. Bernard *et al.* 2004) have found that older people in housing with care settings generally receive considerable and vital support from their families. This raises questions about whether there are 'gaps' in service provision, and what happens to those residents who are not fortunate enough to have access to adequate informal support. Croucher *et al.* (2006) explored a range of models of housing with care for older people and concluded that they do not easily accommodate people with dementia. This was largely because, while the independence and security that these models aim to provide are greatly valued by older people, the provider organization's understanding of the concept of independence in particular was different to that of the older people themselves. As a result, some residents had expected more assistance and support than was available.

Reporting on 'Brighter futures', a study by Kitwood and colleagues (1995) of service provision for people with dementia in residential homes and sheltered housing, Petre (1995) identified a range of challenges for supporting people with dementia in sheltered housing:

- Lack of knowledge about dementia among staff and residents.

- Social isolation as residents with dementia withdraw from social activities and/or are rejected by other tenants.

- The built environment often disadvantages people with dementia, particularly in older buildings.

- Tenants with dementia can cause disruption for other residents.

- Referrers and other professionals may have unrealistic expectations of what sheltered housing can provide.

He concluded that sheltered housing can offer a positive environment to people with dementia, provided that appropriate opportunities for social interaction are available.

The overall aim of housing with care is to promote quality of life for older people by supporting independence, maximizing health and well-being and providing opportunities for ageing in place. We will now examine the evidence for the extent to which these can be achieved for people with dementia.

Promoting independence

One of the main aims of housing with care is to help residents maintain their independence. By providing residents with their own front door and self-contained accommodation, the most recent models such as extra care housing/assisted living and retirement villages offer an environment that has the potential to maximize independence. Other features that are key to independence include flexible care packages, accessible design, and an active social life. However, there are a number of specific challenges to supporting independence for people with dementia in this setting.

One such challenge is providing the right care in the most appropriate way. There is evidence that good quality person-centred care can be effective in managing the behavioural symptoms of people with dementia in housing with care settings (Fossey *et al.* 2006). 'Brighter futures' (Kitwood *et al.* 1995), reported that the role of the warden/manager was key, particularly in terms of determining the attitudes of other residents to those with dementia. Since Kitwood's study the role of 'warden' has altered considerably (Parry and Thompson 2005), partly due to recent changes in the Supporting People Programme. This has led to the introduction of new models for delivering services to older people, often called 'floating support'. This term covers a range of models that offer services by support workers who are not tied to specific accommodation, as many wardens/housing managers previously were, but now have centralized office bases instead.

Vallelly *et al.* (2006) found that the skills and experience of managers in terms of dementia were also one of the main determinants of the extent to which extra care housing/assisted living residents with dementia were integrated. The model of care in operation was also central to supporting independence. The flexible care packages were found to be particularly important for meeting the needs of people with dementia, which could change considerably and often. Many schemes or programmes had the flexibility in their care contracts with the local authority to change the care package without obtaining formal agreement in advance. Systems supporting person-centred care also appeared to offer significant advantages to residents with dementia, particularly in terms of providing continuity of care and opportunities for developing good relationships with staff.

Box 18.1   Case example

An extra care housing tenant with mild dementia, whom we will call Albert, had previously lived in a maisonette (duplex). He began to find the stairs difficult to manage, which prevented him from going out much and put him at increased risk of isolation. His ground floor flat in an extra care housing scheme was much more suitable. As Albert put it: 'They put me on a level that was much more convenient for me and I can get out of the door quick.' He appreciated the independence that this gave him and spent a lot of time out walking in the local area, sometimes with other residents but usually on his own. Albert got on all right with the other tenants but he placed great value on having the privacy of his own flat. 'Oh yes, if I know anybody I'll stop and talk but I am a bit of a loner. I stay here nodding off, go for a walk and then it's time for dinner.'

Albert summed up the sense of independence that he experienced in extra care housing in the following way: 'Nobody bothers you, you come and go as you want but I've never stayed out late.'

Another important consideration is how staff perceive and manage risk. People who live in extra care housing have the legal right as tenants to come and go as they please and to decide who visits them. However, for staff supporting people with dementia this can present challenges in terms of maintaining a balance between autonomy and security. In an article based on the Opening Doors project, Evans and Means (2006) reported that extra care staff often considered people with dementia to be more at risk than other tenants. A number of potential risks were identified by care staff, such as so-called 'wandering'. This was perceived by care staff as a significant challenge to supporting people with dementia in extra care housing, although there were few actual examples of its being a problem. This highlights the importance of providing care and support staff with the appropriate training to support people with dementia. This is particularly important in housing such as extra care or assisted living, where staff are likely to have come from residential care environments or nursing homes that were not so focused on promoting independence. Vallelly *et al.* (2006) found that few staff had received dementia-specific training and that this limited the effectiveness of the support they provided. There are currently no statutory dementia training and qualification guidelines in the UK for housing with care settings.

There is substantial evidence to support the potential for telecare and assistive technology to promote independence for people with dementia generally, including the management of risk. For example, the Safe at Home scheme in Northamptonshire found that a range of technologies can help people with dementia remain in their own homes by reducing levels of risk, helping people feel safer and supporting relatives and carers, as well as being cost-effective (Woolham 2006). Another project, ENABLE, explored the impact of a range of devices in the homes of people with dementia across five European countries, including cooker monitors, bath monitors and picture telephones. The researchers concluded that such devices could improve the quality of life for both users and their informal carers (Hagen *et al.* 2005).

There is considerable evidence that the built environment is a major factor in the extent to which a housing with care environment can promote independence (e.g. Parker *et al.* 2004). There has also been much debate about what aspects of building design can support people with dementia, particularly in terms of maximizing independence, enhancing self-esteem and reinforcing personal identity. The Housing Corporation (2003) have developed quality indicators that are used to benchmark extra care housing across a range of internal and external design factors. These include location, integration with the local community, the provision of facilities and accessibility, all of which are particularly important to residents with dementia. Many good practice checklists have been developed, listing principles and features for designing home and care environments in a way that supports people with dementia (Judd *et al.* 1998; Suffolk County Council www; Utton 2007). The actual evidence base regarding design for dementia is relatively small, but there is considerable 'common sense' consensus on the overall principles of design that can be effective. These include:

- creating small, familiar environments
- incorporating unobtrusive safety features
- providing different rooms for different functions
- good signage
- the use of colour and architectural landmarks to aid orientation and way-finding.

The importance of good design has been highlighted by Vallelly *et al.* (2006). They concluded that many extra care housing schemes incorporated features that supported residents with dementia in terms of orientation and way-finding.

This included the use of indoor streets or malls, which provide an environment that is dry, level and secure. This enables access for people with dementia to a range of facilities that are crucial to their independence, such as shops, restaurants and communal areas. Table 18.2 lists some of the design features that were used to support people with dementia in extra care housing.

Table 18.1 Models of housing with care and residential care

	Extra care housing	Retirement village	Sheltered housing	Residential care
Also known as	Very sheltered housing; category 2.5; integrated housing with care; close care	Continuing care retirement village; retirement community	Category 1, 1.5, or 2; retirement housing court; supported housing	Category 3; care home; rest home; elderly mental infirm (EMI) unit; nursing home
Key features	Typically 40 or more self-contained flats with ensuite facilities Fully wheelchair-accessible and inclusive design standards Some schemes have 'specialist clusters' of flats for people with dementia	100 or more houses, apartments or bungalows Many have a care home on site; a few have dementia units	Typically clusters of 30–40 flats, bedsits or bungalows; mostly self-contained; designed to meet accessibility standards	Residential care homes typically have a number of rooms, some with private bathrooms and kitchenettes, on-site catering facilities and resident lounges
Provided by	Mostly housing associations, some local authorities Increasingly private sector developers are building extra care 'villages'	Not-for-profit organizations, housing associations and private developers	Local authorities, housing associations (social rented), and some private developers	Mostly local authorities and private care companies

	Extra care housing	**Retirement village**	**Sheltered housing**	**Residential care**
Tenure options	Social rent, shared ownership, outright sale and mixed tenure Assured tenancy rights	Some for private ownership, some mixed tenure (private ownership, shared ownership and renting) Assured tenancy rights	Much stock is social rented, but new build is for outright sale or leasehold Assured tenancy rights	Most 'placements' are paid for by local authorities or privately No tenancy rights
Typical facilities	Communal lounge; catering; shop; beauty salon; day centre; activities room; internet room	Communal lounge; catering; shop; activities room; beauty salon; internet room; gym; swimming pool; jacuzzi	Communal lounge; laundry	Communal lounges; catering
Care and support	Emergency alarm system. 24 hour on-site care and support (including at least one 'waking carer' during the night)	Emergency alarm system Most have flexible packages that can be purchased from care team and out of hours emergency provision	Emergency alarm system Most have on-site or visiting warden. Residents can access domiciliary care in the same way as anyone living in their own home	On-site care staff 24 hours a day, 7 days a week Registered with Commission for Social Care Inspection
Provision in England	30,000 units in 2006	Not known	Half a million units in 2006	476,200 registered care home places in 2005

Table 18.2   Examples of design strategies for people with dementia

Colour schemes. Some courts have colour-coded corridors whereby paintwork, carpets, etc. are all of a similar colour to aid recognition. Some courts also use a range of bright, easily identified colours for the recesses that form the entrance to each flat off the main corridors. These can also be personalized by the use of photographs, artefacts, etc.
Defining spaces. Most courts incorporate a small 'pod' lounge area as part of each corridor. This aims to define local areas within the overall court and can be enhanced by the use of visual landmarks such as plants and artwork.
Signage. The use of large, clear and colourful signs for court facilities has been employed to increase their visibility to tenants with dementia.
Overall design of flats. Some newer courts have incorporated barrier-free design in tenants' flats. This provides good visual access between rooms so that, for example, a tenant lying in bed can see and therefore find the bathroom during the night.
From the 'Opening Doors' study (Vallelly *et al.* 2006)

Promoting health and well-being

Many residents with dementia in housing with care settings also have complex health care needs. Vallelly *et al.* (2006) found that these needs were more likely to be met where service provision was part of an overall strategy across housing, health and social care. They concluded that providing access to appropriate health care is one of the key challenges for extra care housing. Some schemes had good links with local general practitioners but in others the on-site consulting rooms and other facilities provided were under-used. Extra care housing has a major preventative role to play in terms of maximizing health. For example, there is a growing amount of research into the potential for people with dementia to benefit from rehabilitative activities (Jorm 1994). There is considerable scope for these to be provided in housing that include care, although Vallelly *et al.* (2006) found limited evidence of this happening so far.

There is considerable evidence to suggest that personal relationships and social interaction are important factors in quality of life for older people (Age Concern 2006; Phillipson 1997). Social well-being was found to be important in housing with care settings by Evans and Vallelly (2007), who interviewed staff and residents in six extra care schemes across England. They found that people with dementia were particularly at risk of social exclusion in this setting and identified six key factors that can impact on social well-being:

- friendship and social interaction
- engaging with the wider community
- the importance of design
- the role of family carers

- staffing and the culture of care

- providing facilities.

Their respondents valued the opportunity to mix with other tenants and it was therefore important to provide opportunities for developing and maintaining social networks. The provision of appropriate facilities and activities was particularly important in this respect and the schemes that took part in the study offered a range of activities for residents, including exercise classes, memory groups, art and craft projects, games and trips. However, there were significant variations in the number and scope of activities, often due to the systems in operation. In some instances, care staff organized activities, often in their spare time, putting extra demands on staff who were already busy. In other places, they employed part-time activity coordinators, funded by the local authority through Supporting People, a centrally funded scheme that provides services to help vulnerable people live independently in their accommodation. In a third model, a committee of residents took responsibility for raising funds and organizing events. While social activities were important, some residents valued the option of spending time alone in their own flats.

Vallelly *et al.* (2006) found that prejudice among other residents was a potential barrier to social integration for residents with dementia, largely due to lack of information and understanding. Kitwood *et al.* (1995) found that people with dementia were often a focus for resentment and tended to be scapegoats for a range of problems. They suggested that residents were more supportive of others if they had developed dementia since moving into a scheme, compared to those who had dementia when they moved in. This was largely because they had already become part of social networks and were therefore less disadvantaged by their reduced social skills. Croucher *et al.* (2006) reported that the old and frail, and particularly those with dementia, were consistently on the margins of social networks and were excluded from many social activities. This supports Oldman's view (2000) that there can be a contradiction between what people want for themselves and what they think should happen to other residents who become increasingly frail or cognitively impaired.

Exercise 18.2 Variations in housing and services

Pick a few communities in your country and in other countries. Explore the levels of housing with care provision they offer and the extent to which this appears to meet the needs of people with dementia.

Do they specifically address care of people with dementia? What indication do they give about whether they might provide a home for life?

You might want to start with some web resources: in the UK (www.eac.org.uk); in the US (http://www.assistedlivinglocators.com/facilities/); (http://www.assistedlivinginfo.com/); in Canada (http://assisted-living-directory.com/canada.cfm)

Ageing in place and a home for life

In recent years much emphasis has been placed on providing housing options for older people and their right to 'age in place'. This contrasts with traditional models where older people are required to move to a different housing setting, often a residential home, in order to have their care needs met. This led to the concept of a 'home for life' or 'ageing in place'. However, this has proved to be a major challenge, particularly for residents with dementia, and some providers have now realized that it can be problematic and even unrealistic, as have numerous writers (e.g. Bernard *et al.* 2004; Croucher *et al.* 2003; Oldman 2000). The review by Croucher *et al.* (2006) did not find any examples where residents could age in place under any circumstances. They concluded that while the evidence seems to suggest that housing with care can accommodate people with mild to moderate cognitive impairment, there is no evidence available to suggest that these residents can be supported over the full course of their illness.

Dementia is highlighted by several studies as a major reason for residents having to move on to other care settings. For example, Vallelly *et al.* (2006) reported that worsening dementia was recorded as a factor for 41% of residents who moved to nursing care. However, the average length of tenancy was very similar for all tenants, whether they had dementia or not, at just over two years. The complexities of long-term care funding also present a challenge to achieving a home for life, as shown by the case study in Box 18.2.

Box 18.2   Case example

An 87-year-old woman who had been diagnosed with dementia was referred to a housing scheme by social services so that she could have her health needs met while being close to her family. She moved into the scheme, which was part sheltered and part extra care.

She was later diagnosed as being terminally ill with cancer and was thought to have only a few weeks to live. At this point the local authority was keen to refer her to a hospice so that responsibility for funding would transfer from the social services budget to 'continuing care'.

The resident's GP, her family and the court manager all felt that an enforced move was not in her best interests because, although her physical health had deteriorated, her quality of life had improved since she moved into the scheme. Negotiations between health and social care providers and the housing association led to her staying in the scheme, supported by Macmillan nurses, until she died later that year.

This case study illustrates the difficulties of implementing a complex continuing care policy across housing, health and social care. However, achieving this can be crucial to providing dignity and choice for older people with dementia in housing with care settings.

> **Exercise 18.3** Exploring services in your local community
>
> Examine the housing strategy developed by your local authority.
>
> Does it have a range of housing with care options?
>
> What is the approach to supporting people with dementia and does it consider integrated and specialist provision?

A study of Hartrigg Oaks, a retirement village operated by the Joseph Rowntree Foundation (Croucher *et al.* 2003) found that despite the presence of an on-site care home, residents with more advanced dementia were usually found alternative placements in specialist dementia care homes. However, a number of larger developments now include specialist dementia services. For example, Westbury Fields retirement village operated by the St Monica Trust in Bristol, England, has a dementia unit within its on-site care home. In their report on a study of Westbury Fields, Evans and Means (2007) found that this was greatly valued by the spouses of village residents who developed dementia because it meant that they could continue living in the village while supporting their partners in the specialist unit. It is also important to emphasize that, while extra care residents do have the legal protection of assured tenancies, it is still possible for the landlord to evict them under certain circumstances, including 'anti-social' behaviour. In this situation, the landlord is required to make alternative living arrangements.

Although most extra care housing schemes aim to integrate people with dementia within the overall scheme, one extra care housing scheme included in the study by Vallelly *et al.* (2006) included a specialist dementia unit. While acknowledging the potential benefits of this arrangement in terms of targeting specialist services, the study identified a number of challenges, which are outlined in Box 18.3.

Box 18.3 Case example

Oak House, an extra care housing scheme run by Housing 21, has 38 self-contained flats, eight of which are in a separate unit designed to meet the specific needs of people with dementia. This unit is accessed from the main building via a keyfob protected door and has its own dining area and residents lounge. The 'Opening doors' study identified a range of issues that created challenges for the specialist unit:

When a couple move in and one partner has dementia but not the other, should they live in the main scheme or the dementia unit?

It is not easy to assess who should live in the unit because many residents have cognitive impairment but no diagnosis of dementia.

What happens when someone living in the scheme develops dementia, do they stay in their flat or move into the dementia unit?

Does a specialist unit increase stigma and prejudice in relation to dementia by reducing contact with other residents?

Debates and controversies

A number of issues remain unresolved in terms of the best ways of supporting people with dementia in housing and care settings. These include:

- Some developments support people with dementia within the main housing scheme (an integrated approach) while others have dementia clusters, units or wings. Which works best in terms of quality of life, quality of care and cost effectiveness?

- A range of design features are used to support orientation and independence for people with dementia but which, if any, really work?

- Housing with care schemes aims to promote diversity but there is evidence of prejudice against people with dementia and relatively few residents from black and ethnic minority groups.

Conclusion

Recognition of the need to provide a range of housing options for the increasing numbers of older people has led to the development of new models of housing with care. However, there is a lack of detailed evidence for the extent to which these meet the needs of people with dementia. The research that has been carried out so far suggests that housing with care settings can support quality of life and independence for people with mild to moderate dementia, as long as a range of factors are taken into account. These include design of the built environment, models of care, staff training, the provision of facilities, social well-being, a balanced approach to risk and the appropriate use of assistive technologies. However, there are serious questions about the ability of housing with care to support residents as their dementia becomes more advanced.

Further information

The Housing Learning and Information Network (LIN) site for housing and dementia. This website addresses housing and disabilities with a specific section on housing and dementia. The focus is on extra care housing.

The Elderly Accommodation Counsel provides information about housing, care and support for older people.

The Alzheimer's Society has a website that includes information on: housing adaptations, design improvements and repairs for people with dementia.

The Care Services Improvement Partnership website provides a range of information on dementia, including housing and design.

References

Age Concern (2006) *Promoting Mental Health and Well-being in Later Life.* London: Age Concern.

Bellantonio, S., Kenny, A., Fortinsky, R., Kleppinger, A., Robison, J., Gruman, C., Kulldorff, M. and Trella, P. (2008) Efficacy of a geriatrics team intervention for residents in dementia specific assisted living facilities: effect on unanticipated transitions. *Journal of the American Geriatrics Society.* Available at: https://wiscmail.wisc.edu/attach/ch 18.doc?sid.

Bernard, M., Bartlam, B. and Biggs, S. (2004) *New Lifestyles in Old Age: Health, Identity and Well-being in Berryhill Retirement Village.* Bristol: Policy Press.

Cox, S. (1998) *Housing and Support for People with Dementia.* London: HACT.

Croucher, K., Hicks, S.L. and Jackson, K. (2006) *Housing with Care in Later Life: A Literature Review.* York: Joseph Rowntree Foundation.

Croucher, K., Pleace, N., and Bevan, M. (2003) *Living at Hartrigg Oaks. Resident's Views of the UK's First Continuing Care Retirement Community.* York: Joseph Rowntree Foundation.

Darke, J. (1994) Women and the meaning of home. In: R. Gilroy and R. Woods (eds) *Housing Women.* London: Routledge: pp. 11–30.

Department of Health (2008) *The National Dementia Strategy for England.* London: Department of Health.

Evans, S. and Means, R. (2006) Perspectives on risk for older people with dementia in extra care housing in the UK: findings from a longitudinal study. *International Journal of Disability and Human Development,* 5(1): 77–82.

Evans, S. and Means, R. (2007) *Balanced Retirement Communities? A case Study of Westbury Fields Mixed Tenure Retirement Village.* Bristol: St Monica Trust.

Evans, S. and Vallelly, S. (2007) *Promoting Social Well-being in Extra Care Housing.* York: Joseph Rowntree Foundation.

Fossey, J., Ballard, C., Juszczak, E., James, I., Alder, N. and Jacoby, R. (2006) Effect of enhanced psychosocial care on antipsychotic use in nursing home residents with severe dementia: cluster randomised trial. *British Medical Journal,* 332(7544): 756–61.

Hagen, I., Cahill, S., Begley, E., Macijauskiene, J., Gilliard, J., Jones, K., Topo, P., Saarikalle, K., Holthe, T. and Duff, P. (2005) Assessment of usefulness of assistive technologies for people with dementia. In: A. Pruski, and H. Knops (eds) *Assistive Technology: From Virtuality to Reality.* Amsterdam: IOS Press.

Heywood, F., Oldman, C. and Means, R. (2002) *Housing and Home in Later Life.* Philadelphia: Open University Press.

Housing Corporation (2003) *Scheme Development Standards*. 5th ed. London: HMSO.

Jorm, A.F. (1994) Disability in dementia: assessment, prevention, and rehabilitation. *Disability and Rehabilitation*, 16(3): 98–109.

Judd, S., Marshall, S. and Phippen, P. (1998) *Design for Dementia*. London: Hawker Publications.

Kitwood, T., Buckland, S. and Petre, T. (1995) *Brighter Futures: A Report on Research into Provision for Persons with Dementia in Residential Homes, Nursing Homes and Sheltered Housing*. Oxford: Anchor Trust.

Masotti, P., Fick, R., Johnson-Masotti, A. and MacLeod, S. (2006) Healthy naturally occurring retirement communities: a low cost approach to facilitating healthy aging. *American Journal of Public Health*, 96(7): 1164–70.

Means, R. (1997) Housing options. In: M. Evandrou (ed.) *Baby Boomers: Ageing in the 21st Century*. London: Age Concern.

Oldman, C. (2000) *Blurring the Boundaries: A Fresh Look at Housing and Care Provision for Older People*. York: Joseph Rowntree Foundation.

O'Malley, L. and Croucher, K. (2005) Housing and dementia care – a scoping review of the literature. *Health and Social Care in the Community*, 13(6): 570–7.

Parker, C., Barnes, S., McKee, K., Morgan, K., Torrington, J. and Tregenza, P. (2004) Quality of life and building design in residential and nursing homes for older people. *Ageing & Society*, 24: 941–62.

Parry, I. and Thompson, L. (2005) *Sheltered Housing and Retirement Housing: A Good Practice Guide*. Coventry: Chartered Institute of Housing.

Petre, T. (1995) People with dementia in sheltered housing. In: T. Kitwood and S. Benson (eds) *The New Culture of Dementia Care*. London: Hawker Publications, pp. 58–61.

Phillipson, C. (1997) Social relationships in later life: a review of the research literature. *International Journal of Geriatric Psychiatry*, 12(5): 505–12.

Rasin, J. and Kautz, D. (2007) Knowing the resident with dementia: perspectives of assisted living facility caregivers. *Journal of Gerontological Nursing*, 33(9): 30–6.

Sikorska-Simmons, E. and Wright, J. (2007) Determinants of resident autonomy in assisted living facilities: a review of the literature. *Care Management*, 8(4): 187–193.

Suffolk County Council. *The Suffolk Extra Care/Dementia Design and Management Guide*. Available from: www.changeagentteam.org.uk/_library/docs/ExamplesOfStrategyAndPolicies/extracare-dementia.pdf (accessed 5 December 2007).

Tinker, A., Wright, F. and Zeilig, H. (1995) *Difficult to Let Sheltered Housing*. Age Concern Institute of Gerontology, King's College London. London: HMSO.

Utton, D. (2007) *Designing Homes for People with Dementia.* London: Hawker Publications.

Vallelly, S., Evans, S., Fear, T. and Means, R. (2006) *Opening the Doors to Independence: A Longitudinal Study Exploring the Contribution of Extra Care Housing to the Care and Support of Older People.* London: Housing Corporation and Housing 21.

Woolham, J. (2006) *Safe at Home: The Effectiveness of Assistive Technology in Supporting the Independence of People with Dementia: The Safe at Home Project.* London: Hawker Publications.

Zimmerman, S., MItchell, C., Chen, C., Morgan, L., Gruber-Baldini, A., Sloane, P., Eckert, J. and Munn, J. (2007) An observation of assisted living environments: space use and behavior. *Journal of Gerontological Social Work,* 49(3): 185–203.

19

Care homes

Jane Fossey

Learning objectives

By the end of this chapter you will:

- understand the factors which influence how a person with dementia experiences a care home

- understand different approaches to care which can meet residents' physical, psychological and social needs

- understand how training, supervision and consultation can enhance care practices

---

Introduction

Many people with dementia continue to live in their own homes (see Chapter 16). However, a significant number are living in some type of care home. This chapter will address the care of people with dementia who are living in care homes. As the care issues are quite similar across the different types of care homes, they will be treated as a group (Bebbington *et al.* 2001; Rothera *et al.* 2003; Quinn *et al.* 2003). The chapter encompasses all residents with cognitive and functional difficulties requiring a sensitive and specialized understanding and response from care staff, regardless of whether they have a formal diagnosis of dementia.

While the number of people with dementia living in all types of care homes is not known, it is substantial. In nursing homes, where the majority of residents are over the age of 85 (Bajekal 2002), estimates of the percentage with dementia have ranged between 50% and 75% in the UK (MacDonald *et al.* 2002). In Australia (Jones *et al.* 2007) and in the USA (Zimmerman *et al.* 2003), residential settings for lower levels of care, such as hostels and assisted living, also have many residents with dementia. In the USA, it is estimated that 23–42% of residential community/assisted living residents have moderate to severe dementia (Zimmerman *et al.* 2003). In addition to dementia, many of these people have multiple physical, cognitive and mental health difficulties. Moves to care homes are related to a variety of conditions (see Figure 19.1), with many people experiencing more than one kind of difficulty at the time they move.

In most instances the decision to move is distressing for both the person with dementia and their family carers (Davies and Nolan 2003; Caron and Bowers 2003). This is especially difficult when the person with dementia

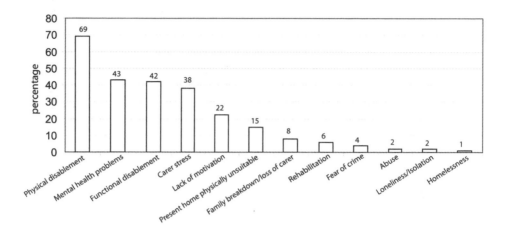

Figure 19.1 Reasons for admission to care home
Source: Office of Fair Trading (2005).

requires, but does not recognize that they need, more assistance than a family carer alone can provide. Until recently there has been little help available for family carers in thinking about whether moving to a care home is the best option (Baldwin *et al.* 2005). Family carers often make decisions about moving to a care home based on what they believe is in the best interest of the person they are caring for (Davies and Nolan 2004) carefully considering the impact on the person with dementia, in particular their quality of life in a care home.

Although 'quality of life' is difficult to define, it is generally believed to include physical, social and psychological dimensions of a person's experience (Gerritson *et al.* 2004). Often, quality of life is the result of the interaction among these three dimensions. For example, people with cognitive or a sensory perceptual impairment (such as reduced ability to understand what is said to them due to dysphasia or hearing impairment), may find their ability to participate in activities restricted, leading to social isolation and a reduced sense of self-worth (Flannery 2002).

People with dementia retain many more abilities and sensitivities than is generally known (see Chapters 7, 9, 12). The things that are important to everyone, are also important to people with dementia (see Chapters 3, 4), for example, being recognized as a unique individual, maintaining independence and the ability to make choices, having friends, having privacy and dignity, participating in leisure and community activities and being able to assess and take risks in a supported way. Specialized expertise is required to conduct individualized assessments and to identify activities that reflect individual preferences (Brooker and Woolley 2006).

One way of maintaining quality in care homes is through standard setting. In many nations, governmental standards for care homes have been developed and systems have been established to investigate whether standards are being met. In the UK, the National Minimum Standards for care homes provide a point of reference for homes to relate to and from which they can assess their ability to meet the standards (see CSCI website). However, as Briggs and Bachelor (2004) point out, it is important not to define care only by what is measurable but to also address what is important from the perspective of individuals with dementia.

This chapter examines some current thinking about practices which promote a positive transition for people moving from their own homes into a care home. It also considers staff and environmental factors which contribute to the experience of a good quality of life for residents living in care homes in terms of their physical, psychological and social well-being.

Moving into a care home

Research on the impact of moving into a care home has focused on three main areas: the experience of relocation for the person with dementia; the impact of the decision-making process for relatives and carers of the person with dementia; and the role of professionals in supporting and guiding the process.

Relocation has been shown to have a negative effect on the abilities and well-being of a person with dementia. A study by MacDonald and Philpot (2004) compared an 'intermediate care' home from which people were expected to be discharged back home with a 'home for life' or permanent care home. While abilities and well-being declined for residents in both settings, those in 'intermediate care' declined more than those in the permanent setting as indicated by fewer behavioural symptoms and less use of neuroleptic medication. The authors suggest that the possibility that several moves, as occurred for those in intermediate care, result in worse outcomes than does a permanent move to a nursing home. Studies investigating the impact of moves between homes have indicated that people who are moved by themselves experience higher rates of mortality and depression, than those who move as part of a group and along with the staff who care for them (Day *et al.* 2000). The implication of this is that familiarity and continuity of social support networks are important when considering a move.

A study conducted by Davies and Nolan (2004) shows that older people and their relatives are often ill-prepared for making an informed choice about a move. Forming a partnership that includes the person who is moving, health and community professionals, and their family will lead to more positive experiences of the decision-making process in which they feel supported and involved (Sandberg *et al.* 2001, 2002).

Some general guidelines have been produced to help health and social care professionals avoid 'taking over' from the family and leaving both the person with dementia and their family isolated as they try to deal with the emotional impact (Alzheimer's Scotland 2005). Research also suggests that it is helpful for the new resident if staff understand what the move means for the resident in terms of losses, fears, hopes and expectations. This can help them deal with the move, and offer residents support to cope with the impact of the move and to maintain existing positive relationships (Oleson and Shadick, cited in Davies

2001). The decision-making process and transition experience also have a significant impact on family carers (Davies and Nolan 2004) (see Chapter 5).

This clearly points to the need for homes to develop supportive assessment processes which recognize the emotional impact of the move and ensure that the potential resident and their family can be fully involved before the person moves to the care home. A biographical 'life history' approach to understanding what matters to individuals, their values and wishes is now common in admission assessment procedures and development of care plans. (see Chapter 10). It is a means for staff to get to know the person and their preferences and can be a key to establishing relationships through sharing past and present experiences (McKee *et al.* 2005). It also provides an opportunity to engage with family members and a means by which families can contribute to ongoing care as their role in direct care delivery changes (Gaugler *et al.* 2004).

A plan of care can be made jointly with the person and their family. Examples of places to start include developing a 'Getting to know you' booklet (Ashburner 2005), creating life diaries (Cole and Williams 2004), and life history boxes which contain personally significant items. These can provide important links to meaningful experiences and people. While this guidance is sound, it can be difficult for staff with little training in care and perhaps even less in providing psychological support, to respond in a way which has lasting impact, unless ongoing support and supervision are available (Eyers 2000; Moniz-Cook *et al.* 1998; see Chapters 3, 4).

Knowing about an individual is a good starting point in helping to maintain their identity. However, it is important to consider how this knowledge can be used on a day-to-day basis to influence the routines and lifestyle. For example, recognizing that someone has worked night shifts throughout their life suggests that they may be awake and need to be occupied at night, sleeping in the afternoons.

Exercise 19.1 Recognizing the importance of individual habits

Imagine you developed dementia and needed to move to a care home.

Make a list of the things that it would be important for staff to know about you in order for you to feel relaxed living there.

When you have made the list, consider which of these things only you know and which someone else close to you would be able to convey.

Think about what your life would be like if there was no one to do that for you. What would you miss? What would be most upsetting? What might frighten you? What might comfort you?

Factors which influence a person's experience of care

Concern about the quality of care in care homes has been expressed from many places, residents, families, advocates, health and social care professionals and politicians (Train *et al.* 2005). Research in several countries and in all types of care homes confirms that there are widespread problems with the quality of care. An evaluation of care quality for people with dementia across three health authorities in the United Kingdom, using dementia care mapping, revealed a great need for improvement in all the homes studied. Residents were spending more than 80% of their time either socially withdrawn or not engaged in any activity (Ballard *et al.* 2001).

Basic principles of care

Person-centred dementia care principles provide a good starting point for high quality care. These principles have been laid out in the National Service Framework (Department of Health 2001) and are described in detail in Chapters 3, 4, 7 and 14. These principles reflect the increasing evidence that people with dementia are able to continue with their emotional lives and experience pleasure and distress in response to things they enjoy or dislike (Bryden 2005; Kitwood 1997). Person-centred dementia care principles include:

- valuing the person and their family

- treating the person as an individual

- taking the perspective of the person when planning and providing care

- ensuring that a positive social environment exists in which the person can experience relative well-being (Brooker 2007).

However, these principles need to be adopted and adapted by homes to make them a reality for residents. A checklist of how these principles may appear in practice was developed as one of a number of activities, in a study to see whether using psychosocial practices could reduce the use of neuroleptic medication for people with dementia in care homes (Fossey *et al.* 2006). It has been produced by the Alzheimer's Society and is available for relatives and staff (Fossey and James 2008). The checklist describes observable areas of practice which indicate positive personal relationships, environment and activities. Some important things to consider are:

- Are residents wearing make-up or jewellery (a sign that there is attention to detail and responsiveness to individual preferences)?

- Are staff speaking to residents not only when they are delivering physical care?

- Do the rooms in the home allow residents to have both communal and private space during the day?

- Are individual and group activities available?

- Are there links to the wider community in terms of trips out or visitors being invited into the home?

The answers to these questions can provide some insight into basic quality of life issues for residents. Positive responses give some assurance that person-centred principles are in operation.

Resonant with Kitwood's work on psychological needs (1997), Nolan *et al.* (2001) has developed the 'Senses Framework' as a way to think about the psychological needs of people with dementia, family carers and staff in care homes. (See Chapter 24.) The six senses are:

- sense of security
- sense of continuity
- sense of belonging
- sense of purpose
- sense of achievement
- sense of significance.

Promoting positive interpersonal relationships

It has been suggested that the relationships that the person with dementia has are the most important features maintaining well-being (Robinson and Banks 2005; Werezak and Morgan 2003; Zgola 1999).

An organizational aspect of enabling close relationships to build and communication between staff and individual residents to develop requires a consistent staff assignment. It also maximizes people's ability to build trusting relationships. People with dementia are often faced with increasing levels of dependency and therefore need dependability and reliability in care staff, who can, through regular contact, develop a responsiveness to their needs and individualize care systems on a personal basis.

It can be useful to consider providing person-centred care within the broader social context. Adams (2005) has suggested that considering the importance of the interpersonal interactions in 'relationship-centred' practice can help staff to engage with family members more easily. Simple everyday interaction which supports friendships is a vital component in sustaining well-being for people in care homes.

Staff's role in introducing residents to each other, helping with phone calls and letter writing to maintain existing relationships and making time to chat need to be recognized as useful interventions in themselves in maintaining well-being (Cole and Williams 2004; Davies 2001). Communication between care staff and residents with dementia may require a great deal of skill to support people who have receptive or expressive dysphasia.

Interactions require greater attentiveness on the part of the carer and the development of skills which include active listening to and observation of non-verbal signs from residents and the use of gestures, pictures, photographs and personal objects to support carers' verbal communication (Powell 2000). Many people with dementia also have sensory disabilities which affect their ability to form relationships. Staff can modify the way they communicate to enhance their ability to interact effectively with residents by, for example, ensuring that they face a resident and have light on them rather than behind them, so their face is not in shadow and can be more easily seen; by using gestures which are consistent with their verbal message; and by presenting information simply – one idea at a time – so that the recipient is not overwhelmed. (see Chapter 12).

Exercise 19.2   Recognizing the power of social interaction

1   List all the people you meet or speak to today.

2   Think of a person with dementia whom you know, and list who they have met or spoken to today.

Are there differences in the types of contact you and they have with other people?

An aspect of personal relationships which is often neglected in care homes is that of a person's sexuality. The public nature of many care homes' living space makes it difficult for moments of intimacy, posing a challenge to maintaining both privacy and dignity. It is important for homes to address these issues by considering how couples can have privacy during visits, or share rooms and also the provision of sofas as well as single chairs to allow for normal affectionate contact in a natural setting. Sexuality is a sensitive subject and training which explores people's knowledge, attitudes and develops skills in talking with residents about it is often required (Gordon and Sokolowski 2004; Heymanson 2003).

Opportunities to create relationships which enable residents to give as well as receive care also have a positive impact on well-being. This can involve interaction between residents and between residents and staff. In addition pets provide an opportunity to give affection and attention and can provide purpose and comfort beyond that of human visitors alone (Lutwack-Bloom *et al.* 2005).

Encouraging family involvement in care home life

Most family members want to maintain their relationship with their relative after they move into a care home. It is helpful if the family can build a relationship with the staff and work in partnership with them. However, in many homes, working with family is rarely acknowledged as part of care staffs' role. Consequently, family carers often feel they have to take the initiative if they wish to remain involved in the care of their relative (Train *et al.* 2005). Families can provide a rich source of support for their own relative and for staff in understanding the most helpful ways of interacting with the person who has dementia. Good practice requires family involvement in the development and review of the person's care plan (Gaugler *et al.* 2004). Having open discussions about concerns and areas of potential risk can be particularly helpful in keeping the person's best interests at the fore. One common issue is about the residents who enjoy walking but are at risk of falling. Discussions about the degree to which they can be accompanied, areas of the home and grounds which may reduce the risk, and the use of aids such as hip protectors to reduce the possible impact should a fall occur, can facilitate the individual in having a greater freedom of movement around the home than might otherwise be immediately possible.

It is important to recognize what families have to offer, as consultants on providing direct care, on the social component of the person's life, through advocacy, and by providing feedback and suggestions on how to organize care to create a welcoming and comfortable ambience. For example, one home organized a 'Friends' group which meets monthly both to provide information and support for new families and also for the 'friends' to organize additional activities with residents to bring the local community into the home and take residents out to local events.

Exercise 19.3 Recognizing the value of supportive relationships

Lucy, a woman with dementia in a care home, is visited every day by her husband, Harry. Recently she has not recognized him on his visits but has appeared to find his company acceptable. Harry has told staff that he thinks it is no longer worth him coming in to see Lucy as it 'does no good'.

Considering the 'Senses' framework described earlier:

What benefits might there be for Lucy, if Harry continues his visits?

Are there any disadvantages for her?

What support might Harry need in deciding whether to continue visiting?

How else might he remain involved in her care?

Supporting personal identity of the resident

Helping people to maintain their identity is closely linked to self-esteem and quality of life in care homes (Davies 2001; McKee *et al.* 2005). To address this, biographical approaches such as reminiscence, life story work and oral history can act as a basis to develop plans to provide personally meaningful activity for individuals within the home and to affirm their identify. It enables people to engage in previously enjoyed activities or link new activities to significant events or aspirations from the past (see Chapter 10).

Specific psychosocial and creative therapies (see Table 19.1 for examples) can also be used to promote meaningful occupation for the person, affirming identify, increasing self-expression, improving communication skills, and providing opportunities to enhance a person's identity and self-esteem. A review of 33 studies (Marshall and Hutchinson 2001) evaluating social, creative and physical activities with people with Alzheimer's Disease concluded that purposeful, organized activity can make a positive contribution to enhancing social interaction.

Table 19.1 Psychosocial approaches to care

Reality orientation See Spector (2000) and Verkaik (2006)	Uses rehearsal and physical prompts to improve cognitive functioning related to personal orientation

Cognitive stimulation therapy See Spector (2006)	Derived from reality orientation, focuses on information processing rather than rehearsal of factual knowledge
Reminiscence therapy and life review See Woods (2005)	Involves discussion of past experiences individually or in a group of people. Photographs, familiar objects, music, or sensory items prompt recall
Validation therapy See Neal and Barton Wright (2003)	Based on the general principle of acceptance of the reality of the person and validation of their experience and incorporates a range of specific techniques
Behavioural management techniques See Maniz-Cooke (1998)	Based on learning theory and utilizes the antecedents and consequences of behaviour to elicit change in an individual
Music/music therapy See Vink (2003)	Includes playing and listening to music as a way of generally enhancing well-being or can be more goal-directed with specific activities being used for a clearly defined therapeutic purpose
Creative therapies See Wilkinson (1998) and James (2006)	Drama, art, toys, dance all offer creative ways of communicating, facilitate verbal and non-verbal self-expression and aim to improve well-being
Snoezelen/multisensory stimulation See Burns (2002)	Stimuli such as light, sound and tactile sensations often in specially designed rooms, aim to increase the opportunity for communication, and improved quality of experience
Simulated presence therapy See Peak (2002)	An audiotape of positive memories and experiences compiled in a conversational style by family members or friends is played to the person to provide reassurance, information and stimulation
Structured activity/interaction programmes See Cohen-Mansfield (2000)	Formal sessions of interaction using a structured conversational format, photos and pictures as discussion items aim to improve engagement and involvement
Exercise See Hokkanen (2003)	Involving walking or group activity has been used to address depression and behavioural difficulties

Environmental manipulation See Day (2000)	Cues such as colour and textural coding in rooms and furnishings, clear signage to private, communal and outdoor areas, planned furniture and building layout facilitates communication, exercise and pleasure and reduces disorientation
Animal-assisted activity or therapy See Kastinas (2000)	Involves animals visiting people (or vice versa) to provide opportunities for social, motivational, recreational or therapeutic benefits to enhance quality of life
Psychotherapies See James (1999, 2003a)	Cognitive-behavioural therapy for anxiety or depression for carers and clients in early stages of illness. Personal construct and brief psychotherapy to address emotional adjustment and self-esteem
Psycho-education with paid and family caregivers See Burgio (2002)	Promotes understanding of the medical and non-medical factors, communication skills, behaviour management strategies, environmental modification, ethical issues, ways of involving families, stress management, practical and legal issues

Knowing an individual's story and beliefs also enables homes to address their needs to maintain their spiritual life, either through the provision of pray areas or through attending to practices such as at mealtimes, providing or avoiding food consistent with the person's faith, recognizing days of celebration or enabling residents to participate in particular seasonal activities and rituals.

Culture and ethnicity can be basic to a person's identity. Therefore, cultural awareness is an important issue in all aspects of dementia care, both to provide overseas staff with knowledge of everyday practices concerning food and drink, local customs and sayings, and important historical and current events to which clients might relate. Some homes provide language tuition for their staff and it can also be helpful to work with a tutor to ensure that useful vocabulary is identified, also to support all staff in meeting the needs of minority ethnic residents for whom Mold's (2005) systematic review of care has shown that there are a number of difficulties in delivering culturally appropriate care and that language and communication difficulties arise which need to be addressed.

Providing an enabling physical environment

The physical environment of a care home also has an impact on the well-being of individuals. Evidence suggests that the design of a home can improve the living experience of people with dementia by, for example, increasing participation in activities and reducing time spent alone, and by providing safe space for residents to walk and thus have less restriction on their freedom (Reimer *et al.* 2004). A review of the design of therapeutic environments for people with dementia recommended that they be small in size and have separate facilities for people with cognitive impairment and those without, be non-institutionalized in décor and provide some environmental stimulation such as ornaments, plants and varied furnishings. In particular, older people need two to three times the amount of light to see as younger people and are more sensitive to glare. They need to have light coloured walls and floors to increase inter-reflected light, and the use of translucent shades to shield the glare from light bulbs. Increasing the contrast colours between features such as doorframes also improves visibility. Creating consistent levels of light between rooms and hallways helps people to move around the home independently (Poole 2006). Clear signage helps people to orient themselves to bathrooms, bedrooms and communal spaces (Day *et al.* 2000).

A similar level of reflection is needed in planning the outside environment for people with dementia who have described how the outdoor environment plays a significant role in their quality of life by providing opportunities for increased personal space, fresh air, exercise, stimulation for conversation, contact with nature, and chance to engage with neighbours (Chalfont 2005). The use of paths to lead residents around areas of interest, clear focal points, and planting which enables a stimulation of the senses through scent or edibility of the plants, all promote well-being (Poole 2006).

The Eden Alternative is a comprehensive model for transforming the physical, interpersonal, psychosocial and spiritual environment, and organizational culture of homes. It is based on the assumption that caregivers will treat residents as they would like to be treated and are empowered to make decisions about care. It involves the introduction of plants and resident animals and activities into the care environment to help create a sense of a spontaneous and natural environment. It has reported benefits in terms of decrease in medication use, infection rates, accidents and pressure ulcers (Thomas 1996). The methods are in use in the USA and Australia and in fewer settings in the UK. To provide any benefit, the GREENHOUSE principles must be implemented comprehensively as superficial adoption reduces the possibility of benefit (Hinman and Heyl 2002).

Practices such as locking doors to prevent people from wandering off are still used in many homes, despite the ethical concerns this practice has raised. In some instances, modification of the environment through the use of signs, the use of patterned floor covering to create a visual guide for people and the use of cloth barriers can overcome the need for more restrictive interventions to ensure physical safety (Feliciano and Vore 2004). However, interventions such as the use of sedating medication, locking doors, using restraints, tagging a person by using an electronic tracking device to monitor their whereabouts, and modifications to the environment to limit a person's freedom have potentially adverse consequences for an individual. The use of neuroleptic medication in particular is associated with an increased risk of falls and an increased incidence of a number of health conditions such as parkinsonian symptoms and stroke, and an overall increased mortality risk (Ballard and Howard 2006). The use of these, or the use of modifications to the environment, to curtail freedom often appears to 'solve' the immediate matter of concern to staff, but in doing so discourages care practice which takes the perspective of the resident into account by seeking to understand the reasons they may have for acting in a certain way, and their needs and wishes. This may in turn limit the range of potential activities a resident can engage in and the possibility of building relationships which might enhance the person's life. The debate generally focuses on the rights of the individual and the right to take risks (Welsh *et al.* 2003). Reaching a decision about an acceptable way to keep people safe requires a good understanding of what they are trying to achieve. Knowing this will allow care staff, in collaboration with the family and the person with dementia, to determine an appropriate course of intervention (Hughes and Louw 2002). (See Chapter 6.)

Supporting staff practice

Within care homes there are both qualified, usually from the nursing profession, and unqualified, staff. Providing long-term care requires staff to be able to work at an emotional level as well as addressing physical care needs. It can, at times, be stressful as they are faced with dealing with residents' distress, confusion and communication which may not be easy to interpret. It requires them to have knowledge about dementia care, a positive attitude to their work and also to develop communication skills to support their practice. For many care staff, the relationship with residents is the most important work issue and a major reason for staying in their job (Parsons *et al.* 2003) and a lack of opportunity to build personal attachments is a strong predictor of staff burnout and turnover (Sumaya-Smith 1995).

It has been suggested that the way people are treated (Sabat 1994) can result in behavioural and emotional difficulties, increasing their degree of disability (see Chapter 4). Staff often take over tasks that individuals are still capable of engaging with because of the focus on efficiency and 'getting the job done' (Jirovec 1991). This can result in 'learned helplessness' for the resident, an induced dependency in which it becomes easier to be a recipient of care than to try to maintain independence (Flannery 2002). Letting go of independence in this way poses a risk to self-concept and autonomy (Shook and Beck 1991). However, by training staff in behavioural strategies it is possible to promote independence in activities of daily living without staff spending a significantly greater amount of time in the activity (Beck *et al.* 1997).

Pulsford (1997) notes that care staff can often adopt an 'all or nothing' approach by which they design elaborate activity programmes which are too ambitious for the majority of residents. This 'failure' leads staff to the conclusion that 'therapeutic activities just can't be done here'. Moniz-Cook *et al.* (1998) proposed that care staff should be given increased opportunity and recognition to use their own initiative and ideas. In their investigation of staff burnout and staff–patient interactions Jenkins and Allen (1998) found that the degree to which staff perceive themselves to be involved in decisions about their work was a 'powerful predictor of resident orientated care'. This highlights the importance of setting realistic goals with staff and providing good supervision structures within the home to ensure that difficulties can be resolved in a timely way.

Despite guidance about the required training level for staff in the National Minimum Standards for Care Homes for Older People in the UK, there is evidence that many services are not meeting the 50 per cent target for staff National Vocational Qualification levels (CSCI 2005). In the USA, despite the requirement for staff certification and training, there is considerable evidence that staff are not receiving sufficient training for their work. They may have little guidance about appropriate ways of working with residents and so do 'what seems best' based on their own judgements and life experience (Spilsbury and Meyer 2004). For example, the controversial use of deceptive practices when interacting with residents seems to be widespread. A survey of care staff showed that 'lying' was a strategy commonly used, often intended kindly, to ease the distress of residents (James *et al.* 2003b). Care staff perceived situations in which lying could be an appropriate therapeutic response in which 'the ends justify the means' (Tuckett 2004), in order to gain compliance or immediately pacify a person in distress. Whether this approach is of benefit or of harm to recipients in the longer term is yet to be ascertained. Guidance within homes about their policy and detailed individual care plans can be helpful for staff to clarify how they are expected to behave in circumstances of residents' distress.

In an attempt to improve care, a number of small-scale research studies have evaluated a range of specific interventions such as staff training in psychosocial skills (Proctor *et al.* 1999), communications (Pillemer *et al.* 2003; Tappen *et al.* 2001), emotion-oriented care (Schrijnemaekers *et al.* 2002), and multi-sensory stimulation and multi-faceted interventions from specialist teams providing training in behavioural and other psychosocial approaches (Rovner *et al.* 1996; Opie *et al.* 2002). A recent evidence-based review (Tilly and Reed 2004) has emphasized the limited number of adequate studies, disappointing outcomes and the need to develop work in the area of interventions focused on preserving daily living skills. Although some of the interventions outlined above have been shown to benefit individual residents with specific behavioural problems, at an organizational level the effect has been far more modest.

Almost 20 years ago, Burgio and Burgio (1990) suggested that organizational practices need to change if care practices are to improve. If training is to have a real impact on how staff work and on care practices, the culture of care and the home as a whole needs to change (Innes *et al.* 2006). Change can cause a sense of uncertainty and anxiety and, for many organizations, maintaining the status quo feels safer than implementing change. Enabling staff to use the knowledge and skills they develop through training requires attending to the difficulties they encounter when attempting to change their practice, ensuring that systems are in place to support practice changes (Fossey and James 2008). Guiding principles for organizational change include (Burgio and Burgio 1990):

- Have clear goals and therapeutic direction to work towards, which all staff are aware of.

- Obtain support from the relevant administrative and professional hierarchies, and to make staff participating in training or supervision aware of this.

- Elaborate on already existing systems which are in place (e.g. build in additional topics to an induction programme).

- Involve staff in the development and planning of the training or supervision.

- Ensure that there is agreement about when staff can practise skills learned in training.

- Identify a support and supervision structure to maintain knowledge and skills developed in training.

- Keep the programme simple and proceed slowly.

- Remain flexible and maintain a dynamic intervention.

- Feed back positive observations and changes to staff to help maintain motivation.

Exercise 19.4 Recognizing opportunities to enable learning

Consider care staff who come from overseas and for whom English is not their first language or native culture.

What cultural experiences do you think it is important for overseas staff to know about when caring for people with dementia?

List the way that the manager can ensure that these staff are supported during training.

Working with the wider health care team

People with dementia often receive less effective medical and mental health services than those in the community (Fahey *et al.* 2003). For example, in terms of physical health, geriatricians' ability to diagnose pain in people with greater levels of cognitive impairment was found to be poor (Cohen-Mansfield and Lipson 2002). However, there is no evidence to suggest that people with dementia experience pain levels that are less than any other group of people (Horgas and Elliott 2004). Given that a person with dementia may have reduced abilities to communicate their specific needs, it is important that care staff are aware of the signs to look out for. Among care homes, there is considerable variability on relationships with local GP practices and physical and mental health teams. There is considerable evidence that good practice requires multidisciplinary consultation and that liaison services should extend to care homes to deliver advice and treatment (Glendinning *et al.* 2002; Hancock *et al.* 2006).

Debates and controversies

From a philosophical point of view there has been a significant shift in the approach to care for people for people with dementia in care homes. However, in practice the change in approach has been developing much more slowly. One of the key areas of debate is about the skill-mix of staff in homes since recruitment and retention continue to be a significant challenge and there is a limited amount of literature which relates the skills of staff to outcomes and quality of life of residents (Kane 2004; Schnelle *et al.* 2004).

Allied to the debate about skill-mix is the training needs of staff and how this can best be provided in-service and through formal educational routes. The role of management practices and leadership style have also been identified as key to influencing resident outcomes (Anderson *et al.* 2003) but are only starting to receive attention from academics and policy-makers recently.

An ongoing debate is whether the specialist provision of dementia care in homes provides a higher quality of care for residents than in homes which accept residents both with and without dementia. The practical and ethical challenge arises when people develop dementia after moving into a non-specialist home. The question arises whether their needs are better met by remaining in their current residence or moving to another home with a 'specialist' status.

Conclusion

Despite an increasing focus on therapeutic interventions for people with dementia, the integration of these practices is by no means universal. As previously highlighted, there are concerns about the current standards of dementia care in relation to meeting the psychosocial needs of residents with dementia. It is therefore important to attend to the 'real world' contexts within which these interventions are taking place and the possible barriers which arise (Jacques and Innes 1998).

Long-term care for older people with dementia is a diverse and complex service. The funding of care home places, and transition from family home to care home, are major issues. Procedures vary around the UK as they do across many different countries. For practice to develop and for residents to achieve a good quality of life, adequate resources and the development of a skilled and specialist workforce need to be addressed. In the UK the National Minimum Standards have set out a clear framework for homes to follow in their delivery of care in line with person-centred principles. The implementation of regular inspection and monitoring processes both of care delivery and of the minimum standards of training for staff in care practices can help to improve quality. However, the framework for training does not address the need for specific dementia training. Although this has been taken up by a number of charitable organizations such as the Alzheimer's Society, Age Concern and Help the Aged through programme development and the production of guidance for best practice, without some statutory regulation it is unlikely that all care homes will address this learning need.

There is also evidence that people in care homes are not receiving the same levels of health care service as those in the community, despite having significant and complex health care needs. There is potential in both NHS policy and practice to create better liaison services with care homes to ensure that residents receive both physical and mental health care services and rehabilitation to support their remaining independence. There is also scope for policy within individual care home organizations to be proactive and address the ways in which homes try to engage with their local health care providers.

Although the principles of person-centred care have been developing over the last ten to fifteen years, research has lagged behind in taking the person with dementia's perspective on their experience of care home life, focusing rather on symptom reduction and the observable outcomes of a variety of different practices. In order for research to adopt person-centred principles in a way which is encouraged in care practice, questions which address the individual's personal experience need to be explored. An obvious starting point is the experience of people with dementia, for which there is a paucity of information compared with the research on family carers.

In increasingly multicultural societies there is also a need for research to address the effects that the different cultural perspectives of both staff and residents have on the quality of care and quality of life in order to inform future education and training of the workforce to deliver excellence in dementia care (see Chapter 3 and Chapter 24).

Further information

The Alzheimer's Society has a website covering a range of topics. Included are several reports that address various aspects of living in a care home and working in care home.

The Royal National Institute of Blind People has a website that includes reports and discussions about working with people who are blind and have dementia.

The Royal National Institute of Deaf People has a website addressing hearing loss in general. As hearing loss is common in older adults, this information will pertain to many people with dementia.

The Commission for Social Care Inspection in England has a website for consumers that addresses a wide range of care home issues.

Help the Aged and **Age Concern** maintain websites for consumers that include a wide array of topics relevant to older people. This includes pensions, lifelong learning, and a number of papers and discussion related to dementia. This website would be useful to people with dementia, carers and professionals.

The National Institute for Health and Clinical Excellence (NICE) maintains a website that addresses many health issues, including dementia. It is primarily for professionals.

References

Adams, T. (2005) From person-centred to relationship-centred care. *Generations Review*, 15: 4–7.

Alzheimer Scotland (2005) *Letting Go Without Giving Up: Continuing to Care for the Person with Dementia*. Edinburgh: Alzheimer Scotland.

Anderson, R., Issel, L.M. and McDaniel, R.R. (2003) Nursing homes as complex adaptive systems: relationship between management practice and resident outcomes. *Nursing Research*, 52(1): 12–21.

Ashburner, C.H. (2005) Person-centred care: change through action research. Unpublished doctoral thesis. London, City University.

Bajekal, M. (2002) *Health Survey for England 2000: Care Homes and their Residents*. London: The Stationery Office.

Baldwin, C., Hope, T., Hughes, R., Jacoby, R. and Ziebland, S. (2005) *Making Difficult Decisions: The Experience of Caring for Someone with Dementia*. London: Alzheimer's Society.

Ballard, C. and Howard, R. (2006) Neuroleptic drugs in dementia: benefits and harm. *Nature Reviews Neuroscience*, 7(6): 492–500.

Ballard, C.G., Margo-Llana, M., Fossey, J., Reichelt, K., Myint, P., Potkins, D. and O'Brien, J. (2001) A one year follow up study of behavioural and psychological symptoms in dementia among people in care environments. *Journal of Clinical Psychiatry*, 62: 631–6.

Bebbington, A., Darton, R. and Netten, A. (2001) *Care Homes for Older People*. Volume 2. *Admissions, Needs and Outcomes*. Canterbury: PSSRU.

Beck, C., Heacock, P., Mercer, S., Walls, R.C., Rapp, C.G. and Vogelpohl, T.S. (1997) Improving dressing behaviour in cognitively impaired nursing home residents. *Nursing*, 46: 126–32.

Briggs, K. and Bachelor, J. (2004) What are the core values of care? *Journal of Dementia Care*, 12: 14–15.

Brooker, D. (2007) *Person-centred Dementia Care: Making Services Better*. University of Bradford. London: Jessica Kingsley.

Brooker, D. and Woolley, R. (2006) *Enriching Opportunities. Unlocking Potential: Searching for the Keys. Summary of a Developmental Evaluation*. Bradford: Extra Care Charitable Trust and Bradford Dementia Group.

Bryden, C. (2005) *Dancing with Dementia: My Story of Living Positively with Dementia*. London, Jessica Kingsley.

Burgio, L.D. and Burgio, K. L. (1990) Institutional staff training and management: a review of the literature and a model for geriatric, long term care facilities. *International Journal of Aging and Human Development*, 30: 287–302.

Burgio, L.D., Stevens, A., Burgio, K.L., Roth, D.L., Paul, P. and Gerstle, J. (2002) Teaching and maintaining behaviour management skills in the nursing home. *The Gerontologist*, 42: 487–96.

Burns, A., Byrne, J., Ballard, C. and Holmes, C. (2002) Sensory stimulation in dementia. *British Medical Journal*, Clinical Research Edition, 325: 1312–13.

Caron, C. and Bowers, B. (2003) Deciding whether to continue, share, or relinquish caregiving: caregiver views. *Qualitative Health Research*, 13: 1252–71.

Chalfont, G. (2005) *Architecture, Nature and Care: The Importance of Connecting to Nature with Reference to Older People and Dementia*. Sheffield: School of Architecture, University of Sheffield.

Cohen-Mansfield, J. (2000) Use of patient characteristics to determine non-pharmacological interventions for behavioural and psychological symptoms of dementia. *International Psychogeriatrics*, 12(1): 373–80.

Cohen-Mansfield, J. and Lipson, S. (2002) Pain in cognitively impaired nursing home residents: how well are physicians diagnosing it? *Journal of the American Geriatrics Society*, 50: 1039–44.

Cole, A. and Williams, H. (2004) Life story work, an aid to well-being. *Signpost*, 9: 14–18.

CSCI (2005) *The State of Social Care in England 2004–2005*. London: Commission for Social Care Improvement.

Davies, S. (2001) The care needs of older people and family caregivers in continuing care settings. In: M. Nolan, S. Davies and G. Grant (eds) *Working with Older People and their Families*. Buckingham: Open University Press.

Davies, S. and Nolan, M. (2003) 'Making the best of things': relatives' experiences of decision about care home entry. *Ageing and Society*, 23: 429–50.

Davies, S. and Nolan, M. (2004) 'Making the move': relatives' experiences of the transition to a care home. *Health and Social Care in the Community*, 12: 517–26.

Day, K., Carreon, D. and Stump, C. (2000) Therapeutic design of environments for people with dementia: a review of the empirical research. *The Gerontologist*, 40: 397–416.

Department of Health (2001) *National Service Framework for Older People*. London: Department of Health.

Eyers, I. (2000) Education and training – do they really really want it? A comparative study of care home staff in England and Germany. *Education and Ageing*, 15.

Fahey, T., Montgomery, A.A., Barnes, J. and Prothero, J. (2003) Quality of care for elderly residents in nursing homes and elderly people living alone: controlled observational study. *British Medical Journal*, 326: 580–3.

Feliciano, L. and Vore, J. (2004) Decreasing entry into a restricted area using a visual barrier. *Journal of Applied Behaviour Analysis*, 37: 107–10.

Flannery, R.B. (2002) Treating learned helplessness in the elderly dementia patient: preliminary enquiry. *American Journal of Alzheimer's Disease and Other Dementias*, 17: 345–9.

Fossey, J., Ballard, C.G., Juszczak, E., James, I.A., Alder, N., Jacoby, R. and Howard, R. (2006) Effect of enhanced psychosocial care on antipsychotic use in nursing home residents with severe dementia: cluster randomised trial. *British Medical Journal*, 332: 756–8.

Fossey, J. and James, I. (2008) *Evidenced Based Approaches to Improving Dementia Care in Care Homes.* London: Alzheimer's Society.

Gaugler, J.E., Anderson, K.A., Zarit, S.H. and Pearlin, L.I. (2004) Family involvement in nursing homes: effects on stress and well-being. *Aging and Mental Health,* 8: 65–75.

Gerritson, D.L., Steverink, N., Ooms, M.E. and Ribbe, M.W. (2004) Finding a useful conceptual basis for enhancing the quality of life of nursing home residents. *Quality of Life Research,* 13: 611–24.

Glendinning, C., Jacobs, S., Alborz, A. and Hann, M. (2002) A survey of access to medical services in nursing and residential homes in England. *British Journal of General Practice,* 52.

Gordon, M. and Sokolowski, M. (2004) Sexuality in long term care: ethics and action. *Annals of Long-term Care,* 12(9): 545–8.

Hancock, G., Woods, B., Challis, D. and Orrell, M. (2006) The needs of older people with dementia in residential care. *International Journal of Geriatric Psychiatry,* 21: 43–9.

Heymanson, C. (2003) Sexuality and intimacy in care homes. *Journal of Dementia Care,* 11(5): 10–11.

Hinman, M.R. and Heyl, D.M. (2002) Influence of the Eden Alternative on the functional status of nursing home residents. *Occupational Therapy in Geriatrics,* 20: 1–20.

Hokkanen, L., Rantala, L. Remes, A.-M., Harkonen, B., Viramo, P. and Winbald, I. (2003) Dance/movement therapeutic methods in management of dementia. *Journal of the American Geriatrics Society,* 51(4): 576–7.

Horgas, A. and Elliott, A. (2004) Pain assessment and management in persons with dementia. *Nursing Clinics of North America,* 39: 593–608.

Hughes, J.C. and Louw, S.J. (2002) Electronic tagging of people with dementia who wander. *British Medical Journal,* 325: 847–8.

Innes, A., MacPherson, S. and McCabe, L. (2006) *Promoting Person-centred Care at the Front Line.* York: Joseph Rowntree Foundation.

Jacques, I. and Innes, A. (1998) Who cares about care assistant work? *Journal of Dementia Care,* 6: 33–7.

James, I.A. (1999) Using a cognitive rationale to conceptualise anxiety in people with dementia. *Behavioural and Cognitive Psychotherapy,* 27(4): 345–51.

James, I.A., MacKenzie, L. and Mukaetova-Ladinska, E. (2006) Doll use in care homes for people with dementia. *International Journal of Geriatric Psychiatry,* 21: 1093–8.

James, I.A., Postma, K. and MacKenzie, L. (2003a) Using an IPT conceptualisation to treat a depressed person with dementia. *Behavioural and Cognitive Psychotherapy,* 31(3): 451–6.

James, I.A., Powell, I., Smith, T. and Fairbairn, A. (2003b) Lying to residents: can the truth sometimes be unhelpful for people with dementia? *PSIGE Newsletter*, 82: 26–8.

Jenkins, H. and Allen, C. (1998) The relationship between staff burnout/distress and interactions with residents in two residential homes for older people. *International Journal of Geriatric Psychiatry*, 13: 466–72.

Jirovec, M.M. (1991) Effects of individualised prompted toileting on incontinence in nursing home residents. *Applied Nursing Research*, 4: 188–91.

Jones, T., Matias, M., Powell, J., Jones, E., Fishburn, J., and Looi, J. (2007) Who cares for older people with mental illness? A survey of residential aged care facilities in the Australian Capital Territory: Implications for mental health nursing. *International Journal of Mental Health Nursing*, 16: 327–37.

Kane, R.L. (2004) Commentary: Nursing home staffing – more is necessary but not necessarily sufficient. *Health Service Research*, 39(2): 251–2.

Katsinas, R.P. (2000) The use and implications of canine companion in a therapeutic day programme for nursing home residents with dementia. *Activities, Adaptation and Ageing*, 25: 13–30.

Kitwood, T. (1997) *Dementia Reconsidered: The Person Comes First*. Buckingham: Open University Press.

Lutwack-Bloom, P., Wijewickrama, R. and Smith, B. (2005) Effects of pets versus people visits with nursing home residents. *Journal of Gerontological Social Work*, 44: 137–59.

MacDonald, A. and Philpot, M. (2004) An attempt to determine the benefits of a 'home for life' principle in residential care for older people with dementia and behavioural problems: a comparative cohort study. *Dementia and Geriatric Cognitive Disorders*, 18: 6–14.

Macdonald, A.J.D., Carpenter, G.I., Box, O., Roberts, A. and Sahu, S. (2002) Dementia and use of psychotropic medication in non 'Elderly Mentally Infirm' nursing homes in South East England. *Age and Ageing*, 31: 58–64.

Marshall, M.J. and Hutchinson, S.A. (2001) A critique of research on the use of activities with persons with Alzheimer's Disease: a systematic literature review. *Journal of Advanced Nursing*, 35: 488–96.

McKee, K., Downs, M., Gilhooly, M., Gilhooly, K., Tester, S. and Wilson, F. (2005) Frailty, identity and the quality of later life. In: A. Walker (ed.) *Understanding Quality of Life in Older Age*. Maidenhead: Open University Press.

Mold, F., Fitzpatrick, J.M. and Roberts, J.D. (2005) Minority ethnic elders in care homes: a review of the literature. *Age and Ageing*, 34(2): 107–13.

Moniz-Cook, E., Agar, S., Silver, M., Woods, R., Wang, M., Elston, C., Win, T. and Holderness Community Health NHS Trust (1998) Can staff training reduce behavioural problems in residential care for the elderly mentally ill? *International Journal of Geriatric Psychiatry*, 13: 149–58. http://www inter-science wiley com/jpages/0885-6230/

National Research Ethics Services (2007) http://www.nres.npsa.nhs.uk/ (accessed 4 April 2008).

Neal, M. and Bartonwright, P. (2003) Validation therapy for dementia. *Cochrane Database of Systematic Reviews,* 3: CD001394 DOI:10.1002/14651858.CD001394.

Nolan, M., Davies, S. and Grant, G. (2001) *Working with Older People and their Families: Key Issues in Policy and Practice.* Buckingham: Open University Press.

Office of Fair Trading (2005) *Care Homes for Older People in the UK: A Market Study.* London: Office of Fair Trading.

Opie, J., Doyle, C., O'Connor, D.W. (2002) Challenging behaviours in nursing home residents with dementia: a randomised controlled trial of multidisciplinary interventions. *International Journal of Geriatric Psychiatry,* 17: 6–13.

Parsons, S., Simmons, W., Penn, K. and Furlough, M. (2003) Determinants of satisfaction and turnover among nursing assistants: the results of a statewide survey. *Journal of Gerontological Nursing,* 29: 393–410.

Peak, J. and Cheston, R.I.L. (2002) Using Simulated Presence Therapy with people with dementia. *Ageing and Mental Health,* 6(1): 77–81.

Pillemer, K., Suitor, J., Henderson, C.R., Meador, R., Schultz, L., Robinson, J. and Hegeman, C. (2003) A comparative Communications Intervention for nursing home staff and family members of residents. *The Gerontologist,* 43: 96.

Poole, J. (2006) *The Alzheimer's Society Guide to the Dementia Care Environment.* London: Alzheimer's Society.

Powell, J.A. (ed.) (2000) *Care to Communicate.* London, Jessica Kingsley.

Proctor, R., Burns, A., Stratton Powell, H., Tarrier, N., Faragher, B. and Richardson, G. (1999) Behavioural management in nursing and residential homes: a randomised controlled trial. *Lancet,* 354: 26–9.

Pulsford, D. (1997) Therapeutic activities for people with dementia – what, why ... and why not? *Journal of Advanced Nursing,* 26: 704–9.

Quinn, M.E., Johnson, M.A., Andress, E.L. and McGinnis, P. (2003) Health characteristics of elderly residents in personal care homes: dementia, possible dementia, and no dementia. *Journal of Gerontological Nursing,* 29: 16–23.

Reimer, M.A., Slaughter, S., Donaldson, C., Currie, G. and Eliasziw, M. (2004) Special care facility compared with traditional environments for dementia care: a longitudinal study of quality of life. *Journal of the American Geriatrics Society* 52(7): 1085–92.

Robinson, J. and Banks, P. (2005) *Care Services Enquiry: The Business of Caring.* London: King's Fund.

Rothera, I., Jones, R., Harwood, R., Avery, A. and Waite, J. (2003) Health status and assessed need for a cohort of older people admitted to nursing and residential homes. *Age and Ageing,* 32: 303–9.

Rovner, B.W., Steele, C., Shmuely, D.S.W. and Folstein, M.E. (1996) A randomised trial of dementia care in nursing homes. *Journal of the American Geriatrics Society,* 44: 7–13.

Sabat, S.R. (1994) Excess disability and malignant social psychology – a case study of Alzheimer's Disease. *Journal of Community and Applied Social Psychology,* 4: 157–66.

Sandberg, J., Lundh, U. and Nolan, M.R. (2001) Placing a spouse in a care home: the importance of keeping. *Journal of Clinical Nursing* 10: 406–16.

Sandberg, J., Nolan, M.R. and Lundh, U. (2002) Entering a new world: Empathic awareness as the key to positive family/staff relationships in care homes. *International Journal of Nursing Studies,* 395: 507–15.

Schnelle, J.F., Simmonds, S.F. Harrington, C., Cadogan, M., Garcia, E. and Bates-Jenson, B.M. (2004) Relationship of nursing home staffing to quality of care. *Health Service Research,* 39(2): 225–50.

Schrijnemaekers, V., Vanrossum, E., Candel, M., Fredericks, C., Derix, M., Sielhorst, H. and van Denbrandt, P. (2002) Effects of emotion oriented care on elderly people with cognitive impairment and behavioural problems. *International Journal of Geriatric Psychiatry,* 17: 926–37.

Shook, E.J. and Beck, C.M. (1991) Impaired mind vs impaired body. *Geriatric Nursing,* 12: 185–7.

Spector, A., Orrell, M., Davies, S. and Woods, B. (2000) Reality orientation for dementia. *Cochrane Database for Systematic Reviews,* 3: CD001119.DOI:10.1002/14651858.CD001119.pub2.

Spector, A., Thorgrimsen, L., Woods, B. and Orrell, M. (2006) *Making a Difference: An Evidence Based Group Programme to Offer Cognitive Stimulation Therapy (CST) to people with dementia.* London: Hawker Publications.

Spilsbury, K. and Meyer, J. (2004) Use, misuse and non-use of health care assistants: understanding the work of health care assistants in a hospital setting. *Journal of Nursing Management,* 12: 411–18.

Sumaya-Smith, I. (1995) Caregiver/resident relationships: surrogate family bonds and surrogate grieving in a skilled nursing facility. *Journal of Advanced Nursing,* 21: 447–51.

Tappen, R.M., Williams, C.L., Barry, C. and Disesa, D. (2001) Conversation intervention with Alzheimer's patients: increasing the relevance of communication. *Clinical Gerontologist,* 24: 63–75.

Thomas, W. (1996) *Life Worth Living.* Acton, MA: Vanderwyk & Burnham.

Tilly, J. and Reed, P. (2004) *Evidence on Interventions to Improve Quality of Care for Residents with Dementia in Nursing and Assisted Living Facilities.* Washington, DC: American Alzheimer's Association.

Train, G., Nurock, S., Kitchen, G., Manela, M., Livingston, G. (2005) A qualitative study of the views of residents with dementia, their relatives and staff about work practice in long term care settings. *International Psychogeriatrics,* 17: 237–51.

Tuckett, A. (2004) Truth-telling in clinical practice and the arguments far and against: a review of the literature. *Nursing Ethics,* 11: 500–13.

Verkaik, R., van Weert, J. and Franke, A. (2006) The effects of psychosocial methods on depressed, aggressive and apathetic behaviours of people with dementia: a systematic review. *International Journal of Geriatric Psychiatry,* 20: 301–14.

Vink, A.C. and Birks, J.S. (2003) Music therapy for people with dementia. *The Cochrane Database Reviews.*

Welsh, S., Hassiotis, A., Mahoney, G. and Deahl, M. (2003) Big brother is watching you – the ethical implications of electronic surveillance measures in the elderly with dementia and in adults with learning difficulties. *Aging and Mental Health,* 7: 372–5.

Werezak, L.J. and Morgan, D.G. (2003) Creating therapeutic psychosocial environments in dementia care. a preliminary framework. *Journal of Gerontological Nursing,* 29: 18–25.

Wilkinson, N., Srikumar, S., Shaw, K. and Orrell, M. (1998) Drama and movement therapy in dementia: a pilot study. *Arts in Psychotherapy,* 25(3): 195–201.

Woods, B., Spector, A., Jones, C., Orrell, M. and Davies, S. (2005) Reminiscence therapy for dementia. *Cochrane Database of Systematic Reviews,* 2: CD001120.DOI:10.1002/14651858.CD001120.pub2.

Zgola, J.M. (1999) *Care that Works: A Relationship Approach to Persons with Dementia.* Baltimore, MD: Johns Hopkins University Press.

Zimmerman, S., Gruber-Baldini, A.L., Sloane, P.D., Eckert, J.K., Hebel, J.R. and Morgan, L.A. (2003) Assisted living and nursing homes: apples and oranges? *The Gerontologist,* 45: 107–17.

20

End of life care

Jane Wilcock, Katherine Froggatt and Claire Goodman

Learning objectives

By the end of this chapter you will:

- recognize that people living with dementia also die with dementia, even if this is not the primary cause of death

- understand the current policy and service context that shape the provision of end of life care for people with dementia

- identify the challenges associated with the provision of end of life care for people with dementia

- critically review the evidence base for the provision of supportive and palliative care for people with dementia and their families towards the end of life

---

Introduction

Facing and experiencing dying are inevitable for a person given a diagnosis of dementia, whatever the cause of death. People can live many years with dementia, eventually dying from the sequelae of dementia or from many other causes. The nature and timing of that death are difficult to predict. End of life care therefore needs to be considered as a broad approach over many years that addresses the needs of person with dementia, their families, and the health and social care staff who engage with them. All care workers who engage with people with dementia need to be aware of this final outcome, as at any point in the illness there may be requests for information about end of life issues or the need for support from people with dementia and their family members. If health and social care staff are not able to recognize when this issue is present, and/or are uncomfortable with the topic, this may lead to less than adequate care at the time, or later on, as the person's health deteriorates.

In this chapter we provide some working definitions on end of life care and describe what dying with dementia might refer to. This chapter will provide an account of the broader social and policy contexts that determine the current features of service provision for people with dementia towards the end of life. We describe ways in which the experience of people with dementia, and their family members, with respect to end of life issues is less than optimal. Drawing on a systematic review of the evidence regarding palliative care interventions and service provision at the end of life for people with dementia and their families, we illustrate some of the complexities of this provision. We consider, in more detail, evidence about two issues: prognostication for people with dementia and the management of pain. The amount and nature of the evidence available regarding the efficacy of care interventions for people with dementia towards the end of life are limited and further areas for research are identified.

Defining 'end of life' care

In this chapter we acknowledge that predominantly end of life care is provided as a person is dying, but we also recognize that interventions and support pertaining to the end of life may be required earlier, from the time of diagnosis onwards (Small *et al.* 2007). End of life care is a contested term and we use the term in this chapter to mean an approach to care over a long time period which encompasses both palliative care and terminal care. We recognize that different understandings for this term exist between health care and social care professionals within countries (Froggatt and Payne 2006), and between countries, which can lead to different emphases in care provision.

End of life care is a broader term that encompasses more than the terminal care phase. This term originates from North America and has been used particularly in the context of the care for older people:

> End of life care for seniors requires an active, compassionate approach that treats, comforts and supports older individuals who are living with, or dying from, progressive or chronic life-threatening conditions. Such care is sensitive to personal, cultural and spiritual values, beliefs and practices and encompasses support for families and friends up to and including the period of bereavement.

(Ross *et al.* 2000)

For the person with dementia this encompasses a period of time that could potentially begin at diagnosis, as future planning about care preferences may be engaged with then. The principles of treatment, comfort and support promoted by the palliative care movement are appropriate at any time when a person with dementia requires support and assistance with unmet needs.

End of life care, as we define it, encompasses palliative care. Palliative care focuses upon the support of people as they live and die with life-limiting illnesses. The origins of palliative care lie with the modern hospice movement. Since the 1960s, in the UK, a range of hospice and palliative care services have developed, including inpatient, day and home care services. The hospice movement initially addressed the needs of people with cancer, but recent expansion and diversification in the specialty have sought to address the needs of people dying with other conditions including dementia (Addington-Hall and Higginson 2001).

Palliative care is defined by the World Health Organization (WHO) as:

An approach that improves the quality of life of patients and their families facing the problems associated with life-threatening illness, through the prevention and relief of suffering by means of early identification and impeccable assessment and treatment of pain and other problems, physical, psychosocial and spiritual.

(Sepulveda *et al.* 2002: 91–6)

This WHO stance on palliative care adopts a public health perspective. There is a distinction between generalist and specialist palliative care (Australian Government Department of Health and Aging 2006). Generalist palliative care is provided by health and social care professionals to individuals in whatever care settings they are situated. This is the type of palliative care that all people living with dementia could expect to receive, as their needs change, from their usual care providers. For people with dementia, this may be mental health professionals, health and social care staff supporting them at home or in a long-term care setting. It will also include their general practitioner who provides the medical advice and treatments.

Specialist palliative care teams meanwhile can support these generalist staff to deliver this care. Professionals who specialize in palliative care provide specialist palliative care for people with unresolved symptoms, or complex psychosocial, end of life or bereavement issues. Specialist palliative care may be provided in dedicated settings such as hospices, but also in hospitals, people's homes and long-term care facilities. The engagement between these specialist palliative care practitioners and the usual providers of care to people with dementia is increasingly on a partnership model, as the expertise of both parties is required to ensure that the specific needs of a person with dementia with respect to their condition and their dying are appropriately addressed.

Terminal care is another term used with regard to care provision for people who are dying, usually associated with the last few days and hours of life, and based upon the knowledge that the individual is dying. In this chapter we do not focus upon this time period imminently before the physical death of a person, but do identify some tools and interventions that have been developed to meet the needs of people specifically at this time.

Living and dying with dementia

End of life care needs to be considered for people with dementia because a diagnosis of dementia for a person will lead to their dying with dementia, regardless of the primary cause of death. The median length of survival from diagnosis to death is eight years (Hofman *et al.* 1991). While dementia has been identified as one of the leading causes of death (Foley and Carver 2001), it is difficult to ascertain exact figures for the numbers of deaths from dementia, as it is under-reported on death certificates (Morgan and Clarke 1995). Estimates from the UK suggest that approximately 100,000 people with dementia die each year (Bayer 2006). In 2005, dementia was the fourth leading cause of death among females and the ninth leading cause of death among males in the UK (Office for National Statistics 2006).

Cox and Cook (2002) identify three ways in which people with dementia can die. First, there are people who have a diagnosis of dementia, but their death is caused by another medical condition, for example, cancer or heart disease. Second, people may die from the interplay of another illness and dementia, where the dementia has not impacted greatly on their functioning. Third, there are people who are described as having end-stage dementia, where the associated consequences of the dementia impact upon all domains of their life and they ultimately die of the complications of this condition. Each of these different ways will directly influence the place and experience of death for an individual and their family members.

As the illness progresses for people with dementia, so the increased need for physical care and greater accommodation of behavioural changes may necessitate a change in the place of residence and care. Some people with severe dementia may need to move into long-term care facilities such as nursing homes or residential care homes (Matthews and Dening 2002). In the UK, over half of all people with dementia live in care homes (MacDonald and Cooper 2007). In 1996, 42–48% of residents in a range of care home settings demonstrated mild cognitive impairment, and a further 19–44% of residents demonstrated severe impairment (Darton *et al.* 2003). Care homes rely on primary care services for medical support and specialist nursing care; however, older people in care homes have variable and often inequitable access to state health services such as allied health support such as physiotherapy and occupational therapy (Jacobs *et al.* 2001). There are also regional variations with regard to hospice and palliative care services for this population, often reflecting differences in local policies and funding. The need for a more strategic proactive approach when providing end of life care in these settings has been highlighted (Froggatt *et al.* 2002; Goodman *et al.* 2003a, 2003b).

Some individuals even as they become frailer and more cognitively impaired may be able to remain in their own homes, but are increasingly reliant on the availability of formal and informal sources of community support. The provision of palliative care for older people with dementia in primary care is provided by a range of nursing services working in collaboration with general practitioners and consultants in palliative medicine (Goodman *et al.* 1998).

The policy context of palliative care and dementia

In recent years across many Western countries there has been a significant increase in the policy and guidance produced that directly influences the organization of end of life care for people with non-malignant disease and by implication dementia. This has occurred in recognition of the increasing numbers of people with dementia in the population, the range of settings where they receive care, the lack of knowledge of practitioners, and the experiential and research evidence that people with dementia have inequitable access to care and inappropriate treatments (Lloyd-Williams and Payne 2002).

Initiatives that have been developed to specifically seek to meet the end of life needs of people with dementia originated in the United States in the 1980s onwards, primarily from the world of dementia services (Volicer 1986). Only recently in the UK has mainstream palliative care begun to address these issues (National Council for Palliative Care 2006), with similar interests developing in old age psychiatry (Hughes *et al.* 2005; Robinson *et al.* 2005). These initiatives have to date been small scale and have often focused on the advanced stages of the condition (Small *et al.* 2007).

Guidance from the National Institute for Health and Clinical Excellence in collaboration with the Social Care Institute for Excellence (NICE-SCIE 2007), in the UK, has identified the key principles for palliative care and dementia. Although wide-ranging and non-controversial, these guidelines set out important benchmarks for care planning and implementation. They emphasize that end of life care in dementia concerns the time from diagnosis to death; that people with dementia should live and die with dignity in the place of their choice; and that the emphasis at the end of life should be on quality of life and carers should be supported.

The consequences of this guidance for service providers are potentially far-reaching. These guidelines presuppose there will be an understanding of when someone is dying, that mechanisms are in place to make sure the person receives symptom relief, continuity of care is provided and the avoidance of unplanned acute admission or unwanted transfer to another unfamiliar setting is observed. For health and social care professionals working with people with dementia, this requires them to be aware and addressing end of life issues, such as decision-making, in advance of the time when it is more difficult for the person with dementia to make their preferences clearly understood.

In the UK, the Department of Health's End of Life Care programme (http://www.endoflifecare.nhs.uk/eolc) has provided both guidance and resources to help commissioners and practitioners reduce the known unpredictability and shortcomings of service provision. This includes the needs of people dying from non-malignant disease whose trajectory to death is characterized by progressive and incremental frailty and dependency, as for many people with dementia. For example, there is the development of modified mainstream palliative care frameworks that provide quality standards and checklists which aim to identify those people with chronic diseases most likely to benefit from end of life care. The intention is that, through planning and coordination between different providers it is possible to make explicit the priorities of care and how multidisciplinary teams can work together. The most common initiatives in use are the primary care-based Gold Standards Framework (also adapted for use with care homes), the Liverpool Care Pathway and the Preferred Priorities of Care (Table 20.1). This includes guidance on prognostic indicators for people with dementia (Table 20.2), which, while not prescriptive, encourages practitioners to review treatment decision-making. Further service-based initiatives include the establishment of end of life care networks, investment in rapid response teams, hospice-at-home services, and expanding training programmes.

Table 20.1   Aims of the Gold Standards Framework, Liverpool Care Pathway and Preferred Priorities of Care tools

Gold Standards Framework (GSF)

Aims to improve community-based care for those with chronic and terminal diseases with an emphasis on continuity, communication and coordination of care (www.goldstandardsframework.co.uk)

Liverpool Care Pathway (LCP)

Focuses on the end stage of a patient's life (last 48–72 hours), strives to provide a pain-free death, and tries to address the psychological and spiritual needs of patient and family at this time (www.lcp-mariecurie.org.uk)

Preferred Priorities of Care (PPC)

Helps to initiate and develop the sensitive conversation around preferred place of care and death between patient, carer and health care professionals to achieve a greater likelihood of fulfilling the patient's wishes (www.cancerlancashire.org.uk/ppc).

Adapted from http://www.endoflifecare.nhs.uk/

Table 20.2   Dementia Prognostic Indicator Guidance, Gold Standard Framework (Department of Health 2005)

- Unable to walk without assistance
- Urinary and faecal incontinence
- No consistently meaningful communication
- Unable to dress without assistance
- Barthel score < 3
- Reduced ability to perform activities of daily living
- Plus any of the following: 10% weight loss in previous six months without other causes, pyelonephritis of UTI, serum albumin 25g/l

In other countries we see similar national programmes that have implications for the care for people with dementia towards the end of life. In Australia, a set of national evidence-based guidelines has been developed to support the provision of a palliative approach in residential aged care facilities (equivalent to care homes and nursing homes) (Australian Government Department of Health and Aging 2006). Although addressing the needs of all residents who live in such institutions, there is also specific attention paid to the needs of people with advanced dementia (Table 20.3).

Table 20.3 Guidelines for a palliative approach in residential aged care (Australian Government Department of Health and Aging 2006)

The development of a palliative approach in residential aged care facilities (long-term care facilities for older people) has been supported in Australia by the development and dissemination of evidence-based guidelines. These guidelines address the following issues:

- A palliative approach
- Dignity and quality of life
- Advance care planning
- Advanced dementia
- Physical symptom assessment and management
- Psychological support
- Family support
- Social support, intimacy and sexuality
- Aboriginal and Torres Strait Islander issues
- Cultural issues
- Spiritual support
- Volunteer support
- End of life (terminal) care
- Bereavement support
- Management's role in implementing a palliative approach.

Exercise 20.1 Determining people's need for end of life care

You have been asked to serve on a regional group of care providers to develop guidelines for end of life dementia care. The following questions have been put to your committee. What would your initial responses be?

At what point in time should end of life services be available to people with dementia and their carers?

Are services needed by people across settings or only to people at home?

What sort of assessment should be recommended for people to determine their end of life care needs?

Should separate guidelines be created for people in different settings? If so, what are the major differences between the needs of people in aged care settings and those at home or in hospital?

Would you recommend any training in end of life care for professional or family carers?

Discuss why you answered the way you did and how your recommendations might differ from what is currently done or currently available.

Challenges in the provision of end of life care

A number of challenges in the provision of end of life care for people with dementia have been identified. These include communication issues, the failure to recognize dementia as a terminal illness, and clinical challenges of care delivery (Robinson *et al.* 2005). The recognition that the nature and timing of death are difficult to predict for any individual can lead to problems of knowing when to commence or desist in the delivery of specific treatments and interventions. How people with dementia are helped to retain autonomy and exercise choices about their care, treatments and place of death, as emphasized within the UK choice agenda present in current palliative care programmes, is also challenged by communication issues for people with dementia and raises questions about the basis on which such agendas are premised (Small *et al.* 2007).

Just as challenges arise due to the particular needs of people living and dying with dementia, there are also challenges that arise from the ways services have been developed. The UK initiatives described above are grounded in practice but they nevertheless draw on cancer models of care and have a limited evidence base about the needs of people with dementia. There is also a concern that these frameworks may lead to an increasing 'routinization' of care and an increase of the professional surveillance of people at the end of life (Clark 2004). Many of these initiatives also require different practitioners to have facilitator and key worker/champion roles that may in the long term be difficult to sustain. In care homes for many older people with dementia, dying is the expected final outcome, but not the reason for receiving care and support. There is a possible tension between setting up systems that improve access to palliative care and ensuring that different views and needs can be accommodated. Any structured tool therefore needs to be sufficiently flexible to account for the complex interplay between the physical symptoms of dying (which may or may not be caused by having dementia), the longer time periods that people with dementia at the end of their life require help and care for, and the involvement of family members and family carers.

Quality of end of life care for people with dementia and their carers

Another challenge that faces care providers in looking after people with dementia and their families concerns the nature of the evidence that they can draw upon to inform their practice. For over ten years research evidence and policy-makers have highlighted that there are many issues in the care of patients with dementia that parallel palliative cancer care. There is evidence that dementia is under-detected and sub-optimally managed in primary care (Bamford *et al.* 2004; Iliffe *et al.* 1990) and such difficulties in making and conveying a diagnosis to the person and their family mean that effective discussion and planning for future treatment and care cannot take place (Bamford *et al.* 2004; Downs *et al.* 2002; Iliffe *et al.* 1999).

Still relatively few patients with dementia currently access palliative care (Davies and Higginson 2004; House of Commons Select Committee 2004; McCarthy *et al.* 1997; Volicer *et al.* 1994). Research reviews that compare different approaches to palliative care for older people and include patients with dementia suggest that the amount of robust, high quality research on palliative care interventions for this patient group is small (Ahmed *et al.* 2004; Oliver *et al.* 2004; Salisbury *et al.* 1999; Sampson *et al.* 2005). For example, in a systematic review of palliative care interventions for people with dementia dying in a hospital, only two interventions (US based) were identified (Sampson *et al.* 2005).

The majority of research on palliative care with people who have dementia has been undertaken in specialist units and hospice settings (Hughes *et al.* 2005). Less is known about providing palliative care for this population when they are being supported at home or in care home settings or whether the findings from specialist settings are transferable for implementation in primary care. The following summary and discussion of some of the available evidence focus on what can be learnt from studies about supporting older people with dementia and their carers at home, in non-specialist and non-acute care environments.

A recent review of palliative care for community-dwelling older people with dementia, which did not just focus on intervention-based studies, found over 7,500 articles and papers (Goodman *et al.* 2007). While not all of these were research based, this volume of evidence emphasizes the degree to which clinicians and researchers are engaged in and challenged by end of life issues for dementia, and reflects the increasing level of interest and debate. In this review it was clear that the identification of good quality outcome indicators for this population is problematic. The most robust measures available were in the areas of symptoms and symptom control, quality of life and satisfaction. Significant gaps existed in the evidence base on continuity of care, advance care planning, spiritual needs, and caregiver well-being. We reviewed 84 intervention studies in which 135 patient-centred outcomes were assessed by 97 separate measures. Of these, 80 were used only once and only eight measures were used in more than two studies. In general, most measures have not undergone rigorous development and testing. Development of quality indicators in end of life care should focus on areas with identified gaps, and testing should be done to facilitate comparability across the care settings, populations, and clinical conditions. Intervention research should use robust measures that adhere to these standards.

Against this backdrop of a limited body of evidence, the complexity and challenges of meeting the needs of people with dementia towards the end of life can be further explicated by considering two key issues: first, prognostication and the importance placed upon predicting the approach of death for people with dementia; and second, meeting the pain needs of people with dementia. Both these areas illustrate the limited evidence that is currently available.

Exercise 20.2 Finding out more

You have been asked to head the team that will determine the direction of a large international research effort. Your first step is to decide the most important areas of research for end of life care for people with dementia.

Identify the three areas that you believe are most pressing and why you think this is so.

How do you think the research you have chosen will affect the lives of people with dementia? The lives of their family carers?

Predicting the approach of death for people with dementia

As already indicated, people with dementia are not a homogeneous group and have different patterns of dying. However, the ability to recognize the dying process has implications for when and how palliative care services are provided. For patients with dementia the uncertainty associated with knowing when a person stops living with dementia and starts dying from it and difficulty in predicting survival time pose problems for care settings such as hospices who provide time-limited support (Hanrahan and Luchins 1995). It is striking that much of the work in this aspect of end of life care has been done in North American environments where knowing when someone may die directly influences financial decision-making about access to specialist end of life care. In North America prognostic indicators are available for determining hospice admission six months pre-death (National Hospice Organization Medical Guidelines Task Force 1995). One study examined the factors associated with six-month mortality in nursing home residents where a risk score based on a series of 12 variables was shown to estimate six-month mortality for nursing home residents with advanced dementia with greater accuracy than existing prognostic guidelines. The final model included the variables: Activities of Daily Living score of 28, male sex, cancer, the need for oxygen therapy, congestive heart failure, shortness of breath, no more than 25% of food eaten at most meals, an unstable condition, bowel incontinence, bedfast, older than 83 years, and not awake most of the day (Mitchell *et al.* 2004a).

Prognostic indicators were also examined in a two-year longitudinal cohort study undertaken to determine survival time among dementia patients who met the criteria for Medicare hospice benefit while testing the National Hospice Organization (NHO) guidelines. The investigators found that patients who met the hospice enrolment criteria predicted a median survival time of 4 months and a mean survival time of 6.9 months; 38% of these patients survived for more than 6 months. FAST (Functional Assessment Staging) scores (Reisberg 1988), on which the NHO criteria rely, and mobility ratings, were significantly related to survival time. However, 41% could not be scored on the FAST as their disease progression was not ordinal and when the palliative care plans were examined, less aggressive care plans resulted in shorter survival times, $p < 0.01$. Although the FAST score can identify a subgroup of appropriate candidates for hospice admission, sole reliance on this measure was cautioned as it may decrease access to hospice care for many dementia patients (Hanrahan *et al.* 1999; Luchins *et al.* 1997). This work underlines how in addition to decision-making about the allocation of limited resources a reliance on scoring systems to decide types of care should be used with caution. This second study illustrates this point well.

Further research, undertaken in the USA, to assess the validity of the Medicare hospice eligibility guidelines for dementia patients, revealed no significant relationship between the Medicare guidelines, or any component of the guidelines, and survival. The results indicated that the Medicare guidelines were not valid predictors of survival in hospice patients with dementia. Advanced age, impaired nutritional and functional status were associated with shortened survival (Schonwetter *et al.* 2003). Care therefore needs to be taken in using such guidelines for people with dementia, as they are not dementia specific. A more helpful set of findings arose from a prospective study that set out to develop a statistical model for predicting short-term survival in patients with Alzheimer's. The main outcome measure was six-month survival following a fever episode. Older age and higher severity of Alzheimer's at the time of the fever episode, palliative care, and hospital admission for long-term care within six months prior to the fever were found to be positively associated with likelihood of mortality within six months of the fever onset (Volicer *et al.* 1993).

Research on prognostication demonstrates that checklists of clinical indicators may provide useful guidelines for clinicians and help to inform decision-making, shared-care planning and joint provision, but their accuracy in terms of predicting death is not high.

Exercise 20.3 Recognizing dying and providing end of life care

Consider the people with dementia you know, or work with, who have died.

At what point did you know they were dying? How did you know they were dying – what cues were relevant for you to make this judgement?

What changes when you know someone is dying, in terms of the care you provide? Would any of these aspects of care have been relevant earlier in the illness and if so, what do we need to change to make this possible? For example, are there health professionals with other types of expertise that could be involved in the care situation earlier on in the illness?

Pain assessment and management

The dementia illness trajectory is one of progressive deterioration with acute episodes of care and patients at the end of their life frequently requiring 24-hour care either in long-stay hospital wards or in nursing homes (Davies and Higginson 2004; Lloyd-Williams and Payne 2002; Lyn and Adamson 2003). Studies have shown that patients with dementia are often subject to painful and unnecessary investigations and treatments during the terminal phase of their illness, are likely to experience symptoms (including pain) that persist for longer and are more likely to be untreated in the last six months of life compared to those with cancer (Evers *et al.* 2002; McCarthy *et al.* 1997; Morrison and Siu 2000).

The prevalence of pain in elderly nursing home residents is estimated to be 40–80% (Blomqvist and Hallberg 2001; Ferrell *et al.* 1995; Marzinski 1991; Proctor and Hirdes 2001; Zwakhalen *et al.* 2006). Pain assessment in people with dementia can be complicated by memory loss, personality changes, and loss of judgement, abstract thinking and communication skills. Additionally, behaviours commonly associated with pain may be absent or difficult to interpret (Herr 2002; Regnard *et al.* 2003). Conversely, aggressive behaviours may be a response by people with dementia who are not able to articulate their pain verbally (Feldt *et al.* 1998). There is evidence that pain assessment is inadequate and that people with dementia are being under-treated (Ferrell *et al.* 1995; Horgas and Tsai 1998; Hurley *et al.* 1996; Kovach *et al.* 2001; Loeb 1999; Proctor and Hirdes 2001; Scherder *et al.* 2005; Sentagen and King 1993).

Hirakawa *et al.* (2006) in a study of people with dementia at home compared symptom experience and end of life care received by home patients based on cognitive function. After controlling for age and other differences in baseline characteristics, dementia was determined to be a significant independent predictor of incontinence or uncontrolled pain. After controlling for age, other differences in baseline characteristics and symptom experience, dementia was determined not to be a significant independent predictor of use of antibiotics or opioids. People with dementia may be unable to inform nurses and professionals about levels of pain, dehydration or discomfort and these should be monitored as a matter of course.

Studies have also pointed to what appears to be a lack of adequate professional training for pain management. In a survey of 68 UK nursing homes, 69% per cent of nursing homes did not have a written policy regarding pain management and 75% did not use a standardized pain assessment tool. Forty per cent of qualified staff and 85% of care assistants had no specialist knowledge regarding the management of pain in older people (Allcock *et al.* 2002).

The optimal pain assessment would be self-reported but this is not always possible with people with dementia and proxy accounts from carers are often used. Recent research into pain assessment among elderly people with severe dementia has focused on understanding non-verbal expressions (Ferrell *et al.* 1995; Herr 2002; Parke 1998). Zwakhalen *et al.* (2006) undertook a systematic review to ascertain which behavioural pain assessment tools are available to assess pain in elderly people with dementia and what the psychometric qualities of these tools were. Twenty-nine publications reporting on behavioural pain assessment instruments were selected. Twelve observational pain assessment scales were identified (DOLOPLUS2; ECPA; ECS; Observational Pain Behavior Tool; CNPI; PACSLAC; PAINAD; PADE; RaPID; Abbey Pain Scale; NOPPAIN; Pain assessment scale for use with cognitively impaired adults). The review found that most observational scales are still under development. Based on psychometric qualities, and criteria sensitivity and clinical usefulness criteria, the authors concluded that PACSLAC and DOLOPLUS2 were the most appropriate scales currently available. Further research needs to improve these scales by further testing their validity, reliability and clinical utility. Although such assessment tools exist for people with dementia, people are still suffering unnecessarily (Aminoff and Adunsky 2004) and clear treatment guidelines and training in pain management are required.

Exercise 20.4   Pain in people with dementia at end of life

You have just taken the post of staff educator in a care home for older people. Like many other homes, about 65% of your residents have dementia. You are determined that residents' pain will be adequately assessed and that residents in your care home will have their pain effectively managed.

What are three things you will do to improve the pain management of residents?

Say why you chose those particular areas to focus on and how you will know if you have been successful.

Debates and controversies

In considering the provision of excellent end of life care for people with dementia and their family carers a number of issues can be debated.

We have promoted a view of end of life care that encompasses the whole time a person with dementia lives with this condition. Is it inappropriate to be raising issues of mortality and dying when a person is only just coming to terms with a diagnosis of dementia? However, not raising and addressing the implications of living and dying with a life-limiting illness can ultimately result in the person with dementia and their family carers receiving a poorer quality of care when dying, that is less likely to reflect that person's values and wishes. How clinicians and care staff manage the timing and way in which these discussions are undertaken, is still being discussed.

We have identified that in some approaches to palliative and hospice care for people with dementia a great emphasis is placed upon prognostication and knowing when a person is dying. This can lead to an over-reliance on this type of knowledge to initiate or withdraw particular types of treatment and intervention. The challenge for care professionals is to consider why knowing someone is dying changes what care is provided. Could some of these treatment and care decisions have been made without the prognostication process?

A large number of outcome measures are used in research studies and are not used consistently across these studies, so comparisons are difficult and the relevance for care providers is not clear. Their appropriateness for this population needs further examination.

The evidence for effective care interventions is not yet strong for people with dementia towards the end of life. Reliance solely on evidence about individual people's experiences, while important, may avoid addressing wider system issues of care provision, policy and funding. Evidence for culture change of care environments and wider health and social care systems is also required, but how can a case be made for the funding and resourcing of this type of work?

Future directions

We know less about the extent to which families provide end of life care at home as it is not reported in the academic literature. It is not known what kind of interventions and support are needed for people caring for people with dementia at home who are at the end of their life. Few studies address carers' needs and assess carers' input, issues of the environment, the possibilities and experiences with home care and overall decision-making processes.

The methodological challenges of researching end of life support mean that evaluations usually rely upon post-bereavement views of relatives and secondary analysis of patient notes. Prognostication and the management of specific symptoms appear to be given greater weight than a focus on a holistic process and care planning for a good ending. An emphasis on survival analysis and prognostication has also meant that little is known about how individuals themselves engage with the anticipation of dying.

Although there are significant ethical and methodological challenges of undertaking research with people with dementia, the scope and range of evidence that is able to directly influence practice are disappointing. There are a lack of intervention-based studies, lack of consistency across studies as to definitions of end of life care, and very few examples of evidence from people with dementia themselves with an over-reliance on proxy or retrospective accounts and data. End of life care for someone with dementia is as likely to involve decision-making about not doing things, for example, aggressively treating certain conditions, as acting upon specific symptoms. Although this is extensively discussed in practice and professional literature, there is minimal research that makes explicit how this is addressed and the consequences for patients and carers. This ambiguity may lead to unclear pathways for care and sub-optimal distribution of resources. The consequences of a lack of evidence may contribute to a poor quality of life for people with dementia and their carers, inappropriate and costly responses to the problems that emerge at the end of life which can then result in hospital admissions, and further disablement. In order to ensure that the needs and expectations of people with dementia and their families are met, and that good quality end of life care is provided, there is a need for further research and staff training across and between dementia and specialist palliative care.

Conclusion

As illustrated by a consideration of the evidence concerning the pain needs of people with dementia, current evidence levels fall short of describing, assessing and meeting the experiences and expectations of people with dementia and their family carers. The evidence shows that older people in care homes have variable and often inequitable access to health services (Jacobs *et al.* 2001) and the need for a more strategic proactive approach when providing palliative care in these settings has been highlighted by the findings from studies on the type and frequency of current palliative care provision (Froggatt *et al.* 2002; Goodman *et al.* 2003a, 2003b). Evidence from carers and professionals has highlighted that barriers exist to the provision of good quality support for people with dementia who are coming to the end of their lives (Diwan *et al.* 2004; Mitchell *et al.* 2004b). Good information and support for coping with behavioural and functional problems, provision of emotional support, improved communication with and between professionals and facilitating social support networks are needed.

Further information

The National Council for Palliative Care initiated a dementia project in 2007. Their reports on dementia can be found on their website. This organization also sponsors workshops on palliative care and has speakers' presentations available to view.

The Hospice Foundation of America provides general support and information regarding hospice care for people of all ages. However, they have published a report that is exclusively about hospice care for someone with dementia. This report can be found on their website.

The Dying Well organization provides general advice on living to the fullest until the end of life. It is operated by Dr Byock, MD, and includes a collection of his articles. Dr Byock has been involved in hospice care since 1978. He is known for founding a hospice for indigent people in Fresno, California. He has received many awards for his work in hospice care.

End of Life Care Programme is an organization devoted to maximizing the choices people have at the end of life. While it does not specifically address issues for people with dementia, it has recently published a report on improving end of life care in care homes.

The Palliative Care and Long-term Care Settings for Older People Worldwide Resources website is an international organization that provides resources and information on end of life care. An outcome of the European Association of Palliative Care conference in Budapest in June 2007, this web-based resource was designed for care providers, educators and researchers interested in palliative care in long-term care settings. The purpose of the website is to support the establishment of contacts and information exchange worldwide.

Acknowledgements

The literature review was supported by a project grant from NoCLoR, the North Central London Research Consortium. We would like to thank the rest of the review team: Dr Steve Iliffe, UCL; Ms Maggie Bissett, Camden PCT; Professor Vari Drennan, St George's Medical School/Kingston University; Dr Martin Blanchard, UCL; and Dr Elizabeth Sampson, UCL.

References

Addington-Hall, J.A. and Higginson, I. (2001) *Palliative Care for Non-Cancer Patients*. Oxford: Oxford University Press.

Ahmed, N., Bestall, J.C., Ahmedzai, S. H., Payne, S.A., Clark, D. and Noble, B. (2004) Systematic review of the problems and issues of accessing specialist palliative care by patients, carers and health and social care professionals. *Palliative Medicine*, 18(6): 525–42.

Allcock, N., McGarry, J. and Elkan, R. (2002) Management of pain in older people within the nursing home: a preliminary study. *Health and Social Care in the Community*, 10(6): 464–71.

Aminoff, B.Z. and Adunsky, A. (2004) Dying dementia patients: too much suffering, too little palliation. *American Journal of Alzheimer's Disease and Other Dementias*, 19(4): 243–7.

Australian Government Department of Health and Aging (2006) *Guidelines for a Palliative Approach in Residential Aged Care.* Canberra: Rural Health and Palliative Care Branch, Australian Government Department of Health and Aging.

Bamford, C., Lamont, S., Eccles, M., Robinson, L., May, C. and Bond, J. (2004) Disclosing a diagnosis of dementia: a systematic review. *International Journal of Geriatric Psychiatry,* 19: 151–69.

Bayer, A. (2006) Death with dementia – the need for better care. *Age and Ageing,* 35(1): 1–12.

Blomqvist, K. and Hallberg, I.R. (2001) Recognizing pain in older adults living in sheltered accommodation: the views of nurses and older adults. *International Journal of Nursing Studies,* 38: 305–18.

Clark, D. (2004) History, gender and culture. In: S. Payne, J. Seymour and C. Ingleton (eds) *Palliative Care Nursing: Principles and Evidence for Practice.* Buckingham: Open University Press.

Cox, S. and Cook, A. (2002) Caring for people with dementia at the end of life. In: J. Hockley and D. Clark (eds) *Palliative Care for Older People in Care Homes.* Buckingham: Open University Press: 86–103.

Darton, R., Netten, A. and Forder, J. (2003) The cost implications of the changing population and characteristics of care homes. *International Journal of Geriatric Psychiatry,* 18: 236–43.

Davies, E. and Higginson, I. (2004) *Better Palliative Care for Older People.* Copenhagen: World Health Organization.

Diwan, S., Hougham, G. and Sachs, G. (2004) Strain experienced by caregivers of dementia patients receiving palliative care: Findings from the Palliative Excellence in Alzheimer Care Efforts (PEACE) Program. *Journal of Palliative Medicine,* 7(6): 797–807.

Downs, M., Clibbens, R., Rae, C., Cook, A. and Woods, R. (2002) What do general practitioners tell people with dementia and their families about the condition? A survey of experiences in Scotland. *Dementia,* 1: 47–58.

Evers, M.M., Purohit D., Perl D., Khan K. and Marin, D.B. (2002) Palliative and aggressive end of life care for patients with dementia. *Psychiatric Services,* 53: 609–13.

Feldt, K.S., Ryden, M.B. and Miles, S. (1998) Treatment of pain in cognitively. impaired compared with cognitively intact older patients with hip-fracture. *Journal of the American Geriatrics Society,* 46: 1079–85.

Ferrell, B.A., Ferrell, B.R. and Rivera, L. (1995) Pain in cognitively impaired nursing home patients. *Journal of Pain and Symptom Management,* 10: 591–8.

Foley, K.M. and Carver, A.C. (2001) Palliative care in neurology: an overview. *Neurology Clinics,* 19: 789–99.

Froggatt, K. and Payne, S. (2006) A survey of end-of-life care in care homes: Issues of definition and practice. *Health and Social Care in the Community*, 14(4): 341–8.

Froggatt, K.A., Poole, K. and Hoult, L. (2002) The provision of palliative care in nursing homes and residential care homes: A survey of clinical nurse specialist work. *Palliative Medicine*, 16: 481–7.

Goodman, C., Knight, D., Machen, I. and Hunt, B. (1998) Emphasising terminal care as district nursing work: a helpful strategy in a purchasing environment? *Journal of Advanced Nursing*, 28(3): 491–8.

Goodman, C., Wilcock, J., Froggatt, K., Blanchard, M., Sampson, E., Drennan, V., Iliffe, S. and Bisset, M. (2007) *Review of the Literature on Palliative Care Interventions for Community Dwelling Older People with Dementia*. CRI-PACC: University of Hertfordshire.

Goodman, C., Woolley, R. and Knight, D. (2003a) District nurses' experiences of providing care in residential homes: issues of context and demand. *Journal of Clinical Nursing*, 12(1): 67–76.

Goodman, C., Woolley, R. and Knight, D. (2003b) The district nursing contribution to palliative care for older people in care homes. *International Journal of Palliative Nursing*, 9(12): 521–7.

Hanrahan, P. and Luchins, D.J. (1995) Access to hospice programs in end-stage dementia: a national survey of hospice programs. *Journal of the American Geriatrics Society*, 43(1): 56–9.

Hanrahan, P., Raymond, M., McGowan, E. and Luchins, D.J. (1999) Criteria for enrolling dementia patients in hospice: a replication. *American Journal of Hospital Palliative Care*, 16(1): 395–400.

Herr, K.A. (2002) Pain assessment in cognitively impaired older adults. *American Journal of Nursing*, 102: 65–7.

Hirakawa, Y., Masuda, Y., Kuzuya, M., Kimata, T., Iguchi, A. and Uemura, K. (2006) End-of-life experience of demented elderly patients at home: findings from DEATH project. *Psychogeriatrics*, 6(2): 60–7.

Hofman, A., Rocca, W., Brayne, C., Breteler, M., Clarke, M., Cooper, B., Copeland, J., Dartigues, J., da Silva Droux, A. and Hagnell, O. (1991) The prevalence of dementia in Europe: a collaborative study of 1980–1990 findings. Eurodem Prevalence Research Group. *International Journal of Epidemiology*, 20: 736–48.

Horgas, A.L. and Tsai, P.F. (1998) Analgesic drug prescription and use in cognitively impaired nursing home residents. *Nursing Research*, 47: 235–42.

House of Commons Health Select Committee (2004) *Palliative Care. Fourth Report of Session 2003–04*. London: House of Commons.

Hughes, J., Robinson, L. and Volicer, L. (2005) Specialist palliative care in dementia. *British Medical Journal*, 330: 57–8.

Hurley, A.C., Volicer, B.J. and Volicer, L. (1996) Effect of fever-management strategy on the progression of dementia of the Alzheimer type. *Alzheimer's Disease and Associated Disorders*, 10(1): 5–10.

Iliffe, S., Booroff, A., Gallivan, S., Goldenberg, E., Morgan, P. and Haines, A. (1990) Screening for cognitive impairment in the elderly using the mini-mental state examination. *British Journal of General Practice*, 40(336): 277–9.

Iliffe, S., Eden, A., Downs, M. and Rae, C. (1999) The diagnosis and management of dementia in primary care: development, implementation and evaluation of a national training programme. *Aging and Mental Health,* 3: 129–35.

Jacobs, S., Alborz, A., Glendinning, C. and Hann, M. (2001) *Health Services for Homes: A Survey of Access to NHS Services in Nursing and Residential Homes for Older People in England and Wales*. Manchester: NPCRDC, University of Manchester.

Kovach, C.R., Noonan, P.E., Griffie, J., Muchka, S. and Weissman, D.E. (2001) Use of the assessment of discomfort in dementia protocol. *Applied Nursing Research*, 14(4): 193–200.

Lloyd-Williams, M. and Payne, S. (2002) Can multidisciplinary guidelines improve the palliation of symptoms in the terminal phase of dementia? *International Journal of Palliative Nursing*, 8(8): 370–5.

Loeb, J.L. (1999) Pain management in long-term care. *American Journal of Nursing*, 99: 48–52.

Luchins, D., Hanrahan, P. and Murphy, K. (1997) Criteria for enrolling dementia patients in hospices. *Journal of American Geriatrics Society*, 45: 1054–9.

Lyn, J. and Adamson, D.M. (2003) *Living Well at the End of Life: Adapting Health Care to Serious Chronic Illness in Old Age*. Arlington, VA: Rand Health.

MacDonald, A. and Cooper, B. (2007) Long-term care and dementia services: an impending crisis. *Age and Ageing*, 36: 16–22.

Marzinski, L.R. (1991) The tragedy of dementia: clinically assessing pain in the confused non-verbal elderly. *Journal of Gerontological Nursing,* 17: 25–8.

Matthews, F.E. and Dening, T. (2002) Prevalence of dementia in institutional care. UK Medical Research Council Cognitive Function and Ageing Study. *Lancet,* 20: 360(9328): 225–6.

McCarthy, M., Addington-Hall, J. and Altmann, D. (1997) The experience of dying with dementia: a retrospective study. *International Journal of Geriatric Psychiatry,* 12: 404–9.

Mitchell, S.L., Kiely, D.K., Hamel, M.B., Park, P.S., Morris, J.N. and Fries, B.E. (2004a) Estimating prognosis for nursing home residents with advanced dementia. *Journal of the American Medical Association*, 291(22): 2734.

Mitchell, S.L., Morris, J.N., Park, P.S. and Fries, B.E. (2004b) Terminal care for persons with advanced dementia in the nursing home and home care settings. *Journal of Palliative Medicine,* 7(6): 808–16.

Morgan, K. and Clarke, D. (1995) To what extent is dementia underreported on British death certificates? *International Journal of Geriatric Psychiatry,* 10: 987–90.

Morrison, R.S. and Siu, A.L. (2000) A comparison of pain and its treatment in advanced dementia and cognitively intact patients with hip fracture. *Journal of Pain and Symptom Management,* 19(4): 240–8.

National Council for Palliative Care (2006) *Exploring Palliative Care for People with Dementia: A Discussion Document.* London: National Council for Palliative Care.

National Hospice Organization Medical Guidelines Task Force (1995) *Medical Guidelines for Determining Prognosis in Selected Non-cancer Diseases.* Arlington, VA: National Hospice Organization.

National Institute for Clinical Excellence (NICE) (2004) *Guidance on Cancer Services. Improving Supportive and Palliative Care for People with Cancer.* London: NICE.

National Institute for Health and Clinical Excellence/Social Care Institute for Excellence (NICE-SCIE) (2007) *A NICE-SCIE Guideline on Supporting People with Dementia and their Carers in Health and Social Care.* National Clinical Guideline No. 42. London: British Psychological Society and Gaskell.

Office for National Statistics (2006) *Health Statistics Quarterly 30,* Spring (2006) London: Palgrave Macmillan.

Oliver, D.P., Porock, D. and Zweig, S. (2004) End of life care in US nursing homes: a review of the evidence. *Journal of the American Directors Association,* 5(3): 147–55.

Parke, B. (1998) Gerontological nurses' ways of knowing: realizing the presence of pain in cognitively impaired older adults. *Journal of Gerontological Nursing,* 24: 21–8.

Proctor, W.R. and Hirdes, J.P. (2001) Pain and cognitive status among nursing home residents in Canada. *Pain Research and Management, The Journal of the Canadian Pain Society,* 6: 119–25.

Regnard, C., Mathews, D., Gibson, L., Clark, C. and Watson, B. (2003) Assessing distress in people with severe communication problems: Piloting the Northgate DisDAT. *International Journal of Palliative Nursing,* 9: 173–6.

Reisberg, B. (1988) Functional Assessment Staging (FAST). *Psychopharm Bulletin,* 24: 653–9.

Robinson, L., Hughes, J., Daley, S., Keady, J. Ballard, C. and Volicer, L. (2005) End-of-life care and dementia. *Reviews in Clinical Gerontology,* 15: 135–48.

Ross, M., Fisher, R. and MacLean, M. (2000) *A Guide to End-of-Life Care for Seniors.* Ottawa: Health Canada.

Salisbury, C., Bosanquet, N., Wilkinson, E.K., Franks, P.J., Kite, S., Lorentzon, M. and Naysmith, A. (1999) The impact of different models of specialist palliative care on patients' quality of life: a systematic literature review. *Palliative Medicine,* 13(1): 3–17.

Sampson, E., Ritchie, C., Lai, R., Raven P. and Blanchard, M. (2005) A systematic review of the scientific evidence for the efficacy of a palliative care approach in advanced dementia. *International Psychogeriatrics,* 17(1): 31–40.

Scherder, E., Oosterman, J., Swaab, D., Herr, K., Ooms, M., Ribbe, M., Segeant, J., Pickering, G. and Benedetti, F. (2005) Recent developments in pain in dementia. *British Medical Journal,* 26(330): 461–4.

Schonwetter, R.S., Han, B., Small, B.J., Martin, B., Tope, K. and Haley, W.E. (2003) Predictors of six-month survival among patients with dementia: an evaluation of hospice Medicare guidelines. *American Journal of Hospital Palliative Care,* 20(2): 105–13.

Sentagen, E.A. and King, S.A. (1993) The problems of pain and its detection among geriatric nursing home residents. *Journal of the American Geriatrics Society,* 41: 541–4.

Sepulveda, C., Marlin, A., Yohida, T. and Ullrich, A. (2002) Palliative care: the World Health Organization's global perspective. *Journal of Pain and Symptom Management,* 24(2): 91–6.

Small, N., Froggatt, K.A. and Downs, M. (2007) *Living and Dying with Dementia: Dialogues about Palliative Care.* Oxford: Oxford University Press.

Volicer, B.J., Hurley, A., Fabiszewski, K.J., Montgomery, P. and Volicer, L. (1993) Predicting short-term survival for patients with advanced Alzheimer's disease. *Journal of the American Geriatrics Society,* 41(5): 535–40.

Volicer, L. (1986) Need for hospice approach to treatment of patients with advanced progressive dementia. *Journal of the American Geriatrics Society,* 34(9): 655–8.

Volicer, L., Collard, A., Hurley, A., Bishop, C., Kern, D. and Karon, S. (1994) Impact of special care unit for patients with advanced Alzheimer's disease on patients. *Journal of the American Geriatrics Society,* 42(6): 597–603.

Zwakhalen, S.M., Hamers, J.P., Abu-Saad, H.H. and Berger, M.P. (2006) Pain in elderly people with severe dementia: a systematic review of behavioural pain assessment tools. *BMC Geriatrics,* 27(6): 3.

21

Grief and bereavement

Jan Oyebode

Learning objectives

By the end of this chapter you will:

- be aware of the ways in which impaired cognitive functioning may affect responses to bereavement in people with dementia
- know about ways to support people with dementia who are bereaved
- be aware of the particular influences of anticipatory grief, chronic sorrow, caregiving and separation through institutional care on spouses and on adult children who experience the death of a relative with dementia
- know about strategies that can be used at the time of death (and post-bereavement) that may help to promote good adaptation
- be aware of ways to help those who are more vulnerable through a difficult period of adjustment

---

Introduction

The purpose of this chapter is to address how the best possible care and support can be provided to people with dementia who experience bereavement, and people who are bereaved of a relative with dementia. The chapter considers special needs of people with dementia who are bereaved as well as the complex, unique situation of those who are bereaved of a relative with dementia.

The first section of the chapter addresses the responses and needs of people with dementia following bereavement, and then considers the particular nature of bereavement when it is someone with dementia who has died. Included is a discussion about the ways people may react and the factors that influence how people respond to bereavement. Finally, the chapter considers the role of professionals in providing support or care for families

The experience of bereavement for people with dementia

People with dementia who are bereaved of someone close to them may react in a range of ways that are influenced by how their cognitive impairment affects their ability to understand and process the event and its consequences. In responding, we need to bear in mind a primary goal of enabling the person to feel secure and supported. This primary goal informs whether and how we work to enable the person to take in the news; whether we facilitate expression of feelings, and how we help the person to establish a new routine.

As recently as 2005, Rentz and colleagues declared that: 'There has been no coherent, comprehensive description of the grief response and mourning process of the person with dementia at any phase of the illness' (2005: 166). This is an area which has not been well researched but about which there is a good deal of clinical knowledge. It is a field in which person-centred understanding and care can make a great deal of difference to the well-being of a person with dementia.

Rentz *et al.* (2005) and Grief and Myran (2006) both provide a series of descriptions from cases in clinical practice about ways in which people with dementia respond to bereavement. Most are similar to how any of us might respond to the loss of someone close to us, but with the complicating layer of the bereavement having to be absorbed through additional filters of cognitive impairment.

One possible reaction is that the person will fail to take in the loss and hence continue to live life as if the other were still alive. While we may all have periods of disbelief or denial following bereavement, this response may be longer lasting and more severe for a person with memory impairment. The person with dementia may respond with renewed grief on every occasion that their bereavement becomes apparent, as they repeatedly experience being confronted with bad news.

There is also a possibility that the bereaved person will invent an alternative explanation for the non-appearance of their dead relative. This again may be explained by the processes of denial, complicated by poor memory and 'confabulation' (i.e. making up a plausible story to fill the memory gap). The person with dementia may reduce the confusion and distress associated with the non-appearance of their relative by either inventing a plausible explanation (they are at work) or by jumping to conclusions that reflect their underlying fears (they have been kidnapped or murdered).

Another response, resulting from a combination of memory loss and inability to recognize people accurately, is that the person with dementia may mistake someone else for the relative who has died, for example, mistaking their son for their husband, or mistaking a fellow resident in a nursing home for their deceased spouse.

It has also been noted that the person with dementia may dwell or ruminate upon certain events or conversations. Grief and Myran (2006) describe this as occurring more frequently in early dementia. This response may be explained by organic damage that causes perseveration of ideas and difficulty shifting from one track of thinking to another. Also due to the brain changes of dementia, a person may have trouble in regulating and modulating emotional responses. Emotions such as sorrow or anger, which are usually restrained, may be openly and deeply expressed. Finally, Rentz *et al.* (2005) suggest that people with dementia who are losing the ability to express themselves directly, may use metaphor to express their sense of loss.

We see from this list that the cognitive impairment of dementia affects the response to bereavement in a number of ways. It may interfere with the person's usual means of coping; it may disturb their ability to accept the death on either a cognitive or an emotional level and it may leave the bereaved person unable to vocalize their distress and possibly unable to recall occurrence of death (Grief and Myran 2006; Rentz *et al.* 2005).

Supporting people with dementia who are bereaved

It is unlikely that models of understanding and recovery from bereavement can be fully transferred to people with dementia. It may be that rather than trying to enable a bereaved person with dementia to come to terms with bereavement through the usual cognitive and emotional channels, we should instead consider promoting different adaptive strategies with the primary goal of enabling the person to feel secure and supported.

Worden's (1991) grief work hypothesis suggests that there are four tasks to be addressed in adjusting to bereavement. These are: taking in the reality of the loss, experiencing the pain of separation, learning to live without the deceased, and emotionally relocating the deceased so as to be able to move on with life. The first three of these are considered below in relation to those with dementia, whilst the consideration of the fourth is integrated throughout the discussion.

Taking in the reality of the loss

Whether and how to tell a person with dementia that their friend or relative has died is a difficult decision which may influence whether the person with dementia is enabled to attend the funeral, wake or other rituals. In some cases it seems that relatives, and care providers, disenfranchise the person with dementia from grieving, treating them as if they are already 'socially dead' (Sweeting and Gilhooly 1997) and therefore not including them in the family and societal response to the death. Rentz and colleagues (2005) point out that caregivers may be anxious about telling the person with dementia of a death as they do not know how the news will be received. If the news is not given, and rituals are not attended, the person will not have the chance to take in this reality, thus blocking the start of the usual process of grieving.

Generally, in early dementia, it is appropriate to tell the person and then to see whether or not they are able to absorb the news. The issue becomes more acute if the person, having been told, appears to forget and reacts with distress on being told again. In trying to help someone to acknowledge their loss, we may repeatedly confront them with news that they remain unable to take in, exposing them and ourselves to repeated distress (Grief and Myran 2006). Rentz and colleagues (2005) suggest it may be more important to consider the relief of sorrow even at the expense of the truth. In later dementia, it is very unlikely the person will be able to take in the news, so it may not be appropriate for them to be told. Professionals involved in the person's care may be able to help families to think through this dilemma and accept that there is only a good enough, not a perfect, solution.

Where it is important for the person to recognize and absorb that they have been bereaved, then techniques used to address learning in dementia may be applied (see Chapter 9). It is possible that reminders of the funeral, such as the order of service, or photographs of the event or the grave, shown and discussed in a supportive and sympathetic atmosphere, may be helpful in enabling the person to absorb the news. Lewis and Trzinski (2006) describe the application of a spaced retrieval paradigm to help an elderly woman realize that her niece had died. This technique involves enabling a person to rehearse important information at gradually increasing intervals of time as a way of helping them to consolidate the information in memory. They felt her recognition of the death helped to reduce high anxiety that was linked to the idea that 'someone' had died. Appreciating whose death it was enabled her to make use of further emotional therapy techniques that she would not otherwise have been able to benefit from.

Experiencing the pain of bereavement

Pain associated with bereavement is seen as a process that helps us to separate emotionally from the deceased. However, the notion that *everyone* needs to grieve has been questioned for those without (Bonanno *et al.* 2002) and those with dementia (Rentz *et al.* 2005). Where someone with dementia is not grieving, we may not have any justification for trying to prompt them to express their emotions. On the other hand, a person with dementia may show problematic behaviour that indicates their distress, due to an inability or lack of opportunity to express their feelings. Where this is the case, it may be helpful to carry out some systematic observation to see if there are particular factors triggering or maintaining grief (Rentz *et al.* 2005; see Chapter 11). Identification of such factors might allow changes to be made either to avoid the triggering of painful grief or to enable a more appropriate expression of grief. For example, an elderly woman with dementia whose husband has died starts to scream whenever her son comes to see her. Staff think this may be because the sight of him, looking so much like his father, reminds her of her bereavement. Staff speak with her son and between them they decide on a response that might allow the woman concerned to express her pain in a more acceptable way. They arrange that they will take her to her own room prior to her son's arrival so that the two of them have a private space. They agree to talk with her to tell he that he is coming. They show her his photo and remind her who he is. When he arrives, he is ready to acknowledge her feelings by talking with her about her deceased husband, thus allowing both of them space to reminisce together and to weep should they feel the need.

More psychotherapeutically based approaches may also be helpful. People with dementia may not be able to benefit from support groups or counselling sessions but it may be possible to use creative techniques to enable expressions of sadness and loss. One such technique, using 'group buddies', is described by Lewis and Trzinski (2006). The group buddies are soft toys used in therapeutic play. Lewis and Trzinski observed that following a bereavement, group members gained comfort from hugging their soft toy and seemed more able to express their feelings when holding the toy. Other creative techniques could include the use of art or music, though there do not seem, to date, to be any reports on evidence for their effectiveness. It may also be important to consider how to enable the person to find alternative ways of meeting their attachment needs whether through the use of substitute relationships, comfort objects or spiritual means such as prayer.

Learning to live without the deceased

Learning to live without the deceased can be understood using the 'dual process model' (Stroebe and Schut 1999). This model, which has become prominent in making sense of grief, suggests that there are two major strands of response to bereavement and that as we make sense of bereavement we move between the two. On the one hand there are 'loss-oriented' processes which focus on the emotional consequences of losing the relationship and on the other hand there are 'restoration-oriented' processes which focus on the practicalities of living life without the deceased. This stance recognizes that when we are bereaved, not only do we need to look back to the lost relationship, grieve and re-form it for the future but we also need to look ahead and learn new ways of living. This is a useful and necessary focus of work with people with dementia who have been bereaved, particularly those in the community. For those who lived with a carer who has now died, there may be a complete change in their living situation. They will need to develop a new structure in their day-to-day life (Rentz *et al.* 2005), possibly in a new living situation and will require assistance and guidance to achieve this.

Exercise 21.1   Deciding what and how much to tell someone with dementia

Dorothy is a 73-year-old woman with moderate Alzheimer's disease. She has been living at home with support from her husband. She manages daily life quite well with his assistance though she has not shopped alone or cooked independently for quite some time. She has always recognized her husband but sometimes gets mixed up about the identity of her two sons and her daughter. Her husband was admitted to hospital with an exacerbation of chronic obstructive airways disease two days ago and died on the day of admission. Although her daughter told her what had happened, the following day she was shocked to find her mother asking when he would be home. The family ask your advice on how to proceed and you are due to meet them in an hour's time.

Bearing this in mind, write out three points indicating issues or advice you would raise in discussion with the family in order to help them find a way forward.

Think of two possible advantages of the family sensitively repeating to her that her husband will not be coming home and that he has died.

Think of two possible barriers or risks associated with telling her.

Now think of two possible advantages or gains from **not** repeating to Dorothy that her husband has died and think of two possible disadvantages.

It is hoped that Exercise 21.1 has prompted you to think clearly about the pros and cons of telling people with dementia about the death of someone close. It may have helped you to realize that there is no single correct way to proceed. It may also have made you think empathically about the positions of both Dorothy and her daughter, while also considering how to tackle a very emotional issue in a sensitive way.

Family bereavement of a person with dementia

Overall, those whose relative dies of dementia may be at no greater risk of difficulty adapting than those accommodating to other deaths, yet a minority may be more vulnerable. There is some evidence that those who do not acknowledge or express grief in response to ongoing and anticipated losses during dementia caregiving may be vulnerable, as are those who have become very exhausted or depressed during caregiving. Lack of social support during caregiving also predicts a struggle after bereavement. Preventive interventions to address these areas may be helpful.

One of the early studies of loss and grief among family caregivers of people with dementia, points out that this is a unique and complex situation (Collins *et al.* 1993). In this section I will try to give some explanation of why this is so and suggest ways in which, as service providers, we can be aware of and respond to relatives' needs.

This section starts with a description of what is known about the way that people respond to the death of a relative with dementia. It then considers the influence of three particular issues: anticipatory grief, caregiving and institutionalization. The chapter concludes with a summary of the implications for service provision.

Responses to bereavement of a relative with dementia

In Western society, spouses and adult children are the major groups of kin who provide care to relatives with dementia. The position of each is quite different and this appears to be reflected in responses to bereavement. Spouses seem more likely to experience a sense of grief during caregiving which continues after the person has died, whereas adult children report feeling worn down by extended caregiving and may experience an initial sense of relief after bereavement, although this can give way to a resurgence in grief over the following months (Meuser and Marwit 2001; Mullan 1992). The themes of relief and grief as well as an added theme of guilt/regret are echoed in work by Collins and colleagues (1993) and Almberg *et al.* (2000).

The death of the person with dementia, especially after a lengthy period of caregiving, may represent the end of a major episode of life and may be seen as a turning point. Skaff *et al.* (1996) say that the death may provide a renewed opportunity for the individual to reaffirm or rediscover their own identity and achieve personal growth. Skaff and colleagues quote from a daughter who says: '[I am] at a turning point, crossroads … But whatever, I am going to be doing things I want at my pace. Because for the last six years I lost control' (1996: 255), and from a wife: 'My life at this point is a real learning experience because I have never before been totally independent' (1996: 255).

This transition may bring improvements in quality of life and functioning. Schulz *et al.* (1997) undertook a comprehensive review of bereavement and caregiving. They found that bereavement had few negative effects and actually had some positive aspects compared with caregiving.

Despite this relatively optimistic picture, however, some people find it more difficult to adjust. Schulz *et al.* (2006) found that 20% of their 217 bereaved caregivers had high levels of complicated grief and depression 15 weeks after the death. However, these rates decreased dramatically over the following 6–12 months. This seems to indicate that grief may be very intense for quite a proportion of the bereaved, but it may also be reasonably short-lived. By contrast, however, two studies have reported elevated levels of depression in caregivers up to four years after bereavement (Bodnar and Kiecolt-Glaser 1994; Kiecolt-Glaser *et al.* 1991). It has been found that between 11.5% (Bradley *et al.* 2004) and 30% (Schulz *et al.* 2003) of bereaved caregivers experience depression 12 months after the death. Table 21.1 shows factors drawn from research findings that give some indication of those who may be at risk of a difficult period of adjustment.

Thus the results of research to date indicate differences in the bereavement responses of spouses and adult children, with grief possibly being predominant for spouses while offspring may experience relief mixed with some intense grief that may lift fairly quickly. There are likely to be gains in some aspects of life for the bereaved compared with the burden of caregiving. Yet a substantial minority of those whose relative with dementia dies will find it hard to adjust to living without them.

Table 21.1 Factors shown to be associated with, or to predict, complicated grief after bereavement of a person with dementia

---

- Being a spouse rather than an adult child (Boerner *et al.* 2004; Schulz *et al.* 2006)

- Having a relative with more severe dementia (Schulz *et al.* 2006)

- Having poor physical or mental health, especially depression, prior to bereavement (Almberg *et al.* 2000; Boerner *et al.* 2004; Schulz *et al.* 2006)

- Gaining benefit and satisfaction from caregiving (Boerner *et al.* 2004; Schulz *et al.* 2006)

- Having poorer perceived support prior to bereavement (Bass *et al.* 1991)

- Being dissatisfied with aspects of nursing home care (Bass *et al.* 1991)

- Not being able to think about, plan for or grieve for the death in advance (Owen *et al.* 2001)

- Not being able to acknowledge pre-death losses or associated grief (Collins *et al.* 1993; Mullan 1992)

- Being unable to say goodbye (Almberg *et al.* 2000)

- Having a shorter time since the death (Boerner *et al.* 2004)

- Being unable to access any positive memories (Almberg *et al.* 2000)

There are three aspects in particular that make losing a person with dementia distinctive. Each of these will now be considered.

Anticipatory grief and chronic sorrow

People anticipating bereavement may experience grief in advance of the death. This is thought to mean that some of the process of coming to terms with loss takes place ahead of time, possibly leading to an easier adjustment after the event. However, the nature of dementia may make anticipatory grief different from grief that occurs in other circumstances. It can be hard to disinvest emotions while providing personal care, and the level of care may not leave time for a social life or the formation of new relationships. In addition, unlike the situation of caring for someone with a terminal illness and intact cognitive functioning, there is no longer the chance to finish unfinished business (Almberg *et al.* 2000). An interesting research report by Owen *et al.* (2001) highlights some of the impact of anticipatory grief. They found that anticipatory grief in dementia carers lessened grief after bereavement in comparison with those who did not acknowledge or experience anticipatory grief.

There is another layer of complexity to consider because dementia in itself leads to the loss of many aspects of the person. This means that, in addition to anticipatory grief, actual grief is experienced during caregiving. Although these ongoing losses are not bereavements by death, they may still provoke feelings of grief, as evidenced in the moving accounts provided by Meuser and Marwit (2001). Sanders and Corley (2003) found that over two-thirds of caregivers saw themselves as grieving, with a focus on current loss of intimacy and past roles the person with dementia had fulfilled. Lindgren and colleagues (1999) suggest that this type of grief might be referred to as 'chronic sorrow'.

The relationship between chronic sorrow and adaptation to bereavement is not entirely clear. However, as with anticipatory grief, there is some research which suggests that acknowledgement of loss and sorrow during caregiving may lighten the degree of grief after bereavement (Collins *et al.* 1993; Mullan 1992). On the other hand those who have high levels of depression before bereavement have also been found to have sustained depression afterwards (Schulz *et al.* 2006). It may be that while grieving during caregiving lessens grief of bereavement after death, becoming depressed during caregiving is a different matter. Depression therefore needs to be clearly distinguished from grief in caregivers as different responses are probably required.

Caregiving and the subsequent response to bereavement

For spouses of those with dementia, caregiving almost inevitably precedes widowhood. Quite a lot of work aiming to understand the impact of prior caregiving on responses to bereavement has looked at predictions derived from the 'stress-process model' of caregiving (Pearlin *et al.* 1990). The stress-process model of dementia provides a helpful framework for understanding the way that caregiving affects responses to bereavement. Primary stressors and secondary role strains are relieved by the death of the person but secondary intra-psychic strains and resources may be affected both positively and negatively by prior caregiving. This model is more fully described in Chapter 5 which addresses the family experience of dementia. In brief, the model proposes that the well-being of carers is determined by the interplay of several factors:

- primary stressors (stresses directly caused through caring for someone)

- secondary role strains (the 'knock-on' effects of primary stressors on other roles and relationships)

- secondary intra-psychic strains (the impact of primary stressors and secondary role strains on one's self-esteem and sense of self).

These factors interact with each other to impact on well-being with their effect being lessened by the mediating effects of resources, including both inner strength and external social support.

Using this model, Mullan (1992) proposes that caregiving will affect bereavement to the extent that it decreases the primary stressors inherent in caregiving and has an impact on secondary strains and resources.

Primary stressors and secondary strains

When caregiving ceases, former carers are released to pick up the reins of other areas of life and report a number of positive changes that can be seen as resulting from the decrease in primary stressors and secondary role strains. However, the loss of involvement and investment in caregiving and the loss of any associated satisfaction may leave former carers initially feeling empty and devoid of purpose, thus causing secondary intra-psychic strain. It seems that those who invest most in caregiving and gain satisfaction from it suffer from a greater loss of identity when the person is no longer there (Boerner *et al.* 2004; Mullan 1992; Schulz *et al.* 2006).

In addition, there may be intra-psychic strain in the form of guilt post-bereavement (Mullan 1992). This seems to derive from the tensions inherent in providing intensive levels of care which lead to ambivalence and mixed emotions. The caregiver may want to care for their loved one yet find it so hard that at times they will have become impatient, maybe even abusive, and may have wished the whole ordeal to be over. After the person dies they may feel guilty about their care having been less than perfect.

The impact of caregiving on resources can also bring both benefits and disadvantages to the bereaved. On the positive side, some aspects of caregiving may provide experiences that enable carers to develop skills and resources which engender resilience following bereavement (Skaff *et al.* 1996; Wells and Kendig 1997). On the negative side, the more the strain and exhaustion of caregiving, the more the carer may find their personal resources and resilience depleted on bereavement (Almberg *et al.* 2000; Bass and Bowman 1990; Schulz *et al.* 2006).

Support from wider family and friends may be helpful after bereavement (Almberg *et al.* 2000) yet many carers will have inevitably neglected others or been neglected by others during the period of providing intensive care. On bereavement they may find themselves with a smaller social network than they had prior to their period of caregiving.

Thus overall, we see that caregiving leaves a unique imprint on the experiences of caregivers after bereavement. There is an immediate release from primary stressors and secondary role strain but there is a mixed impact on secondary intra-psychic strain and resources. As professionals, we need to ensure that we do not let the knowledge that there is relief from caregiving burden overshadow the fact that former carers may be left exhausted, with a risk of depleted social networks and a possible crisis of identity.

Exercise 21.2   When someone with dementia dies: helping carers to adjust

Pauline cared for her husband, Jack, who had increasingly severe dementia over about eight years before his recent death a few days after admission to hospital with a chest infection. She was at his side when he died.

Pauline and Jack had a long and close marriage. Although exhausted by the physical effort involved in 24-hour care and vigilance, Pauline took pride in looking after Jack. She liked to show visitors a photo of them together at their golden wedding and felt she ensured he continued to look just as smart as he had done in that photo. The couple's only son has a responsible job and when talking to him Pauline has always minimized Jack's problems and her own 'care-giving burden', feeling her son should not have to worry about them.

Think about and list factors that may predispose Pauline to finding adjustment to the death of her husband difficult.

Think about and list factors that may help Pauline to adjust.

It is hoped that undertaking Exercise 21.2 may have given you an opportunity to think about how anticipatory grief, chronic sorrow and caregiving may affect grief. The exercise should also have given you a chance to increase your familiarity with the stress-process model of caregiving. You should have been able to use the concepts of primary and secondary stressors, resources and intra-psychic strains to help with your listing of factors that might make it more or less difficult for Pauline to adjust.

Institutionalization

For some, the experience of caregiving is followed by a period of institutionalization. Some research indicates that those who place their relative with dementia in a nursing home may experience greater sadness and guilt than those who are able to keep their relative at home (Rudd *et al.* 1999). This may then lead to increased feelings of guilt and regret after bereavement. The carer's appraisal of the quality of nursing home care has, understandably, been found to be related to the level of emotional distress after bereavement. Where relatives have had concerns about the quality of care, then distress levels are higher after bereavement (Bass *et al.* 1991).

It might be expected that when a person with dementia moves into a nursing home, their relatives could start to re-establish an independent way of life that will prepare them for bereavement. This appears to be the case for adult children but not for spouses. Meuser and Marwit (2001) found that spouse caregivers who had placed the person with dementia in a nursing home had intense feelings of loss, grief and guilt. They remained emotionally attached to their spouse, impeding their ability to adapt to living alone.

Thus letting the person with dementia move into nursing home care may lead to a greater sense of regret and guilt following bereavement, especially if the relatives had doubt about the standards of care. While for many adult children, a period of institutionalization may allow re-establishment of other roles, for spouses it seems to remain an emotionally difficult time and it may not help the later bereavement response.

Implications for services

There appear to be few services for caregivers of people with dementia following bereavement (Murphy *et al.* 1997) and little research into best practice.

In the general population there are indications that it is not helpful to offer professional bereavement counselling routinely to all who have been bereaved. Identifying those who may be vulnerable to a complicated response and undertaking targeted preventive interventions are more appropriate. Where problems develop after bereavement, despite or due to lack of preventative interventions, then therapeutic intervention is indicated (Schut *et al.* 2001). This is also likely to be the case for those who have cared for someone with dementia.

All those who are later bereaved may be helped by caregiver interventions that promote skills and resources prior to bereavement. These may give rise to a greater sense of mastery, less regret or guilt, and better social support after bereavement. There is evidence that relatives benefit from an opportunity to say goodbye to the person with dementia and that they may find it helpful to be offered a post-bereavement meeting with professionals who knew their relative.

Interventions for all who are bereaved

During caregiving

We have seen how responses to bereavement are influenced by the experiences of caregiving and institutionalization and by the degree to which the carer has grieved ongoing and anticipated losses during these periods. Thus it follows that interventions during caregiving may prove helpful to carers after bereavement (Mullan 1992). Indeed, Shulz and colleagues (2006) found that participating in a 6-month psychosocial and skills-based intervention made a significant contribution to lower levels of complicated grief post-bereavement.

At the time of death

Around the time of death, research shows that it is helpful for subsequent well-being for relatives to have a chance to say goodbye. The more services can recognize and offer this, the better the outcome is likely to be for carers (Almberg *et al.* 2000).

Following bereavement

Almberg *et al.* (2000) found that almost a third of caregivers in their Swedish sample spoke of missing professional support after the death of their relative with dementia, a view echoed in the themes found by Collins *et al.* (1993) in the accounts of caregivers following the death of the person with dementia. In view of this, it would seem appropriate that professionals who have been involved in the person's care offer to meet at least once after the death with family members. This may be seen as akin to review or 'debriefing' rather than 'therapy'. Offering the family a single appointment after their relative's death might be of benefit in several ways. It would give an opportunity for the family to talk with someone who knew their relative in his or her last days and knew the circumstances of their death. It would give the opportunity to ask questions thus possibly dispelling misconceptions and guilt, and it would mark the end of contact by design rather than by circumstance, allowing relatives to feel cared for rather than abandoned.

Almberg *et al.* (2000) were surprised to find, in the largely secular society of Sweden, that a number of participants in their research reported spiritual support as being very helpful after bereavement. This reminds us to consider spiritual well-being as well as secular practical and emotional support.

Preventative interventions for those at risk of complicated responses to bereavement

Research tells us that caregivers who are isolated or whose resources are depleted may struggle to come to terms with bereavement. Almberg *et al.* (2000) suggest that drawing the family together to formulate care plans during the period of caregiving may mobilize family resources and be helpful after bereavement. This might also be a vehicle for addressing the unfinished business that can no longer be addressed directly with the person with dementia.

Those who do not acknowledge or express loss during caregiving have greater emotional distress after bereavement and it may be that if professionals can offer the opportunity to caregivers to talk about ongoing and anticipated losses during caregiving this would be helpful afterwards (Collins *et al.* 1993).

We have also seen how carers who have been depressed during caregiving are at risk of being depressed after bereavement. Thus distinguishing depression from grief and recognizing and offering interventions to alleviate depression may also be expected to make a difference (Schulz *et al.* 2006).

Exercise 21.3 Teaching staff to support families in bereavement

You are asked to provide a two-hour training session for staff working in a nursing home that cares for a lot of people with dementia on how to support families whose relative has died there.

Give three learning objectives you might have for this session, along the lines of:

- for staff to _____
- for staff to _____
- for staff to _____

List three pieces of information you might include to address one of these learning objectives.

Describe a discussion point or interactive exercise you could use to address another of your three learning objectives.

Thinking about how to teach others tends to make us think very clearly about what we understand about a topic. This exercise was intended to help you to consolidate what you have learned about how to provide excellent care for relatives who have lost a loved one from dementia.

Debates and controversies

Perhaps in relation to bereaved people with dementia, the greatest dilemma is whether to try and enable them to understand that a person they know and care about has died. Telling may provoke upset in ourselves and in the person with dementia, yet not telling may add to their social exclusion and cheat them of the chance to grieve.

There are also dilemmas in relation to service provision for those whose relative dies because of dementia. In a service system that focuses on 'the patient' and which is short of resources, then is it possible and appropriate for services to provide for family members, especially after the death of the 'identified patient'? It seems that the answer to this is partly to focus on providing good family and relationship-centred support and care during the whole of the dementia journey, thus helping to ensure that its ending does not leave behind a wake of severe and lasting distress.

Conclusion

Adaptation to bereavement for someone with dementia is greatly complicated by cognitive impairment. The person's ability to take in and accommodate the news will vary according to the degree of impairment. Knowing how to help a bereaved person with dementia challenges us to think carefully about the ethical and moral basis of how we respond.

For the relative of someone with dementia, bereavement is the final phase in the dementia journey, the phase in which they are left travelling alone. This chapter has considered the complex ways in which actual and anticipatory grief prior to bereavement impact on the process of adaptation. It has also looked at the ways in which caregiving and institutionalization are intertwined with what happens after the person with dementia dies. It seems that the death of a relative with dementia may differ for spouses, who are often exhausted and full of grief, and adult children who may experience a mixture of relief, grief and regret. Overall, those whose relative dies of dementia may be at no greater risk of difficulty adapting than those accommodating to other deaths, yet a minority are more vulnerable. The chapter suggests strategies during dementia care, at the time of death and post-bereavement that may help to set a trajectory that promotes good adaptation. It also suggests ways of intervening during dementia care that may be helpful to those who are more vulnerable.

There is a need for further research to document the interventions that are being used both with bereaved people with dementia and those bereaved of a relative with dementia in order to find out more about their effectiveness.

People with dementia who lose someone close to them may react in a range of ways that are influenced by their struggle with cognitive impairment. In this situation, we need to bear in mind a primary goal of enabling the person to feel secure and supported, letting this inform whether we work to enable the person to take in the death; whether we facilitate expression of emotions and how we help the person to establish a new routine. There is a need for further research in this area to document the interventions that are being used and find out more about their effectiveness.

These topics of dementia and bereavement are under-researched and service responses are often inadequate. Small steps can be taken which are likely to make a great difference to the outcomes whether for bereaved people with dementia or bereaved caregivers.

Further information

General information about bereavement can be found on the **BBC website**. This site provides contacts that might be useful, guidance for people caring for someone with a terminal illness, practical tips concerning funerals, memorials and probate, and help dealing with the physical and emotional aspects of bereavement.

The Department of Health has a website devoted to bereavement. This website includes information on conferences and workshops about bereavement, support and information about dealing with bereavement, and is relevant to consumers and professionals.

The main organization in the UK concerned with bereavement care is **Cruse Bereavement Care,** which exists 'to promote the well-being of bereaved people and to enable anyone bereaved by death to understand their grief and cope with their loss'. CRUSE provides counselling and support and offers information, advice, education and training services.

A UK forum for those interested in bereavement research is the **Bereavement Research Forum** which aims to provide a forum for interested professionals to discuss, promote and develop bereavement research. Their website lists conferences, symposia and research reports that are useful to professionals caring for people during bereavement.

References

Almberg, B.E., Grafstrom, M. and Winblad, B. (2000) Caregivers of relatives with dementia: Experiences encompassing social support and bereavement. *Aging and Mental Health*, 4(1): 82–9.

Bass, D. and Bowman, K. (1990) The transition from caregiving to bereavement: The relationship of care-related strain and adjustment to death. *The Gerontologist*, 30: 35–44.

Bass, D., Bowman, K. and Noelker, L. (1991) The influence of caregiving and bereavement support on adjusting to an older relative's death. *The Gerontologist*, 31: 32–42.

Bodnar, J. and Kiecolt-Glaser, J. (1994) Caregiver depression after bereavement: Chronic stress isn't over when it's over. *Psychology and Aging*, 9: 372–80.

Boerner, K., Schulz, R. and Horowitz, A. (2004) Positive aspects of caregiving and adaptation after bereavement. *Psychology & Aging*, 19: 668–75.

Bonanno, G.A., Wortman, C.B., Lehman, D.R. *et al.* (2002) Resilience to loss and chronic grief: A prospective study from preloss to 18-months postloss. *Journal of Personality and Social Psychology*, 83: 1150–64.

Bradley, E.H., Prigerson, H., Carlson, M.D., Cherlin, E., Johnson-Hurzeler, R. and Kasl, S.V. (2004) Depression among surviving caregivers: Does length of hospice enrollment matter? *American Journal of Psychiatry*, 161: 2257–62.

Collins, C., Liken, M., King, S and Kikinakis, C. (1993) Loss and grief among family caregivers of relatives with dementia. *Qualitative Health Research*, 3: 236–53.

Grief, C. and Myran D. (2006) Bereavement in cognitively impaired older adults: Case series and clinical considerations. *Journal of Geriatric Psychiatry & Neurology*, 19: 209–15.

Kiecolt-Glaser, J., Dura, J., Speicher, C., Trask. J. and Glaser, R. (1991) Spousal caregivers of dementia victims: Longitudinal changes in immunity and health. *Psychosomatic Medicine*, 53: 345–62.

Lewis, M. and Trzinski, A. (2006) Counseling older adults with dementia who are dealing with death: Innovative interventions for practitioners. *Death Studies*, 30: 777–87.

Lindgren, C., Connelly, C. and Gaspar, H. (1999) Grief in spouse and children caregivers of dementia patients. *Western Journal of Nursing Research*, 2: 521–37.

Meuser, T. and Marwit, S. (2001) A comprehensive stage-sensitive model of grief in dementia caregiving. *The Gerontologist*, 41: 658–70.

Mullan, J. (1992) The bereaved caregiver: A prospective study of changes in well-being. *The Gerontologist*, 5: 673–83.

Murphy, K., Hanrahan, P. and Luchins, D. (1997) A survey of grief and bereavement in nursing homes: The importance of hospice grief and bereavement for the end-stage Alzheimer's disease patient and family. *Journal of the American Geriatrics Society*, 45: 1104–7.

Owen, J., Goode, K. and Haley, W. (2001) End of life care and reactions to death in African-American and white family caregivers of relatives with Alzheimer's disease. *Omega*, 43: 349–61.

Pearlin, L., Mullan, J., Semple, S. and Skaff, M.(1990) Caregiving and the stress process: an overview of concepts and their measures. *The Gerontologist*, 29: 583–94.

Rentz, C., Krikorian, R. and Keys, M. (2005) Grief and mourning from the perspective of the person with a dementing illness: Beginning the dialogue. *Omega*, 50: 165–79.

Rudd, M., Viney, L. and Preston, C. (1999) The grief experienced by spousal caregivers of dementia patients: The role of place of care of patient and gender of caregiver. *International Journal of Aging and Human Development*, 48: 217–40.

Sanders, S. and Corley, C. (2003) Are they grieving? A qualitative analysis examining grief in caregivers of individuals with Alzheimer's disease. *Social Work in Health Care*, 37: 35–53.

Schulz, R., Boerner, K., Shear, K., Zong, S. and Gitlin, L. (2006) Predictors of complicated grief among dementia caregivers: A prospective study of bereavement. *American Journal of Geriatric Psychiatry*, 14: 650–8.

Schulz, R., Mendelsohn, A., Haley, W. *et al.* (2003) End of life care and the effects of bereavement among family caregivers of persons with dementia. *New England Journal of Medicine*, 349: 1891–2.

Schulz, R., Newsom, J., Fleissner, K., Decamp, A. and Nieboer, A. (1997) The effects of bereavement after family caregiving. *Aging and Mental Health*, 1: 269–82.

Schut, H., Stroebe, M.S., van den Bout, J. and Terheggen, M. (2001) The efficacy of bereavement interventions: determining who benefits. In: M.S. Stroebe, R.O. Hansson, W. Stroebe and H. Schut (eds) *Handbook of Bereavement Research: Causes, Consequences and Care*. Washington, DC: American Psychological Association, pp. 705–38.

Skaff, M., Pearlin, L. and Mullan, J. (1996) Transitions in the caregiving career: Effects of sense of mastery. *Psychology and Aging*, 11: 247–57.

Stroebe, M. and Schut, H. (1999) The dual process model of coping with bereavement: Rationale and description. *Death Studies*, 23: 197–224.

Sweeting, H. and Gilhooly, M. (1997) Dementia and the phenomenon of social death. *Sociology of Health and Illness*, 19: 93–117.

Wells, Y.D. and Kendig, H.L. (1997) Health and well-being of spouse caregivers and the widowed. *The Gerontologist*, 37: 666–74.

Worden, W. (1991) *Grief Counselling and Grief Therapy: A Handbook for the Mental Health Practitioner*. New York: Springer.

PART FOUR

Embedding excellence in dementia care

22

Involving people with dementia in service development and evaluation

Rachael Litherland

Learning objectives

By the end of this chapter you will:

- know about a range of approaches that can be used to elicit views of people with dementia
- recognize the challenges involved in seeking the views of people with dementia
- have an understanding of service user involvement for people with dementia
- know some of the guiding principles for involving people with dementia as service users

---

Introduction

Considering people with dementia as 'users of services', with an active role to play in their design and delivery, is a relatively recent phenomenon. With a policy imperative, practitioners and professionals are increasingly committed to finding ways to involve people with dementia. This requires both the development of innovative methods to enable people to have a voice and a commitment to acting on what has been heard.

Until relatively recently it was more common to think of people with dementia as passive *recipients* of services rather than active *users* of services. Recent years have witnessed a 'great reappraisal of dementia' (Kitwood 1997: 13). Among other things, this has resulted in a move away from seeing the consequence of dementia as the 'complete annihilation of self' (Beard 2004: 806) to a position that acknowledges the awareness that many people with dementia have about their situation (Clare *et al.* 2005), including the services they use. It is increasingly recognized that people with dementia have something to say and that it is our responsibility to hear the voices of people with dementia (Goldsmith 1996).

The voices of people with dementia can now be heard in a wide range of research on the experience of dementia (e.g. Wilkinson 2002), through personal stories and narratives (e.g. Bryden 2005) and, increasingly, in terms of their experience of health and social care (e.g. Barnett 2000). People with dementia are also beginning to work together to instigate collective action (e.g. the Scottish Dementia Working Group, Dementia Advocacy and Support Network International).

Alongside this emerging perspective are legislative and policy frameworks that vigorously promote user involvement. For example, in the UK, the Health and Social Care Act 2001 states that those in receipt of services should be involved in planning and developing services even if that person needs help to understand or to retain information relevant to the decision.

The purpose of this chapter is to provide an overview of user involvement with particular emphasis on user involvement of people with dementia. This chapter will draw on practice and research to provide guidance on approaches to and principles of involving people with dementia. Some of the challenges involved in this work will be highlighted. Ironically discussions of service user involvement often shift the perspective of service users back to the periphery, focusing instead on the experiences of professionals who *choose* to involve people who use the services. I will therefore attempt to keep the voices of people with dementia central to this discussion by drawing on my previous work through the Alzheimer's Society's 'Living with Dementia' programme.

What does service user involvement mean?

'Service user' has become the recognized term in health and social care to describe people in receipt of services. The term 'service user' suggests that the user is central to shaping service development and delivery, shifting power away from the provider toward the consumer. It suggests that the recipients of service have the right to choose and change services, to better meet their needs.

Involvement has been an objective for a range of groups for many years. The mental health field has seen a change in landscape from the individual achievements of the mental health activists of the 1970s and 1980s to a degree of permanence within the field that acknowledges users as experts (Sainsbury Centre for Mental Health 2005: 74). Similarly, self-organized groups of older people are influencing decisions at the highest level (e.g. Older Persons Advisory Group (OPAG) and older persons forums supported by Help the Aged) with a move away from just consulting with older people towards active partnerships to influence decisions (Reed *et al.* 2006: 5).

Robson *et al.* (2003) distinguished between management-centred and user-centred user involvement. In management-centred user involvement the service user is involved by responding to agendas set by the organization, for example, giving views on an organization's strategic plan. User-centred user involvement, on the other hand, refers to circumstances where service user objectives and priorities become the organization's objectives and priorities, for example, the operation of the Scottish Dementia Working Group, an independent campaigning group formed by people with dementia. The group is supported by a paid coordinator to identify its own objectives and develop a work plan to meet these objectives which have included giving views on a range of health and community care issues such as medication, national templates for dementia services and stem cell research.

Management-centred user involvement, perhaps in response to policy or funding objectives, has been criticized for resulting in a form of 'moral coercion' (Small and Rhodes 2001: 5) where users feel obliged to be involved – maybe as a condition of receiving a service or because of how they perceive the authority of those in charge of services. Research with people who are seriously ill or approaching the end of their lives (Small and Rhodes 2001) concludes that user involvement is not a priority for this group and that such people often have other agendas and more pressing concerns than to be actively involved in service development or evaluation.

An additional critique of user involvement is the potential for it to be a tokenistic exercise. A common experience of service users participating in a management-centred user approach is to be asked for views and then to feel their knowledge is not valued or taken seriously by professionals, policy-makers and services (Branfield and Beresford 2006): 'People think the only thing we know is how to moan. But they are not listening. We know what needs changing; we know what works and what doesn't work. We know this because we live it 24/7, 52 weeks a year with no days off' (2006: 3).

Exercise 22.1   Approaches to involving service users

Research and practice within other fields have been critical of user involvement initiatives based on the agendas of organizations rather than defined and developed directly by service users.

Why do you think management-centred approaches to user involvement have been criticized?

What do you think are the challenges in applying a purely user-centred approach to the involvement of people with dementia?

Involving people with dementia in service development and evaluation

In accepting that a diagnosis of a type of dementia is life-changing rather than life-ending, it is a natural progression to consider ways to involve people with dementia in services that affect their lives. There is now a growing recognition that people with dementia are able to provide accurate and valid reports about services, whether verbally (Bamford and Bruce 2000) or behaviourally (see Chapter 25).

Bamford and Bruce (2000) conducted a small study to determine the feasibility of consulting people with dementia about the outcomes they desired from services. In common with their carers, people with dementia discussed a range of outcomes that were significant to them including access to social contact, company, meaningful activity and stimulation, having a sense of social integration and maximizing a sense of autonomy. Sometimes people with dementia expressed different views to their carers. For example, maintaining a sense of personal identity, 'a sense of oneself as a competent and valued person' (2000: 556) was seen as important by service users but was rarely identified as important by carers.

People with dementia are leading the call for greater involvement in service development asserting their *rights* to be involved in services that affect their lives.

Dementia Advocacy Support Network International (DASNI) successfully lobbied Alzheimer's Disease International (ADI) – the international federation of Alzheimer associations throughout the world – to consider ways it could become more inclusive of people with dementia. (See DASNI website for correspondence on this issue.) Achievements to date have included representatives with dementia on the executive council of ADI, a conference fund to support people with dementia and their care partners to attend ADI conferences, and a strategic commitment to giving people with dementia a greater voice in the decision-making of ADI (personal correspondence).

As people's condition changes, they may use a variety of services (Cheston *et al.* 2000), all of which they can be said to have a stake in as a user or consumer. In theory, service user involvement, in whatever form, should be expected throughout the length of the condition. That said, for many people with dementia there is a 'window of opportunity' (Litherland 2003) – a short period of time before the impact of dementia reduces one's ability to respond to opportunities, and the window is closed. This accelerates the need to find ways to support involvement and can really test an organization's commitment to user involvement, where organizational structures are complex and decision-making is traditionally quite lengthy and management-centred. This challenge is highlighted in *Engaging People with Early Stage Alzheimer's Disease in the Work of the Alzheimer's Society* (2006), a research report commissioned by the Alzheimer Society Canada where urgency to act and adapt is counterbalanced by funding cutbacks, the impact of cognitive decline and the need for internal policies and regulations that support involvement.

Involving people with dementia in a national organization

In April 2000, the national 'Living with Dementia' programme was launched by the Alzheimer's Society in response to contact from an increasing number of people with dementia looking for support to come to terms with their diagnosis and find ways of living as normally as possible for as long as possible. A proportion of people also had a real desire to have their voice heard in an organization that represented their interests: 'Listen to us, hear us, we are here.'

The Living with Dementia programme, now an integrated programme of work, was initially a two-year development project to develop information and support, engage with people with dementia, and test out new ways of involving people with dementia. Its remit may appear broad because it was!

As a starting point, it was useful to consider lessons from initiatives in other fields. However, the specific and variable impact of dementia on people's capacity to be involved relied on developing new practices. The Living with Dementia programme learned how to involve people with dementia by doing just that, by emphasizing the expert role of people with dementia in working out the 'how' of user involvement.

A first challenge was to find people with dementia who wanted to get involved in a national programme. People with dementia were contacted through local support groups and dementia practitioners were asked to identify people whom they thought might like to get involved. As the programme was advertised more widely, people with dementia began to make direct contact.

Initially most of the concerns presented were very individual: 'Support is the key to me leading as normal a life as possible. People knowing and treating me as the person I still am. Giving me room to live.' But as I travelled to meet more people, in their own environments, a critical mass of people who wanted to be part of the programme began to develop. They believed that the views of people with dementia should be heard within the Alzheimer's Society and externally: 'You need to focus on the ability and contribution that we can make, rather than what we can no longer do.'

'User involvement' was not a meaningful way of explaining the purpose of the Living with Dementia programme. Similarly, a user-centred approach (Robson *et al.* 2003), with people with dementia setting their own objectives and priorities, was not an option as a starting point. Most contacts were not used to having their experience listened to, had little confidence in their ability to be involved and had never met anyone else with dementia. Instead, we discussed opportunities that people might like to be involved in. These were concrete examples (e.g. writing a booklet, giving views on making supermarkets easier to use, keeping a photographic diary, recruiting a new member of staff, talking about day support opportunities, speaking at a conference), that were usually time-limited to give people a chance to review their involvement on an ongoing basis. The skills and interests of individuals with dementia were matched with available opportunities – a former GP began to give presentations about life with dementia to the medical profession; a former architect discussed the changes that could be made to an office environment to make it more accessible for people with dementia. Alongside emerging activists was the growth of a movement of people and groups of people with dementia who connected with the aims of the Living with Dementia programme and began to feel supported to 'come out' about their experiences and wishes.

People with dementia said the following practices helped them to get involved:

- being respected and listened to

- a welcoming attitude

- being given encouragement

- a clear and prompt response to questions and concerns

- early diagnosis (leaving more time to be involved)

- acknowledging the diagnosis (not pretending we don't have dementia)

- varied opportunities to get involved

- opportunities to take part without it involving 'consultation'.

They also said that these things made involvement more difficult:

- fear that I will not be taken seriously

- lack of time for people to listen and make relationships

- lack of money

- poor access to transport

- lack of diagnosis

- negative attitudes about the abilities or rights of people with dementia

- being asked about issues that are not relevant

- lack of feedback about what has happened as a result of being involved

- lack of personal identification with issues of 'dementia' or 'Alzheimer's'.

Involvement approaches – ideas from research and practice

Cantley *et al.* (2005) looked at how to involve people with dementia in planning and developing services by reviewing the practice experience of 16 projects and groups. Four projects acted as development sites for the study, where staff and service users were helped to develop specific involvement activities. The focus was on consultation approaches – about home care, services, methods of involvement and quality of life – and a range of involvement methods were used, including individual and group discussions, questionnaires, observation and consultation events. Along with some useful pointers to best support involvement activities (e.g. selecting a venue for a consultation event, questions to consider when planning involvement activities and developing a reflective diary), common features that underpin involvement approaches emerged across project sites. Well-thought-through plans, prior to any involvement activity, are essential to enable people with dementia to fully participate; ethical practice should be paramount, for example, obtaining consent before seeking, recording and using people's views; establishing communication is central and being able to make adjustments in response to individuals' different and varying needs. An important acknowledgement in the study is that the projects relied on the willingness of staff to be innovative and responsive in their approach. In one situation pre-planned consultation questions were abandoned when it became clear that people with dementia could not recollect the topic they were questioned about (information at a local memory clinic). Instead a word (in this case 'information') was written on a large sheet of paper which then triggered other words and discussion and ultimately reminded people of their experiences at the memory clinic (Cantley *et al.* 2005: 37).

A study by Allan (2001) looked at how staff could encourage people with dementia to express views and preferences in the course of day-to-day activities. Allan worked with 40 care practitioners in 10 dementia care settings to consider appropriate techniques for engaging with people with dementia. She found that enabling people to express their views took many forms, with individuals responding to different approaches at different times in different ways. The communication needs of individuals, the person's background and interests, and their relationships with staff needed to be taken into account before identifying the most appropriate consultation approach. Approaches were tested by staff in their care service environment and included observation, verbal exchanges as a part of other activities, the use of pictures to stimulate discussion and indirect discussion where the service user was encouraged to think about what another person's opinions might be. Part of Allan's work was to support staff in recognizing their existing skills and to become more confident about knowing how and when to apply these skills to enable people to express their views. In the service environment, this meant care staff being more alert to everyday situations when consultation might be possible, for example, during personal care tasks.

Allan's work demonstrates the cognizant role that practitioners must adopt, responding to individual need and drawing on a portfolio of techniques. She notes the organizational systems that need to be in place to support practitioners to take on this role, including enough workplace time to allow for reflection and discussion.

Finally, Hubbard *et al.* (2003) suggest we develop a repertoire of strategies to be used with different individuals. They used interviews or observations to determine the experiences of new residents of a care home. Observations removed the constraints of an interview situation, allowing residents to converse in their own way within the context of their immediate environment whilst interviews provided a more focused opportunity allowing residents to discuss their past and to shape the conversation. Sometimes, however, the interview situation presented difficulties such as when people became embarrassed because they could not recall a factual piece of information, and it was thought that a more open approach, combining observation with interviewing, may have been more appropriate.

In the above studies the entrepreneurial nature of involvement work with people with dementia is acknowledged. The key principle that emerges is the need for a flexible approach responsive to individual need. The studies also highlight the considerable skills that workers must be able to access including good preparation, identifying the most appropriate involvement method, being a responsive and sensitive communicator and allocating time for review and reflection. It is also important to be mindful of the organizational context within which user involvement activity occurs. A strategic approach that promotes creativity and innovation supports the recognition and development of staff skills and recognizes the emotional demands of the work will contribute to an environment where the involvement of service users is valued and achievable (Cantley *et al.* 2005).

Exercise 22.2   Skills for involving users

The skills of workers have been highlighted as an important component of a good user involvement approach.

What skills do you think are necessary to support the involvement of people with dementia?

How do you think this might affect the workers?

In thinking about Exercise 22.2, you may want to identify the attributes that a worker could bring to a user involvement situation, such as enthusiasm, patience, creativity and good communication skills. There may also be practical approaches that are relevant such as strategic thinking and the ability to form good relationships with other services. Consider if the required skills are inbuilt of if they can be learned. You may also want to think about the emotional impact of this specialist work on an individual worker and how an organizational environment might help or hinder a worker to implement a user involvement approach.

Policy context

In recent years the government has placed an emphasis on empowering patients and the public to have a greater say in the services they use. As a result, health and social care practitioners increasingly expect and are expected to work alongside people with dementia as stakeholders (an individual or organization that has a direct interest in a service) for example, through Local Involvement Networks (LINks). A change in working cultures is also promoted with those who deliver services having a responsibility to listen and act on the user voice. This voice is encouraged and supported to develop through initiatives such as the Expert Patients Programme – a self-management training programme delivered to people living with a long-term condition by volunteer tutors who themselves have a long-term condition. It offers a portfolio of techniques for managing the condition and aims to improve quality of life and increase people's confidence to manage their own condition.

Finding out what people with dementia think of the service they use

If we think of involvement as a process rather than a one-off event, then the techniques and approaches we choose are just one step on the journey.

Answering the following questions will help to ensure the most appropriate choice of approach:

- How will you identify people who wish to be involved?

- How can you best support people to identify their own needs and set their own priorities?

- Know your purpose: why do you want to involve people with dementia, what is it you want to know/what activities do they want to engage in? What might be the best techniques for finding out? Is it relevant to people with dementia?

- What issues might emerge during involvement activities? What measures can you put in place to deal with these issues? Do you have a contingency plan?

- Do you have the right skill set to support a particular involvement initiative? If not, who else should you ask to support the initiative?

- Are there lessons you can draw on from other practice examples? If so, what adaptations would you need to make?

Direct approaches: talking to people

Interviews

Successful interviews are dependent on successful communication between the interviewer and interviewee. As we have seen in the chapter on communication and relationships (see Chapter 12), there is much that the interviewer can do to enable effective communication. Dewing (2002) suggests that the complexity of the questions needs to be set at a level that the person finds comprehensible and recommends 'dementia-specific interview methods' (2002: 165) that help enhance understanding about the interview context. These might include a photograph of someone being interviewed or the use of a tape-recorder or video camera for play back. Some participants' ability to communicate verbally can vary from day to day, within the same day and from one week to the next (Hubbard *et al.* 2003). Therefore, multiple interviews over time have been shown to be useful, also helping to improve the skills of the interviewer (Pratt 2002).

Box 22.1 Case example

People with dementia were asked their views on the content and design of the Alzheimer's Society's website. The interviewer showed people the website under discussion and asked people to think about a website as a giant library containing all the information in the world. People were then invited to think of questions they had about dementia. A variety of techniques were used depending on individual need – using the website as a visual tool, using pre-prepared headings written on sheets of paper to help prompt questions, open-ended discussion with the interviewer about issues that were important to them. The interviewer was well known to many of the participants and used her knowledge of people's communication styles to support people to express their views.

The flexible interview approach illustrated in Box 22.1, which was adapted in response to individual need, resulted in a wealth of information about the topic under discussion. The interviewer initially directed the discussion, using questions, prompts and analogies. This seemed to help by keeping people focused on the website and aware of the purpose of their involvement, with the interviewer acting as a memory aid and facilitator.

Group discussions

One-to-one interviews can sometimes feel pressurized and people may worry about the impact of what they say. Group discussions can overcome this by generating a group rather than individual response. Hearing the views of others can help people articulate their own thoughts. Bamford and Bruce (2002), in running focus groups with people with dementia on the topic of the experience of receiving care, however, do note some difficulties. These include lack of respect of viewpoint between participants, constraints of existing social relationships preventing people expressing their viewpoints, and the occurrence of parallel conversations rather than a broader group discussion.

Box 22.2　Case example

Up to seven people attended Living with Dementia meetings in London. Members of the group came up with the following terms of conduct:

● Distribute easy to understand agendas before meetings. This gives us a chance to prepare and write down our thoughts.

● Meetings should be short, with only one or two agenda points. We get tired and find it difficult to concentrate after a while.

● It helps if you give us some ideas. But sometimes we will want to talk about things that are important to us.

● Slow down the pace of discussion to give people time to say what they want to say. Don't talk too much!

● It helps to take turns so that everyone can have their say, even if this is not in words.

● Refreshments are essential. They help us to relax and make our journey worthwhile.

● Send us an easy to understand record of the meeting as soon as possible.

● Send us a reminder just before the next meeting.

There was incredible agreement within the group when setting these ground rules. Some are common to all group situations; many, however, are very particular to the experience of being a group member with dementia. There was recognition of the requirement for meetings to be adapted so that everyone was able to participate as fully as possible. There was also a desire for equity within the group, particularly wanting to make sure that those who had more significant communication difficulties were given time and support to contribute. The importance of the individual within this new group was paramount.

Use of props and prompts

Physical cues and prompts are shown to aid communication during interviews and focus groups, helping people focus on the subject under discussion. Pictures or cards with single emotions written on them have been successfully used to stimulate conversation and discussion (Allan 2001). Dewing (2002) suggests that interactions involving the handling of props can enable the person to feel more confident and therefore respond less hesitantly.

Indirect approaches

Discussion as part of other activities

An exclusive focus on talking may be intimidating or inhibiting for some people with dementia. Conversations can be facilitated through other activities such as going for a walk (Allan 2001). It may be necessary to approach involvement activities in a much more fluid way, 'talking around the research' (Dewing 2002: 12) in an effort to engage with the person, or responding to 'intermittent conversation' (Hubbard *et al.* 2003) which can be less demanding for the person with dementia.

Box 22.3   Case example

'I think we approach user involvement differently to other areas. We maybe don't do it so formally. We do it by listening to the groups, during lunch or whatever ... so we don't really sit down and say, "What would everyone like to do?" because you don't get a direct answer because no one wants to say, "This is what we want to do." We try to listen to the conversations, ask all the workers involved what they think we should be going, and go out and try it. If it is successful we know we've done the right thing. If it is not successful, then that's also telling us it's not the right thing they want. So we try and learn from those sorts of things. It is not really a formal way of approaching it and I don't know if that is right or not ...'

Voluntary organization providing day care, quoted in Cantley *et al.* (2005: 18)

Non-verbal and behavioural communication

Not everyone will be able to or want to communicate. Relying solely on verbal methods of communication is likely to result in a significant proportion of people with dementia being excluded from any involvement process. Researchers often take notes about aspects of non-verbal communication and the emotions of the person with dementia (Allan 2001). Brooker describes the use of observational methods including dementia care mapping for eliciting service users' views on quality in Chapter 26.

Exercise 22.3   User involvement in practice

Imagine you are organizing an event for 30 people with dementia, to find out their views on the best ways to design accommodation for people with dementia.

What would you consider when planning the event?

How would you decide which involvement approaches to use?

What practical adjustments would you make to ensure everyone could be involved?

Guiding principles for involving people with dementia in service development and evaluation

Key principles to successful involvement of people with dementia in service development and evaluation include: building trust; providing enough time and being flexible; deciding whose views to seek; providing a supportive physical and social environment; and having a commitment to acting on the feedback received.

Building trust

Being questioned can be perceived as threatening to someone with cognitive impairment as people with dementia often make mistakes when asked questions (Stalker *et al.* 1999). In a situation where there is often an imbalance of power between people who use a service and those who provide the service, time to build up trust and relationships is essential.

Deciding whose views to seek

Gatekeepers such as a social worker, community psychiatric nurse, care home manager, or family carer, are sometimes relied upon to access service users or to aid communication. Although someone the person knows and trusts can play a role in supporting a person with dementia to understand a process, the potential biases of this situation should be considered. For example, Bamford and Bruce (2000) noted that, when asked for advice on participants for their focus group, staff excluded people with severe cognitive impairment, those with communication difficulties and those who disliked being sedentary.

Having sufficient time and being flexible

The experience of dementia is unique to each person, and a flexible approach to working with people with dementia needs to be taken. As discussed by Oyebode and Clare in Chapter 9, people with dementia process information at a slower rate than those without dementia. People with dementia have highlighted that they need more time to complete tasks and may become anxious if put under undue pressure:

> There are times of course when it is simply impossible for me to take part in anything. Apart from the gradual mental deterioration associated with Alzheimer's I often succumb to sporadic episodes of confusion which may last for just a day, or as much as a week, and to varying degrees of intensity ... On my good days I will give all I've got.

> (Robinson 2002: 104–5)

Providing a supportive social environment

Involvement approaches can be damaged by ignoring social cues. Hubbard *et al.* (2003) noted the feelings of a interviewee with dementia as she struggled to remember facts and reflected that by interjecting or prompting they could have reduced her embarrassment. Public perceptions of dementia can undermine a person's willingness to get involved in decisions or activities. Sharing positive messages and demonstrating the achievements of people with dementia can help to provide a more positive social context for involvement activities.

I went to the Newcastle convention a while ago and was totally amazed at what I saw. It was the first time I had seen people with dementia giving talks about the illness and their lives. Being there made me realise that I was certainly not alone and if other people could do this sort of thing then perhaps I should get involved. My wife said the change in me after this was remarkable ...

Living with Dementia (2006: June/July; 2)

Providing a supportive physical environment

Many people with dementia need environmental cues to understand the nature of what is being discussed (Dewing 2002). Some people find it easier to talk in a quiet, private place while others may be uncomfortable with this level of intensity. Allan (2001) suggests a flexible approach to finding an environment that suits the person.

Having a commitment to acting on the feedback received

People need to know when they have taken the time and trouble to contribute their perspective and be involved that it will be taken into account. The time needed for follow-up action, evaluation and feedback can easily be underestimated in the face of pressing organizational agendas (Cantley *et al.* 2005).

What does user involvement achieve?

In the involvement field in general, providers and researchers have begun to ask what evidence there is that user involvement improves services (Branfield and Beresford 2006) and service users have been questioning the usefulness of getting involved ('what difference does it actually make?'). Meanwhile, for people with dementia, it is a new experience to have their voice 'privileged' (Wilkinson 2002), to be listened to and to be influential. For example, within the Living with Dementia project, one participant said: 'It is nice to speak up for yourself instead of having professionals do it for you.' And staff often find their sense of meaning in the work they do with people with dementia is reinforced: 'You have a better understanding with the client and now have built a better relationship with them' (Allan 2001).

The development of appropriate methods and tools to support and enable service user involvement is still the main focus for researchers and practitioners, with any evaluation assessing the usefulness of methodologies rather than impact. As initiatives become more prevalent, it would be useful for future research to consider the development of outcome measures, in terms of service impact (to avoid tokenistic tick-boxing and the waste of people's time) and, most importantly, the impact for people with dementia, at all stages of their experience.

Debates and controversies

As we have seen in Chapter 3, people with dementia are a heterogeneous group. When seeking to involve people with dementia in service development and evaluation there is a danger that we will assume that all people with dementia have the same experience of a service, what Reid *et al.* (2001) refer to as an assumed 'uniformity of experience'. In addition, we are in danger of relying on those who are more articulate or more able to represent that experience. It is important to acknowledge that different service users will have different experiences of different services. The most effective way to do this is not always clear.

Working with people with dementia as service users can be difficult if people are unaware they have dementia or do not have insight into their condition. However, this can be overcome by using terms preferred by the service user such as 'memory problems' and by discussing a 'representation' (Reid *et al.* 2001) of the aims of the involvement process, for example, in Reid's case asking about what it is like 'being here' rather than discussing the day centre. Any opinions expressed are still credible and valid regarding the issue at hand.

Sometimes we may be unsure as to the meaning of what is being communicated (Dewing 2002). Bamford and Bruce (2002) have cautioned against interpreting metaphors in story-telling, especially as participants did not always recall comments or stories they had told. They also suggest that participation in a focus group or interview may provide a welcome distraction from usual routines and activities and so may result in the expression of predominantly positive views. Group settings can also result in people giving idealized 'public' accounts of their feelings, which are sometimes contradicted in subsequent contributions by the same participant. Using proxies to gain important information must be done cautiously and skilfully. The extent to which proxies are used, and determining the point at which they should be consulted, remain controversial.

Although we have said that involvement should be expected throughout the experience of dementia, the reality is that a lot of involvement activity is with people who are in the earlier stages. There is still much work to be done to ensure that the voice of people throughout their whole experience of dementia is accessed in practice. There remains disagreement about the most effective ways to involve people throughout the course of dementia.

Conclusion

The involvement of people with dementia as service users, although a relatively new area of work, has developed a momentum that is seeing the appearance of a growing amount of innovative practice, led to some extent by people with dementia. Now the 'voice' of the person with dementia has emerged, and there are methods available to ensure that voice is heard, the key will be to take action with or on behalf of those voices. Although the experience of dementia is unique to each individual, there is a collective voice emerging, which expects to be listened to and is beginning to set its own agendas and priorities. Many researchers and practitioners are enthused by the possibilities this presents and will continue to chart new waters, with people with dementia as our teachers: 'Like Columbus, I am on a voyage of discovery. My route is not exact and I must make adjustments as I go along.'

Further information

The Scottish Dementia Working Group, Alzheimer Scotland, is run by people with dementia to campaign to improve services and attitudes towards people with dementia. It also provides information on local services in Scotland. The organization publishes a newsletter, *Dementia in Scotland*, with information on services, issues of importance to people with dementia and their carers, and government initiatives. It also publishes information on new treatments for dementia. The website is separated into three sections: (1) people worried about their memory; (2) people with dementia; and (3) carers (http://www.alzscot.org.uk/pages/sdwg).

The Dementia Advocacy and Support Network international is an international internet-based group of people with dementia. The group formally began in 2000 as an offshoot of the Coping with Personal Memory Loss group. It is primarily a mechanism for disseminating information about and to people with dementia.

The Alzheimer's Society is a membership organization that is working to improve the lives of people affected by dementia. It has 25,000 members including people with personal experience of dementia and professionals who provide or design services for people with dementia and their carers. The organization provides local support in the form of information to people and communities that are affected by dementia. There are similar organizations in most countries and many regions.

The Care Services Improvement Partnership has a useful guide for involving people with dementia called *Strengthening the Involvement of People with Dementia: A Resource for Implementation*. You can download this from their website.

References

Allan, K. (2001) *Communication and Consultation: Exploring Ways for Staff to Involve People with Dementia in Developing Services*. Bristol: Policy Press.

Alzheimer's Society Canada (2006) *Engaging People with Early Stage Alzheimer's Disease in the Work of the Alzheimer's Society*. Toronto: Imagine Canada.

Bamford, C. and Bruce, E. (2000) Defining the outcomes of community care: The perspectives of older people with dementia and their carers. *Ageing and Society*, 20: 543–70.

Bamford, C. and Bruce, E. (2002) Successes and challenges in using focus group with older people with dementia. In: H. Wilkinson (ed.) *The Perspective of People with Dementia: Research Methods and Motivations*. London: Jessica Kingsley.

Barnett, E. (2000) *Including the Person with Dementia in Designing and Delivering Care – 'I Need to Be Me!'* London: Jessica Kingsley.

Beard, R. (2004) Advocating voice: Organisational, historical and social milieux of the Alzheimer's disease movement. *Sociology of Health and Illness*, 26(6): 797–819.

Branfield, F. and Beresford, P. (2006) *Making User Involvement Work: Supporting Service User Networking and Knowledge*. York: Joseph Rowntree Foundation.

Bryden, C. (2005) *Dancing with Dementia: My Story of Living Positively with Dementia*. London: Jessica Kingsley.

Cantley, C., Woodhouse, J. and Smith, M. (2005) *Listen to Us: Involving People with Dementia in Planning and Developing Services*. Northumbria: Dementia North.

Cheston, R., Bender, M. and Byatt, S. (2000) Involving people who have dementia in the evaluation of services: A review. *Journal of Mental Health*, 9(5): 471–9.

Clare, L., Roth, I. and Pratt, R. (2005) Perceptions of change over time in early Alzheimer's disease. *Dementia*, 4(4): 487–520.

Dewing, J. (2002) From ritual to relationship: A person-centred approach to consent in qualitative research with older people who have a dementia. *Dementia*, 1(2): 157–71.

Goldsmith, M. (1996) *Hearing the Voice of People with Dementia: Opportunities and Obstacles*. London: Jessica Kingsley.

Hubbard, G., Downs, M. and Tester, S. (2003) Including older people with dementia in research: challenges and strategies. *Aging and Mental Health*, 7(5): 351–62.

Kitwood, T. (1997) The experience of dementia. *Ageing and Mental Health*, 1(1): 13–22.

Litherland, R. (2003) Listen to us. *Working with Older People*, 7(4): 17–20.

Pratt, R. (2002) Nobody's ever asked how I felt. In: H. Wilkinson (ed.) *The Perspective of People with Dementia: Research Methods and Motivations*. London: Jessica Kingsley.

Reed, J., Cook, G., Bolter, V. and Douglas, B. (2006) *Older People 'Getting Things Done': Involvement in Policy and Planning Initiatives*. York: Joseph Rowntree Foundation.

Reid, D., Ryan, T. and Enderby, P. (2001) What does it mean to listen to people with dementia? *Disability and Society*, 16(3): 377–92.

Robinson, E. (2002) Should people with Alzheimer's disease take part in research? In: H. Wilkinson (ed.) *The Perspective of People with Dementia: Research Methods and Motivations*. London: Jessica Kingsley.

Robson, P., Begum, N. and Locke, M. (2003) *Developing User Involvement: Working towards User Centred Practice in Voluntary Organisations*. Bristol: Policy Press.

Sainsbury Centre for Mental Health (2005) *Beyond the Water Towers: The Unfinished Revolution in Mental Health Services 1985–2005*. London: Sainsbury Centre for Mental Health.

Small, N. and Rhodes, P. (2001) *User Involvement and the Seriously Ill*. York: Joseph Rowntree Foundation.

Stallker, K., Gilliard, J. and Downs, M. (1999) Eliciting use perspectives on what works. *International Journal of Geriatric Psychiatry*, 14: 120–34.

Wilkinson, H. (2002) *The Perspective of People with Dementia: Research Methods and Motivations*. London: Jessica Kingsley.

23

A trained and supported workforce

Barbara Bowers

Learning objectives

By the end of this chapter, you will:

- understand the context within which the dementia care workforce is developing
- know the characteristics of people who work as paid caregivers for people with dementia
- understand paid carers' needs for support and the influence of training on work life quality
- understand the role of training in developing and maintaining a high quality workforce
- understand the components of effective dementia training programmes

Introduction

The preceding chapters clearly demonstrate the importance of skills, knowledge and commitment in providing high quality care for people with dementia, whether paid professionals, support workers, or family members. Although many people with dementia are cared for by family members throughout much of their illness (see Chapter 5), paid caregivers are frequently relied on at some point, sometimes supplementing the care provided by family members and sometimes taking over when families are unable to continue (see Chapters 5, 16 and 19). Despite the tremendous effort by families, as the number of people with dementia increases, the need for paid caregivers is also increasing. Parallel with this increased need is a worldwide shortage in health and social care workers, compounding the difficulty in finding sufficient caregivers for people with dementia (WHO 2006a). As care of older adults with dementia is one of the fastest growing areas of need worldwide, it will likely be one of the most affected by the international health worker shortage.

Recruiting and training skilled and compassionate workers to care for people with dementia has become a serious challenge for many nations (Mathers and Leionardi 2000). While recruiting new workers into the workforce will partially address the worker shortage, the issue is complicated by ongoing difficulties retaining workers, or high worker turnover rates. Although not all countries track worker turnover, the problem has been reported in many countries (Castle 2005; DEST 2008; Dyson 2007; Stack 2003). Increasingly, nations are shifting their focus from recruiting to retaining workers. This shift in focus has led to a greater emphasis on worker training and support.

In addition to finding and keeping a sufficient number of workers to provide care, there is mounting evidence that many dementia care workers may be inadequately trained for the work they do. This chapter will outline: the factors that challenge efforts to recruit dementia care workers; the strategies used to recruit new workers and develop the dementia care workforce; what is known about the workers who care for people with dementia; the experiences of people who provide dementia care; and the impact of education and support on both the quality of care and the quality of the work environment.

The context of workforce development

An international issue

Most nations are experiencing a general ageing of their populations and with it a dramatic increase in the number of people with dementia (Mathers and Leonardi 2000). While dementia is well recognized as an increasing health issue in Western, developed nations, epidemiological data suggest it is distributed equally (geographically) throughout the world and between developed and developing nations. For example, almost half of all people with dementia are living in Asia, while 30% live in Europe and 12% in North America (Anders *et al.* 2003; Mathers and Leonardi 2000; WHO 2006b, see Chapter 1). A comparison between developed and developing nations reveals that an estimated 52% of all people with dementia are currently living in developing nations (Anders *et al.* 2003), making dementia care a global issue.

The worker shortage

> An unprecedented demand for long-term care services, driven in part by the aging of the world's population, is leading to a shortage of supply of workers who can provide care.
>
> (Ladan (2005), President, AARP Global Network)

According to a report from the WHO Global Health Workforce Alliance, there is a serious and rapidly growing international health worker shortage (WHO 2005). As populations continue to age around the world, and the number of people with dementia continues to rise, the availability of an adequate workforce to provide that care will become an increasingly urgent issue. Not all nations are equally affected by the shortage. The worker shortage is most acute in developing nations. This can be partially explained by 'the pull of higher salaries in industrialized countries and the push of poor working conditions at home [which] drive thousands of health workers to jobs abroad each year' (WHO 2005: 8).

Compounding the general shortage of health workers is the almost universal lower remuneration for aged care work compared with work in other health sector jobs as well as the common perception of aged care work as less desirable, and less prestigious than work in other health sectors (Beck *et al.*

1999; Korczyk 2004), an experience common to aged care workers around the world. Not surprisingly then, in many countries the health worker shortage is most acute, in settings that care for people with dementia.

Responses to the workforce shortage

The strategies used to expand the aged care workforce vary. For example, developing nations focus their efforts internally, on improving access to training programmes and improving working conditions, while developed nations are looking abroad, actively recruiting workers from other (mostly developing) nations (Korczyj 2004; WHO 2005).

Recruiting abroad

A growing practice known as 'insourcing' is used, primarily by developed nations, to increase their health workforce (WHO 2005). This involves importing workers from other (generally emerging) nations to address their worker shortage (WHO 2005). A large international industry has developed to assist in this practice. As a result discussions about the ethics of 'poaching' workers from struggling nations have been increasing (DoH 2004; Young 2007).

Recruiting abroad, has consequences for the nations losing workers as well as for the destination countries. The loss of skilled workers has obvious negative consequences for countries of origin and for their ability to meet their own need for workers. There are also consequences for the destination countries such as growing resistance to immigration and to the necessity of immigrant settlement programmes. Resistance is particularly acute in destination countries experiencing high levels of unemployment (Hoppe 2005; Korczyk 2004). One consequence of this is a backlash against immigrants, resulting in political pressures that may undermine the development of effective resettlement services, preventing them from integrating into their new communities (Manteghi 2005).

Recruiting internally

Recruiting internally primarily involves attracting workers already engaged in the same type of work. While this might temporarily improve the situation in a particular organization or area, it is certainly not a long-term solution as it does not create a net addition to the worker pool. This continual recruiting also leads to great mobility among workers. This mobility increases costs and undermines the quality of care. In addition to the high cost of turnover, workforce instability also undermines quality of care and quality of life (Coleman 2003a, b; Fleming *et al.* 2003). More recent programmes have attempted to encourage young people to consider careers in aged care, bring retired workers back into the workforce, and even enlist family caregivers into the paid workforce (Stone *et al.* 2007a).

Attitudes toward aged care and dementia care

Recruiting efforts are undermined by general attitudes toward care of older adults and people with dementia. The same negative attitudes are even reflected among health care professionals: nurses, therapists, medical doctors and social workers where caring for older people is not a popular career choice (Poirrier 1994). One study of Danish health care workers found that only 4% had a positive attitude about caring for people with dementia (Astrom *et al.* 1987; Kim 2006). Surveys of students in health-related occupations around the world reflect similar attitudes (Briscoe 2005; Kim 2006; McLafferty 2004).

Responding to this challenge are studies designed to identify the factors that influence student attitudes and to design programmes that improve attitudes of future health professionals. Educational models that have demonstrated success include scheduling aged care clinical experiences late in the educational programme, using passionate, knowledgeable teachers/mentors who see aged care as exciting and challenging, and ensuring that students will be given sophisticated and challenging work to do during their experiences (Burbank *et al.* 2006; Plowfield *et al.* 2006). These strategies contrast sharply with the common practice of putting beginning students in nursing home experiences and using nursing homes to practise basic skills such as injections and bed baths, leaving students with the impression that care of older adults is simple and unexciting or that not much can be done.

Workers in aged care are also generally paid less than they could earn in other health sector jobs, reinforcing the notion that the work requires less skill. In the USA the low pay is compounded by the frequently poor health insurance coverage for workers, putting them at risk for their own health problems. This is especially true in home care and assisted living (Bowers 2001; Crown *et al.* 1995; GAO 2001).

Dementia care: where is it needed?

A need that crosses settings and specialties

The focus of this chapter is on workers employed in settings specifically designated for older adults. However, it should be remembered that health care workers in all settings (hospitals, clinics, home care, and hospices) and specialty areas (emergency, orthopaedics, surgery, etc.) will be caring for some people who have dementia. For example, in the USA half of hospital days are used by older adults, half of whom are estimated to have some dementia (NHPCO 2007; Silverstein and Maslow 2006; see Chapter 17). Statistics from the USA, Hong Kong, the Netherlands and Nigeria document that a high number of ambulance transfers and emergency care visits, and hospital admissions are for older people (Akande 2004; Lee *et al.* 2001; NCHS 2005; van Charante *et al.* 2007). Therefore, contrary to common assumptions, understanding how to care for people with dementia is relevant to most health care settings and providers, not only those that are specifically aged care.

Dementia care in specialized settings

Assisted living

Assisted living is the fastest growing housing choice for older adults in the USA (Hyde *et al.* 2007; Teri *et al.* 2005) where over 2 million people are currently living. It is estimated that more than half of assisted living residents have some degree of dementia. The number of people in assisted living is expected to increase rapidly, eventually overtaking the number of people living in nursing homes (Teri *et al.* 2005). A report from the Australian Institute of Health and Welfare (2004) suggests a similar situation in Australia, with 50% of residents in low care (less dependent residents) having either probable or possible dementia. In both countries, little is known about the workers who provide care, their level of education, their knowledge of dementia, their attitudes toward people with dementia, their training opportunities after taking the job, or their care practices. One thing we know is that they are less closely supervised than are workers in nursing homes or residential aged care, working in relative isolation, making the adequacy of their training an even more important issue than it is for nursing home workers.

Nursing homes

Once believed to be a phenomenon of Western nations, nursing homes are found increasingly around the world. In Taiwan, for example, numbers of nursing homes increased five-fold between 1996 and 2001 (Tu *et al.* 2006). Korea and Japan have also seen a dramatic rise in the number of nursing homes (Lee 2002; Nagatomo *et al.* 2001). Estimates vary concerning the percentage of older adults in residential aged care who have dementia. However, recent estimates suggest the rate is between 40% and 85% (Cipher *et al.* 2006; Feldman *et al.* 2006).

Home care

While not necessarily considered an aged care work setting, the majority of home care patients are over 65. In the USA, 70% of home care visits are for people over 65, many of who are over 75 (NCHS 2004). This large percentage of older patients reflects, in part, the higher incidence of illness among older adults and the increasing number of older adults. It also reflects efforts by governments around the world to address both the shortage of workers in aged care and the cost of long-term care, by encouraging older people, including people with dementia, to remain at home as long as possible (Korczyk 2004). Even when families are highly involved, many people, and their families, will eventually need help from the formal care network, including home care. Understanding how to care for people with dementia is vital for home care workers as they are a major resource to families and they are working without the benefit of co-workers and supervisors who can provide ready assistance.

Aged care/dementia care workers

Worker characteristics

A WHO report confirms that (with few exceptions) health workers around the world have common characteristics (Spratley *et al.* 2000: WHO 2005). While data on aged care workers (nursing homes, home care, assisted living) in particular, are not widely available, data from the USA suggest that aged care workers differ in several ways from workers in other health sectors. They tend to be older, poorer, less well educated, primarily female (generally 90–95%), often employed part-time, and with unpredictable work hours (Crown *et al.* 1995; Korczyk 2004; GAO 2001; Spratley *et al.* 2000), and in the USA are less likely than other service workers to have health cover (Stone *et al.* 2007b). There is also evidence that many workers in aged care have extremely complicated and stressful personal lives (Tellis-Nayak and Tellis-Nayak 1989).

Worker skill and knowledge

Available evidence suggests that aged care workers have less formal training for their work than do other workers in health-related fields (Beck *et al.* 1999; Korczyk 2004). While some nations, such as Sweden, the Netherlands and Germany, are attempting to increase the basic educational requirements for aged care workers, many nations continue to rely primarily on personal experience (e.g. housewife experience), or more recently on past employment in a similar work setting, as a skill base (Korczyk 2004). This lower level of training both reflects and contributes to the perception that workers in this field are unskilled, which in turn works to keep wages low.

As it becomes more and more apparent that aged care and dementia care require a special skill set, many nations are struggling with questions about how and how much to invest in the development of an appropriate workforce. Many countries still rely on a personal and/or experiential skill base, supplementing this with knowledge or skill deemed to be basic to the work (Korczyc 2004). Whether that supplementary training includes dementia and dementia care varies widely. In some countries workers in aged care are required to complete basic training in dementia and dementia care. For example, in the USA, nurse aides (who provide 80–90% of direct care in nursing homes and most of the direct care in assisted living and home settings) are required to complete a 75-hour general aged care training programme (varying somewhat by state) and to pass a certification exam. The federal government currently mandates some portion of this time be devoted to care of people with 'cognitively impaired individuals' and 'communicating with people who have a cognitive impairments' (Federal Regulations 2005). In other countries, including many developed nations, there are no such requirements (Korczyk 2004).

In discussions about whether training should be mandated, what that training should include, and what experience or skills can be transferred from other types of experience, it is important to determine the basic competencies needed for aged care and dementia care work. There is growing consensus about what competencies are needed for dementia care work. Many of these are outlined in previous chapters. For example, the knowledge areas that are generally considered important for dementia care workers include: understanding the behaviour of people with dementia and knowing how to communicate (see Chapters 3, 4, 11, 12 and 14); understanding person-centred and relationship care (see Chapters 4, 5, 20, 23, 25 and 27); and assessing and promoting the well-being of people who have dementia (see Chapters 2, 8, 11, 13, 14, 15, 17, 19 and 27). Specific competencies identified by international organizations such as Alzheimer's associations and foundations generally include: basic knowledge of dementia, person-centred care and quality of life for people with dementia, communicating with someone who has dementia, and responding to distressing or aggressive behaviour (MDC 2006).

Exercise 23.1   Finding and developing competent dementia care workers: dementia care as an employment programme

You have taken a summer job with your local council. One of the issues they have given you to work on is developing a group of workers who can provide some respite for family carers of people with dementia in your city. So far you have received several suggestions about how to proceed. One particularly influential council member has suggested that your project could solve two problems simultaneously. First, it could help family carers. Second, it could solve an employment problem caused by a recent clothing factory closure.

How will you respond?

Developing and supporting a high quality workforce

The impact of education on quality of work life and quality of care

There is ample evidence that education, if conducted effectively, has a positive impact on the quality of work life and the quality of care provided by dementia care workers (Noel *et al.* 2000). However, the links between education and competencies and between competencies and practice are not necessarily direct. That is, education does not always result in competence and being competent to perform does not ensure a competent performance. Therefore, in determining how to best educate a workforce to care for people with dementia, it would be useful to understand the impact of education on practice. Fortunately there is considerable evidence available (McCabe *et al.* 2007; Sveinsdottir *et al.* 2006).

Focus of educational programmes: behaviours that cause stress for staff

Although there are several generally accepted areas of competence for dementia care workers, most of the dementia education programmes focus on the behaviour that staff find distressing. Significantly, a review of research on staff training programmes to improve the quality of care, focusing on 'behaviour management' concluded that effective educational programmes have significant 'secondary benefits' (Kuske *et al.* 2006; McCabe *et al.* 2007), that is increased staff satisfaction, reduced staff stress and decreased staff turnover. Intervention studies are similar in their emphasis on teaching staff to prevent and respond to distressing behaviours. This is not surprising as the 'behaviour' of people with dementia has been repeatedly identified, by aged care workers around the world, as one of their greatest sources of stress (Beck *et al.* 1999; Brodaty *et al.* 2003; Coogle *et al.* 2007; Davison *et al.* 2007; Nagatomo *et al.* 2001;

Pekkarinen *et al.* 2004; Roper *et al.* 2001). While some of this research looked at resident satisfaction and quality of life, the focus has been on staff stress, increasing job satisfaction and decreasing worker turnover. There is even some evidence that we are losing many of the most caring and committed workers (Bowers and Becker 1992).

More recently, however, there has been greater acknowledgement that the distressing behaviour is often a failed attempt to communicate, and that the distress of the person with dementia can be addressed along with the distress of the worker, by improving the workers' ability to communicate with the person who has dementia. Keep in mind what you learned in Chapters 4 and 11, specifically the importance and effectiveness of reading and understanding 'behaviour' as a way to communicate more effectively with someone who has even advanced dementia. Another important finding is that worker stress strongly influences the quality of interactions between residents and staff (Sourial *et al.* 2001).

The research on residential aged care and dementia care workers has documented a clear relationship between distressing resident behaviours and staff stress. Aggressive resident behaviour, in particular, increases worker stress. The significance of this can be underscored, particularly in nursing home environments, by estimates that 28% of nursing home residents engage in behaviours considered 'seriously' problematic for staff, while an additional 31% engage in behaviours that are at least 'mildly problematic' for staff (Heponiemi *et al.* 2006; Nametz and Jesudason 1990).

The impact of education: what the research suggests

Recognizing the stress associated with the type of work, researchers have conducted many studies to examine the impact of worker knowledge about dementia on worker stress levels. Findings have consistently indicated that lack of knowledge about dementia, particularly how to prevent and respond to 'distressing behaviour', is a common and powerful source of stress for workers (Beck *et al.* 1999; Davison *et al.* 2007; Kim 2006; Palmer and Withee 1996; Ruiz *et al.* 2006). Recently, a number of intervention studies have demonstrated clearly that an effective educational programme on understanding and responding appropriately to aggressive or distressing behaviour will both reduce worker stress and improve the quality of care they provide.

A study conducted in Australia demonstrated both a short- and long-term reduction in worker stress following an 8-session, combined didactic and experiential dementia education programme. Results showed an increase in worker self-efficacy, a dramatic improvement in performance (as assessed by supervisors), and a reduction in resident behaviours that staff found distressing (Davison *et al.* 2007). A study by Chrzescijanski *et al.* (2007) in Australia also found a decrease in resident behaviour that was experienced by staff as distressing, following an educational programme designed to improve staff attitudes toward people with dementia. Specifically, this study found that staff were better able to identify indicators of resident distress, and to respond accordingly after a multi-session, 3-month educational programme.

A study in the USA examined the impact of a computer-based dementia training program on staff attitudes, knowledge and self-efficacy. Using separate modules, a variety of presentation formats designed to target a range of learner styles, and follow-up training, these researchers found improvements in knowledge, attitudes and self-efficacy of workers. In another study conducted in 15 nursing homes, Teri and her colleagues (2005) also demonstrated a positive impact of staff training on worker stress and, significantly, on the quality of care. In particular, improvements in care were documented in relation to prevention of and responses to distressing resident behaviour. As in the study by Davison, this study showed a decrease in resident distress levels following the training programme.

In a study of three nursing homes, using ten one-hour sessions with a psychologist, workers' ability to read emotional cues, both body language and facial expression, greatly enhanced the communication between the person with dementia and the caregiver (Magai *et al.* 2002) One of the most significant findings from the research in this area is the ability of staff, following a carefully designed training programme, to more effectively interpret and respond to resident behaviour. The ability to read resident cues more effectively clearly results in less aggressive behaviour on the part of people with dementia, leading to a better quality of life for them as well as the workers who care for them. This study clearly ties resident distress to staff stress, encouraging workers and researchers to look more closely at the residents' experience and perspective when designing practice change.

What makes a successful educational programme?

Although a number of studies have documented the positive impact of training programmes on worker effectiveness in dealing with behaviour they find distressing, other studies have not shown such positive results. The effectiveness of dementia care training programmes parallels what has been documented about the effectiveness of staff development more generally. This section will briefly review the research on staff development in general and in long-term care before describing the research on training specific to dementia care.

Research on the relationship between education and practice change has come from many fields. A consistent finding is that new knowledge, by itself, rarely results in practice change and almost never leads to sustained changes in practice (Broad 1997). Lasting practice change requires an effective training programme, learner preparation prior to the training, and sustained, targeted support following the educational session (Cromwell and Kolb 2004). While learner characteristics are often assumed to be the primary determinant in whether new learning is applied in the practice setting, research suggests otherwise (Cromwell and Kolb 2004). In a review of research examining the transfer of new learning to work settings, Cromwell and Kolb (2004) conclude that worker intent to use the new knowledge, worker confidence, voluntariness of attendance at the training programme, and support of supervisors and peers, collectively, determine the eventual use of knowledge gained.

While intent-to-use new knowledge, worker confidence and voluntariness of attendance at the educational programme might appear to reflect personal characteristics of the worker, they are also highly related to, and largely determined by, the supervisor and the work environment. For example, the review conducted by Cromwell and Kolb, showed how support and encouragement of supervisors can positively influence both worker intent to use new knowledge and worker confidence. Voluntariness of attendance is also related to supervisor effectiveness in that sending the right worker to the right training programme, matching worker interests with opportunities, increases the voluntariness of attendance and subsequently the likelihood that new learning will be used to improve practice (Cromwell and Kolb 2004).

A review of research on the effectiveness of staff development programmes in long-term care revealed that many training programmes, both dementia-specific and others, were not designed to maximize the transfer of learning back to the practice setting. Half of all dementia-specific staff development studies reported using no preparation or follow-up, significantly diminishing the possibilities for success. Only 5 of 48 educational programmes reviewed in one analysis included workplace reinforcement following the educational programme (Aylward *et al.* 2003; Kuske *et al.* 2006; Stolee *et al.* 2005). Although critical of the general quality of research on staff development in long-term care, Kuske *et al.* (2006) confirmed that preparation of the learner, the use of adult education principles, supervisor support, and worksite reinforcement all contribute to the effectiveness and longevity of training impact. This finding is consistent with the studies reviewed earlier in this chapter concerning the impact of training programmes on communication skill and stress levels of workers. Programmes that were successful were the ones with ongoing reinforcement, supervisor support and careful attention to learning styles.

Exercise 23.2   Characteristics of a good dementia care worker

You are the director of nursing in a residential aged care home. You have recently recruited someone to be in charge of staff development for your organization. Her plans are to develop an extensive orientation programme for people who have no experience in aged care, making sure they know about dementia before they start working. She is also focusing on recruiting people with great interpersonal skills, as she believes they make the best aged care workers. This would also allow her to focus her training efforts on people who don't have these skills.

You have been asked to review her plan. What are your thoughts?

Supporting and retaining dementia care workers

Turnover and retention of workers

Although many countries do not keep national statistics on turnover rates of workers caring for older adults, staff turnover has been consistently identified as a serious challenge to maintaining an adequate and competent workforce in developed nations around the world. Literature from Australia (Chou *et al.* 2002; Moyle *et al.* 2003), New Zealand (Kiata *et al.* 2005) and Taiwan (Sung *et al.* 2005) has also identified staff retention/turnover in aged care and dementia care settings as an ongoing and serious problem. Since the early

1980s the literature on residential aged care has reflected a serious concern over recruiting and retaining a qualified workforce. Since that time, we have learned quite a bit about how to recruit and retain workers, and about the circumstances that promote worker turnover.

In the USA, turnover rates for nurse aides in residential aged care have been well documented, with some reaching over 100% annually (IOM 2001). For supervising nurses, the rate of annual turnover has averaged around 50%. Even managers in residential aged care settings leave their jobs at relatively high rates, around 40% annually (Castle 2005). Although not as high as the figures just provided, non-residential aged care settings and assisted living also experience problems with worker turnover. Turnover is a serious problem for several reasons. First, relationships with care workers have been repeatedly identified by older people receiving services as one of the most important aspects of care quality. In addition to having a worker who is familiar with your preferences and needs, the relationship itself is extremely important for quality of life (Bowers *et al.* 2006; Foner 1994). Second, worker retention has implications for maintaining the workforce skill level as turnover makes it difficult to maintain the necessary skills. Third, high turnover leads to inadequate staffing, which in turn causes worker stress.

Causes of worker turnover

Most of the published research on turnover relates to front-line workers (personal carers/care assistants), those who do the majority of the hands-on work in nursing homes, assisted living and home care. Causes of turnover for these workers are varied and well documented. Workplace stress and turnover are related to some of the issues already discussed such as insufficient skills and knowledge, poor compensation and low status of work. Other factors contributing to turnover, documented in several countries, are: aggression and violence in the work setting; inadequate staffing; not being able to participate in decision-making about care; lack of respect from management/supervisors; physical demands and risks of the work; and poor supervision (Dunn *et al.* 1994; Moyle *et al.* 2003).

Aggression and assaults

According to the US Government Occupational Safety and Health Office (Michael 2002), aged care work has one of the highest rates of worker injury and has been established as one of the most dangerous worksites in the USA (Michael 2002). Data compiled by the Canadian government have also documented a high rate of worker injuries in long-term care settings (Yassi *et al.* 2004). Repeated exposure to aggressive and/or demanding behaviour, from both residents and family, is common in long-term care (Morrison and Siu 2000; Secrest *et al.* 2005; Vinton and Mazza 1994) and has a negative impact on both job satisfaction and job performance (Chappel and Novak 1994). Staff training has been shown to decrease resident aggression and assaults on workers. For example, a study examining the impact of a training programme to teach nurse aides to prevent and deal effectively with aggression, Maxfield *et al.* (1996) documented a reduction in resident aggression following the intervention. The researchers provided two one-hour training sessions with follow-up visits and instruction to improve care particularly during bathing and grooming. Consequently, two hours of training had a significant impact on quality of care and injuries related to resident aggression. Other studies have found similar results (Chrzescijanski *et al.* 2007; Palmer and Withee 1996).

Assaults on workers are also less frequent in specialty dementia care units where workers are likely to be trained in care of people with dementia (Morgan *et al.* 2005; Vinton and Mazza 1994). Worker stress and less training were correlated with a higher incidence of assaults from residents.

Inadequate preparation

Depression

Care workers find it stressful to care for people with chronic depression. As depression is common among nursing home residents, estimated to be somewhere between 10% and 40% (Burgio *et al.* 1988; Nametz and Jesudason 1990), this is probably a significant and widespread source of stress for staff. A study in Japan demonstrated a high correlation between dementia and depression, also finding that people with dementia who are depressed are more likely to engage in behaviours that are stressful for workers (Nagatomo *et al.* 2001). This would indicate that educational programmes for dementia care workers should include the development of skills to identify and respond to depression and that better general treatment of depression would lead to lower levels of stress among workers.

Daily care

Daily care is a common source of difficulty for inadequately trained staff, especially when working with people who have dementia. Several studies have examined the impact of training on bathing, feeding and daily care of residents with dementia. These studies, collectively, show a reduction in aggression, and better resident nutrition when workers are skilled in communicating with people who have dementia (Chang and Lin 2005; Chang and Madigan 2006; Hoeffer *et al.* 2006). Another study (Stevens *et al.* 1998) demonstrated the effectiveness of combined nurse aide training and improved supervision by nurses for increasing resident self-care. This same study demonstrated that a combination of formal training and structured self-monitoring can improve the quality of nurse aides' responses to resident anxiety and distress (Stevens 1998) Effective training can clearly reduce the distress experienced by people with dementia, and as a consequence, their caregivers.

Staffing

Inadequate staffing has been consistently correlated with high levels of stress among workers (Bowers and Becker 2002; Chappel and Novak 1992; IOM 2001) and has been correlated with worker injury rates (Trinkoff *et al.* 2005). Although many nations have now enacted minimum staffing levels for at least high acuity residential aged care settings, many aged care staff find the workload to be extremely heavy, often finding it impossible to complete their assigned work in the time allotted (Bowers 1987; Bowers *et al.* 2001). As a consequence, workers often leave at the end of their shift feeling that they had not provided high quality care, had not met their own expectations or those of their supervisors and co-workers (Bowers 1987; Foner 1994). Inadequate staffing has an impact on care quality (Harrington *et al.* 2000) and is a particularly important issue in dementia care settings where rushing residents and maintaining a rigid schedule can cause resident distress, and as a result, staff stress. Inadequate staffing levels have also been linked to worker injury in residential aged care settings. The relatively older age of the workforce in aged care, as compared to workers in other health care environments, compounds the impact of heavy physical work.

Not feeling valued or respected: the importance of good supervision

Extensive research in residential aged care settings indicates that many workers feel unsupported and devalued, particularly by the professional staff and managers in their work settings and by families of the people they care for (Bowers *et al.* 2003; Brannon *et al.* 2007; Foner 1994; Noelker *et al.* 2006; Ryzin 2007). Not feeling supported or valued by their supervisors is the main reason workers in aged care settings decide to leave their jobs (Bowers *et al.* 2003; McGillis *et al.* 2005). While carers working in aged care, around the world, have identified this as a major source of dissatisfaction, licensed staff and managers in the same environments often speak about the respect and admiration they have for the carers (Bowers *et al.* 2003; Brannon *et al.* 2007; Castle *et al.* 2007). This apparent contradiction seems to be a reflection of the difference between carers and their supervisors about what constitutes a positive work environment and positive relationships between carers and their supervisors. The sources of these differences are discussed below. Managers have been shown to play a pivotal role in the implementation of new practice models in innovative practice such as self-managed work teams (Yeattes and Seward 2000). Worker stress and satisfaction are also directly related to the quality of care (Sikorska-Simmons 2006). Supervisory training has been shown to improve supervisory skills and working conditions (McDonald and Kahn 2007).

Not having a say

Front-line workers (carers, nurse aides) often feel unable to participate in care planning as they are either not invited or are unable to attend care conferences (Gurnik and Hollis-Sawyer 2003; McDonald and Kahn 2007; Stone *et al.* 2002). While supervisors often extend an invitation to carers to attend these meetings, the work demands generally prevent them from participating. Consequently, the invitation is often perceived by carers as disingenuous, creating resentment. In response to this, involving carers more actively and consistently in care decisions is a core goal of the nursing home culture change movement (Kane *et al.* 2007) which has been designed to improve quality of care and quality of work life (see Chapter 26).

Emotional distress

Aged care workers experience a high level of emotional distress. One reason for this is that caring for and becoming bonded to people who are at the end of life, means that workers experience continual loss of people they have become attached to. Workers have described particular emotional turmoil when they believe an older person is dying, not wanting the person to die alone (Parks *et al.* 2005) Seeing residents with untreated pain is also a source of great emotional stress for workers (Cipher *et al.* 2006).

Exercise 23.3   Developing programmes to keep staff

You have just taken a job in the human resources department of an organization that operates a home care programme, two assisted living sites and three nursing homes. Staff turnover has become a serious problem over the past few years, costing the organization quite a bit of money for retraining and orientation. You are asked to head a project designed to retain staff. The first suggestion you receive is to develop an interview guide so that you can screen applicants more carefully.

What is your response?

What workers say about working with people with dementia

Many workers come to think of the people they care for as family, finding great rewards in the relationship and their ability to make a difference in their lives (Foner 1994; Secrest *et al.* 2005) Studies from several countries have validated that workers in long-term care settings, caring for people with dementia, are highly satisfied with their work, whether or not they are happy with their working conditions (Stone *et al.* 2002; Moyle *et al.* 2003). Workers with prior experience caring for family or friends with dementia are even more likely to find their work satisfying (Bowers 1987; Coogle *et al.* 2007; Maas *et al.* 1994)

A survey conducted in Sweden across care environments found that while nurses working in dementia care environments perceived greater emotional conflicts and greater knowledge demands than did nurses in other environments, they also reported a higher sense of support from colleagues than did nurses in other elderly care environments (Josefsson *et al.* 2007). An important finding is that workers with previous rewarding experience caring for friends or family are less likely to remain on their job (Coogle *et al.* 2007). A study of how nurse aides think about their work (Bowers 1987) suggests that it is the inability to provide high quality under adverse working conditions that drives these workers away.

Debates and controversies

Providing effective education and support for workers in dementia care will result in high quality care and workers who are likely to enjoy their work and remain in their jobs. This requires effective educational programmes and effective supervision of dementia care workers. Dementia care educational programmes are too often uninformed by what we know is successful, wasting valuable resources and raising expectations that are not subsequently met.

One of the most important influences on the quality of work life is the quality of supervision. Despite this, there are few serious efforts to develop the skills of supervisory staff or to hold them accountable for effective supervision. Maintaining a competent, stable workforce will require much greater commitment to the improvement of working conditions, such as effective, supportive supervisors.

The level of compensation for workers caring for older people and people with dementia continues to be inadequate. This workforce continues to be paid less than other workers, despite the demanding and stressful working conditions, the emotional and physical challenges of the work, and the difficult home lives of many people in this workforce.

Finally, one of the most contentious issues, worldwide, is the level of staffing in residential settings despite the convincing documentation that inadequate staffing hurts both workers and the people they care for.

Conclusion

Dementia care workers will be needed in increasing numbers around the world. The international competition for health workers, along with high turnover rates, has created workforce instability with negative consequences for both workers and the people they care for. There are reasons to believe that the instability of the workforce can be effectively addressed with high quality educational programmes, improved skills of supervisors, and other consistently favourable working conditions. In particular, research has demonstrated the effectiveness of well-designed educational programmes in improving many of the work-related situations that workers find most stressful. Dementia care workers are generally satisfied with their work, find it rewarding, and are motivated to remain by strong bonds with the people they care for.

Further information

The Pioneer Network Exchange is a network of care homes that are committed to improving the culture of nursing homes, improving care quality and working conditions. It has created a loose affiliation among homes from all over the USA that work together to promote person-centred values in resident care and respect for care providers. It is a grass roots organization started in the 1980s.

The Paraprofessional Healthcare Institute is an organization operated by care workers. It provides a forum for discussing issues, and disseminates reports that are relevant to the working conditions in care homes.

Better Jobs/Better Care was a national initiative funded by the Robert Wood Johnson Foundation that is committed to enhancing both work life for care workers across settings and for the people receiving services. The initiative, housed in the American Association of Homes and Services for the Aging, managed a four-year initiative that included innovative demonstration projects as well as research.

The WHO- Global Workforce Alliance is a WHO-sponsored alliance of worker organizations and governments to track working conditions, need for workers, and the movement of workers around the world. The website keeps up-to-date information from many countries around the world as well as historical reports on workforce changes over time.

References

Akande, T. (2004) Referral system in Nigeria: Study of a tertiary health facility. *Annals of African Medicine*, 3(3): 130–3.

Anders, W., Winblad, B., Aguero Torres, H. and von Strauss, E. (2003) The magnitude of dementia occurrence in the world. *Alzheimer's Disease & Associated Disorders*, 17(2): 63–7.

Astrom, S., Adolfsson, R., Sandman, P.O., Wedman, I. and Winblad, B. (1987) Attitudes of health care personnel towards demented patients. *Comprehensive Gerontology*, 1: 94–9.

Australian Institute of Health and Welfare (2004) *The Impact of Dementia on the Health and Aged Care Systems*. Canberra: AIHW. Available at: http://www.aihw.gov.au/publications/index.cfm/title/10011 (accessed 15 January 2008).

Aylward, S., Stolee, P., Keat, N. and Johncox, V. (2003) Effectiveness of continuing education in long-term care: a literature review. *The Gerontologist*, 43(2): 259–71.

Beck, C., Ortigara, A., Mercer, S. and Shue, V. (1999) Enabling and empowering certified nursing assistants for quality dementia care. *International Journal of Geriatric Psychiatry*, 14(7): 197–212.

Bowers, B. (1987) Intergenerational caregiving: Adult caregivers and their aging parents. *Advances in Nursing Science*, 9(2): 20–31.

Bowers, B. (2001) *The Work of Nurses and Nurse Aides in Long Term Care facilities*. IOM Committee on Work Environments for Nurses and Patient Safety. Institute of Medicine. Washington, DC: National Academy Press.

Bowers, B. and Becker, M. (1992) Nurse aides in nursing homes: The relationship between organization and quality. *The Gerontologist*, 32: 360–6.

Bowers, B., Esmond, S. and Jacobson, N. (2003) Turnover reinterpreted: CNAs talk about why they leave. *Journal of Gerontological Nursing*, 29: 36–43.

Bowers, B., Esmond, S., Norton, S. and Holloway, E. (2006) The consumer/provider relationship as care quality mediator. In: S. Kunkel and V. Wellin (eds) *Consumer Voice and Choice in Long Term Care*. New York: Springer Publishing.

Bowers, B.J., Lauring, C. and Jacobson, N. (2001) How nurses manage time and work in long-term care facilities. *Journal of Advanced Nursing*, 33(4): 484–91.

Brannon, D., Barry, T., Kemper, P., Schreiner, A. and Vasey, J. (2007) Job perceptions and intent to leave among direct care workers. *The Gerontologist*, 47(6): 820–7.

Briscoe, V.J. (2007) The effects of gerontology nursing teaching methods on nursing student knowledge, attitudes, and desire to work with older adult clients. Unpublished doctoral dissertation, Walden University.

Broad, M. (1997) Overview of transfer of training: From learning to performance. *Performance Improvement Quarterly*, 10(2): 7–21.

Brodaty, H., Draper, B. and Low, L. (2003) Nursing home staff attitudes towards residents with dementia: strain and satisfaction with work. *Journal of Advanced Nursing*, 44(6): 583–90.

Burbank, P.M., Dowling-Castronovo, A., Crowther, M.R. and Capezuti, E.A. (2006) Improving knowledge and attitudes toward older adults through innovative educational strategies. *Journal of Professional Nursing*, 22(2): 91–7.

Burgio, D., Jones, L., Butler, F. and Engle, (1988) Behavior problems in an urban nursing home. *Journal of Gerontological Nursing*, 14: 31–4.

Castle, N. (2005) Turnover begets turnover. *The Gerontologist*, 45(2): 186–94.

Castle, N., Engberg, J. and Men, A. (2007) Nursing home staff turnover: Impact on nursing home compare quality measures. *The Gerontologist*, 47(5): 650–61.

Chang, C. and Lin, L. (2005) Effects of a feeding skills training programme on nursing assistants and dementia patients. *Journal of Clinical Nursing*, 14: 1185–92.

Chang, C. and Madigan, A. (2006) The effect of a feeding skills training program for nursing assistants who feed dementia residents in Taiwanese nursing homes. *Geriatric Nursing*, 27(4): 229–36.

Chappel, N. and Novak, M. (1992) The role of support in alleviating stress among nursing assistants. *The Gerontologist*, 32: 351–9.

Chappel, N. and Novak, M. (1994) Caring for institutionalized elders: stress among nursing assistants. *Journal of Applied Gerontology*, 13: 299–315.

Chou, S., Boldy, D. and Lee, A. (2002) Measuring job satisfaction in residential aged care. *Journal for Quality in Health Care*, 14(1): 49–54.

Chrzescijanski, D., Moyle, W. and Creedy, D. (2007) Reducing dementia-related aggression through a staff education intervention. *Dementia*, 6(2): 271.

Cipher, D., Clifford, A. and Roper, K. (2006) Behavioral manifestations of pain in demented elderly. *Journal of the American Medical Directors' Association*, 7: 355–65.

Coleman, B. (2003a). *Consumer-directed Personal Care Services for Older People in the US*. Issue In-Brief Number 64. Washington, DC: AARP Public Policy Institute.

Coleman, B. (2003b) *Consumer-directed Personal Care Services for Older People in the U.S.* Issue In-Brief Number 75. Washington, DC: AARP Public Policy Institute.

Coogle, C., Parham, A. and Young, K. (2007) Job satisfaction and career commitment among nursing assistants providing Alzheimer's care. *American Journal of Alzheimer's Disease and Other Dementias*, 22: 251.

Cromwell, S. and Kolb, J. (2004) An examination of work–environment support factors affecting transfer of supervisory skills training to the workplace. *Human Resource Development Quarterly,* 13(4): 449–71.

Crown, W., Ahlburg, D. and MacAdam, M. (1995) The demographic and employment characteristics of home care aides, hospital aides, and other workers. *The Gerontologist*, 35: 162–70.

Davison, T.E., McCabe, M.P., Visser, S., Hudgson, C., Buchanan, G. and George, K. (2007) Controlled trial of dementia training with a peer support group for aged care staff. *International Journal of Geriatric Psychiatry*, 22: 868–73.

Department of Education, Science and Training (DEST) (2008) *Australian Aged Care Nursing: A Critical Review of Education, Training, Recruitment and Retention in Residential and Community Settings.* Available at: http:// www.dest.gov.au/sectors/higher_education/publications_resources/profiles/ archives/australian_aged_care_critical_review.htm (accessed 31 March 2008).

Department of Health (2004) Commonwealth Code of Practice for International Recruitment of Health Workers. World Health Assembly, Meeting of Commonwealth Health Ministers, 2003, Geneva, Switzerland. Available at: http://www.thecommonwealth.org/shared_asp_files/uploadedfiles/ %7B7BDD970B-53AE-441D-81DB-1B64C37E992A%7D_Commonwealth CodeofPractice.pdf (accessed 31 March 2008).

Dunn, L., Rout, U., Carson, J. and Ritter, S. (1994) Occupational stress amongst care staff working in nursing homes: an empirical investigation. *Journal of Clinical Nursing*, 3: 177–83.

Dyson, R. (2007) Address to aged care delegates (SFUW and NZNO) Wellington, New Zealand, 26 February. Available at: http:// www.beehive.govt.nz/speech/address+aged+care+delegates+sfwu+amp+nzno.

Federal Regulations (2005) *Code of Federal Regulations*, Title 42, Volume 3. Washington, DC: US Government.

Feldman, H., Clarfield, A., Bdodsky, J., King, Y. and Tzvi, D. (2006) An estimate of the prevalence of dementia among residents of long term care geriatric institutions in the Jerusalem area. *International Psychogeriatrics,* 18(4): 643–52.

Fleming, K. C., Evans, J. M. and Chutka, D.S. (2003) Caregiver and clinician shortages in an aging nation. *Mayo Clinic Proceedings*, 78: 1026–40.

Foner, N. (1994) Nursing home aides: Saints or monsters? *The Gerontologist*, 34: 245–50.

General Accounting Office (GAO) (2001) *Nursing Workforce: Emerging Nurse Shortages Due to Multiple Factors (GAO-01–944)*. Washington, DC: GAO.

Gurnik, M. and Hollis-Sawyer, L. (2003) Empowering assisted living front line staff to better care for Alzheimer's and dementia residents. *Ageing International*, 28(1): 82–97.

Harrington, C., Kovner, C., Mezey, M., Kayser-Jones, J., Burger, S., Mohler, M., Burke, R. and Zimmerman, D. (2000) Experts recommend minimum nurse staffing standards for nursing facilities in the United States. *The Gerontologist*, 40(1): 5–16.

Hoeffer, B., Talerico, K.A., Rasin, J., Mitchell, M., Stewart, B.J., KcKenzie, D., Barrick, A.L., Rader, J. and Sloane, P.D. (2006) Assisting cognitively impaired nursing home residents with bathing: effects of two bathing interventions on caregiving. *The Gerontologist*, 46(4): 524–32.

Hoppe, R. (2005) Looking abroad to meet the demands for caregivers. *AARP International*. Available at: http://www.aarpinternational.org/gra_sub/gra_sub_show.htm?doc_id=55377 (accessed 31 March 2008).

Hyde, J., Perez, B. and Forester, B. (2007) Dementia and assisted living. *The Gerontologist*, 47 (Special Issue III): 51–67.

Institute of Medicine (IOM) (2001) *Quality of Care in Nursing Homes*. Washington, DC: National Academy Press.

Josefsson, K., Sonde, L., Winblad, B. and Wahlin, T-B.R. (2007) Work situation of registered nurses in municipal elderly care in Sweden: A questionnaire survey. *International Journal of Nursing Studies*, 44: 71–82.

Kane, R., Lum, T., Culter, L., Dagenholtz, H. and Yu, T. (2007) Resident outcomes in small house nursing homes: A longitudinal evaluation of the initial GREEN HOUSE program. *American Journal of Geriatrics*, 55: 832–9.

Kiata, L., Kerse, N. and Dixon, R. (2005) Residential care workers and residents: the New Zealand story. *New Zealand Medical Journal*, 118(1214): 1–11.

Kim, J. (2006) Effects of gerontological nursing practicum on attitudes toward elders with dementia and elders among Korean nursing students. *Taehan Kanho Hakhoe*, 36(4): 645–51. (In Chinese).

Korczyk, S. (2004) *Long-Term Workers in Five Countries: Issues and Options*. Washington, DC: AARP Public Policy Institute. Available at: http://www.aarp.org/research/longtermcare/trends/aresearch-import-876-2004-07-.html.

Kuske, B., Hanns, S., Luck, T., Angermeyer, M.C., Behrens, J. and Riedel-Heller, S.G. (2006) Nursing home staff training in dementia care: a systematic review of evaluated programs. *International Psychogeriatrics, Review of Nursing Home Training in Dementia Care*, Oct 20: 1–25.

Lee, A., Hazelett, C., Lau, F., Kam, C., Wong, P., Wan, C. and Chow, S. (2001) Morbidity patterns of non-urgent patients attending accident and emergency departments in Hong Kong: cross-sectional study. *Hong Kong Medical Journal,* 7: 131–8.

Lee, G. 2002 The experience of institutionalization of the elderly. *Journal of Korean Community Nursing,* 13(4): 359–65.

Maas, M., Buckwalter, K., Swanson, E. and Mobily, P. (1994) Training key to job satisfaction. *Journal of Long Term Care Administration,* Spring: 23–6.

Magai, C., Cohen, C.I. and Gomberg, D. (2002) Impact of training dementia caregivers in sensitivity to nonverbal emotion signals. *International Psychogeriatrics,* 14(1): 25–38.

Manteghi, L. (2005) *Crossing Borders or Staying in Place? The Long Term Care Workforce Debate.* Washington, DC: AARP Global Network.

Mathers, C. and Leonardi, M. (2000) Global burden of dementia in the year 2000: summary of methods and data sources. *The Lancet Global Mental Health Series.* Available at: http://www.thelancet.com/online/focus/mental_health/collection (accessed 15 February 2008).

Maxfield, M., Lewis, R., and Cannon, S (1996) Training staff to prevent aggressive behavior of cognitively impaired elderly patients during bathing and grooming. *Journal of Gerontological Nursing,* 22: 37–43.

McCabe, M., Davison, T. and George, K. (2007) Effectiveness of staff training programs for behavioral problems among older people with dementia. *Aging & Mental Health,* 11(5): 505–9.

McDonald, I. and Kahn, K. (2007) Respectful relationships. *Future Age,* 6(2): 12–16.

McGillis, L., McGilton, K., Krejci, J., Pringle, D., Johnston, E., Fairley, L. and Brown, M. (2005) Enhancing the quality of supportive supervisory behavior in long term care facilities. *Journal of Nursing Administration,* 35(4): 181–7.

McLafferty, I. and Morrison, F. (2004) Attitudes towards hospitalized older adults. *Journal of Advanced Nursing,* 47(4): 446–53.

Michael, R. (2002) OSHA continues nursing home focus occupational safety and health. *Ergonomics Today,* www.osha.gov (accessed 10 March 2008).

Michigan Dementia Coalition (MDC) (2006) *Knowledge and Skills Needed for Dementia Care: A Guide for Direct Care Workers. Michigan.*

Morgan, D., Stewart, N., D'Arcy, C., Forbes, D. and Lawson, J. (2005) Work stress and physical assault of nursing aides in rural nursing homes with and without special care units. *Journal of Psychiatric and Mental Health Nursing,* 12: 347–58.

Morrison, R. and Siu, A. (2000) A comparison of pain and its treatment in advanced dementia and cognitively intact patients with hip fracture. *Pain and Symptom Management,* 19: 240–8.

Moyle, W., Skinner, J., Rowe, G. and Gork, C. (2003) Views of job satisfaction and dissatisfaction in Australian long-term care. *Journal of Clinical Nursing*, 12: 168–76.

Nagatomo, I., Akasaki, Y., Tominaga, M., Hashiguchi, W., Uchida, M. and Takigawa, M. (2001) Abnormal behavior of residents in a long-term care facility and the associated stress of care staff members. *Archives of Gerontology and Geriatrics*, 33: 203–10.

Nametz, P. and Jesudason, V. (1990) Behavioral problems among nursing home residents: Data from the 1988 Wisconsin annual survey of nursing homes. *Health Data Review*, 4: 1–7.

National Center for Health Statistics (2004) *Home Health Care Patients: Data from the 2000 National Home and Hospice Care Survey*. Available at: http://www.cdc.gov/nchs.

National Center for Health Statistics (NCHS) (2005) *Patient Arrivals by Ambulance at Emergency Departments, by Age Group – United States, 2003*. Available at: http://www.cdc.gov/nchs/about/major/ahcd/ercharts.htm (accessed 2 March 2008).

National Hospice and Palliative Care Organization (NHPCO) (2007) *Facts and Figures: Hospice Care in America*. Available at: http://www.nhpco.org/files/public/public_policy/advocacy/key-facts-figures.pdf (accessed 10 February 2008).

Noel, M.A., Pearce, G.L. and Metcalf, R. (2000) Front line workers in long-term care: the effect of educational interventions and stabilization of staffing ratios on turnover and absenteeism. *Journal of the American Medical Directors Association*, Nov/Dec: 241–7.

Noelker, L., Ejaz, F., Menne, H.l. and Jones, J. (2006) The impact of stress and support on nursing assistant satisfaction with supervision. *Journal of Applied Gerontology*, 25(4): 307–23.

Palmer, A.C. and Withee, B.M. (1996) Dementia care: effects of behavioral intervention training on staff perceptions of their work in veterans' nursing home. *Geriatric Nursing*, 17(3): 137–40.

Parks, S.M., Haines, C., Foreman, D., McKinstry, E. and Maxwell, T.L. (2005) Evaluation of an educational program for long-term care nursing assistants. *Clinical Experience*, January/February: 61–5.

Pekkarinen, L., Sinervo, T., Perala, M.L. and Elovainio, M. (2004) Work stressors and the quality of life in long-term care units. *The Gerontologist*, 44(5): 633–64.

Poirrier, G.P. (1994) The effects of an educational intervention on young adult undergraduate students' stereotypical ageist attitudes toward the elderly. Dissertation, Louisiana State University.

Plowfield, L.A., Raymond, J.E. and Hayes, E.R. (2006) An educational framework to support gerontological nursing education at the baccalaureate level. *Journal of Professional Nursing*, 22(2): 103–6.

Roper, J., Shapira, J. and Beck, A. (2001) Nurse caregiver feelings about agitation in Alzheimer's disease. *Journal of Gerontological Nursing,* 27: 32–9.

Ruiz, J., Smith, M., van Zuilen, M., Williams, C. and Mintzer, M. (2006) The impact of a computer-based training tutorial on dementia in long term care for licensed practice nursing students. *Gerontology and Geriatrics Education,* 26(3): 67–9.

Ryzin, J. (2007) Workplace interventions for retention, quality, and performance. *Future Age,* 6(2): 16–19.

Secrest, J., Iorio, D. and Martz, W. (2005) The meaning of work for nursing assistants who stay in long term care. *Journal of Clinical Nursing,* 14(8b): 90–7.

Sikorska-Simmons, E. (2006) Linking resident satisfaction to staff perceptions of the work environment in assisted living: A multilevel analysis. *The Gerontologist,* 46(5): 590–8.

Silverstein, N. and Maslow, K. (2006) *Improving Hospital Care for Persons with Dementia.* New York: Springer Publishing Company.

Sourial, R., McCusker, J., Cole, M. and Abrahamowicz, M. (2001) Agitation in demented patients in an acute care hospital: Prevalence, disruptiveness and staff burden. *International Psychogeriatrics,* 13: 183–97.

Spratley, E., Johnsom, A., Spchalski, J., Fritz, M. and Spencer, W. (2000) *The Registered Nurse Population: Findings from the National Sample Survey of Registered Nurses.* Washington DC: US Department of Health and Human Services.

Stack, S. (2003) Beyond performance indicators: A case study in aged care. *Australian Bulletin of Labour,* 29(2): 143–61.

Stevens, A., Burgio, L., Bailey, E., Burgio, K., Paul, P.L., Capilouto, F., Nicovich, P.L. and Hale, G. (1998) Teaching and maintaining behavior management skills with nursing assistants in a nursing home. *The Gerontologist,* 38: 379–84.

Stolee, P., Esbaugh, J., Aylward, S., Cathers, T.l., Harvey, D., Hillier, L., Keat, N. and Feightner, J. (2005) Factors associated with the effectiveness of continuing education in long term care. *The Gerontologist,* 45(3): 399–409.

Stone, R., Lipson, D., Barbaratta, L., Bryant, N. and Mosely, N. (2007a) Health insurance coverage for direct care workers: riding out the storm. *Better Jobs, Better Care Issue Brief 3.* Available at: http://www.bjbc.org/content/docs/BJBCIssueBriefNo3.pdf (accessed 9 December 2007).

Stone, R., Lipson, D., Barbaratta, L., Bryant, N. and Mosely, N. (2007b) Family care and paid care: separate worlds or common ground? *Better Jobs, Better Care Issue Brief,* 5. Available at: http://www.bjbc.org/content/docs/BJBCIssueBriefNo5.pdf (accessed 5 December 2007).

Stone, R., Reinhard, S., Bowers, B., Zimmerman, D., Phillips, C. and Hawes, C. (2002) *Evaluation of the Wellspring Model for Improving Nursing Home Quality*. Commonwealth Fund Report. Available at: http://cmwf.org (accessed 3 March 2008).

Sung, H., Chang, S. and Tsai, C. (2004) Working in long term care settings for older people with dementia: nurses' aides. *Journal of Clinical Nursing*, 14: 587–93.

Sveinsdottir, H., Biering, P. and Ramel, A. (2006) Occupational stress, job satisfaction and working environment among Icelandic nurses: a cross-sectional questionnaire survey. *International Journal of Nursing Studies,* 43: 875–89.

Tellis-Nayak, V. and Tellis-Nayak, M. (1989) Quality of care and the burden of two cultures: when the world of the nurse aide enters the world of the nursing home. *The Gerontologist,* 29: 307–13.

Teri, L., Huda, P., Gibbons, L., Young, H. and van Leynseele, J. (2005) STAR: A dementia-specific training program for staff in assisted living residences. *The Gerontologist,* 45(5): 686–93.

The Australian Institute of Health and Welfare (2004) *The Impact of Dementia on the Health and Aged Care Systems* Canberra: AIHW, Cat. No. AGE 37.

Trinkoff, A., Johantgen, M., Muntaner, C. and Rong, L. (2005) Staffing and worker injury in nursing homes. *American Journal of Public Health,* 95(7): 1220–5.

Tu, Y., Want, R. and Yeh, S. (2006) Relationship between perceived empowerment care and quality of life among elderly residents within nursing homes in Taiwan: A questionnaire survey. *International Journal of Nursing Studies*, 43: 673–80.

Van Charante, E., van Steenwijk-Opdam, P. and Bindels, P. (2007) Out-of-hours emergency services: patients' choices and referrals by general practitioners and ambulance services. *BMC Family Practice,* 8: 46.

Vinton, L. and Mazza, N. (1994) Aggressive behavior directed at nursing home personnel by residents' family members. *The Gerontologist*, 34(4): 528–33.

World Health Organization (WHO) (2005) *Global Health Workforce Alliance*. WHO. Available at: http://www.who.int/workforcealliance/en/ (accessed 9 March 2008).

World Health Organization (WHO) (2006a) *World Health Report: Working Together for Health*. Available at: http://www.who.int/whr/2006/chapter1/en/index.html (20 February 2008).

World Health Organization (WHO) (2006b) *Characteristics of the Community-based Aged Care Workforce*. Geneva: WHO.

Yassi, A., Cohen, M., Cvitkovich, Y., Park, I., Ratner, P., Ostry, A., Vilage, J., and Pollak, N. (2004) Factors associated with staff injuries in intermediate care facilities in British Columbia, Canada. *Nursing Research*, 53(2): 87–98.

Yeattes, D. and Seward, R. (2000) Reducing turnover and improving health care in nursing homes: the potential effects of self-managed work teams. *The Gerontologist,* 40(3): 358–63.

Young, R. (2007) *Mobility of Health Professionals in Europe.* UK Case Study. London: Healthcare Workforce, Kings College London.

24

Attending to relationships in dementia care

Sue Davies and Mike Nolan

Learning objectives

By the end of this chapter you will:

- be able to discuss the significance of relationships for people with dementia and their carers
- identify key components which contribute to developing effective partnerships within the context of dementia care
- appreciate the relevance of relationship-centred care and the Senses Framework to achieving excellence in dementia care

---

Introduction

Recent research has highlighted the critical contribution of relationships to creating excellence in dementia care. Furthermore, the notion of working in partnership with service users and carers is now well established, at least at an ideological level. However, historically, the predominant focus in research on caring relationships has been on caregiver stress and how this might be reduced, and we know much less about ways of supporting mutually beneficial relationships that might enhance experiences of caregiving for all concerned. Dementia has been seen as having a largely destructive effect on relationships, and the potential therapeutic value of relationships between people with dementia and their caregivers has been, in the main, neglected. More recently, a number of authors have begun to describe an approach to dementia care that explicitly recognizes the interdependencies of caregiving and the rewards that may be generated for all parties: the person with dementia, their family carer(s) and health and social care providers (Adams and Gardiner 2005). In this chapter, we argue that this approach, termed relationship-centred care (Tresolini and the Pew-Fetzer Task Force 1994; Nolan *et al.* 2006) has the potential to change the culture of dementia care in ways that ensure that the personhood of, and the interdependencies between, *all* stakeholders are protected and enhanced.

In this chapter, we argue that:

- Relationships are central to the care experiences of people with dementia.

- Current approaches in dementia care pay insufficient attention to relationships to ensure excellence in practice.

- New approaches to practice, including relationship-centred care and the Senses Framework, can enhance relationships within dementia care.

Our aim is to highlight the significance of relationships within the context of living with dementia and describe frameworks for practice that explicitly recognize the needs and experiences of all stakeholders within dementia caregiving situations. The following areas will be considered:

- the impact of dementia on relationships

- the importance of relationships to experiences of dementia

- building and maintaining dementia-caregiving relationships

- new approaches to care, including relationship-centred care and the Senses Framework, that explicitly recognize the significance of relationships in dementia care.

We conclude with a practical example of a project that employed these approaches in order to create an enriched environment of dementia care in a nursing home setting.

The impact of dementia on relationships

The impact of a diagnosis of dementia reaches far beyond the person to whom it is given. It permeates through the family system and to relationships outside the boundaries of the family.

(Weaks *et al.* 2005: 149)

The nature of dementia is such that a diagnosis results in major tensions and trials within family relationships. The onset and progression of dementia are characterized by cognitive and communicative impairment, threatening the person's relationships with others, both within and outside the family. The impact on aspects of the marital relationship can be particularly profound, and may include reduced sharing of activities, loss of emotional support between spouses and a diminution in the quality of verbal communication. These effects are likely to have negative consequences for both partners (Baikie 2002), with loss of relationships resulting in depression and distress. If relationships with family and friends are lost or diminished, contact with caregiving staff may have to substitute in assisting the person with dementia to maintain their sense of identity and personhood.

For care-giving staff, relationships can also be challenging, with many practitioners feeling they lack the skills to communicate effectively with people with dementia (Nolan *et al.* 2002a; Tolson *et al.* 1999). As a consequence, the 'inverse-care law' has been identified in some care settings, with people with the most significant degree of cognitive impairment receiving the lowest levels of input in terms of emotional and social support (Bruce *et al.* 2002; Nolan and Grant 1993). Studies have suggested that many practitioners lack a clear sense of what they are aiming for in their day-to-day work with older people with advanced dementia (Marshall 2001), and this inhibits relationships. For example, Bruce *et al.* (2002) found that staff in care homes tended to concentrate their efforts where they could see they were making a difference, and this is more difficult with people with advanced cognitive impairment. Hansebo and Kihlgren (2002) suggest that one of the main challenges for paid carers of people with cognitive frailty is to feel that their communication with residents is worthwhile, which is a prerequisite to experiencing their caring as meaningful. Furthermore, staff need to feel that they are appreciated by service users and their families (Campbell 2003) and this can be difficult in the context of dementia.

All these challenges are of particular concern given the significance of relationships to experiences of dementia and it is to this that we now turn.

The importance of relationships to experiences of dementia

As several authors note, dementia has traditionally been viewed using a largely biomedical model with the primary focus being on the varying types of dementia and their presenting symptoms (Clare 2002; Phinney 1998, 2002; Robinson *et al.* 1997). However, the pioneering work of the late Professor Tom Kitwood introduced a radically new perspective.

According to Kitwood (1990), dementia can be most accurately understood as a socially embedded experience, the result of the complex interactions between neurological impairment, life history, health status, social environment, personality and 'malignant social psychology'. Kitwood (1997) argued that many of the difficulties people with dementia experience are not the result of the disease itself but rather are due to the social environment that is created for them. The observation that relationships are central to the life experiences of people with dementia was instrumental in introducing the concept of 'person-centred care' into care practices. Using this approach, the challenge for both family and paid carers working with people with dementia, is how to create a positive environment in which the quality of life for people with dementia can be enhanced, and their 'personhood' maintained.

A fundamental aspect of maintaining identity and personhood is the ability to form and maintain personal relationships (Tester *et al.* 2004). This is no less significant for people with dementia. The construction of self is never an individual activity, but requires the cooperation and contribution of others (Basting 2003). Studies suggest that most family carers invest considerable efforts in sustaining the self-esteem and sense of agency of the person with dementia, even if their actual contribution to the relationship diminishes over time (Caron and Bowers 2003; Perry and O'Connor 2002). Keady and Nolan (2003) provide a detailed account of the considerable 'work' that family carers invest in trying to 'maintain the involvement' of the person with dementia as an active agent. However, few studies have explored family relationships in dementia from the perspectives of both carers and people with dementia prospectively, over time. Building on the work of Keady and Nolan, Hellström *et al.* (2005) describe how spouse carers and people with dementia both actively work together to create a 'nurturative relational context' in which both partners continue to see themselves as a 'couple' who 'do things together' to maintain a sense of reciprocity and complementarity in their relationship. Such efforts can sustain relationships over a number of years (Hellström *et al.* 2007).

Galvin *et al.* (2005) describe family carers as the 'intimate mediators', suggesting they act as 'bridge-maker' between at least two domains of knowledge. Galvin *et al.* suggest that an insider view is able to facilitate empathic understanding in others (outsiders), resulting in a deeper understanding and more individualized care.

Exercise 24.1   Families and professionals working together

In what ways can professionals assist family caregivers to perform the role of intimate mediator described by Galvin *et al.*, and to ensure the best 'blend' of professional and family expertise?

So far we have focused on the importance of 'dyadic' relationships between the person with dementia and either paid or family carers. Recently research has stressed the importance of looking beyond the dyad to 'triadic' relationships (Clissett 2007; Nolan *et al.* 2002b) that include the person with dementia, family and paid carers. A study of experiences of dementia services in rural Scotland, for example, found that the most frequently mentioned positive aspect of services for both service users and carers was the loving relationship with service providers (Innes *et al.* 2005). In this study, service users and carers were clearly being enabled to continue existing social activities or develop new ones built on positive relationships with care providers. Stimulating and appropriate care created reciprocal relationships between service providers and service users which added to the quality of the service experienced. Clissett (2007) found that paid carers could support the relationship between community-dwelling older people with dementia and their family carers in a number of ways. In particular, professional carers tended to have an influence on decision- making between the family carer and cared for person and on their ability to (re)discover pleasure in each other's company.

It is increasingly recognized that relationships with service users are a crucial component of the experiences of staff who work with people with dementia and their families (see Chapter 23). Ryan *et al.* (2004), for example, identified high levels of job satisfaction among community-based dementia care workers, underpinned by their ability to maintain relationships with people with dementia and their families in the context of triadic relationships, and contribute to enhancing the status and quality of life of people with dementia. There is also evidence that relationships with residents and their families are key factors shaping the work experiences of staff within care home settings (Brown-Wilson 2007; Moyle *et al.* 2003). However, it is vital that the needs of staff members are also taken into account, with Kitwood (1997) asserting that it is not possible to deliver person-centred care unless staff experience a 'staff-centred' work environment (see Chapter 12).

Caring for people with dementia in any care setting, and ensuring that this care is of a high quality, requires a sophisticated level of skill and knowledge and staff need support if disaffection and burnout are to be avoided. Certainly, the contribution of 'emotion work' to the care of people with dementia is emerging as an important area for further research. Berg *et al.*, for example, discuss how nurses described a 'mutual interdependency' with patients with dementia during the caring process resulting in an 'intertwined life' (Berg *et al.* 1998). Similarly, Rundqvist and Severinsson (1999) report that nurses caring for older people with dementia described the most important aspects of their relationships with their patients as touching (including caressing and hugging), confirmation (involving mutuality and sensitivity) and promoting positive values within the caring culture such as consideration, patience and compassion. Such 'emotional labour' can be very demanding and is inevitably linked to the well-being of the care provider (Gattuso and Bevan 2000). It is now widely recognized that positive perceptions of work are far more likely in an environment which has relatively few boundaries, which enables people to feel that they are part of a community, and acknowledges differences of opinion while allowing feelings to be explored (Kitwood 1997; Nolan *et al.* 2002a).

Building and maintaining relationships in the context of dementia

Caregiving is relational and cannot be separated from people's experiences of each other in the past, present, or even the anticipated future.

(Ward-Griffin *et al.* 2007: 13)

As discussed in the previous section, relationships in caring for older people with dementia have been identified as central to positive care experiences (Brooker 2006; Dewing 2004; McCormack 200). However, it is not always clear how enabling relationships are developed (Dewing 2004).

Gallant *et al.* (2002) suggest that enabling partnerships involve power sharing and negotiation, cooperation, openness and respect. The issue of 'power' is particularly relevant within the context of dementia care, as older people with dementia are easily disempowered. For example, Proctor (2001) illustrates vividly how the exercise of power on the part of health and social care practitioners can 'silence' the voices of older women with dementia.

This is not a one-way street and it is increasingly clear that creating meaningful relationships with people with dementia and their families is a highly skilled activity. In attempting to describe some of the skills and strategies that are effective in this regard, Adams and Gardiner (2005) differentiate between 'enabling' and 'disabling' communication within dementia caregiving triads. Enabling dementia communication occurs when family and paid carers either help the person with dementia to express their thoughts, feelings and wishes or represent the person with dementia as someone who is able to make decisions about their own care. Disabling dementia communication, on the other hand, occurs when family carers or health and social care professionals either prevent the person with dementia from expressing their thoughts, feelings and wishes or represent them as unable to participate in decision-making.

Recently there have been calls to create more equitable relationships based on a sharing of power in which the 'expertise' of all parties is more fully recognized. Initiatives such as the 'expert patient' (Department of Health 2001) are based on the premise that people living with long-term conditions have considerable knowledge and skills in how best to manage their condition. Similarly, several years ago Nolan *et al.* (1996) proposed a model of 'carer as expert' in which the expertise of the family carer is used, together with the expertise of paid carers, to identify the best form of care. In most circumstances the person themselves, and/or the family carer, knows best the needs and wants of the person with dementia (person knowledge) However, they may not always know the best way of meeting those needs. Of course it is the person with dementia who holds the most intimate knowledge and whose expertise should be sought wherever possible. Unfortunately, such expertise is often overlooked, despite evidence of the very proactive strategies that people with dementia often adopt to manage their lives (Bryden 2005) and models for professionals to work actively with them (Brooker 2006). By the time formal services are involved, it is often the family carer who is the focus of attention.

Sustaining caring relationships involves supporting carers, (caregivers) morale (among both family and paid carers), and this depends largely on maintaining a sense of accomplishment and a belief that what you are doing has an obvious effect on the cared-for person's well-being. In order to sustain such a perception it is necessary to see small changes as evidence of achievement. This requires practice models that facilitate the identification of such changes.

The need for a new approach

The inter-relationships between the experiences of people with dementia, their families and staff suggested by the research reviewed in this chapter reinforce the value of sharing perspectives and agreeing on goals of care. It is now clear that relational dynamics are essential to creating good care partnerships, and that the best relationships exist when all parties are able to work together, express their opinions and appreciate each other's perspective. Weaks *et al.* (2005) argue that an understanding of the impact of dementia on all relationships and a practice-based supportive framework to support relationships are essential to creating more positive models of care. Nolan *et al.* (2003) propose that 'symmetry' and 'synchronicity' are vital elements within caring relationships. In other words, it is essential that all parties are able to make a contribution that is recognized and valued, and that each party recognizes and respects the perspective of others within the caring relationship in order that care is delivered in the most appropriate way. This is the fundamental basis of the approach known as 'relationship-centred care'.

The term 'relationship-centred care' was first coined by a Task Force in the USA in the early 1990s. The Pew Fetzer Task Force was set up to examine ways of developing curricula across the caring disciplines that would recognize the interaction between biomedical and psychosocial aspects of health care and that would demonstrate an integrated approach. The Task Force concluded that the notion of relationship-centred care should underpin all health interactions, with the significance of this summed up as follows:

> ... relationships are critical to the care provided by nearly all practitioners and a sense of satisfaction and positive outcomes for patients and practitioners. Although relationships are a prerequisite to effective care and teaching, there has been little formal acknowledgement of their importance and few formal efforts to help students and practitioners learn to develop effective relationships in health care.

(Tresolini and the Pew Fetzer Task Force 1994: 1)

In promoting a more holistic vision of health care, the Task Force focused on several areas including: the social, economic, environmental, cultural and political contexts of care; the subjective experience of illness; and the relationships that develop between practitioners, patients, families and the wider community over time. They suggested that the interaction of these factors lies at the heart of relationship-centred care (RCC) and forms the 'foundation' of any therapeutic or healing activity.

The Task Force outlined the basic elements of a system that would promote RCC but recognized that the concept was still emerging, and that further work was needed to operationalize the concept in ways that would ensure an appropriate balance between the needs of all involved in health care relationships. Nolan *et al.* (2006) have applied the concept of relationship-centred care to work with older people and argue that care staff need help to identify ways of interacting with older people and their families that best support relationships. With this in mind, the Senses Framework was developed.

The origins of the Senses Framework can be traced back to work on the relationships between family and professional carers (Nolan *et al.* 1996), and individuals in need of help, including those with dementia (see especially Keady 1999). The framework was then further developed to provide a therapeutic rationale for carers working in continuing care settings (Nolan 1997), and has since been tested in a range of care environments (Aveyard and Davies 2006a; Davies *et al.* 1999; Nolan *et al.* 2006). The framework extends existing ideas about person-centred care to include the needs of families and staff and, in this way, provides a framework for considering how 'relationship-centred care' might be achieved. It suggests that the best care for older people involves the creation of a set of senses or experiences, for older people, for family caregivers and for staff working with them. These are:

- a *sense of security* – of feeling safe and receiving or delivering competent and sensitive care

- a *sense of continuity* – the recognition of biography, using the past to contextualize the present

- a *sense of belonging* – opportunities to form meaningful relationships or feel part of a team

- a *sense of purpose* – opportunities to engage in purposeful activities or to have a clear set of goals to aspire to

- a *sense of achievement* – achieving meaningful or valued goals and feeling satisfied with one's efforts

- a *sense of significance* – to feel that you matter, and that you are valued as a person. (Nolan *et al.* 2006)

A particular advantage of the Senses Framework is that it prompts consideration of the important components of care from the perspective of older people, family members and staff working with them. Furthermore, through linking the experiences of older people, their families and staff, the Senses Framework has the potential to promote understanding of the experiences of others, thus enhancing communication and the ability to work in partnership (Nolan *et al.* 2006). Studies have highlighted the role that the Senses play in helping to create an 'enriched' environment of care (Brown 2006; Nolan *et al.* 2002a, 2006). Such 'enriched' environments ensure that the Senses are met for *all* individuals/ groups in a given care context, including, for example, residents/patients, staff, family carers and students.

The remainder of this chapter describes the application of these conceptual models in the context of a research and development project taking place in a care home for older people with dementia. Information from the evaluation of the project is included to show how use of the models can enhance care experiences for people with dementia, their family caregivers and paid care staff.

Using the Senses Framework to develop partnerships in dementia care

RCC and the Senses Framework have provided the conceptual basis for ongoing development work in several care homes in a large city in the north of England, including a nursing home for older people with dementia (Aveyard and Davies 2006a; Davies *et al.* 2007). In 2002, senior staff within this home had expressed interest in developing the home as a 'teaching nursing home' and began to establish a partnership with researchers at a local university. An exploratory phase involved interviews and questionnaires with staff and relatives, periods of observation within the home and a series of staff 'away days'. On the basis of this information, a number of priorities for development work were identified and fed back in the form of a brief report. Participants were also introduced to RCC and the Senses Framework as the conceptual basis for the project.

Within the initiative, the main mechanism for partnership working was an 'action group' involving relatives, staff and managers, and facilitated initially by the two researchers. Residents were also welcome to attend, but as a result of their advanced cognitive frailty were not regular participants in the meetings, although many contributed actively to the events organized by the group. Meetings of the action group took place monthly and focused on identifying priorities for development work that would improve the experiences of residents, relatives and staff within the home. Action plans for each priority area were devised and the group actively raised funds to support the implementation of their ideas. A number of developments have been implemented by the group which have enhanced the experiences of all stakeholders. For example, an early project involved the development of a welcome booklet including information for new residents, their families and staff (Box 24.1). Some other achievements of the action group are shown in Table 24.1.

Box 24.1   Developing a welcome booklet

During an early meeting of the Action Group relatives identified a need for more relevant information to allow them to make an informed decision when choosing a care home. It was also agreed that there is very little easily accessible information about dementia, and in particular about the impact of caring for someone with this condition. The group generated the idea of a 'welcome booklet' that would capture what was 'special' about 67 Birch Avenue so that potential residents and their families, and new members of staff, would have a clear picture of the home and its philosophy of care, as well as providing useful information about dementia and its effects. Relatives agreed to write about their own experiences of caring for someone with dementia, both before and after admission to the home, and to encourage other members of their families to record their own stories. Staff were encouraged to use the same technique to share their own perspectives. Extracts from the contributions are included below.

> There's a lot of job satisfaction in this work. You've got to have that care because you come into the job to care. We've got to treat the residents as we would want to be treated. I've lived through this with my dad, having to go into a home, so I understand what it's like for relatives.
>
> (Cook)

> My grandmother has Alzheimer's disease. It's tragic and sad and strange, and at the same time, although she is not who she was and does not relate as she used to, she still lives, someone is still there who loves gentle touch. I need to remember her past, alive and holding on to life, being a wonderful and inspiring schoolteacher, a mother of four and a grandmother of many. She was a warm and firm presence.
>
> (Grand-daughter of resident)

As a result, the booklet represents a sharing of experiences of working with and caring for the residents, rather than a simple description of what goes on within the home (Aveyard and Davies 2006b).

Table 24.1   Achievements of the Support 67 Action Group

- Activities programme
- Relatives support group
- Booklet for new residents and relatives
- Fund-raising
- Uniforms for staff
- Education programme

- Skills profile for qualified staff
- PAT dog 'Missie'
- Garden project
- Building modifications project

In early planning meetings, both the Senses Framework and the idea of relationship-centred care were presented as possible underpinnings for the work, and these clearly resonated with staff and relatives. As part of the evaluation for the project, members of the action group were invited to reflect on the extent to which the activities of the group had created or enhanced the 'Senses' for each of the three main stakeholder groups. Results of this exercise are shown in Table 24.1.

The ease with which participants were able to map activities and achievements onto the Senses Framework suggests that this provided a useful, research-based tool to guide developments. Interview data also provided insights into the processes involved in establishing partnership working within a care home environment and highlighted some of the barriers and facilitators to such developments (Aveyard and Davies 2006a; see Box 24.2).

Box 24.2 Barriers and facilitators to partnership working within a nursing home for people with dementia

Facilitators

Opportunities for regular communication

The action group helped to improve communication between relatives and staff. By spending more time together, staff and relatives felt they had developed a greater understanding of each other's needs and there were suggestions that as a consequence, relationships had improved.

Opportunities to demonstrate mutual appreciation

The project had provided opportunities for staff and relatives to recognize and show appreciation for the contribution that each group makes to life within the home. Feedback during group sessions has helped to reinforce to staff that relatives feel they 'do a good job' and provide highly skilled care. Staff were also able to show how much they valued the continuing contribution made by relatives.

Opportunities for joint working

As individual projects developed, staff and relatives found that by working together they had developed into a powerful force for change. A number of participants expressed the view that they were able to exert more influence and promote change by working together.

Providing a mechanism for change

The action group had channelled people's enthusiasm for change, with identification of both immediate and longer-term goals.

Bringing together various kinds of expertise

Staff and relatives were able to share ideas and experiences with positive outcomes. For example, one discussion about visiting at meal-times resulted in joint preparation of guidelines for visitors. The partnership with researchers enabled the advancement of ideas about partnership working in long-term care settings through publications and conference presentations.

Barriers

Difficulties in releasing staff from direct care duties to attend meetings

Although senior staff remained committed to the project and other staff attended meetings intermittently, it was difficult to ensure consistent attendance at meetings. It was therefore important to develop other ways to make sure that staff and relatives were aware of developments and to enable them to contribute their ideas.

Layout of the building

The design of the building in four linked bungalows required high staff/ resident ratios to support adequate care and supervision, limiting staff time for involvement in project activities. The home also lacked a large communal area for events and activities (this became one of the first development priorities).

Difficulties in recruiting new relatives

The number of relatives directly involved in the project fluctuated, but it was sometimes difficult to recruit new members. Altering the format of meetings to make them less formal and advertising them as coffee mornings proved a successful strategy.

Lack of funding for some initiatives

Because the group had so many ideas for improving experiences within the home, funding was often an issue. However, co-opting senior figures within the local community to the action group raised the profile of the home and considerable amounts of funding were secured through access to grant-making bodies and fund-raising events at the home.

Difficulties in involving residents with advanced cognitive frailty

Residents were always welcome at meetings, and attended from time to time, but because of their level of cognitive frailty were unable to participate actively in determining the focus of developments. To a large extent the project depended on staff and relatives to articulate the concerns and experiences of residents on their behalf.

(Adapted from Aveyard and Davies 2006a; Davies *et al.* 2007)

The findings of this project suggest that using the Senses Framework and ideas about relationship-centred care to inform partnership working can make a significant impact on the relationships between people with dementia, family carers and paid staff. Use of the framework has been shown to assist staff, residents and relatives to reach agreement about appropriate goals for care (Aveyard and Davies 2006a). Furthermore, it seems that putting in place initiatives that have benefits for all stakeholders has the potential to promote an increased sense of well-being for all groups. The project provides evidence of the relevance of relationship-centred care as a basis for practice, education and research in the context of dementia care.

Debates and controversies

> **Exercise 24.2** Person-centred and relationship-centred care: similarities and differences
>
> The references below are articles about person-centred and relationship-centred care. In order to complete this activity, you will need to access and read these articles. As you read, make notes about any differences between 'person-centred' and 'relationship-centred care'. Are these approaches mutually exclusive or might one incorporate the other? How could you make use of the Senses Framework in your work?
>
> Nolan, M.R., Davies, S., Brown, J., Keady, J. and Nolan, J. (2004) Beyond 'person-centred' care: a new vision for gerontological nursing. *International Journal of Older People Nursing*, in association with *Journal of Clinical Nursing*. 13(3a): 45–53.
>
> Adams, T. (2005) From person-centred care to relationship-centred care. *Generations Review*, 15(1): 4–7.
>
> Dewing, J. (2004) Concerns relating to the application of frameworks to promote person-centredness in nursing with older people. *International Journal of Older People Nursing* in association with *Journal of Clinical Nursing*, 13(3a): 39–44.
>
> McCormack, B. (2004) Person-centredness in gerontological nursing: an overview of the literature. *International Journal of Older People Nursing* in association with *Journal of Clinical Nursing*, 13(3a): 31–8.

An ongoing debate is the distinction between person-centred and relationship-centred care (Brooker and Nolan 2007). Common characteristics include considering all aspects of the person (biological, psychosocial), preserving and respecting individuality, facilitating choice and negotiation, involvement and relationships. These similarities have led to debates about whether person-centred care and relationship-centred care are one and the same thing or whether one includes the other (Brooker and Nolan 2007). Given the centrality of relationships to the experiences of people with dementia, we would argue that care for people with dementia cannot be person-centred unless it is also relationship-centred. Clark, for example, (Clark 2002) proposes that, if we are to provide meaningful care and services to older people, we need to 'situate' an older person's individual needs within a rich matrix of relationships and socio-cultural beliefs. Similarly, McCormack (2001) suggests that we need to replace an individualistic view of autonomy in later life with one based on 'interconnectedness and partnership'. These perspectives acknowledge the potential of person-centred care, but call for more attention to be paid to the interdependencies that shape our lives (Kelly *et al.* 2005; McCormack 2001). The final exercise in this chapter encourages you to explore these arguments further.

There are also questions concerning the ways in which practitioners use such frameworks in the context of their day-to-day work and whether they highlight the tension between 'how practice could be and how it seems to be' (Dewing 2004: 5). Building and maintaining positive relationships and effective partnerships take an investment of time and skill that is frequently not always available in today's pressured care environments. The need to make sure that the voices of individual partners do not dominate decision-making requires an understanding of interpersonal dynamics and advanced communication skills. Until the complexity of working effectively with people with dementia and their families is recognized and acknowledged in the form of adequate preparation and additional financial remuneration, it is likely that positive partnership working in the context of dementia care will remain a vision rather than a reality. Furthermore, research is urgently needed to address the challenge of involving people with advanced dementia more effectively in the decisions that affect them, and seek ways of enabling people with dementia and their supporters to recognize and value the contribution they make within caring relationships.

Conclusion

The significance of relationships in supporting quality of life for people with dementia and their families is clear from repeated research studies. Furthermore, research is also revealing the importance of relationships to sustaining paid carers who work with people with dementia in their caring role, and ensuring high levels of job satisfaction. It then becomes imperative to identify ways of working that support people with dementia, their family and paid carers to develop and maintain positive relationships. The literature in this field suggests the importance of mutual awareness, respect and appreciation, effective communication and joint decision-making as important components of working together. We have described conceptual models that we feel can assist people with dementia and their carers to translate these core principles into action and described a project that made use of these models to enhance experiences within a nursing home for older people with dementia.

The principles underpinning notions of relationship-centred care suggest that it is only when all participants within caring relationships are able to achieve and recognize reciprocity that the vision of true partnership working will be realized. We believe that the conceptual models described in this chapter represent one small step on the road to excellence in dementia care.

Further information

In the UK, the charity **Help the Aged** is coordinating a campaign entitled My Home Life, which is underpinned by the model of relationship-centred care and the Senses Framework. This initiative is aimed at improving the quality of life of those who are living, dying, visiting and working in care homes for older people.

References

Adams, T. and Gardiner, P. (2005) Communication and interaction within dementia care triads: developing a theory for relationship-centred care. *Dementia*, 4: 185–205.

Aveyard, B. and Davies, S. (2006a) Moving forward together: evaluation of an Action Group involving staff and relatives within a nursing home for older people with dementia. *International Journal of Older People Nursing*, 1: 95–104.

Aveyard, B. and Davies, S. (2006b) The Support 67 Action Group: easing the path into care. *Journal of Dementia Care*, 14(6): 19–21.

Baikie, E. (2002) The impact of dementia on marital relationships. *Sexual and Relationship Therapy*, 17(3): 289–99.

Basting, A. (2003) Looking back from loss: views of the self in Alzheimer's disease. *Journal of Aging Studies*, 17(1): 87–99.

Berg, A., Hallberg, I.R. and Norberg, A. (1998) Nurses' reflections about dementia care, the patients, the care and themselves in their daily caregiving. *International Journal of Nursing Studies*, 35(5): 271–82.

Brooker, D. (2006) *Person-centred Dementia Care: Making Services Better*. Bradford Dementia Group Good Practice Guides. London: Jessica Kingsley.

Brooker, D. and Nolan, M. (2007) Person-centred and relationship-centred care: two sides of the same coin? Symposium presented to the British Society of Gerontology Annual Conference, 7 September, Sheffield.

Brown, J. (2006) Student nurses' experience of learning to care for older people in enriched environments: a constructivist inquiry. Unpublished PhD thesis, University of Sheffield.

Brown-Wilson, C. (2007) Exploring relationships in care homes: a constructivist inquiry. Unpublished PhD thesis, University of Sheffield.

Bruce, E., Surr, C., Tibbs, M. and Downs, M. (2002) Moving towards a special kind of care for people with dementia living in care homes. *NT Research*, 7(5): 337–47.

Bryden, C. (2005) *Dancing with Dementia: My Story of Living Positively with Dementia*. London: Jessica Kingsley.

Campbell, S. (2003) Empowering nursing staff and residents in long-term care. *Geriatric Nursing*, 24(3): 170–5.

Caron, C.D. and Bowers, B.J. (2003) Deciding whether to continue, share or relinquish caregiving: carers' views. *Qualitative Health Research*, 13(9): 1252–71.

Clare, L. (2002) Developing awareness about awareness in early stage dementia. *Dementia*, 1(3): 295–312.

Clark, P.G. (2002) Values and voices in teaching gerontology and geriatrics. *The Gerontologist*, 42: 297–303.

Clissett, P. (2007) A constructivist investigation into relationships between community dwelling older people and their carers. Unpublished PhD thesis, University of Sheffield.

Davies, S., Atkinson, L., Aveyard, B., Martin, U., McCaffrey, S. and Powell, A. (2007) Changing the culture within care homes. In: M. Nolan, E. Hanson, G. Grant and J. Keady (eds) *What Counts as Knowledge, and Whose Knowledge Counts? Realising User and Carer Involvement in Research and Development*. Maidenhead: Open University Press, pp.50–68.

Davies, S., Nolan, M., Brown, J. and Wilson, F. (1999) *Dignity on the Ward: Promoting Excellence in Care*. London: Help the Aged and the Orders of St John Trust.

Department of Health (2001) *The Expert Patient: A New Approach to Chronic Disease Management for the 21st Century*. London: Department of Health.

Dewing, J. (2004) Concerns relating to the application of frameworks to promote person-centredness in nursing with older people. *International Journal of Older People Nursing* in association with *Journal of Clinical Nursing*, 13(3a): 39–44.

Gallant, M.H., Beaulieu, M.C. and Carnevale, F.A. (2002) Partnership: an analysis of the concept within the nurse–client relationship. *Journal of Advanced Nursing*, 40(2): 149–57.

Galvin, K., Todres, L. and Richardson, M. (2005) The intimate mediator: a carer's experience of Alzheimer's. *Scandinavian Journal of Caring Sciences*, 19(1): 2–11.

Gattuso, S. and Bevan, C. (2000) Mother, daughter, patient, nurse: women's emotion work in aged care. *Journal of Advanced Nursing*, 31(4): 892–9.

Hansebo, G. and Kihlgren, M. (2002) Carers' interactions with patients suffering from severe dementia: a difficult balance to facilitate mutual togetherness. *Journal of Clinical Nursing*, 11(2): 225–36.

Hellstrom, I., Nolan, M. and Lundh, U. (2005) We do things together: a case study of 'couplehood' in dementia. *Dementia*, 4(1): 7–22.

Hellstrom, I., Nolan, M. and Lundh, U. (2007) Sustaining 'couplehood': Spouses' strategies for living positively with dementia. *Dementia: The International Journal of Social Research and Practice*, 6(3): 383–409.

Innes, A., Blackstock, K., Mason, A., Smith, A. and Cox, S. (2005) Dementia care provision in rural Scotland: service users' and carers' experiences. *Health & Social Care in the Community*, 13(4): 354–65.

Keady, J. (1999) The dynamics of dementia: a modified grounded theory study. PhD study, University of Wales, Bangor.

Keady J. and Nolan, M. (2003) The dynamics of dementia: working together, working separately or working alone? In: M. Nolan, L. Lundh, G. Grant and J. Keady (eds) *Partnerships in Family Care: Understanding the Caregiving Career*. Maidenhead: Open University Press, pp. 15–32.

Kelly, T.B., Tolson, D., Schofield, I. and Booth, J. (2005) Describing gerontological nursing: an academic exercise or prerequisite for progress? *Journal of Clinical Nursing*, 14(3a): 13–23.

Kitwood, T. (1990) The dialectics of dementia with particular reference to Alzheimer's disease. *Ageing and Society*, 10: 177–96.

Kitwood, T. (1997) *Dementia Reconsidered: The Person Comes First*. Buckingham: Open University Press.

Marshall, M. (2001) The challenge of looking after people with dementia. *British Medical Journal*, 323: 410–11.

McCormack, B. (2001) *Negotiating Partnerships with Older People: A Person-centred Approach*. Aldershot: Ashgate.

Moyle, W., Skinner, J., Rowe, G. *et al.* (2003) Views of job satisfaction and dissatisfaction in Australian long-term care. *Journal of Clinical Nursing*, 12(2): 168–76.

Nolan, M.R. (1997) Health and social care: what the future holds for nursing. Keynote address at Third Royal College of Nursing Older Person European Conference and Exhibition, Harrogate.

Nolan, M., Brown, J., Davies, S., Keady, J. and Nolan, J. (2002a) *Advancing Gerontological Education in Nursing: Final Report of the AGEIN Project*. Report to the English National Board for Nursing, Midwifery and Health Visiting. Sheffield: University of Sheffield.

Nolan, M., Brown, J., Davies, S., Nolan, J. and Keady, J. (2006) *The Senses Framework: Improving Care for Older People through a Relationship-centred Approach*. Getting Research into Practice Series. Sheffield: University of Sheffield.

Nolan, M.R. and Grant, G. (1993) Rust out and therapeutic reciprocity: concepts to advance the nursing care of older people. *Journal of Advanced Nursing*, 18(8): 1305–14.

Nolan, M.R., Grant, G. and Keady, J. (1996) *Understanding Family Care*. Buckingham: Open University Press.

Nolan, M., Grant, G., Keady, J. and Lundh, U. (2003) New directions for partnerships: relationship-centred care. In: M. Nolan, G. Grant, J. Keady and U. Lundh (eds) *Partnerships in Family Care*. Maidenhead: Open University Press.

Nolan, M., Ryan, T., Enderby, P. and Reid, D. (2002b) Towards a more inclusive vision of dementia care practice and research. *Dementia: The International Journal of Social Research and Practice*, 1(2): 193–211.

Perry, J. and O'Connor, D.L. (2002) Preserving personhood, (re)cognising the spouse with dementia. *Family Relations*, 51(1): 55–61.

Phinney, A. (2002) Fluctuating awareness of the breakdown of the illness narrative in dementia. *Dementia*, 1(3): 329–44.

Proctor, G. (2001) Listening to older women with dementia: relationships, voices and power. *Disability and Society*, 16(3): 361–76.

Rundqvist, E.M. and Severinsson, E.I. (1999) Caring relationships with patients suffering from dementia: an interview study. *Journal of Advanced Nursing*, 29(4): 800–7.

Ryan, T., Nolan, M., Enderby, P. and Reid, D. (2004) Part of the family: sources of job satisfaction amongst a group of community-based dementia care workers. *Health & Social Care in the Community*, 12(2): 111–18.

Tester, S., Hubbard, G., Downs, M., MacDonald, C. and Murphy, J. (2004) What does quality of life mean for frail residents? *Nursing & Residential Care*, 6(2): 89–92.

Tolson, D., Smith, M. and Knight, P. (1999) An investigation of the components of best nursing practice in the care of acutely ill hospitalised older patients with coincidental dementia: a multi-method design. *Journal of Advanced Nursing*, 30(5): 1127–36.

Tresolini, C.P. and the Pew Fetzer Task Force (1994) *Health Professions, Education and Relationship-Centred Care: A Report of the Pew Fetzer Task Force on Advancing Psychological Education*. San Francisco, CA: Pew Health Professions Commission.

Ward-Griffin, C., Oudshoorn, A., Clark, K. and Bol, N. (2007) Mother–adult daughter relationships within dementia care: a critical analysis. *Journal of Family Nursing*, 13(1): 13–32.

Weaks, D., Wilkinson, H. and Davidson, S. (2005) Families, relationships and the impact of dementia – insights into the 'ties that bind'. In: L. McKie, and S. Cunningham-Burley, *Families in Society: Boundaries and Relationships*. Bristol: Policy Press.

25

Leadership in dementia care

Tonya Roberts, Kimberly Nolet and Lynda Gatecliffe

Learning objectives

By the end of this chapter you will be able to:

● recognize leadership styles and differences between management and leadership

● identify the roles of leaders in influencing some of today's important issues in dementia care delivery

● identify the challenges facing today's health care leaders

● recognize important skills for health care leaders, including strategic planning, supporting employees and systems thinking

---

Introduction

Person-centred dementia care has become synonymous with quality care for people with dementia (Brooker 2004). One meaning, described by Kitwood (1997), refers to the role of interactions and interpersonal care in maintaining personhood by addressing fundamental human needs. More recently, person-centred care has been adopted in 2001 by the National Health Service (NHS) as a core standard in the National Services Framework for Older People (Department of Health 2001). Its meaning here pertains more to the ability of people with dementia to be involved in planning and evaluating their needs and priorities for care (Nolan *et al.* 2003).

In the USA, Australia and the UK, person-centred care is also rapidly replacing traditional approaches in many nursing homes. Residents in these nursing homes often report a better quality of life than those living in traditional nursing homes (Fagan 2004) and family satisfaction is often higher (Tellis-Nayak 2007). Additionally, many nursing homes practising person-centred care experience lower rates of staff turnover and higher rates of job satisfaction (Berkhout *et al.* 2004) which has important implications for the staff–resident relationships at the core of person-centred care (Bowers *et al.* 2003) as well as other resident outcomes (Castle and Engberg 2005).

Delivering quality person-centred dementia care, however, is difficult. There are barriers to success both in the external health care environment and from within organizations. Globally the health care environment is continually changing in response to an increasing demand for quality services and the increasing need to be efficient in the use of resources. Places in which dementia care is often delivered, such as nursing homes, assisted living facilities, or at home with home care services, are particularly challenged by these demands. Largely reimbursed with public funds, resources are typically poor in these environments. At the same time, regulations and consumers demand a high level of quality services. The strain makes it difficult to provide an environment that can support the creativity and flexibility needed to deliver person-centred dementia care. Within an organization, there are often misperceptions among stakeholders that undermine efforts to transform or sustain person-centred care practices. Organizational decision-making structures further complicate the process. However, providers and organizations working with persons with dementia and delivering person-centred care have had success. A key component of this success is effective leadership.

This chapter begins by defining leadership and its various approaches. Global health care challenges facing leaders in dementia care and specific challenges to leaders implementing person-centred care within organizations are then discussed. The need for effective leadership in dementia is outlined with examples of a leader's influence on staff and the work environment in an organization. The chapter ends with the specific skills effective leaders have that successfully influence staff and patient outcomes.

Defining leadership

Defining leadership is often difficult and its meaning can vary in different contexts and across theories or approaches. The definition of leadership is often confused with management. In Table 25.1, Rost (1991) provides a comparison of leadership and management.

Table 25.1 Distinguishing leadership from management (Rost 1991)

Leadership	Management
Influence relationship	Authority relationship
Leaders and followers intend real change	Managers and subordinates produce and sell goods and/or services
Intended changes reflect mutual purposes	Goods/services result from coordinated activities

Other authors provide a similar dichotomous view of leadership and management (Goodwin 2006). Viewing the two terms in this way often leads to the assumption that leadership is good and management is bad. However, this is not true. Each serves a different purpose and the two are not necessarily mutually exclusive. In effectively led organizations, good leadership and good management must work together in tandem (Goodwin 2006).

Various theories of leadership define the concept in different ways by describing the set of traits, skills or behaviours that a leader does or should possess. There is a competing assumption across these theories about whether leaders are born or made. For example, trait theory and contingency theory presuppose that leaders are born. Trait theory assumes that personal qualities or traits of an individual determine their effectiveness as a leader. Contingency theory posits that a leader's style should be contingent upon the situation one finds him or herself in. These styles cannot be changed and so are only effective when the situation matches. On the other hand, situational leadership theories assume leaders can be made. According to a situational leadership theory, one particular set of skills or behaviours is not deemed best; rather different situations require different types of leadership. In these theories, the leader is believed to be able to adjust their behaviour accordingly to the needs of their staff.

Global challenges facing health care leaders

Global health care is in a state of flux. A myriad of demographic, social, political and economic forces are responsible for either an increase in demand for health care services or a call for improved delivery of services that is changing the nature of health care systems throughout the world (Hyrkas *et al.* 2005; Kizer 2001). Specifically, the ageing of the global population, advances in information and medical technology, trends in health care costs, and the call for evidence-based medicine are discussed below.

Several factors have increased or are predicted to increase demand for health services. Specifically, there is an increase in the number of consumers and a change in the nature of how they consume. Both the ageing of the global population and the increased prevalence of chronic diseases are rapidly becoming an area of concern in health care. By 2045 the number of adults over the age of 60 is projected to be over 1.5 billion, outnumbering children globally for the first time in history (United Nations 2007). Life expectancy is increasing (United Nations 2007) and the prevalence of chronic diseases is on the rise most rapidly in developing countries (Yach *et al.* 2004).

Concurrently, demand for services from an increasingly well-informed consumer is changing the nature of the health care encounter. Overall, patients are becoming activists in their care, demanding and using their information in care decisions. Media and information technology have aided patients and consumers to be more knowledgeable about illnesses and treatments (Institute of Medicine 2001; Kizer 2001). Approximately 70 million Americans used the internet for health information. Advances in medical technology have raised consumer expectations for care. However, the rate of development of these advances has outpaced the ability of providers to safely, efficiently and effectively deliver them (Institute of Medicine 2001).

At the forefront of these demographic and social changes just described is the need for more efficient, improved delivery of services. In most developed countries health care is the largest industry and employs a significant proportion of the population. From 1990 to 2004, health care spending has grown faster in each of the 30 countries in the Organization for Economic Co-operation and Development (OECD) except Finland (OECD 2007). For example, in 2004, the USA spent 15.3% of their gross domestic product (GDP) on health care. Switzerland spent 11.6%, Australia 9.2%, and the UK 8.3% (OECD 2007). Though the funding systems for health care differ between countries, spending on health care continues to increase at unsustainable rates in many countries (Kotlikoff and Hagist 2005). In both the USA and the UK, measures are continually being implemented to reduce ever growing costs. Recent attempts to control costs in the USA involve increased cost-sharing (Anderson *et al.* 2005). The NHS is undergoing restructuring to allow market competition to play a role in reducing cost (Fotaki and Boyd 2005).

In addition to soaring costs, inconsistencies in the way services are delivered have put great pressure on providers to be accountable for their practice and decisions. Evidence-based practice is becoming the benchmark for care decisions, further changing how care is delivered. In the UK, evidence-based practice is a consistent theme in health policy (Walshe and Rundall 2001). For example, the UK government has developed national frameworks for defining how services should be delivered, promoting the creation of performance measures, and the elimination of unjustified variations in practice (Department of Health 1998). Additionally, in both the USA and the UK, there has been an increased investment in health care research and establishments of databases and registers to nationally track all health projects (Adelman *et al.* 2000; Swales 1998).

Organizational challenges

Forces internal to an organization can also influence the ability to implement person-centred dementia care successfully. These difficulties arise in response to defining what person-centred care is and how it will be implemented, as well as the relationships among staff members and the structure of the organization. There is often a lack of clarity or consistency in the way person-centred care is defined. A lack of a clear vision or explicit expectations and role descriptions leaves staff, residents and families often very confused about what the changes will mean for them and how the changes will influence care (Scalzi *et al.* 2006). Implementation is often met with resistance and some unsure stakeholders may even actively undermine efforts. For example, those who have had a long tenure or a position of authority in the organization may resist adoption of person-centred care principles. Direct care workers may be uncomfortable with exerting authority and be unsure how to manage it. Management staff may be threatened by relinquishing power.

With managers trying to manage budgets and meet regulations, and direct care staff providing hands-on care, there is often discrepancy in the way managers and staff view the work environment (Chenoweth and Kilstoff 2002). This increases stress levels and results in staff feeling their work is unsupported, undervalued and unappreciated (Muntaner *et al.* 2004). Problems also arise when different staff members have varying abilities and knowledge to perform person-centred care. Training and ongoing education are often thought as sufficient for staff to implement knowledge into practice. However, systems are often not in place to allow this to happen. For example, staff who learn how to effectively communicate with an agitated resident cannot practise the skill on the floor if they are not given the time to do so. Additionally, decision-making structures are often not conducive to person-centred dementia care (Chenoweth and Kilstoff 2002). Workers in direct contact with persons with dementia often do not have authority to make decisions about care or work practices, hindering their ability to meet the needs and preferences of the person with dementia.

Consequences for organizations, caregivers and consumers

Staff are in the complicated position of providing quality care in more efficient ways and being accountable, while meeting rising consumer expectations. Staff can become frustrated, confused, uncertain, and have low morale. Workers do not trust what they know because the future is not predictable. There is a general feeling of a loss of power to make choices and practise effectively (Laschinger and Finegan 2005). These conditions are very stressful, and in fact, health care staff experience levels of stress at higher rates than other members of the workforce (Wall *et al.* 1997). Work stress is also found to be associated with job satisfaction, and job satisfaction, in general, is found to be a significant predictor of absenteeism, burnout, turnover and intention to quit (Lu *et al.* 2005). Consider direct care workers in the US long-term care industry as an example. Workers are charged with providing high quality of care in a tightly regulated, resource-poor environment. Stress levels are high among workers, and these direct care workers experience some of the highest health care turnover rates of over 100% in some places (Decker *et al.* 2003).

Caregiver stress can be linked to poor care. For example, a qualitative study of doctors' perceptions of stress and its impact on care showed errors from simple to fatal which were attributed to overwork, exhaustion, lack of support and symptoms of depression (Firth-Cozens and Greenhalgh 1997). Furthermore, Westwood and colleagues (2001) found that levels of stress among nurses were related to the number of patient incidents. A shortage in nursing staff could also be related to physical injury and decreased patient satisfaction. Additionally, high levels of turnover disrupt the continuity of care needed to provide person-centred dementia care. Relationships between the staff and residents cannot develop and the communication to support the needs and preferences of the residents does not occur, resulting in frustration, confusion and agitation for residents.

The role of effective leadership

Effective leaders are increasingly being looked to as essential components in managing and sustaining an organization in turbulent times. Leaders are responsible for the effective allocation of resources (Hyrkas *et al.* 2005) and improving service to consumers. Possibly more importantly, effective leadership has also been shown to successfully improve health care worker job satisfaction and the working environment. Pearson and colleagues (2007) performed a comprehensive review of nursing leadership and its role in fostering a healthy work environment in health care. Several of the studies included found that leadership style can affect staff job satisfaction. Specifically, leaders who empower staff were shown to improve job satisfaction. Good leadership is related to better working environments and lower staff turnover (Scott-Cawiezell 2005).

Leaders shape the environment to attain the above outcomes in key ways. Jim Collins, author of one of the defining leadership books of the new millennium, *Good to Great* (2001), found one of the biggest differences among companies that truly made real, sustained financial turnaround over a fifteen-year period was the leadership of the companies and the corporate culture those leaders created. These leaders were able to propel transition and sustain changes. Collins (2001) and others (Yukl 2006) have found that great leaders couple professional will with personal humility. A great leader shows resolve to do anything that gets long-term results, sets the standards of excellence for the rest of the organization, and will not blame others for poor results. In addition, the great leader will be modest, act with quiet determination, channel ambition to the organization and credit others with success (Collins 2001).

The culture that leaders create within an organization has been shown to be particularly important in person-centred dementia care. Many of the organizations that have undergone changes to implement person-centred care have described the role of leadership as vital to the continued success of efforts. The text *Culture Change in Long-Term Care* (Weiner and Ronch 2003) gives a multitude of examples and case studies of how leadership drives the environment and effectively promotes the provision of person-centred care through actions, words and vision. Effective leadership in a person-centred care organization will reduce resistance, produce opportunities for staff to obtain and use new skills and knowledge, and provide clarity of the concepts and values underpinning the organization's model of dementia care. Staff become more satisfied and have a sense of pride in their jobs.

Several domains of key leadership actions have been shown to be most successful in improving job satisfaction and creating the culture Collins described. Particularly in a person-centred dementia care environment where numerous departments must systematically interact to provide care, these include: 1) strategic planning; 2) developing and embedding a shared vision; 3) meeting employee expectations, trust, credibility, communication; 4) supporting employees; and 5) systems thinking (Senge 1990; Yukl 2006). The rest of the chapter discusses these four key domains and their implications for overcoming the challenges facing an organization providing person-centred dementia care.

Strategic planning

> Being a visionary leader is about solving day-to-day problems with my vision in mind.
>
> (Bill O'Brien, in Senge 1990: 217)

Strategic planning has an important impact on how the overall organization operates and determines what priorities drive decision-making and resource allocation. In dementia care, where resources are scarce, regulation is tight, and personhood is being increasingly valued, the importance of strategic planning cannot be understated.

Strategic planning is proactive, long-range planning that addresses an issue that concerns the entire organization. Strategic planning can:

- help address external and internal factors during times of change and turbulence

- help plan and use staff and other resources most effectively and efficiently

- help focus the organization's culture and its customer base

- build consensus about where an organization is going.

Strategic planning is an opportunity to be a proactive leader and influence organizational culture (Zuckerman 2006). By involving multiple levels of staff in the planning phase, you tend to maximize communication, buy-in and dissemination of efforts across the organization. For example, if providing state-of-the-art dementia care is part of an organization's mission, formulating strategy around the mission can provide an opportunity for leaders to bring together nursing staff, engineering staff, dietary staff, social workers, families of patients, communications staff, staff developers and physical therapists to form an inclusive strategy. If each shares a piece of strategy, it will more likely be comprehensively disseminated and appreciated across the organization.

Models of strategic planning

Generally, all traditional models of strategic planning have the following steps (Charney 1995; Mintzberg 2000):

- assess the current state of the organization/unit

- develop a vision (purpose) of where to go

- determine the 'gap' between current state and the vision

- set a direction, including baseline goals, to close the 'gap'

- implement the strategic plan

- evaluate the strategic plan periodically.

New models have developed that are more specific (McNamara 2003). Issue-based models emphasize a one-year plan and budget in the context of the long-term strategic plan. Alignment planning examines things that are working well in an organization and how they can be adjusted to make vision and strategy. Scenario planning is often used in conjunction with other models and focuses on systems thinking, considering how each strategy could best and worst impact the organization.

In the 1990s, a popular performance measurement framework was developed by Kaplan and Norton (1996) called the 'balanced scorecard'. This framework has since developed into a full strategic planning model and is commonly used by organizations, including health care, in several countries. The balanced scorecard approach combines vision statements with objectives, measures, targets, and initiatives in four categories: 1) customer, 2) learning and growth, 3) internal processes and 4) financials. Kaplan and Norton argue many organizations rely primarily on financial data only to drive strategy, and tout their approach as providing a more balanced, multi-perspective look at the past, present and future. The balanced scorecard approach shares four primary processes, common to most strategic planning models, however, the balanced scorecard approach emphasizes linking individual performance to vision and goals, and using learning and feedback (rather than relying on data) to evaluate and adjust strategy. A criticism of the balanced scorecard approach is, ironically, that it does not actually give a score. Jensen (2001) argues there is no theory-based bottom-line score, and thus managers cannot obtain an objective view of performance.

With a few exceptions, health care organizations see strategic planning as a project rather than a constant management process (Zuckerman 2006). Zuckerman argues the complex, changing conditions in health care would benefit from using more flexible, dynamic processes. Emerging models of strategic planning emphasize a less formalized process. Mintzberg (2000) claims traditional strategic planning cannot succeed because it is mainly an assessment activity, leaving little room for synthesis of ideas and creative plans. He suggests a more informal, hybrid process called 'strategy making' where few commitments are made, as the future is fairly unpredictable. Another more fluid system suggested by scholars is called 'organic planning' where shared dialogue sessions are consistently held without formalizing a linear plan. Story-boarding, learning, and discussions of current processes are common techniques used by this model (McNamara 2003).

Components of strategic planning

Although forms of strategic planning have differences, it is useful to look at the core, common components of most models to produce an operable plan. Assessment of the organization, building vision and mission, creating and evaluating a plan will be briefly explored below.

Assessment

The SWOT (developed by Stanford professor Albert Humphrey in the 1970s) and Environmental Scan (groundwork laid by Francis Aguilar in the 1960s and refined over decades) are two common tools used to assess the current state of an organization. Items such as consumer perception of the organization, position in the marketplace relative to competition, strengths and weaknesses within the organization, and areas for growth can be assessed using these models. It should be noted that these models are ways to organize information for analysis, but will not tell an organization the best way to collect the data. Employee surveys and interviews, consumer surveys and interviews, marketplace and financial data, and performance indicators are a few items an organization may use to help inform the assessment. The SWOT and Environmental Scan models are valuable, yet some have argued they are too cumbersome, time-consuming and too analytical (Hill and Westbrook 1997; Scott-Armstrong 1982). Alternative methods are just beginning to emerge for organizations to assess and strategic plan, however, none have emerged as gold standards such as the SWOT and Environmental Scan models have in the past.

Building shared vision and mission

Strategic planning is central to leading organizations, and through that process a vision and mission are built. Vision and mission should be used to guide daily activities in an organization. However, there exists a lack of clarity about what visions and mission are and how to execute them via strategy and action. Often 'vision statement' and 'mission statement' are used interchangeably; however, there is a distinct difference. A vision statement pushes an organization toward a future achievement, while a mission statement guides current organizational behaviour.

In dementia care, focusing on individual needs and personhood exist at the core of a vision and mission statement. For example, a vision statement might be 'Smith Home will become a national exemplar for providing person-centred dementia care.' A mission statement could then be, 'Smith Home recognizes the individual lives and needs of residents and strives to create a homelike environment for each person. By showing respect, sharing in their past, present and future, developing significant relationships, and nurturing interests, staff will nurture residents in maintaining meaningful lives.'

Once a vision is created and a mission statement produced, leaders must then bring the vision and mission alive in the organization. Senge (1990) argues the shared vision can be 'exhilarating' to employees. It can foster innovation and can increase employee commitment. To achieve these benefits, a leader must move to spread and operationalize vision and mission throughout the organization. If communicated and modelled effectively, employees should be able to explain and elaborate on the vision and mission to outsiders and new employees, further driving the vision into the organization and community. Dolak (2001) outlines several steps leaders can take to infuse vision and mission throughout the organization:

- create a simple statement called a 'strategic principle' (Gadiesh and Gilbert 2001) that is simple and memorable to employees

- insist all managers model behaviours consistent with the vision

- share the vision at every opportunity, internally and externally

- design communication (email footer, newsletters, advertising, etc.) to always include elements of the vision

- set the expectation that all employees will share the vision

- consistently act in accordance with the behaviour expected of others.

Additionally, there may be systems, policies and/or investments that need to be examined to carry out vision and mission. This leads into the next topic of creating a plan to progress towards the mission and vision.

Exercise 25.1   Developing mission and vision

Lakeview is a 98-bed nursing home that has seen an increase in dementia patients over the last five years. The director of nursing's (DON) father in another city recently was diagnosed with dementia, and upon choosing a long-term care facility for him, she found herself drawn to facilities with special dementia care units. She brought this up in a meeting with the administrator, inquiring if she could explore the idea of having a specialized unit at Lakeview. She'd like to provide other families with the same comfort she had, knowing staff were well trained for caring for dementia residents. The administrator and DON visit a few other facilities with these units and gather some readings. They agree it is the right direction for Lakeview to go, but have some concerns about implementing such a change. How will they decide which staff to assign to the unit? Can the facility afford to make some minor remodelling changes for a special unit? Will other residents feel neglected with this new focus? Will they have enough dementia residents on a consistent basis to fill the unit? Staff at the facilities visited appear to need more time with residents in dementia care units, yet Lakeview's staffing budget is already stretched thin.

According to the stages of strategic planning, how might they proceed? What types of information might they need to gather as part of strategic planning? What might a mission and vision statement look like for the facility?

Creating and implementing the plan

While vision and mission guide the 'big picture' in an organization, developing goals and objectives are steps to action. Developing goals and objectives, and the strategies to meet those, are at the heart of the strategic plan.

Goals are 'specific statements of what is to be achieved' according to the mission and vision of the organization (Sullivan and Decker 2001). Objectives are 'statements of achievement specific to abilities within the organization' (Sullivan and Decker 2001). The key differing point is that goals are outcome-oriented and at the organizational level, while objectives are sub-units of goals and are process-oriented and met at the individual or unit level. Goals are measurable, but are often only measured as met/not met. Objectives will likely have quantifiable results that can be measured for progress. For example, a home care agency wants to help those with dementia stay in their homes, and knows managing medication is necessary for that to happen. A goal might be 'Each person with dementia receiving our services will have a medication dispensing system in their homes to allow for better tracking and management of their medications.' Objectives for this will be measurable in increments, such as, 'Monthly totals of persons with dementia owning a medication dispensing system will increase.'

Strategies will need to be developed for meeting goals and objectives. Effective leaders will necessarily approach this with a varied team of employees. The process of strategic planning will, at minimum, need to include willing individuals that share common vision at the following levels (Sullivan and Decker 2001): 1) top-level administrators, 2) representatives of those closest to the work (e.g. frontline caregivers, social workers), and 3) staff to collect data and distribute information. Sullivan and Decker argue in the early stages of planning, it's important to only include staff that 'buy in' to the vision and mission. Naysayers 'can be included once some parts of the plan are formulated' to increase buy-in (Sullivan and Decker 2001: 27).

Evaluating the plan

Evaluating the success of the strategic plan can happen at multiple levels. Evaluating individual strategies can be done efficiently if clear objectives have been developed. Input at multiple levels (data, interviews with staff and consumers) is important to include (McNamara 2003; Zuckerman 2006). However, it is important to have a dynamic process where the objectives, goals and even sometimes mission can be adjusted as time evolves.

Exercise 25.2   Developing goals and objectives

Refer back to Exercise 25.1. The administrator and DON have several concerns about how they will implement the new dementia care unit at Lakeview. One of their concerns is that residents and family in the non-dementia unit might feel treated unequally because dementia unit residents will have remodelled space and staff will be given extra training and time to work with residents.

Try to identify a possible goal and objective around this issue. Keep in mind this goal and objective should be compatible with mission and values.

Who would need to be involved in developing these goals and objectives, as well as planning strategies to ensure the goal is met?

How leaders meet employee expectations

In a study by Kouzes and Posner (1993), employees stated the most important thing for leaders to do is 'do what they say they will do', 'practise what they preach', or 'walk the talk'. Other research concurs, indicating employees expect credibility, honesty, support, visibility, passion, collaboration, flexibility and/or competence from leaders (Bowers *et al.* 1999; Upenieks 2003).

Credibility

A leader's most arduous task may be continually trying to build credibility with employees. Kouzes and Posner (1993) found that employees perceiving high credibility of their managers have a high sense of pride in their workplace, have higher commitment to the organization and have a consistent sense of team spirit. When they see managers as having low credibility, employees may be less productive, are motivated primarily by money and have a low sense of commitment to the organization.

Assuring management has credibility with staff can mean deliberate change in systems and leadership practices. Credibility is earned through engaging in two-way communication, displaying competence and integrity (Kouzes and

Posner 2003). If a leader verbalizes commitment to a respectful work environment, yet keeps a verbally abusive nurse around because there is a nurse shortage, credibility can be lost.

Communication

Communication patterns between leadership and staff exponentially impacts organizational climate and effectiveness (Forbes-Thompson *et al.* 2006; Schein 2004). If you were to look at an organizational chart for your facility and consider all the places (within and outside) that information flows, you would probably find, at minimum, these key places:

- all departments and staff
- patients
- families
- board of directors
- corporate staff
- public/potential consumers
- trade associations.

Examining which direction the communication flows between entities and how consistent the communication is can provide a snapshot of where an organization stands in pursuit of a good communication structure.

Research has highlighted the poor perceptions staff hold regarding communication from their leaders (Forbes-Thompson *et al.* 2006; Schein 2004). Anecdotally, leaders also cite their desire to hear better communication from their staff. Many leaders and managers will say they wish employees would bring issues and discuss solutions more often. Getting employees to give constructive feedback or raise issues can be challenging.

Some suggested strategies for enhancing safe two-way communication are assuring staff have a venue to celebrate accomplishments and having more frequent, smaller meetings with frontline staff. Creating safe systems for complaints is also important, but can take time, cultivation of relationships and several efforts to develop. Anonymous suggestion boxes and frequent one-on-one meetings are two common strategies.

Integrity

> ... leadership is part vision, part art, part science, part experience, part faith and part know-how, all bound together in an ironclad package called integrity.

(Howard Adamsky)

Integrity can simply be defined as 'honouring one's word' and can provide an actionable path to gaining employees' trust (Erhard *et al.* 2007). Integrity is an issue heard often as chief executive officers are making unethical decisions and the term 'toxic leadership' becomes popular in organizational literature (Lipman-Blumen 2005). Leaders can influence employee perceptions by considering several factors: 1) knowing what commitments he/she has made and demonstrating those commitments have been met and addressing failed commitments (Garman *et al.* 2006) and 2) modelling behaviour congruent with his/her own expectations such as arriving on time for meetings, pitching in to help staff as needed and communicating problems (Scanlan 2006).

As noted by Garman and colleagues (2006) above, respect is an important component of successfully relating to employees. Respect is recognizing the value or excellence of a person or ability. Engaging in collaborative activities with staff, such as serving on committees or helping with meal delivery, is an excellent way for leadership to show respect and value for employee work and input. Acknowledging employee participation in the process, sharing the workload, and giving specific feedback on how the employees made a clear difference will show respect to those involved. A simple 'thank you' is somewhat meaningful, but a specific thank you, made public, can have significantly larger impact (Bowers 2004).

Employees place a very high value on the fairness displayed by leaders (Feltner *et al.* 2008). Perceived fairness has been associated with decreased burnout, decreased turnover and increased productivity across sectors (Heponiemi *et al.* 2007). Leaders can look for ways to increase perceived fairness in the work environment, such as enlisting employees' help in designing guidelines for conduct, performance evaluations and reward/discipline structures.

Communicating clear expectations to staff can also lead to perceived fairness. If employees are not clear about expectations, each may not have an equal opportunity to meet or exceed those expectations. In turn, leaders may seem to 'play favourites' and be seen as 'unfair' by other staff. There are several questions a leader can ask to determine if he/she is displaying fairness in the workplace: 1) Are you expecting more of some, and if so, are they being fairly compensated (financially or otherwise) for the extra responsibility? 2) Are you unfairly holding a problem employee to a lower standard of expectations because you are frustrated and unsure how to handle it? For example, if an exemplary social worker is called upon to mentor all the new social workers, are they given a new job title, or mentor pay? Or are they recognized and paid the same as others who do not provide these additional duties? Leaders and managers should examine their practices to gain a clearer picture of how fairness might be currently perceived and amended accordingly.

Supporting and empowering employees

Employee 'empowerment' can be a rather ambiguous term in health care. Many leaders are unsure what constitutes empowering their staff. To some, they consider verbal encouragement the equivalent of empowerment. While verbal support is important, structures for decision-making and encouragement at all levels are important.

Kanter (1993) asserts empowerment from organizational structures enables employees to be satisfied and more effective in their jobs, yet nurses still feel lack of control over their nursing work (Manojlovich 2007). Empowerment is seen from coming from two primary sources: environment (Kanter 1993) and personal psychological state (Manojlovich 2007). Empowerment from one's environment is often referred to as 'structural empowerment' (Laschinger and Havens 1996), and includes (Kanter 1993):

- having actual structures for advancement opportunities

- organizational awareness of worker contributions

- access to resources, information and support.

Leaders can have a direct impact on structures to empower staff. Providing career ladders, mentor programmes, and providing adequate resources for staff are all leadership tasks, yet providing all of these is not always simple. Resources, particularly in dementia care, are often lacking. Leaders must creatively look for ways to maximize effectiveness of current resources. Some examples of ways health care organizations have maximized current resources:

- more/redesigned space for facility operations

- incentive programmes for employees

- career ladders for employees

- redesign of patient living and social environments

- staff training/education in primary areas of concern

- technology to help staff do jobs efficiently

- alternative staffing models that create efficiency.

Leaders need not approach finding resources in isolation. Internal teams can assemble to identify resource needs, anticipate future needs and consider ways to address those needs.

Systems thinking

Current leadership knowledge addresses the need to focus on the systems around which an organization operates (Senge 1990; Sullivan and Decker 2001). Systems thinking is a unique approach to problem solving that views problems as a part of the overall system and if focusing on individual problems, rather than the system, it will further exacerbate the problem (McDermott and O'Conner 1997). All behaviour in organizations is affected by the system in which the behaviour occurs. For example, when the staff is trying to be more responsive to patients who are wandering, there will be many 'systems' factors that influence success of that effort. Safety measures, family involvement, social worker perspective, fall prevention programmes, the general staff knowledge, and the systems of accountability for responding to patients are only a few of the systems issues that influence management of wandering. Looking only at the responsiveness of a particular nurse, or the ability of a particular certified nurse assistant (CNA), to keep track of a resident will not go very far to address the problem. It might improve the situation for one resident at one time, but is unlikely to have any impact beyond that. Implementing an accountability system for pain management will, on the other hand, affect many patients, influence all shifts and all levels of staff.

While it is ideal if all staff can learn to think about the system influences on how they provide care, and how the work gets done, the leaders in the organization are the ones who need to take the lead. It is important that leaders respond (and are seen to respond) to problems by looking at system contributors as well as other more local factors.

Exercise 25.3 Systems thinking

Albert Thorpe has just had particularly difficult cataract surgery and is staying overnight at the hospital. The physician knows Albert also has very mild dementia. The morning after his surgery, a staff nurse comes to take Albert's vital signs, and Albert starts to yell at the nurse, insisting he wants to leave and nobody is to touch him. The startled nurse goes to the door and calls for another nurse to help. Within seconds, Albert is trying to climb out of his bed and falls, while still yelling. Meanwhile, Albert's daughter happens to arrive for his discharge and is upset to find her father in such distress. Albert eventually calms down and they get him back in to bed, as he appears to be unaffected by the fall. The charge nurse, recalling the note of dementia in his chart, informs Albert's daughter that hospitalizations and surgery can sometimes trigger more severe episodes of dementia. The staff nurse who took his vital signs is embarrassed, as she did not realize Albert had dementia, and might have approached him a bit differently had she known (although she does not really know how she would have done it differently, she just knows people with dementia have special care and communication needs). Albert's daughter is still upset, as she now has more than his vision to worry about when he gets home. She has only dealt with Albert's mild dementia and is now worried he will not know his family and accept their help.

How might hospital staff help prepare Albert's daughter for caring for his dementia needs upon discharge? Consider the roles of the social worker, discharge nurse, physician, and pharmacist, particularly.

Not all staff knew the patient had dementia, and seemed unprepared to work with dementia patients. What systems issues should be addressed to prevent future problems?

Debates and controversies

Leadership theories continue to evolve as technology, consumer preferences and economic realities shift in the business world. Health care has been a slow adopter of changes, particularly in long-term care environments. As contemporary leaders begin to sit at the heads of health care organizations, debates and controversies in leadership styles and methods will continue to emerge. Some current considerations for health care leaders include:

- How can consumer preferences be honoured in a tightly regulated environment? How will we manage risk?

- How can organizations provide modern, person-centred care given scarce financial and staff resources?

- How will education of leaders evolve and how will success be measured? Is it worthwhile to invest in developing a leader who does not have natural skills?

- Will established methods of strategic planning and assessment give way to more efficient methods, and how will that influence the work environment, consumer satisfaction, and long-term planning?

Conclusion

Global and organizational challenges to the delivery of person-centred dementia care have resulted in an environment in which staff are stressed, confused and dissatisfied, influencing the continuity and quality of person-centred dementia care. Leadership is becoming recognized as a key factor in overcoming these challenges, although health care has been slow to adapt. In recent years, however, groups caring for persons with dementia have been focusing on instilling person-centredness throughout their organizations. This creates a situation ripe for leaders to embrace strategic planning as a tool to enhance both the work and care environment.

Across varying approaches to leadership, different skills and abilities are emphasized as being important. However, the culture leaders create is pivotal in many environments and key skills and strategies that have been implicated in the success of creating this culture include a leader's ability to develop and implement a vision for the organization, create supportive staff relationships, and think at a system level. These essential ingredients, when present, can greatly enhance the delivery of person-centred care.

Further information

The **Mind Tools** web site provides management, leadership and career training.

The **Center for Strategic Planning** has a useful website.

References

Adelman, N., Chester, L. and Slack, K. (2000) The HSRProj database: update on health services research in progress. *Health Affairs,* 19(4): 257–8.

Anderson, G.F., Hussey, P.S., Frogner, B.K. and Waters, H.R. (2005) Health spending in the United States and the rest of the industrialized world. *Health Affairs,* 24(4): 903–14.

Berkhout, A.J., Boumans, N.P., Van Breukelen, G.P., Abu-Saad, H.H. and Nijhuis, F.J. (2004) Resident-oriented care in nursing homes: effects on nurses. *Journal of Advanced Nursing,* 45(6): 621–32.

Bowers, B.J. (2004) Reality, not rhetoric, empowers this staff. *BEST Practices,* 3(1): 6–10.

Bowers, B., Esmond, S. and Canales, M. (1999) Approaches to case management supervision. *Administration in Social Work,* 23(1): 29–49.

Bowers, B.J., Esmond, S. and Jacobson, N. (2003) Turnover reinterpreted: CNAs talk about why they leave. *Journal of Gerontological Nursing,* 29(3): 36–43.

Brooker, D. (2004) What is person-centred care in dementia? *Reviews in Clinical Gerontology,* 13(3): 215–22.

Castle, N.G. and Engberg, J. (2005) Staff turnover and quality of care in nursing homes. *Medical Care,* 43(6): 616–26.

Charney, C. (1995) *The Manager's Tool Kit.* New York: American Management Association.

Chenoweth, L. and Kilstoff, K. (2002) Organizational and structural reform in aged care organizations: Empowerment towards a change process. *Journal of Nursing Management,* 10(4): 235–44.

Collins, J.C. (2001) *Good to Great: Why Some Companies Make the Leap – and Others Don't.* New York: Harper Business.

Decker, F.H., Gruhn, P., Matthews-Martin, L., Dollard, K.J., Tucker, A.M. and Bizette, L. (2003) *Results of the 2002 AHCA Survey of Nursing Staff Vacancy and Turnover in Nursing Homes.* Washington, DC: American Health Care Association.

Department of Health (1998) *National Service Frameworks.* Available from: http://www.dh.gov.uk/en/Publicationsandstatistics/Lettersandcirculars/ Healthservicecirculars/DH_4004836 (accessed 25 January 2008).

Department of Health (2001) *National Service Framework for Older People.* Available from: http://www.dh.gov.uk/en/Publicationsandstatistics/Publications/ PublicationsPolicyAndGuidance/DH_4003066 (accessed 25 January 2008).

Dolak, D. (2001) Creating and communicating vision: The business leader's primary responsibility. Available from: http://www.davedolak.com/articles/ dolak5.htm (accessed 19 January 2008).

Erhard, W., Jensen, M. and Zaffron, S. (2007) Integrity: A positive model that incorporates the normative phenomena of morality, ethics and legality. 07–01 Harvard NOM Working Paper. Available at: http://www.ssrn.com/link/ HBS-NOM-Unit.html

Fagan, R.M. (2004) Pioneer network: Changing the culture of aging in America. In: A.S. Weiner and J.L. Ronch (eds) *Culture Change in Long-term Care.* Binghamton, NY: Haworth Social Work Practice Press.

Feltner, A., Mitchell, B., Norris, E. and Wolfle, C. (2008) Nurses' views on the characteristics of an effective leader. *Association of Operating Room Nurses AORN Journal,* 87(2): 363.

Firth-Cozens, J. and Greenhalgh, J. (1997) Doctors' perceptions of the links between stress and lowered clinical care. *Social Science & Medicine,* 44(7): 1017–22.

Forbes-Thompson, S., Gajewski, B., Scott-Cawiezello, J. and Dunton, N. (2006) An exploration of nursing home organizational processes. *Western Journal of Nursing Research,* 28(8): 935.

Fotaki, M. and Boyd, A. (2005) From plan to market: a comparison of health and old age care policies in the UK and Sweden. *Public Money & Management,* 25 (4): 237–44.

Gadiesh, O. and Gilbert, J.L. (2001) Transforming corner-office strategy into frontline action. *Harvard Business Review,* May: 73–9.

Garman, A.N., Fitz, K.D. and Fraser, M.M. (2006) Competencies: Communication and relationship management. *Journal of Healthcare Management,* 51(5): 291.

Goodwin, N. (2006) *Leadership in Health Care: A European Perspective.* London: Routledge.

Heponiemi, T., Elovainio, M., Laine, J., Pekkarinen, L., Eccles, M., Noro, A., Finne-Soveri, H. and Sinervo, T. (2007) Productivity and employees' organizational justice perceptions in long-term care for the elderly. *Research in Nursing and Health,* 30(5): 498–507.

Hill, T. and Westbrook, R. (1997) SWOT analysis: It's time for a product recall. *Long Range Planning,* 30(1): 46–52.

Hyrkas, K., Appelqvist-Schmidlechner, K. and Kivimaki, K. (2005) First-line managers' views of the long-term effects of clinical supervision: how does clinical supervision support and develop leadership in health care? *Journal of Nursing Management,* 13(3): 209–20.

Institute of Medicine (IOM) (2001) *Crossing the Quality Chasm.* Washington, DC: National Academy Press.

Jensen, M. (2001) Value maximization, stakeholder theory, and the corporate objective function. In: J. Andriof *et al.* (eds) *Unfolding Stakeholder Thinking.* Sheffield: Greenleaf.

Kanter, R.M. (1993) *Men and Women of the Corporation.* New York: Basic Books.

Kaplan, R.S. and Norton, D.P. (1996) *The Balanced Scorecard: Translating Strategy into Action.* Boston, MA: Harvard Business School Press.

Kitwood, T. (1997) *Dementia Reconsidered.* Buckingham: Open University Press.

Kizer, K.W. (2001) Establishing health care performance standards in an era of consumerism. *Journal of the American Medical Association,* 286(10): 1213–17.

Kotlikoff, L.J. and Hagist, C. (2005) *Who's Going Broke? Comparing Growth in Healthcare Costs in Ten OECD Countries.* NBER Working Paper No. W1(1833). Available from: www.nber.com (accessed 28 January 2008).

Kouzes, J.M. and Posner, B.Z. (2003) *Credibility: How Leaders Gain it and Lose it, Why People Demand it.* San Francisco, CA: Jossey-Bass.

Laschinger, H.K.S. and Finegan, J. (2005) Using empowerment to build trust and respect in the workplace: a strategy for addressing the nursing shortage. *Nursing Economics,* 23(1): 6.

Laschinger, H.K. and Havens, D.S. (1996) Staff nurse work empowerment and perceived control over nursing practice: conditions for work effectiveness. *Journal of Nursing Administration,* 26(9): 27.

Lipman-Blumen, J. (2005) *The Allure of Toxic Leaders: Why We Follow Destructive Bosses and Corrupt Politicians – and How We Can Survive Them.* Oxford: Oxford University Press.

Lu, H., While, A.E. and Barriball, K.L. (2005) Job satisfaction among nurses: a literature review. *International Journal of Nursing Studies,* 42(2): 211–27.

Manojlovich, M. (2007) Power and empowerment in nursing: Looking backward to inform the future. *Online Journal of Issues in Nursing,* 12(1).

McDermott, I. and O'Conner, J. (1997) *Practical NLP for Managers.* Aldershot: Gower.

McNamara, C. (2003) *Field Guide to Non-Profit Strategic Planning.* Minneapolis: Authenticity Consulting.

Mintzberg, H. (2000) *The Rise and Fall of Strategic Planning.* Toronto: Prentice-Hall.

Muntaner, C., Li, Y., Xue, X., O'Campo, P., Chung, H.J. and Eaton, W.E. (2004) Work organization, area labor-market characteristics, and depression among US nursing home workers: A cross-classified multilevel analysis. *International Journal of Occupational & Environmental Health,* 10(4): 392–400.

Nolan, M., Grant, G., Keady, J. and Lundh, U. (2003) New directions for partnerships: relationship-centred care. In: M. Nolan, G. Grant, J. Keady and U. Lundh (eds) *Partnerships in Family Care.* Maidenhead: Open University Press.

Organization for Economic Cooperation and Development (OECD) (2007) *OECD in Figures 2006–2007.* OECD Observer. Available from: http://www.oecdobserver.org/news/fullstory.php/aid/1988/OECD_in_Figures_2006–2007.html (accessed 28 January 2008).

Pearson, A., Laschinger, H., Porritt, K., Jordan, Z., Tucker, D. and Long, L. (2007) Comprehensive systematic review of evidence on developing and sustaining nursing leadership that fosters a healthy work environment in healthcare. *International Journal of Evidence-based Healthcare,* 5(2): 208–53.

Rost, J. (1991) Leadership and management. In: G.R. Hickman (ed.) (1998) *Leading Organizations: Perspectives for a New Era*. Thousand Oaks, CA: Sage Publications.

Scalzi, C.C., Evans, L.K., Barstow, A. and Hostvedt, K. (2006) Barriers and enablers to changing organizational culture in nursing homes. *Nursing Administration Quarterly*, 30(4): 368–72.

Scanlan, L. (2006) Leadership and management. Expectations without accomplishment. *Healthcare Financial Management*, 60(1): 100.

Schein, E.H. (2004) *Organizational Culture and Leadership*. San Francisco, CA: Jossey-Bass.

Scott-Armstrong, J. (1982) The value of formal planning for strategic decisions: Review of empirical research. *Strategic Management Journal*, 3: 197–211.

Scott-Cawiezell, J. (2005) Are nursing homes ready to create sustainable improvement? *Journal of Nursing Care Quality*, 20(3): 203–7.

Senge, P.M. (1990) *The Fifth Discipline: The Art and Practice of the Learning Organization*. New York: Doubleday/Currency.

Sullivan, E.J. and Decker, P.J. (2001) *Effective Leadership and Management in Nursing*. Upper Saddle River, NJ: Prentice Hall.

Swales, J. (1998) Culture and medicine. *Journal of Social Medicine*, 91(3): 118–26.

Tellis-Nayak, V. (2007) A person-centred workplace: the foundation for person-centred caregiving in long-term care. *Journal of the American Medical Directors Association*, 8(1): 46–54.

United Nations (2007) *World Population Prospects: The 2006 Revision. Fact Sheet Series A*. Population Division, Population Estimates and Projections Section, Department of Economic and Social Affairs. Available from: http://www.un.org/esa/population/publications/wpp2006/FS_ageing.pdf (accessed 28 January 2008).

Upenieks, V. (2003) Nurse leaders' perceptions of what compromises successful leadership in today's acute inpatient environment. *Nursing Administration Quarterly*, 27(2): 140.

Wall, T.D., Bolden, R.I., Borrill, C.S., Carter, A.J., Golya, D.A., Hardy, G.E., Haynes, C.E., Rick, J.E., Shapiro, D.A. and West, M.A. (1997) Minor psychiatric disorder in NHS trust staff: occupational and gender differences. *British Journal of Psychiatry*, 171: 519–23.

Walshe, K. and Rundall, T.G. (2001) Evidence-based management: from theory to practice in health care. *Milbank Quarterly*, 79(3): 429–57.

Weiner, A.S. and Ronch, J.L. (2003) *Culture Change in Long-term Care*. New York: Haworth Social Work Practice Press.

Westwood, M., Rodgers, M. and Sowden, A. (2001) *Patient Safety: A Mapping of the Research Literature*. Report from NHS Centre for Reviews and

Dissemination, University of York and Centre for Clinical Psychology and Health Care Research. Available from: http://66.102.1.104/scholar? (accessed 25 January 2008).

Yach, D., Hawkes, C., Gould, C.L. and Hofman, K.J. (2004) The global burden of chronic diseases: overcoming impediments to prevention and control. *Journal of American Medical Association,* 291(21): 2616–22.

Yukl, G.A. (2006) *Leadership in Organizations.* New York: Prentice-Hall.

Zuckerman, A. (2006) *Raising the Bar: Best Practices for Healthcare Strategic Planning.* Philadelphia: Health Strategies and Solutions, Inc. and SHSMD of the AHA.

26

Quality: the perspective of the person with dementia

Dawn Brooker

Learning objectives

By the end of this chapter you will:

- know why it is essential that evidence on quality includes the perspective of the person with dementia

- know that there are a variety of ways in which evidence can be gathered: through interviews and structured questionnaires, through use of proxy reports and through observation

- know that each of these has strengths and limitations so that a combination of approaches is optimal

- know that gathering evidence on quality from the point of view of the person with dementia is not a trivial process and due care needs to be taken to ensure the evidence is of good integrity

---

Introduction

When people are very dependent on care services, quality of life becomes inextricably linked with quality of care. With chronic progressive disabilities such as dementia, with which people live for a very long time, quality of life may be *the* most important goal. As dementia progresses, the ability of individuals to secure help in their own right, or to assert their best interests in the face of poor service quality, becomes increasingly difficult. Unless the person with dementia is blessed with a strong family support structure they may have very few advocates who will act solely in their best interests. Because of this, their citizenship rights are easily violated. This renders them extremely vulnerable to abuse – be it financial, physical, sexual or psychological.

Individuals living with dementia are likely to find it difficult to complain directly about poor quality of care because of the nature of cognitive disability that is part and parcel of dementia. In addition, many family members are worried that if they complain, services will be taken away from them or that there will be repercussions for their loved ones. Performance on many aspects of health and social care is routinely monitored by central government in the UK and other countries. However, routine monitoring of quality of life or quality of care is challenging. The tendency can be to monitor the aspects of care that are easy to measure, such as room size or prescribing. As quality reviewers, inspectors and surveyors move to focus more on outcomes of care (CSCI 2006), monitoring quality of care from the perspective of the service user with dementia becomes increasingly important.

A major barrier to hearing the voice of people with dementia is society's response in not valuing their opinion. It is more straightforward to provide services or to conduct research without seeking the viewpoint of people living with dementia. From an ethical point of view, however, it is now difficult to exclude the viewpoint of people who use health and social care services. There has been an increasing emphasis on consumerism and user involvement in health and social care over the past 20 years. The political activity of people living with physical disabilities has paved the way for the empowerment of those with learning disabilities and mental health problems.

The purpose of this chapter is to describe how evidence is gathered about quality of life and quality of care from the perspective of the person living with dementia. The chapter begins by considering the challenges inherent in accessing the perspective of people with dementia. Most of the chapter is devoted to describing three main ways of gathering information from the perspective of a person with dementia – interviews including use of structured questionnaires, proxy reports, and observation – and recommending a combination of such approaches.

The challenge of taking a user perspective about quality in dementia care

Providing evidence about service quality or quality of life is a complex process. Everyone thinks they know good quality when they see it and everyone agrees that good quality is what they want, but actually describing the different dimensions of quality can end up being a difficult and complex process.

In taking a user perspective of quality, the most direct way is to ask for the service user's opinion of their current lifestyle or their opinion of a particular service that they have used. This method poses a problem for people with dementia in that the ability to recall events and feelings from the very recent past is impaired from early on in most dementias. Questions about opinions that have been held for the person's whole adult life (such as what political party they support or how they like their eggs cooked) are relatively straightforward and reliable over time (Feinberg and Whitlach 2001). If, however, the aim is to find out what someone with dementia thinks about a day care service, this is more of a challenge. Questions like this may be met with a response of 'What day care service?' Alternatively, the person may search their memories of long ago for something that sounds like day care, and use these memories as a basis for their comments. Their responses may reflect past experiences rather than current ones.

A further challenge is that the ability to articulate judgements is increasingly compromised as expressive speech becomes more difficult. The person with dementia may have quite complex feelings about a particular service. The ability to describe complex feelings in a straightforward way is difficult for people with dementia. Likewise, the ability to appreciate the consequences of talking about judgements is increasingly compromised. Continuing with the example of asking someone with dementia about a day care service, they may quickly lose the context of why the interviewer is asking them about it. For example, they may tell the interviewer about how they dislike a service without being able to keep in mind other reasons why they might moderate their complaints. A person without cognitive disability might decide to put up with a poor day care service because it represents the lesser of two evils. They are able to keep in their mind that the alternative could mean their wife would not be able to carry on caring for them without a break.

There are also cultural and cohort-related differences in complaining. Speaking out and complaining for the current cohorts of people over 80 years old is considered bad manners and not good form. So, although the person with dementia might think the service is terrible, politeness may stop them from saying so.

Another way of gathering evidence about service quality is to look at what their behaviour, as a consumer, tells us. For example looking at how many times an individual used the day centre could be an indicator that they thought it was of good quality. However, the choice to be a consumer of a particular service is usually not the person's with dementia. Very often another person such as a relative or a health or social care professional will have instigated the service and may also be responsible for arranging transport and attendance. So, the fact that a person with dementia uses a particular day care service five days per week does not necessarily mean they think the service is good.

Ways to include the perspective of the person with dementia

There are a number of different reasons for wanting to gather evidence that informs us about the perspective of people with dementia. Researching people's experience of life is of intrinsic interest. Research on a range of questions and evaluation of innovative interventions or service provision are other reasons. From a practice perspective, having user experience as a central focus for quality assurance or clinical governance is important. Practitioners are often faced with making decisions about whether a particular placement or service is meeting people's needs. Similarly inspectors and surveyors need to know whether services are really meeting the needs of service users. In the following section the different routes to gather the experience of people living with dementia is not differentiated between these different areas of work. The author's reflection is that, having gathered evidence from the perspective of service users with dementia as a researcher, a clinician, a quality assurance manager and a collaborator with inspectors, that the general issues cut across the different purposes.

Interviews, focus groups and structured questionnaires

People living with dementia are identified at a much earlier stage in the disease process than they were ten years ago and hence are more able to speak out on their own behalf. This has resulted in a growing number of first-hand accounts from people living with dementia. The empowerment of people living with dementia, speaking out on their own behalf and helping set the agenda is a relatively new phenomenon. In response to this, the Alzheimer societies and associations worldwide have moved from organizations that primarily support family carers to ones that support and represent people living with dementia directly as well.

Many accounts of living with dementia have come directly from interviews with people who have dementia, speaking about their own experience. Useful guidance about how best to interview people living with dementia or to help them participate in focus groups are now available (Bamford and Bruce 2002; McKillop and Wilkinson 2004; Murphy 2007). This guidance emphasizes the idea of partnership, the importance of building a relationship and rapport between the interviewer and the person with dementia, being proactive in maximizing the likelihood of good communications, and in attending carefully in interpreting what is being communicated. For example, if a participant begins to relate a story that appears unrelated to the topic under discussion, it is worth attending carefully to the emotional content of such a story to see if the person with dementia is trying to relate how they feel in the here and now. Often, audiotaping and transcription can bring to light insights of this nature that might have been missed on first hearing.

The relationship of the person with dementia to the interviewer or focus group facilitator is key. If the interviewer is also responsible for providing that person with a service, it may be difficult for the interviewee to express dissatisfaction and the interviewer may find it difficult to hear negative feedback. On the other hand, being familiar with the day-to-day workings of a service may mean that the interviewer is more able to make sense of what is being said and could help the person with dementia express their thoughts more fully than could an interviewer without such extensive 'insider' knowledge.

On a day-to-day basis, people with dementia can express preferences (Feinberg and Whitlatch 2001). People with dementia may need extra help to express an opinion and must be given time to respond. They may not always express their feelings in a straightforward verbal way, but family members and attentive care staff often grow to know what constitutes a 'yes' and a 'no' for individuals experiencing even advanced dementia.

Over recent years there has been a plethora of dementia-specific quality of life questionnaires published. Many of these involve the person with the dementia completing the questionnaire as part of a structured interview with a researcher. Scholzel-Dorenbos *et al.* (2007) reviewed nine instruments for rating quality of life for people with dementia, three of which were dementia specific. These were the DQol (Brod *et al.* 1999) the QOLAD (Logsdon *et al.* 1999) and the DEMQOL (Smith *et al.* 2005). Evidence is provided that these can be used reliably with people with mild to moderate dementia.

Learning the necessary skills to interview people with dementia takes time. Reading the guidelines provided by McKillop and Wilkinson (2004) and Murphy (2007) are useful even to those using structured interviews as a starting point. It is recommended that providing adequate time for rapport building and for checking out meanings and interpretations needs to be taken into consideration when engaging in this type of evaluation.

From the author's experience of supervising staff engaged in interviewing, the strength of feelings evoked by conducting interviews can take both care practitioners and researchers by surprise. Recently, having key workers sit in during research interviews using the QOLAD with residents, the disclosures during these interviews affected how the key workers felt about the residents being interviewed. It made them realize, possibly for the first time, that their residents had an internal emotional life in the same way that they have themselves. Researchers undertaking qualitative interviews have reported being moved to tears or anger about what they are told by people with dementia during the interviews. If practitioners and researchers are not supported to work through these feelings, they may not be able to use the evidence in the most constructive way. Practitioners and researchers have often built up unconscious defences about seeing people with dementia as people like themselves. Talking through experiences that challenge these defences can help care practitioners and researchers become more sensitive to the needs of people with dementia. If these feelings are not addressed, however, it may set up a pattern of avoidance whereby the practitioners and researchers avoid any future emotional contact with people with dementia.

Direct feedback from people living with dementia can be influenced by many things in addition to cognitive impairment. Interviews are often limited to some extent by a person's desire to please the interviewer. Many people will have had the experience of being asked in a restaurant whether a meal is satisfactory and answering in the affirmative. It is often the case that true feelings about the quality of a meal are not revealed by asking people directly. The same is true of health and social care. People may claim to be satisfied when all other indicators provide evidence that the quality of care is very poor. Relying solely on what people say about their experience of a service as evidence that it is of good quality is of doubtful validity in almost all contexts.

Gathering evidencing about quality from proxies

A subset of people living with dementia, particularly in long-term care, will not be able to express themselves meaningfully verbally. In some respects, this would not be so much of a problem if the experience of those who could speak out was similar to those who cannot. For example, in a long-term care setting if the residents who can take part in interviews are reporting high levels of satisfaction then it might be reasonable to assume that people with advanced dementia were also happy. There is evidence to suggest, however, that residents who are able to participate in an interview have very different experience of care than do people with advanced dementia (Thompson and Kingston 2004). Within a care-home setting, for example, those residents who are more socially able are likely to have more staff and visitor contact. The person who finds it difficult to achieve eye-contact and who has very limited capacity for speech is likely to attract less attention.

When people have difficulty speaking for themselves about their situation it is common practice to ask someone who knows them well to speak on their behalf. In the case of people living with dementia this is often the person's next of kin or, failing this, a health or social care worker who has knowledge of their current situation. This is generally known as a proxy opinion. While proxies may be able to provide answers that would concur with the person with dementia on some occasions, there are many reasons why this might not be the case.

Exercise 26.1 Who would I choose as my proxy?

Write down quickly and honestly the three activities that give you most pleasure in your life.

Ask your life partner (if you have one) or closest friend to do the same on your behalf.

Ask your eldest child (if you have one) to do the same on your behalf.

Ask someone who regularly provides you with a service, for example, mechanic, domestic help, hairdresser, server at a favourite restaurant or shop to do the same on your behalf.

Exercise 26.1 helps to identify some of the reasons why proxy opinions are problematic. The face individuals present to different people is often very specific to that relationship. What people disclose to their partners, their close friends, their children and their service providers varies a great deal. Also certain proxies have a vested interest in highlighting certain things and not others. For example, a person's hairdresser may be more likely to put going to the hairdressers in the top three activities.

There is a body of evidence to suggest that family carers often have significantly different views of quality of care and quality of life to people with dementia (Aggarwal *et al.* 2003). There is also a fairly consistent finding that residents in nursing homes rate their quality of life as better on a variety of dimensions than staff do when asked to rate quality of life as a proxy on behalf of residents. Mittal *et al.* (2007) systematically investigated factors that widened the gap between resident-rated and staff proxy-rated quality of life. interestingly, a key finding was that higher job satisfaction on the part of the staff meant that they were more sensitive in rating their residents' quality of life than they would themselves. The implication of this is that if we are relying on proxy staff ratings, the validity of these may be at risk particularly where job satisfaction is poor.

Advocacy for people living with dementia is a possible alternative. Advocates are more independent proxies than family carers or professionals and may be able to get a closer approximation to the viewpoint of the people living with dementia, although the practice is complex (Cantley and Steven 2004). Further research is required to elucidate this complexity and demonstrate best practice models. Those appointed as Independent Mental Capacity Advocates under the new UK Mental Capacity Act 2005 may be asked to make judgements on quality of life issues by proxy.

Some of the structured quality of life instruments have versions of the same instrument that can be completed both by the person with dementia and their proxy – either family member or key worker. This is true both of the QOLAD (Logsdon *et al*, 1999) and the DEMQOL (Smith *et al.* 2005). The participant and proxy versions of these tools are not interchangeable. They offer different perspectives and both are important to track over time if they are to be used to evidence the impact of interventions or services. For example, if the tools were being used to evaluate quality of life over a period of several years it may be that the participant version is more valid early on, while the proxy version is more valid as the dementia progresses.

Some structured quality of life instruments ask proxies – usually either care workers or professionals – to rate how a person has felt over the past few weeks and what their activities and patterns of behaviour have been like. In the ADRQL, the trained interviewer asks the proxy raters about their observations of the person with dementia over the past few weeks and then summarizes these. The QUALID (Weiner *et al.* 2000) is a brief scale filled in by a proxy focusing on activity and emotional state. Ettema *et al.* (2007) describes the QUALIDEM, which is also rated by professionals from care-giver reports. The Psychological Well-being in Cognitively Impaired Persons (PWB-CIP) (Burgener *et al.* 2005) and the Well-Being Profile tool (Bruce 2000) provide proxy measures of an important aspect of quality of life. The advantage of these proxy-rated measures is that they can be used across a wider range of cognitive disability and can be used to track changes over time. Some of these, such as the ADRQL (Rabins *et al.* 1999) also require the person administering them to undergo training.

Observation as evidence

Observation is a basic part of care and of human interaction. As well as listening to what people say, human beings are programmed to observe body language and behaviour. In a research context observation forms the basis of scientific method. Participant observation is a well used method in qualitative research.

Observational methods can be helpful in assessing what happens to people with dementia who are receiving services and in assessing their reaction to different situations when people find it difficult to speak about those reactions. Observation can be either structured or unstructured, systematic or casual.

Structured observational methods developed specifically for evidencing quality in long-term care settings have been around for many years. As far back as 1995 Brooker reviewed a number of such methods namely patient engagement (McFayden 1984); the Short Observation Method (SOM) (MacDonald *et al.* 1985); the Patient Behaviour Observation Instrument (PBOI) (Bowie and Mountain 1993); the Quality of Interactions Schedule (QUIS) (Dean *et al.* 1993) and Dementia Care Mapping (DCM) (Kitwood and Bredin 1992). Later observational methods in the dementia care field include the DS-DAT (Volicer 1999), which is a direct observation scale to assess direct signs of comfort/discomfort in people with severe dementia. The Affect Rating Scale (Lawton 2001) has been utilized widely in the USA. These observational methods all offer a structured way of observing and assessing the experience of people with dementia living in formal care settings or using services. They are only of use in communal care settings where the observer can 'fade' into the background.

Observational methods provide the opportunity to include the perspective of those who cannot speak for themselves. They provide evidence of what happens to people with dementia in communal areas of formal care settings and evidence of how people spend their time, and of how they are treated by staff and professionals. There is always a trade-off between utilizing a structure that enables behaviour and events to be captured systematically and having a code in place for the seemingly infinite variety of events that can occur. Some methods are more complex than others. No structured method can describe every situation. In some situations with some particaulr person in some particular context there will be something that does not fit into a coding system. Note-taking and contextual qualification are always necessary to capture the many exceptions to the rules.

There has probably been more published on DCM than any other single dementia specific observation tool (Brooker 2005). The late Professor Tom Kitwood developed Dementia Care Mapping as an attempt to represent the standpoint of the person with dementia in service evaluations. Kitwood described DCM as 'a serious attempt to take the standpoint of the person with dementia, using a combination of empathy and observational skill' (Kitwood 1997: 4).

DCM was developed in an era when it was thought that people with dementia could not provide reliable accounts of their own experience. The motivation for its development, however, as the quote from Kitwood suggests, was so that the standpoint of the person with dementia was represented. The development of DCM and subsequent guidance for its use in practice and research have emphasized the centrality of people with dementia in this process. There is a concern that observations may in themselves diminish the quality of life of people with dementia by making them feel intimidated. Brooker and Surr (2005) provide various ways to ensure that observations include both service users and staff so they do not feel marginalized or intimidated by the process.

The structured observational methods that seek to clarify the experience of care generally require training and practice if they are to provide reliable evidence. DCM, the Affect Rating Scale and the DS-DAT all require structured training. Bradford Dementia Group has spent many years standardizing training in DCM and making it easy to learn. Over the years, the basic training course has increased from two to four days. Even with a standardized training programme, the inter-rater reliability of practitioners using DCM in regular practice is not high (Thornton *et al.* 2004). Those who have used DCM for research purposes can achieve good reliability (Sloane *et al.* 2007).

More recently within the context of researching people's experience in care homes, video and digital recording have also been used in care settings and with individuals. Such recordings provide the advantage of being able to replay and provide very fine-grained analysis (Cook 2002). This enables in-depth observation to occur without the imposition of predetermined categories. Video evidence can be particularly valuable when working with people with very advanced dementia whose speech on first listening seems meaningless – but on repeated replay shows clear attempts at communication (e.g. Killick and Allan 2006).

Just as interviewing can be an emotional experience for the interviewer, observing in a care setting can be a challenging experience. Innes and Kelly (2007) describe the difficult emotions involved in observing poor care practice. It brings observers face to face with shortcomings in a service they may previously have thought was good and may evoke feelings of inadequacy that they have not intervened when practice is poor.

Combining forms of evidence

Given the limitations of all the ways of gathering information about quality of life and quality of care, a combination of approaches is recommended. Providing evidence of quality relies on multiple methods and multiple perspectives, not on a single source of evidence (Innes and Kelly 2007; Murphy 2007). It needs to provide evidence of the different perspectives from interviews with people with dementia, with staff and family carers, questionnaires and of observation of practice and non-verbal behaviour and the physical and social environment. Interviews and observation together provide a very rich data set used with service users and staff teams to get their views on quality improvements (Barnett 2000). One method is not a substitution for the other. They should be seen as complementary to each other. This is reflected in a number of developments and systems to assist care providers in seeking evidence from these different perspectives (e.g. Brooker 2007; Faulkner *et al.* 2006; Poole 2006).

Another example of using observational data in combination with other sources of evidence includes the new method of inspecting the standards of care in English care homes for people with dementia. The Short Observation Framework for Inspection (SOFI) was developed by the author in collaboration with the Commission for Social Care Inspection (CSCI) who have responsibility for monitoring standards in residential and nursing homes (Brooker *et al.* 2007). SOFI involves structured observation of a sample of five residents in a communal area, often over a lunch time period, usually for a period of a couple of hours. Although the observation time is relatively brief, inspectors have the advantage of doing this as part of an in-depth evaluation in which they can interrogate other records in a care home, interview staff and residents and seek to triangulate evidence and explore themes through case tracking. SOFI was not designed as a stand-alone measure. It is always used in conjunction with other inspection tools such as interviewing service users, staff, significant others and a review of records. Through using SOFI, the inspector attempts to tune into the residents' experience, something that is often not possible through interviewing people over such a short time period. It can be thought of as providing information, which forms part of a jigsaw or picture about what the residents experience. Such a picture can enable inspectors to drill down to practice issues such as care culture, staff training and over-use of medication.

Deciding on how to gather information

From this overview, it can be seen that there are many tools to choose from. Choosing the most appropriate tools will be determined by a number of considerations. Some of these are outlined in Exercise 26.2.

Exercise 26.2   Questions to help you to identify which tools you need

1   What is the question I want to answer?

2   How much time have I got?

3   Do I want to know about relatively few people in a great deal of depth?

4   Do I want to survey a larger number of people?

5   Do I want to demonstrate change over time?

6   How able are the people with dementia that I want to gather evidence from?

7   Do they have the cognitive capacity to answer the questions I need to ask verbally? Are there ways I can assist them to answer?

8   Do they have the understanding of language to cope with my questions and the ability to express themselves in my area of enquiry? Are there less taxing ways of helping them to answer my questions?

9   Do they have eyesight and hearing problems that may hinder them taking part? Are there things I can do to alleviate these?

10   What is the quality of the support networks around the people I want to gather evidence from?

11   How reliable would family members be in being able to comment on the part of the person with dementia? How reliable would friends be in being able to comment on the part of the person with dementia?

12   How reliable would care staff be in being able to comment on the part of the person with dementia?

13   What is the context in which I will collect the evidence?

- people's own homes
- care home
- housing scheme
- hospital ward
- club

14.   Do I have the necessary skills and experience to gather this evidence?

15.   Do I have the necessary skills and experience to analyse this evidence?

16.   What instruments and processes will help to provide best evidence?

Being clear at the outset about the reasons for collecting evidence will help in the choice of the optimal combination of tools. Evaluating the impact of an activity programme will give rise to a different approach than evaluating outcomes in an acute hospital setting. Recognizing whether it is important to know about changes over time will also influence which tools are selected.

If the purpose of using these tools is within a quantitative research context, then it is worth bearing in mind that many of the tools have been fairly recently developed. Consequently, the data on what represents a significant change are only just emerging. Currently the QOLAD (Logsdon 1999), DCM (Brooker 2005) and ADRQL (Lyketsos *et al.* 2003) have data available suitable for power calculations. This is likely to change as more studies are published.

The amount of time available to gather evidence is important. Providing evidence from the perspective of the service user is particularly labour-intensive with people with dementia. To ensure that an interview or observation process is relatively enjoyable, is ethical and provides meaningful information takes more time than getting key workers to fill in a questionnaire.

Quality of life and quality of care are influenced by the cultural background and current situation in which the person with dementia finds themself. Likewise the tools that are used to evidence quality are determined in part by the culture of the people who developed them. Caution is required when using tools developed in one country to assess quality of services in another country. Even if translation is not an issue, the same words in the English language can have different meanings in different English-speaking countries and indeed in different parts of the same country. This has implications when using structured questionnaires containing statements that people with dementia are asked to agree or disagree with. Having the experience of working with DCM across many different counties and continents, the author reflects that although some things, such as the importance of being shown respect, are universal, the ways in which this is expressed are very much determined by cultural rules. These rules are difficult to access unless one is part of that culture.

Providing evidence about quality when people are living in their own home, in extra care housing or in a care home will determine both the instruments that are chosen and the processes you choose to collect evidence. Using structured observation in domestic settings is problematic. Likewise, if people are ill in hospital then their perceptions about quality of life are likely to be different than when their health is stable. Some methods and processes will work in some settings but not in others.

As a generalization, questionnaires and interviews with people with mild to moderate dementia are likely to be more straightforward than with people who have more advanced dementia. The author's experience, however, is that there are many people with dementia who seemingly have very limited cognitive capacity but who can sum up what is going on around them using a few very carefully chosen words. As a general rule though, observational and proxy measures will be easier to use with those in moderate or advanced stages.

Observational tools are sometimes promoted because there is an expectation that they will perform in a more uniform manner across the spectrum of dependency. However, in DCM there is much evidence to suggest that low well-being scores are more likely in people with greatest dependency needs. On the other hand other researchers have found the opposite or no correlation between level of cognitive impairment and well-being scores. The correlations between low scores and high dependency may of course be related to a third factor of poorer quality of psychosocial care for people with dementia who have high dependency needs (Brooker 2005). From Mittal's (2007) research we now also have the possibility that this may be related to the job satisfaction among staff.

Dementia is an umbrella term that covers different disease processes in people who are often experiencing a wide range of co-morbid acute and chronic health problems. Having a single tool that will produce standardized results across all the diagnostic categories and all the degrees of disability is not possible.

To help readers think through some of the process issues in planning to collect evidence of quality it is suggested they use the example in Exercise 26.3.

Exercise 26.3 Identifying which tools and processes to use

In response to the way in which older people are treated in hospital and care homes, the UK government launched the Dignity in Care campaign (Department of Health 2006) to ensure older people were treated with dignity in hospital and in care homes.

If you wanted to systematically gather evidence from the perspective of people with dementia on this theme, how would you go about it?

What instruments would you use?

What might the impact be of your report?

Debates and controversies

The reliability and validity of different instruments claiming to measure quality of life and quality of care are an ongoing issue. All of the formal standardized measures cited here have evidence about the reliability of the method used by different raters across time. Most of the statistics that are quoted about reliability for any of the instruments reviewed in this chapter will have been carried out under research conditions, not regular practice. The observation of the author is that in a complex field such as dementia care people have a habit of changing measures to fit their specific purpose and this can weaken reliability and validity. Some tools that were developed primarily for research such as the QUIS are now used in practice to improve quality of care. Other tools such as DCM, which were developed primarily as a way of developing care practice, have been utilized in research. This is an issue that practitioners need to be aware of if they are relying on scores as evidence of quality in dementia. The awareness that scores can be deflated or inflated depending on how the tool is applied appears to be limited. If this information is collated to inform policy decisions, the errors can multiply exponentially.

There is also the question of how different instruments relate to each other and which provide the most valid evidence for quality from the perspective of the person with dementia. It has been argued in this chapter that, in part, we attempt to compensate for the shortfalls in all these measures by triangulating each with the other. Edelman *et al.* (2004) demonstrated a moderately significant correlation between DCM scores and the proxy QOLAD/Staff (Logsdon *et al.* 1999) and the proxy Alzheimer's Disease-Related Quality of Life – ADRQL (Rabins *et al.* 1999) in adult day care. This study did not demonstrate a correlation between any of these measures compared to direct quality of life interviews with a less cognitively impaired sub-group. In his multi-method study, Parker (1999) noted that during interviews, people with dementia rated their quality of life as better than their DCM scores would suggest. The relationship between these different types of evidence requires further research.

Conclusion

Evidencing quality from the perspective of the person living with dementia is complex both conceptually and practically. There is an inherent tension in providing standardized measures of quality of life and quality of care for such a heterogeneous group of people living out their lives in a multiplicity of ways. Yet unless there are standardized measures of these important outcomes and processes, then practitioners, inspectors, researchers and policy-makers will continue to rely on the easy-to-measure such as cognitive status or compliance with health and safety regulations. There are more ways of evidencing the personal perspective for people with dementia in health and social care than ever before but it still remains a time-consuming and resource-heavy process if the evidence is to have any validity. Is the cost of providing this evidence worth the benefits that will accrue from having it? There is evidence going back for a very long time that many people living with dementia experience poor quality care that impacts adversely on their quality of life. Having more tools to describe this does not change the situation. It is a necessary but in and of itself insufficient condition for change. This situation will only change when there is a political and societal will to address it.

Further information

Dementia and Advocacy Support Network International (DASN) is an organization by and for people who have been diagnosed with dementia. The organization is entirely internet-based with participants from around the world. The purpose of the organization is to promote the dignity of people with dementia, to provide a forum for exchange of information and to advocate for people with dementia.

The Bradford Dementia Group maintains a comprehensive list of articles related to Dementia Care Mapping.

The Relatives and Residents Association is an organization that champions the rights and well-being of people with dementia who are going into care homes or live in care homes. It is a resource on care home standards and is designed to assist relatives to determine the quality of care homes.

The Commission for Social Care Inspection England (CSCI) is a website for consumers and relatives that addresses how quality of care homes is determined. It tells consumers how to find the information they need on particular homes.

References

Aggarwal, N., Vass, A.A., Minardi, H.A., Ward, R., Garfield, C. and Cybyk, B. (2003) People with dementia and their relatives: personal experiences of Alzheimer's and the provision of care. *Journal of Psychiatric and Mental Health Nursing,* 10: 187–97.

Bamford, C. and Bruce, E. (2002) Successes and challenges in using focus groups with older people with dementia. In: H. Wilkinson (ed.) *The Perspectives of People with Dementia: Research Methods and Motivations.* London: Jessica Kingsley.

Barnett, E. (2000) *Including the Person with Dementia in Designing and Delivering Care – 'I Need to Be Me!'* London: Jessica Kingsley.

Bowie, P. and Mountain, G. (1993) Using direct observation to record the behaviour of longstay patients with dementia. *International Journal of Geriatric Psychiatry,* 8: 857–64.

Brod, M., Stewart, A.L., Sands, L. and Walton, P. (1999) Conceptualization and measurement of quality of life in dementia: the dementia quality of life instrument (DQoL). *The Gerontologist,* 39(1): 25–35.

Brooker, D. (1995) Looking at them, looking at me. A review of observational studies into the quality of institutional care for elderly people with dementia. *Journal of Mental Health,* 4: 145–56.

Brooker, D. (2005) Dementia care mapping: a review of the research literature. *The Gerontologist,* 45 (special issue 1): 11–18.

Brooker, D. (2007) *Person Centred Dementia Care: Making Services Better.* London: Jessica Kingsley.

Brooker, D., May H., Walton, S., Francis, D. and Murray, A. (2007) Introducing SOFI: A new tool for inspection of care homes (Short Observation Framework for Inspection). *Journal of Dementia Care,* 15(4): 22–3.

Brooker, D. and Surr, C.A. (2005) *Dementia Care Mapping: Principles and Practice.* Bradford: University of Bradford, p. 155.

Bruce, E. (2000) Looking after well-being: a tool for evaluation. *Journal of Dementia Care,* 8(6): 25–7.

Burgener, S.C., Twigg, P. and Popovich, A. (2005) Measuring psychological well-being in cognitively impaired persons. *Dementia,* 4(4): 463–85.

Cantley, C. and Steven, K. (2004) 'Feeling the way': Understanding how advocates work with people with dementia. *Dementia,* 3(2): 127–43.

Commission for Social Care Inspection (CSCI) (2006) *Inspecting for Better Lives: A Quality Future.* Available from: http://www.csci.org (accessed 7 February 2008).

Cook, A. (2002) Using video observation to include the experiences of people with dementia in research. In: H. Wilkinson (ed.) *The Perspectives of People with Dementia: Research Methods and Motivations.* London: Jessica Kingsley.

Dean, R., Proudfoot, R. and Lindesay, J. (1993) The Quality of Interactions Scale (QUIS): Development, reliability and use in the evaluation of two Domus units. *International Journal of Geriatric Psychiatry*, 8: 819–26.

Department of Health (2006) Dignity in care campaign. Available from: http://www.dh.gov.uk/en/Policyandguidance/Healthandsocialcaretopics/Socialcare/Dignityincare/index.htm (accessed June 2007).

Edelman, P., Fulton, B.R. and Kuhn, D. (2004) Comparison of dementia-specific quality of life measures in adult day centres. *Home Health Care Services Quarterly*, 23(1): 25–42.

Ettema, T.P., Droes, R-M., de Lange, J., Mellenbergh, G.J. and Ribbe, M.W. (2007) QUALIDEM: Development and evaluation of a dementia specific quality of life instrument. Scalability, reliability and internal structure. *International Journal of Geriatric Psychiatry*, 22: 549–56.

Faulkner, M., Davies, S., Nolan, M. and Brown-Wilson, C. (2006) Development of the combined assessment of residential environments (CARE) profiles, *Journal of Advanced Nursing*, 55(6): 664–77.

Feinberg, L.F. and Whitlatch, C.J. (2001) Are persons with cognitive impairment able to state consistent choices? *The Gerontologist*, 41(3): 374–82.

Innes, A. and Kelly, F. (2007) Evaluating long stay settings; reflections on the process with particular reference to DCM. In: A. Innes and L. McCabe (eds) *Evaluation in Dementia Care*. London: Jessica Kingsley.

Killick, J. and Allan, K. (2006) The Good Sunset Project: Making contact with those close to death. *Journal of Dementia Care*, 14(1): 22–4.

Kitwood, T. (1997) *Dementia Reconsidered*. Buckingham: Open University Press.

Kitwood, T. and Bredin, K. (1992) A new approach to the evaluation of dementia care. *Journal of Advances in Health and Nursing Care*, 1(5): 41–60.

Lawton, M.P. (2001) Quality of care and quality of life in dementia units. In: L.S. Noelker and Z. Harel (eds) *Linking Quality of Long-term Care and Quality of Life*. New York: Springer Publishing Company.

Logsdon, R.G. (1999) *Assessing Quality of Life in Alzheimer's Disease*. New York: Springer Publishing Company, pp. 17–30.

Logsdon, R.G., Gibbons, L.E., McCurry, S.M. and Teri, L. (1999) Quality of life in Alzheimer's disease: Patient and caregiver reports. *Journal of Mental Health and Aging*, 5: 21–32.

Lyketsos, C.G., Gonzales-Salvador, T., Chin, J.J. *et al.* (2003) A follow-up study of change in quality of life among persons with dementia residing in a long-term care facility. *International Journal of Geriatric Psychiatry*, 18: 275–81.

MacDonald, A.J.D., Craig, T.K.L. and Warner, L.A.R. (1985) The development of a short observation method for the study of activity and contacts of old people in residential settings. *Psychological Medicine*, 15: 167–72.

McFayden, M. (1984) The measurement of engagement in institutionalised elderly. In: I. Hanley and J. Hodge (eds) *Psychological Approaches to Care of the Elderly*. London: Croom Helm.

McKillop, J. and Wilkinson, H. (2004) Make it easy on yourself! Advice to researchers from someone with dementia on being interviewed. *Dementia*, 3(2): 117–25.

Mittal, V., Rosen, J., Govind, R. *et al.* (2007) Perception gap in quality-of-life ratings: An empirical investigation of nursing home residents and caregivers. *The Gerontologist*, 47(2): 159–68.

Murphy, C. (2007) User involvement in evaluations. In: A. Innes and L. McCabe (eds) *Evaluation in Dementia Care*. London: Jessica Kingsley.

Parker, J. (1999) Education and learning for the evaluation of dementia care: the perceptions of social workers in training. *Education and Ageing*, 14(3): 297–314.

Poole, J. (2006) Best practice in dementia care. Improving the health and well-being of older people with mental health needs. *Journal of Care Services Management*, 1(1): 16–33.

Rabins, P., Kasper, J.D., Kleinman, L., Black, B.S. and Patrick, D.L. (1999) Concepts and methods in the development of the ADRQL. *Journal of Mental Health and Aging*, 5 (1): 33–48.

Scholzel-Dorenbos, C.J.M., Ettema, T.P., Bos, J. *et al.* (2007) Evaluating the outcome of interventions on quality of life in dementia: Selection of the appropriate scale. *International Journal of Geriatric Psychiatry*, 22: 511–19.

Sloane, P., Brooker D., Cohen, L., Douglass, C., Edelman, P., Fulton, B.R., Jarrott, S., Kasayka, R., Kuhn, D., Preisser, J.S., Williams, C.S. and Zimmerman, S. (2007) Dementia care mapping as a research instrument. *International Journal of Geriatric Psychiatry*, 22: 580–99.

Smith, S.C., Lamping, D.L., Banerjee, S. *et al.* (2005) Measurement of health related quality of life for people with dementia: development of a new instrument (DEMQOL) and an evaluation of current methodology. *Health Technology Assessment*, 9(193): III–IV.

Thompson, L. and Kingston, P. (2004) Measures to assess the quality of life for people with advanced dementia: Issues in measurement and conceptualisation. *Quality in Ageing*, 5(4): 29–39.

Thornton, A., Hatton, C. and Tatham, A. (2004) Dementia care mapping reconsidered: exploring the reliability and validity of the observational tool. *International Journal of Geriatric Psychiatry*, 19: 718–26.

Volicer, L., Hurley, A.C. and Camberg, L. (1999) A model of psychological well-being in an advanced dementia. *Journal of Mental Health and Aging*, 5: 83–94.

Weiner, M.F., Martin-Cook, K., Svetlik, D.A., Saine, K., Foster, B. and Fountaine, C.S. (2000) The Quality of Life in Late stage dementia (QUAL-ID) Scale. *Journal of the American Medical Directors Association*, 1: 114–16.

27

Reframing dementia: the policy implications of changing concepts

Jesse F Ballenger

Learning objectives

By the end of this chapter you will:

- understand the basic historical development of dementia as a public health issue in the twentieth century

- understand how that history has shaped politics and policy

- understand the implications of that history for the structure of public policy and policy debate on dementia, in particular, why research efforts for prevention or cure of dementia have been so much better funded than policies to support caregivers, particularly in the United States

---

Introduction

Politics and policy for age-associated progressive dementia revolve around two imperatives: funding for research into prevention or cure, and funding for programmes to support professional and family caregivers of people with dementia. While on the face of it these two imperatives would not seem inevitably to conflict, in policy discourse in the United States at least they have typically been pitted against each other, even by advocates who recognize the need for both research and care. The result of this contest has been that research has generally enjoyed significantly more public funding than innovative programmes to support care. This chapter examines the history of advocacy efforts for Alzheimer's disease (AD) in the United States to help explain why the drive to cure has trumped the need for quality care in terms of public funding, and consider what would be necessary for change.

To be sure, the United States, like other comparably developed countries, spends enormous sums on dementia care through Medicaid and Medicare, programmes created in 1965 that pay for health care to the indigent and elderly respectively. In 2005, Medicaid paid $21 billion for nursing home care for people with AD. While Medicare does not generally pay directly for dementia care, health care for people with dementia costs much more because people with dementia are more likely to require hospitalization or other expensive care arrangements for treatment of concurrent illnesses; a study funded by the Alzheimer's Association estimated that Medicare spends nearly three times more for beneficiaries with dementia than those without – costs amounting to

$91 billion in 2005. And of course with the ageing of the baby boom generation, Medicaid and Medicare spending on dementia is projected to increase to truly monumental proportions in the coming decades (Alzheimer's Association 2007).

But by all accounts this spending is hardly adequate to meet the needs of people with dementia and those who care for them. Medicaid requires that patients (and their spouses) spend down their savings to poverty levels before it will begin to pay for residential care, and many expenses associated with dementia care are not covered by either programme – thus adding financial stress rather than relieving it. More importantly, both Medicare and Medicaid were structured around meeting the needs of people suffering from acute illnesses; they do not provide or encourage the development of services and programmes that would be most helpful and appropriate to people with dementia and their families. There is no comprehensive network of programmes to support quality care for people with dementia or, more generally, older people with chronic illnesses. Family members shouldering the physical and emotional burdens of caregiving find it difficult to find and access what services do exist to help them, and continue to struggle to piece together the fabric of care.

The federal government spends relatively little on care programmes specifically designed for dementia. The 2008 federal budget allocated only about $13.4 million for dementia caregiving programmes – most of it for a matching grants programme that provides funds to states for developing innovative programmes aimed at influencing broader health care systems and providing community-based services for those with AD and their caregivers. The proposed 2009 budget, currently being negotiated in Congress, would eliminate this programme completely. By contrast, funding for biomedical research on Alzheimer's disease (along with biomedical research in general) has grown tremendously and remains stable throughout two decades of budgetary constraint in the United States. In 1976, the federal government spent less than a million dollars on AD research. The 2008 budget allocated about $645 million, which represented a slight decline from a peak of $658 million in 2003. This followed similar growth in overall spending for biomedical research at the National Institutes of Health (NIH), which grew from about $2.3 billion in 1976 to about $28.5 billion in 2005, where it has remained for the past several years.

This chapter does not argue that we are spending too much for research, but that we cannot expect that potential breakthroughs in medical treatment on the distant horizon can solve the problems people with dementia and their families face today or in the near-term future. Policies that support caregivers and enrich the environment of dementia patients can have a dramatic impact on the quality of life of patients now. It is long past time to redress the imbalances in the way the two policy imperatives are approached, and that this will require re-framing the problem in a way that does not pit them against each other.

Framing dementia in history

The politics and policy of dementia have been dominated by the emergence of AD, its most prevalent form, as a major public issue since around 1980. The seemingly rapid rise at that time of AD from an obscure entity known only to specialists, to a household word and object of a massive research programme is typically represented as a result of scientific progress. But the emergence of AD involved much more. The basic biological, clinical and epidemiological facts of AD had been established and widely accepted since the early twentieth century: neuritic plaques and neurofibrillary tangles associated with memory loss and cognitive deterioration, occurring sometimes in people in their 50s and early 60s but much more often in older people. To be sure, there has been significant scientific progress in understanding age-associated progressive dementia between Alois Alzheimer's first description of AD in 1906 and the present. But these basic facts did not change in the 1980s, nor have they changed since. What has changed – significantly – is the cultural framing of dementia.

Frames are the concepts and metaphors that allow human beings to understand reality, transforming the indecipherable complexity of raw experience into a comprehensible pattern that we can recognize. Frames shape what counts as common sense, and as a result they shape our goals, and our plans and actions for reaching them. In politics, frames shape social policy and the social institutions we form to implement policy (Lakoff 2004).

In the late 1970s, a group of neuroscientists, family members, and policy-makers successfully reframed age-associated, chronic, progressive dementia as the product of discrete disease processes rather than an outcome of ageing. By 1980 as we shall see, AD, as the most common and devastating of the disease processes producing dementia, came to dominate the politics and policy of dementia, driving an emphasis on biomedical research over caregiving.

Of course, this was only the latest of several major re-framings of dementia that have occurred over the past century. It is useful to divide the modern history of dementia into three periods, as indicated in Table 27.1. In the first period, the basic clinical, biological and epidemiological facts of AD were established. Subsequent historical periods involved less a dramatic change in our understanding of those facts than a change in the way those facts have been framed with relation to broader issues of ageing: how researchers, policy-makers and the general public thought dementia was related to ageing, and why it was important to pay attention to dementia. Table 27.1 shows the successive reframing of age-associated progressive dementia since its basic clinical and pathological features were established by Alzheimer and Kraepelin at the beginning of the last century.

Table 27.1 Three periods in the modern history of dementia

Period	Frame
1900–1929	Alzheimer, Kraepelin and the foundations of Alzheimer's disease *Frame: AD as a prototypical brain disease*
1930–1969	American psychiatry, social gerontology and the fight against senility *Frame: Dementia as a problem of ageing*
1970–present	Emergence of Alzheimer's Disease as a public issue *Frame: AD as the dread disease afflicting an ageing society*

The next three sections discuss the development and framing of dementia in each historical period.

Exercise 27.1   Don't think of an elephant

Try the following simple thought experiment: Don't think of an elephant! Whatever else you do, do not think of an elephant. Of course, it is impossible to meet this challenge, for the word *elephant* itself evokes the image of an elephant. Cognitive linguist George Lakoff uses this example to explain the power of cognitive frames: 'Every word, like *elephant,* evokes a frame, which can be an image or other kinds of knowledge: Elephants are large, have floppy ears and a trunk, are associated with circuses, and so on. The word is defined relative to that frame. When we negate a frame, we evoke the frame' (Lakoff 2004).

What does this thought experiment say about the power of frames, and what are the implications for the politics and policy of dementia?

Alzheimer, Kraepelin and the foundations of Alzheimer's disease

German psychiatrist Alois Alzheimer and his mentor Emil Kraepelin are generally held to have established the foundations of AD as a diagnostic category one hundred years ago after Alzheimer's brief report of the case of a 51-year-old woman who developed progressive dementia, accompanied by focal signs, hallucinations and delusions. On post-mortem, her brain was found to contain numerous senile plaques and neurofibrillary tangles, which were made visible to microscopic observation through a newly developed silver-staining technique. In 1910, on the basis of this case and a handful of others, Alzheimer's mentor and boss Emil Kraepelin bestowed the eponym in the 8th edition of his influential psychiatric book. Alzheimer and Kraepelin's work provided a unified description of the clinical symptoms of AD and its essential pathological features – the plaques and tangles that are found in the brain at autopsy – that remains the basis of the AD concept today (Ballenger 2000).

From our vantage point today, what perhaps seems most surprising about the early history of the AD concept was that it seemed relatively insignificant to Alzheimer, Kraepelin and their contemporaries. Alzheimer's initial report drew no enthusiastic reaction from the audience of psychiatrists who heard him give it, nor did its publication in 1907 draw any significant attention (Maurer and Maurer 2003), and Kraepelin himself devoted only a few pages of a massive book to it. After Alzheimer's death in 1915, almost none of the many tributes to him written by his colleagues even mentioned AD. Alzheimer was remembered by his contemporaries, including Kraepelin, for his clinical and histopathological acumen and intensive work ethic, not for having discovered the 'disease of the century' for which his name is a household word today (Maurer and Maurer 2003).

AD did not seem significant to Alzheimer, Kraepelin and their contemporaries because they framed it terms of the problems psychiatry faced at the time. At the turn of the twentieth century, the feeling was widespread that clinical psychiatry was far behind other fields of medicine that were increasingly able to identify the pathogenesis and aetiology of discrete disease entities through bacteriological and pathological research (Rosenberg 1992). Psychiatry by contrast seemed only able to explain mental illness in terminology that seemed more metaphysical than scientific. The one exception was the discovery by German psychiatrists in 1857 that 'general paresis', one of the most common forms of insanity, was connected to syphilitic infection. The recognition that general paresis was in fact tertiary syphilis raised new hope that clinical–pathological correlations would lead to etiological theories, and ultimately therapeutic interventions, for other forms of mental illness (Engstrom 2003; Shorter 1997).

Kraepelin and Alzheimer were interested in AD because it seemed a good candidate to be the second major mental disorder for which a clear pathological basis had been established. Ultimately, it was not accepted as such because it could not be disentangled from ageing. Though they established a clear clinical picture with a basis in brain pathology, they could not decisively determine whether the clinical symptoms and pathological structures constituted a disease entity or a part of the normal processes of ageing, as remains the case today. Ironically, Kraepelin, known as the Linnaeus of psychiatry because he established a simple and rational nosological system based on careful observation of the natural history of mental diseases, exacerbated the confusion by creating the entity 'AD' to distinguish the relatively rare cases in which dementia developed before the age of 65 (pre-senile dementia) from the common occurrence of dementia in more advanced ages (senile dementia). Kraepelin made this distinction despite the fact that the pathological hallmarks, clinical symptoms and natural history of both pre-senile and senile dementia were virtually identical. Age of onset appeared to be the only criterion on which the distinction was made. In grappling with Kraepelin's classification of the dementias, subsequent researchers had to puzzle not only about the relationship of senile dementia to the normal processes of ageing, but about the relationship between Alzheimer's pre-senile dementia to senile dementia, and whether it was related to ageing in the same way or at all (Beach 1987).

So why then did Kraepelin create the new entity? He may have done so for a variety of reasons, but it seems clear that for him it made no sense to call senile dementia a disease. The pathological processes of old age that produced senile dementia were understood to be on the extreme end of 'normal', while dementia occurring at earlier ages, even though associated with the same brain pathology, seemed to suggest a disease (Ballenger 2006a). As many historians have pointed out, this assumption that mental and physical deterioration were normal in old age was deeply embedded in medicine and Western culture more broadly, and remains powerful today (Haber 1983; Katz 1996). This assumption remained powerful, and seemed to be the reason that the psychiatric literature maintained the distinction between AD as a rare disorder distinct from senile dementia through the 1970s, despite the fact that researchers were well aware of and puzzled by its apparent similarity to senile dementia (Holstein 1997, 2000). As framed by Alzheimer and Kraepelin, age-associated progressive dementia was interesting to the degree that it could be seen as a disease distinct from ageing; to the degree that it was connected with ageing processes, its status as a disease was doubtful and significance minimal.

Framing dementia as a problem of ageing in mid-century American psychiatry

The first challenge to this framing of dementia within medicine was the work of American psychiatrists in the 1930s, whose interest in it grew precisely because it was so strongly associated with ageing. For American psychiatrists in the 1930s, age-associated progressive dementia posed a daunting problem. In the late-nineteenth century, reforms in public policy made care of the mentally ill the responsibility of state rather than local governments. An unintended result of this was that local welfare officials were given a strong financial incentive to regard the old people who could no longer live independently in the community as insane so that they would be institutionalized in the state mental hospitals at the expense of state governments As a result, both the absolute and proportional number of aged patients admitted to the state hospitals increased dramatically, and the mental hospitals remained the institutional centre of psychiatry in the United States during this period (Grob 1983; 1986). Because psychiatry regarded senile dementia as incurable, its rising prevalence in the state mental hospital patient population undermined the therapeutic environment that the state hospitals were supposed to provide. Because the population in society as a whole was ageing, the problem was regarded by many as an impending crisis – a demographic avalanche that would bury the state hospital as a viable institution, and the professional legitimacy of psychiatry along with it (Ballenger 2000).

American psychiatrists reacted to this problem in two ways. Some argued that since senile dementia was not a proper psychiatric condition, alternative care arrangements ought to be found for patients with dementia who were clogging the state hospital system. This was accomplished in 1965 through provisions in the Medicare and Medicaid legislation that made the federal government responsible for funding nursing-home care of the elderly, resulting in the shift of many thousands of elderly patients out of the mental hospitals and into nursing homes and various community care arrangements that were created in response (Grob 1991).

But another group, led by David Rothschild of the Worcester State Hospital in Massachusetts, developed a new theory of dementia that emphasized psychosocial factors over brain pathology in the aetiology of dementia – thus bringing the age-associated dementias into the mainstream psychiatry of the time. The basis of this re-conceptualization was the imperfect correlation between dementia and brain pathology; in some cases, the senile plaques and neurofibrillary tangles that were found in the brains of patients suffering from dementia were also found in the brains of patients who had shown no sign of dementia in life. In other cases, the brains of patients who died severely demented were found at autopsy to be relatively intact. For Rothschild and his followers, this lack of correlation between clinical and pathological data was the most interesting aspect of dementia because it suggested that individuals possessed a differing ability to compensate for organic lesions. Seen this way, age-associated dementia was more than the simple and inevitable outcome of a brain that was deteriorating due to disease and/or ageing. Rather, dementia was a dialectical process between the brain and the psychosocial context in which the ageing person was situated. Factors such as pre-morbid personality structure, emotional trauma, disruptions of family support, and social isolation were regarded as at least as important in explaining dementia as the biological processes within the brain that produced plaques and tangles (Ballenger 2000).

For psycho-dynamically oriented American psychiatrists, the psychodynamic approach was a more satisfying theory of dementia, and provided a logical basis for making meaningful therapeutic interventions, and there was a surge of interest in age-associated dementias within American psychiatry during this period. In the 10 years from 1926 to 1935, there had only been nine articles concerning senile dementia and/or Alzheimer's disease published in the *American Journal of Psychiatry* and the *Archives of Neurology and Psychiatry*, the two leading professional journals; in the following decade, 36 articles appeared. Much of this literature concerned the use of therapies that had previously been considered inappropriate for aged patients – including psychotherapy, electroconvulsive therapy, hormones, vitamins and other drug treatments. From 1935 to 1959, 35 articles reporting on the use of therapies, including group psychotherapy and hormone treatments, appeared in these two journals. These reports were generally enthusiastic about the results, but this may say as much about how badly clinicians wanted meaningful treatments for dementia as about their efficacy. In any case, these positive results were generally not replicated when randomized controlled studies began to be conducted on many of these treatments in the 1970s (Ballenger 2000).

But the psychodynamic model offered more than a rationale for the therapeutic efforts of desperate psychiatrists in the state hospitals. It also seemed to provide insight into the entire experience of ageing in post-World War II America. In the 1940s and 1950s, virtually all American psychiatrists working on senile dementia, including Rothschild himself, who had developed his model on extensive post-mortem evidence, stopped investigating brain pathology. Nor did they attempt to delineate various disease entities based on pathological lesions, but folded Alzheimer-type dementia, cerebral arteriosclerosis and functional mental disorders into a broad concept of senile mental deterioration, whose pathological hallmarks were not brain deterioration but modern social relations. The locus of senile mental deterioration was no longer the ageing brain, but a society that, through mandatory retirement, social isolation and the disintegration of traditional family ties, stripped the elderly of their role in life. Bereft of any meaningful social role and suffering the effects of intense social stigma, it was not surprisingly that the mind of the elderly began to deteriorate. As Rothschild argued:

in our present social set-up, with its loosening of family ties, unsettled living conditions and fast economic pace, there are many hazards for individuals who are growing old. Many of these persons have not had adequate psychological preparation for their inevitable loss of flexibility, restriction of outlets, and loss of friends or relatives; they are individuals who are facing the prospect of retirement from their life-long activities with few mental assets and perhaps meagre material resources. (Rothschild 1947: 125)

Other American psychiatrists in this period pushed the turn to the social much further than Rothschild, going so far as to argue that that social pathology should in fact be regarded as the *cause* of brain pathology. Maurice Linden and Douglas Courtney argued that 'senility as an isolable state is largely a cultural artifact and that senile organic deterioration may be consequent on attitudinal alterations' (Linden and Courtney 1953: 912), though the authors acknowledged that this hypothesis was difficult to prove. David C. Wilson was less circumspect, arguing that the link between social pathology and brain deterioration was simply a matter of waiting for 'laboratory proof' to support what was adequately demonstrated by clinical experience – that the 'pathology of senility is found not only in the tissues of the body but also in the concepts of the individual and in the attitude of society'. Wilson cited the usual evidence of pathological social relations in old age: the break-up of the traditional family, mandatory retirement and social isolation. 'Factors that narrow the individual's life also influence the occurrence of senility,' he asserted. 'Lonesomeness, lack of responsibility, and a feeling of not being wanted all increase the restricted view of life which in turn leads to restricted blood flow' (Wilson 1955: 905). Social pathology could even be discerned, it seemed, within the constricted blood vessels of the ageing brain.

By bringing together cultural anxieties about the isolation, emptiness and stigma of ageing in modern society with the frightening symptoms of dementia, the psychodynamic approach to senile mental deterioration contributed to a broad reframing of ageing that was taking place in post-World War II American society. The psychodynamic figured especially in popular and professional discourse that sought to make retirement a meaningful and desirable stage of life by making it financially secure and emotionally satisfying. To the emerging field of social gerontology, the high prevalence of senile mental deterioration, as construed by psychiatrists like Rothschild, was an indictment of society's failure to meet the needs of the elderly (Ballenger 2006b).

The 'adjustment' of the individual to ageing was the key concept for social gerontologists in the 1940s and 1950s. This adjustment could be negative, resulting in senile mental deterioration, or it could be positive, resulting not only in the preservation of mental health, but the discovery of new and satisfying interests and activities to replace those that had been lost with age (Ballenger 2000). Though adjustment to old age was ultimately a personal matter, prominent gerontologists argued that 'in modern America the community must carry the responsibility of creating conditions that make it possible for the great majority of older people to lead the independent and emotionally satisfying lives of which they are capable' (Havighurst 1952: 17). The community's responsibility went beyond altruism, for if their needs were not met, the burgeoning ageing population would result in a catastrophic increase in senility. As Jerome Kaplan, an advocate for recreation programmes argued, 'with the number of people who are over 65 increasing significantly each year, our society is today finding itself faced with the problem of keeping a large share of its population from joining the living dead – those whose minds are allowed to die before their bodies do' (Kaplan 1953: 3). The solution was a programme to provide older people with meaningful activities to fill the remainder of their lives.

Broadly construed, this was the programme of social gerontology for reconstructing old age. And whatever the scientific merits of this model of the social production of 'senility' as an account of the pathogenesis of dementia, those who framed dementia this way were generally successful in winning a series of significant policy changes that helped to transform the experience of ageing in America. By the 1970s, much of this programme had in fact been accomplished. The material circumstances of old age had been markedly improved (though not to an equal extent for all older people); significant legal protections had been won against age discrimination; negative stereotypes in popular and professional discourse were increasingly challenged, and, perhaps most importantly, the elderly themselves organized for effective political advocacy an action on their own behalf (Haber and Gratton 1994). In this context, the problem of age-associated dementia became more visible and tragic. As noted above, after 1965 deinstitutionalization increased the burden that dementia posed to communities and families, while heightened expectations for old age made senile dementia an even more devastating prospect (Ballenger 2006b).

Reframing senility as Alzheimer's disease

This framing of dementia as part of a broad category of senility that had been the basis of psychodynamic psychiatry and gerontology in the 1940s and 1950s began to seem inappropriate for the new era of ageing that was taking shape in the 1960s and 1970s. Ageism was now the key term in social gerontology for a more aggressive and politicized generation. Ageism was coined by Robert Butler in 1968 to describe the 'process of systematic stereotyping of and discrimination against people because they are old, just as racism and sexism accomplish this with skin colour and gender' (Butler 1975: 12). One of the worst aspects of ageism was the belief that ageing entailed inevitable physical and mental decline, and Butler and other gerontologists argued that virtually all of the physical and mental deterioration commonly attributed to old age was more properly understood as the product of disease processes distinct from ageing. 'Senility', in the view of gerontologists like Butler, was not a medical diagnosis, but a 'wastebasket term' applied to any person over 60 with a problem, and rationalized the neglect of those problems by assuming that they were inevitable and irreversible. ' "Senility" is a popularized layman's term used by doctors and the public alike to categorize the behaviour of the old,' Butler argued. 'Some of what is called senile is the result of brain damage. But anxiety and depression are also frequently lumped within the same category of senility, even though they are treatable and often reversible.' Because both doctors and the public found it so 'convenient to dismiss all these manifestations by lumping them together under an improper and inaccurate diagnostic label, the elderly often did not receive the benefits of decent diagnosis and treatment'

(Butler 1975: 9–10). Butler did not discount the reality of irreversible brain damage, as had an earlier generation of psychiatrists. Rather, he argued that the refusal to systematically distinguish the various physical and mental disease processes from each other and from the process of ageing itself was a manifestation of the ageism that kept society from taking the problems of older people seriously. In this context, a group of clinical neurologists and psychiatrists, neuropathologists and biochemists who entered the field in the 1960s and 1970s worked to reframe age-associated dementia in old age as a number of disease entities distinct from ageing.

These researchers produced significant gains in scientific knowledge about dementia in the 1960s and 1970s: the British research group of Martin Roth, Gary Blessed and Bernard Tomlinson put the connection between pathology and the clinical manifestation of dementia on a firmer foundation by developing a technique of quantifying plaques in the brain and correlating them with scores on standardized dementia scales; Robert Terry and Michael Kidd separately used electron microscopy to study the plaques and tangles, providing important clues to their molecular structure; three separate research groups in the United States and the United Kingdom identified a deficit in the neurotransmitter acetylcholine as a central feature of AD. But none of this research was sufficient to resolve the central question of whether AD and other dementias were connected to the process of ageing or not. A reasonable case could – and still can – be made either way. On the one hand, no pathological, biochemical or clinical markers existed or yet exist which qualitatively differentiate AD from an extreme form of normal ageing. If AD were a distinct disease entity, one would expect a number of these markers to be distributed in a bimodal pattern throughout the ageing population, differentiating the diseased from the normal. But every potential marker for AD more closely follows a linear distribution ascending with age, suggesting that AD is the end point of a continuum. One could suppose, as proponents of a disease model, that real markers have simply not been identified yet or cannot yet be measured with sufficient accuracy to reveal the expected distribution, but such suppositions are far from persuasive evidence. There are also problems in viewing AD as but an extreme point on the continuum of ageing. From the continuum model, it would follow that everyone who lived long enough would develop AD, and it ought to be possible to establish an age limit beyond which all survivors are demented. While the prevalence of AD clearly climbs with age, there are many well-established cases of people living to be very old – well past a hundred years – with little cognitive impairment. If the endpoint of such a continuum is well beyond the human lifespan, conceptualizing AD this way becomes virtually meaningless. One could suppose that individuals age at different rates, but this would lead back towards viewing those who aged 'prematurely' as suffering from a distinct disease (Huppert and Brayne 1994).

Though conclusive evidence was lacking, the question was too important to be ignored since many researchers seemed to feel that the issue called into question the value of their enterprise. AD research had to be about more than an investigation into one of the many effects of ageing; to ascribe an aetiological role to ageing, it seemed, was to associate research with a fanciful pursuit of the fountain of youth. AD was definitively reframed by American neurologist Robert Katzman in a 1976 editorial in the *Archives of Neurology*, in which he argued that distinction between AD and senile dementia should be dropped since at both the clinical and pathological level they were identical. This dramatically increased the number of cases of AD. Extrapolating from a number of small community studies that had been done in the 1950s and 1960s, Katzman estimated that there were as many as 1.2 million cases of AD in the United States in 1976, and 60,000–90,000 deaths a year from it – making it the fourth or fifth leading cause of death in the United States (Katzman 1976). In 1978, Katzman along with Robert Terry and Katherine Bick enlisted the support of the directors of the National Institute of Neurological Disorders and Stroke, the National Institute of Mental Health, and the newly established National Institute on Aging (NIA) to convene a major workshop conference on AD to address nosological issues and encourage talented researchers from a variety of fields to begin working on the disease. An essential outcome of Katzman's editorial and the conference was consensus not only that AD and senile dementia were a unified entity – Senile Dementia of the Alzheimer Type – but that this entity was not part of the normal ageing process. Rather, it was a disease whose mechanisms could be unravelled through basic research leading eventually to effective treatments and ultimately prevention (Katzman and Bick 2000).

Exercise 27.2 Cultural framing and the experience of dementia

We have examined the ramifications of historical shifts in the framing of dementia for politics and policy. But such shifts in frame probably had an impact on the direct experience of dementia for both caregivers and people with dementia. For example, a different framing of dementia may make the condition more or less stigmatizing. An interesting source for further exploring this issue are autobiographies. As Alzheimer's disease emerged as a major public issue, autobiographical accounts by caregivers became a popular resource for better understanding the experience of dementia. Notable caregiver accounts include Shanks (1999), Bayley (1999) and Levine (2004) – though many have appeared. Perhaps more interesting still, a number of autobiographies have been published by people with dementia, for example, Henderson (1998), DeBaggio (2002) and Taylor (2006). It is difficult to compare the experiences described in these books to the experience of dementia in earlier historical periods because such memoirs simply did not appear prior to the emergence of AD as a major public issue. But, reading these autobiographical accounts, the struggle with stigma and fear are certainly dominant themes.

In what ways might the different historical frames described in this chapter have affected the experience of dementia for caregivers and people with dementia?

Framing cure versus care in Alzheimer's disease advocacy

The reframing of AD was politically powerful, allowing researchers, ageing advocates and policy-makers committed to AD research to make a convincing case that public resources should be allocated for research into AD. Perhaps the most prominent advocate for AD research was Robert Butler, who was appointed the first director of the National Institute on Aging (NIA) when it was established in 1974. Butler made AD the focal point of the fledgling institute, following a disease-specific lobbying strategy that had worked for other institutes within the National Institutes of Health. Butler knew that it would be much easier to sell to Congress on the need for research on a dread disease than on the basic science of ageing (Fox 1989). Butler's strategy was highly successful; by the end of the 1980s, the NIA budget for AD research had increased more than 800%. Federal funding for AD research has continued to grow, even in an era characterized by budgetary constraints, reaching a plateau of over $600 million by the first decade of the twenty-first century.

But the reframing of dementia as AD and the disease-specific lobbying strategy built around it have had negative albeit unintended consequences for advocacy efforts to win support for caregivers, an imperative that most involved in the AD field recognize and endorse. This can be seen in the early history of the Alzheimer's Association, the leading advocacy organization for age-associated progressive dementia in the United States, whose commitment to support of caregivers cannot be questioned. Yet the Association's decision to focus exclusively on AD meant it would be a much more effective advocate for research than for caregiver support. The national organization was formed as the Alzheimer's Disease and Related Disorders Association (ADRDA – later shortened to Alzheimer's Association) in 1979 by the merger of seven local grassroots organizations, but in 1980 conflict among these groups arose over whether the organization should advocate for all sorts of brain conditions, and two of the organizations left when the national organization resolved to focus public education and advocacy efforts exclusively on AD (Fox 1989). If the primary goal of the organization was to increase the level of federal support for biomedical research, then the narrow focus on AD was the perfect strategy and the Alzheimer's Association became a highly effective advocate for increasing AD-specific research funding for the NIA. But if the primary goal was to increase the level of support for caregivers, the disease-specific strategy was counterproductive. Programmes and services that would help AD victims and their families would help victims and caregivers struggling with the effects of any type of brain impairment, and some policies dearly sought by AD families, such as long-term care insurance, would benefit those struggling with virtually any chronic disabling illness. If increasing support for caregivers had been the primary goal of the Association, the logical course would have been to create a broader constituency of people affected by the many diseases that would have benefited from the same policies.

The marginalization of care can also be seen in the rhetoric of AD advocates which frequently posited a trade-off – albeit usually implicitly – between support for research and support for caregiving. AD advocates ostensibly endorsed with equal vigour an increase in federal money to support both research and caregiving. But in describing the 'disease of the century', they forged a link between the costs of caregiving and the need for research that undermined the plausibility of arguments that could be made for major social policy initiatives to address the problems of caregivers. In making the case for research funding, AD advocates emphasized the tremendous economic burden the disease placed on society for items like nursing home care – costs which would dramatically increase if a treatment or cure for the disease were not found. In so doing, they also underscored the degree to which policy changes that would substantially benefit caregivers would be prohibitively expensive. For example, in the mid-1980s, the ADRDA's first president Jerome Stone frequently decried what he saw as the imbalance between the amount of money spent on research and the amount of money spent on care. In the ADRDA's first annual report (1984), he noted that 'our nation still spends 800 times more to care for our nearly three million Alzheimer's victims than it allocates for research. Federal and private insurance programmes still pay little or none of the staggering costs of Alzheimer's patient care' (ADRDA 1984: 2). Stone is not trying to marginalize the need for caregiver support here, but that is the effect. In such formulations, these two policy goals stand in an uneasy relationship. Caregiving is positioned as an unfortunate and unnecessary burden – the price we pay for our failure to commit enough resources to find a cure.

The unintentional marginalization of caregiving in the rhetoric of AD advocates is perhaps most explicit in the frequent comparisons made between AD and polio, thus invoking one of the triumphal moments of modern medical science. For example, when ADRDA board member Lonnie Wollin was asked in his 1985 testimony before Congress to prioritize funding for caregiving vs. funding for research, he found it difficult to choose. 'There are people calling our office who are frightened. They need respite and care,' he noted. 'On the other hand, if you don't fund substantial research, you will have this problem for a long time. The only analogy would be polio. Had the money gone into treatment, we would have a magnificent portable iron lung, but no cure for the disease. I think the dollars that are available have to be spread out between the immediate respite care and research' (US House of Representatives, Select Committee on Aging 1986: 24). Wollin was clearly trying to balance the two policy goals equally, but for Members of Congress the power of the polio analogy surely tipped the balance in favour of research. The polio analogy was a rhetorical trump card, making funding for biomedical research a moral imperative in its ability to relieve suffering, and the most sensible fiscal policy because it would dramatically lower the costs of caring for disease victims. If polio was indeed the 'only analogy', then, whether Wollin explicitly said so or not, research had to be the number one priority.

Exercise 27.3   Reframing dementia

In order to win broader support for innovative public programmes to support care for people with dementia it will be necessary to reframe dementia as something other than a degenerative brain disease.

What concepts, images, and metaphors would allow this kind of reframing of dementia?

Debates and controversies

There are many reasons why it has been difficult to win support for dementia caregiving in the United States, but its marginalization within AD advocacy discourse has surely not helped. To move the politics and policy of dementia care forward, we will need to create new meanings and possibilities for dementia care. In part, this will require setting aside the logic of the disease-specific strategy to forge alliances between larger constituencies for policies that would aid caregivers for all sorts of chronic disorders. It will also require creating a new language for caregiver that lifts it free from an association with the goal of finding a cure or prevention for dementia that inevitably marginalizes care. These meanings have begun to emerge through innovative programmes like Dementia Care Mapping and the Timeslips storytelling project, which utilizes storytelling to transform the relationship between people with dementia and professional caregivers. The values embodied in these programmes must be translated into the language of advocacy, so that dementia care can begin to be seen as a good in itself rather than simply a burden that we must shoulder in the absence of medical breakthroughs. Finally, some in the AD field argue that we may need to challenge the framing of dementia as a medical entity itself and adopt a less rigid understanding of the experience of dementia that accepts not only the obvious losses, but recognizes the possibilities for meaning and enjoyment that can remain and perhaps even be enhanced (Whitehouse and George 2008).

Conclusion

In the USA, funding for research into prevention and cure of dementia has received significant government support, with evidence suggesting that this support is increasing. Far less has been expended on research or the development of programmes to support family and professional caregivers who provide the bulk of care for people with dementia. This trend in funding is compounded by the ongoing discrepancy in government health funding for acute versus chronic care. That is, funding for acute care is considerably greater than is funding for chronic conditions. As a chronic condition, dementia care programmes fall into this less supported care category One consequence is that family members who have long shouldered the burdens of caregiving are finding it difficult to access services that would help them continue to provide care. This chapter has outlined the history of developments in the USA that have led to these funding differences and the efforts to shift more dollars in the direction of developing care programmes for people with dementia and their caregivers.

Further information

Timeslips Storytelling Project is a project which is actively engaged in reframing dementia by emphasizing the creativity and imagination that remain in people with dementia through a creative storytelling method designed for people with dementia and their caregivers.

Anne Basting, the creator of the Timeslips Project, has a blog called 'Forget Memory' that is broadly aimed at 'imagining a better life for people with memory loss'.

The Rockridge Institute is a non-profit, non-partisan think tank devoted to deepening and broadening public understanding of the worldviews, values and ideas that drive the political process. Rockridge's approach is rooted in the theory of cognitive frames that informs this chapter.

The Alzheimer's Association is the leading health care voluntary association in the United States advocating for public policy related to AD and related forms of dementia.

Alzheimer's Disease International (ADI) is a federation leading health voluntary associations from 77 different nations advocating for public policy related to AD and related forms of dementia.

References

Alzheimer's Association (2007) *Alzheimer's Disease Facts and Figures* (2007) Chicago: Alzheimer's Association.

Alzheimer's Disease and Related Disorders Association (1984) *ADRDA 1984 Annual Report*. Chicago: Alzheimer's Disease and Related Disorders Association.

Ballenger, J.F. (2000) Beyond the characteristic plaques and tangles: mid-twentieth century US psychiatry and the fight against senility. In: P. Whitehouse, K. Maurer and J.F. Ballenger (eds) *Concepts of Alzheimer Disease: Biological, Clinical and Cultural Perspectives*. Baltimore, MD: Johns Hopkins University Press.

Ballenger, J.F. (2006a) Progress in the history of Alzheimer's disease: The importance of context. *Journal of Alzheimer's Disease,* 9: 1–9.

Ballenger, J.F. (2006b) *Self, Senility and Alzheimer's Disease in Modern America*. Baltimore, MD: Johns Hopkins University Press.

Bayley, J. (1999) *Elegy for Iris*. New York: St. Martin's Press.

Beach, T.G. (1987) The history of Alzheimer's disease: Three debates. *Journal of the History of Medicine and Allied Sciences*, 42: 327–49.

Butler, R.N. (1975) *Why Survive? Being Old in America*, 1st edn. New York: Harper and Row.

DeBaggio, T. (2002) *Losing My Mind: An Intimate Look at Life with Alzheimer's*. New York: Free Press.

Engstrom, E.J. (2003) *Clinical Psychiatry in Imperial Germany: A History of Psychiatric Practice*. Cornell Studies in the History of Psychiatry, 1st edn. Ithaca, NY: Cornell University Press.

Fox, P. (1989) From senility to Alzheimer's disease: the rise of the Alzheimer's disease movement. *Milbank Quarterly*, 67(1): 58–102.

Grob, G. (1983) *Mental Illness and American Society, 1875–1940*. Princeton, NJ: Princeton University Press.

Grob, G. (1986) Explaining old age history: the need for empiricism. In: D.D. Van Tassel and P.N. Stearns (eds) *Old Age in a Bureaucratic Society*. New York: Greenwood Press.

Grob, G. (1991) *From Asylum to Community: Mental Health Policy in Modern America*. Princeton, NJ: Princeton University Press.

Haber, C. (1983) *Beyond Sixty-five: The Dilemma of Old Age in America's Past*. Cambridge: Cambridge University Press.

Haber, C. and Gratton, B. (1994) *Old Age and the Search for Security: An American Social History*. Bloomington, IN: Indiana University Press.

Havighurst, R. (1952) Social and psychological needs of the aging. *Annals of the American Academy of Political and Social Science*, 279: 11–17.

Henderson, C.S. (1998) *Partial View: An Alzheimer's Journal*. Dallas, TX: Southern Methodist University Press.

Holstein, M. (1997) Alzheimer's disease and senile dementia, 1885–1920: An interpretive history of disease negotiation. *Journal of Aging Studies*, 11(1): 1–13.

Holstein, M, (2000) Aging, culture, and the framing of Alzheimer Disease. In: P.J. Whitehouse, K. Maurer and J.F. Ballenger (eds) *Concepts of Alzheimer Disease: Biological, Clinical and Cultural Perspectives*. Baltimore, MD: Johns Hopkins University Press.

House of Representatives, Select Committee on Aging (1986) 99th Congress, *Alzheimer's Disease: Burdens and Problems for Victims and their Families*. Washington, DC: US Govt. Printer.

Huppert, F. and Brayne, C. (1994) What is the relationship between dementia and normal aging? *Dementia and Normal Aging*. New York: Cambridge University Press.

Kaplan, J. (1953) *A Social Program for Older People*. Minneapolis: University of Minnesota Press.

Katz, S. (1996) *Disciplining Old Age: The Formation of Gerontological Knowledge, Knowledge, Disciplinarity and Beyond*. Charlottesville, VA: University Press of Virginia.

Katzman, R. (1976) Editorial: The prevalence and malignancy of Alzheimer disease. A major killer. *Archives of Neurology*, 33(4): 217–18.

Katzman, R. and Bick, K. (2000) *Alzheimer Disease: The Changing View*. San Diego, CA: Academic Press.

Katzman, R., and Bick, K.L. (2000b) The rediscovery of Alzheimer Disease during the 1960s and 1970s. In *Concepts of Alzheimer Disease: Biological, Clinical and Cultural Perspectives*. P. Whitehouse, K. Maurer and J. F. Ballenger, Baltimore, MD: Johns Hopkins University Press.

Lakoff, G. (2004) *Don't Think of an Elephant: Know Your Values and Frame the Debate*. White River, VT: Chelsea Green.

Levine, J. (2004) *Do You Remember Me? A Father, a Daughter, and a Search for the Self.* New York: Free Press.

Linden, M. and Courtney, D. (1953) The human life cycle and its interruptions: a psychologic hypothesis. *American Journal of Psychiatry,* 109: 906–15.

Maurer, K. and Maurer, U. (2003) *Alzheimer: The Life of a Physician and the Career of a Disease.* New York: Columbia University Press.

Rosenberg, C.E. (1992) *The Crisis in Psychiatric Legitimacy: Reflections on Psychiatry, Medicine, and Public Policy. Exploring Epidemics and Other Essays in the History of Medicine.* New York: Cambridge University Press.

Rothschild, D. (1947) The practical value of research in the psychoses of later life. *Diseases of the Nervous System,* 8: 123–8.

Shanks, L.K. (1999) *Your Name is Hughes Hannibal Shanks: A Caregiver's Guide to Alzheimer's.* New York: Penguin.

Shorter, E. (1997) *A History of Psychiatry: From the Era of the Asylum to the Age of Prozac.* New York: John Wiley and Sons.

Taylor, R. (2006) *Alzheimer's from the Inside Out.* Baltimore, MD: Health Professions, Press.

Whitehouse, P.J. and George, D. (2008) *The Myth of Alzheimer's: What You Aren't Being Told About Today's Most Dreaded Diagnosis.* New York: St. Martins Press.

Wilson, D.C. (1955) The pathology of senility. *American Journal of Psychiatry,* 111: 902–6.

28

The history and impact of dementia care policy

Jane Gilliard

Learning outcomes

By the end of this chapter, you will:

● understand the impact of public policy on provision of care for people with dementia

● understand the historical shifts in defining dementia and how these shifts have influenced care and services

● be familiar with strategies for implementing public policy at the local and organizational levels

● understand the importance of integrating mental health and older people's services to achieve quality care for people with dementia

Introduction

While it is important to target dementia care practice improvements at both the individual and organizational levels, pervasive and lasting practice change requires a broader approach, including changes in public policy. We have seen elsewhere in this book how new ideas and the implementation of a different way of working can enhance the lives of people with dementia. This chapter will describe how policy changes and the initiatives they generate can support or undermine efforts to improve the lives of people with dementia and their carers.

Using England as an exemplar, this chapter traces the history and impact of public policies related to care and services as well as care environments for people with dementia. It reviews policy developments over the past decade up to the current development of a National Dementia Strategy. Many of the changes in public policy concerning dementia care and services can be traced to indecision about whether dementia should be considered an ageing or a mental health issue, and consequently, how services should be organized, where they should be located and who is primarily responsible for them.

As a consequence of comprehensive policy changes in England, the English health and social care systems have undergone enormous changes in the past few years. For some, these changes have been welcome while other agencies and individuals have found them more challenging. For some, it means great uncertainty and insecurity. For others, it marks a time of opportunities and a way to move forward. Effective policy change implies careful attention to all the impediments along the way.

The English policy context

An historical and ongoing challenge for those who commission and provide services for people with dementia has been where to locate their services within the organizational structure. Should services for people with dementia be located within the mental health structure? Or in the older people's services structure? This decision has significant consequences. If the former, people with dementia are likely to lose resources to services for adults aged between 18 and 65. If the latter, attention is often focused on mainstream services for older people which may not meet the needs of people with dementia or may even exclude them. The simple act of choosing between these two possibilities has consequences. As Benbow notes:

> One of the dilemmas is whether Older People's Mental Health should 'sit' in mental health services or older people's services. It should not be an 'either, or' but must be both. OPMH is part of mental health (and that must be valued and respected) but has to work across all the places where older adults with mental health problems may be found, and therefore has to relate to, work within and work with older people's services, acute hospitals and the whole of residential and nursing care. To see it as one or the other is to deny the challenge of working across both service areas.

> (Benbow 2006)

The gap between mental health services and older people's services became increasingly evident as policy emerged. In 1999, a National Service Framework (NSF) for Mental Health was published (Department of Health 1999). Explicit within this NSF was an age cut-off at 65. Service development recommendations for older people (and younger people with dementia) would be in a forthcoming NSF for Older People. Funding to support the implementation of the NSF for Mental Health was made available, and a new body – the National Institute for Mental Health in England – was established to work with local health and social care organizations on its implementation in practice.

In 2001, a National Service Framework for Older People was published (Department of Health 2001). This contained eight standards to improve care and quality of life for older people. Standard Seven specifically addressed the care of people with dementia and with depression. Disappointingly, there was no funding attached to the NSF for Older People. Organizations had to seek creative ways to meet the milestones and standards that were laid down, and significant achievements were made. These achievements often involved significant changes in service design to free up resources in one area and move them across for reinvestment elsewhere.

This divergence between the two NSFs led to particular challenges in delivering better services for people with dementia. Further attention was given to the organization of services for people with dementia by a contemporaneous report from the Audit Commission in 2000. The *Forget-me-Not* report (Audit Commission 2000) demonstrated that general practitioners felt a sense of helplessness when they had a patient with dementia and that only 50% believed that it was important to look actively for early signs of dementia and to make an early diagnosis. Many of the others said they saw no point in looking for an incurable condition – even though carers could be helped by early advice. A follow-up report, *Forget-me-Not 2*, published in 2002 (Audit Commission 2002), reported that disappointingly little had changed in the two years since the publication of the first report.

Specifically recognizing dementia as relevant to both ageing and mental health expertise and services, the Department of Health published a vision statement, *Securing Better Mental Health for Older Adults* (Department of Health 2005a) in June 2005. This was a landmark publication in which the National Directors for Mental Health and for Older People promoted a joint vision for improving services for people with dementia. Their vision included:

- services to be based on needs, not age

- all services to view people as a whole, taking into account their physical as well as their mental health needs

- organizations working together to provide best quality care

- skilling up all staff who work with older people so that they have an understanding of mental health in later life and can recognize when they should refer on to specialist services

- investment in older people's mental health service provision.

Recognizing the challenges in implementing the vision the Department of Health followed up this visionary document with a service development guide – *Everybody's Business: Integrating Mental Health Services for Older Adults* (Department of Health 2005b). This publication describes a service which is fit for purpose as one which:

- recognizes the dignity of individual service users. It respects and values their diversity as well as acknowledging their major role in the process of planning and developing services

- is grounded in respect for all those who engage with these services, not only those using them but also their supporters and carers

- provides the practical advice and information service users and their carers need as well as developing a consistently high quality, comprehensive package of care and support which minimizes bureaucracy

- makes sure that the best and most effective treatments are widely and consistently available

- is open to everyone. It responds to people on the basis of need not age and ensures that wherever older people with mental health problems are in the system they are not discriminated against and have their mental health needs met.

The purpose of *Everybody's Business: Integrating Mental Health Services for Older Adults* was to inform local discussions about commissioning and providing services, to provide best practice guidance, and some key health economics data. It gives pointers to a number of policy drivers which offer the hooks and levers to develop better services for older people with mental health problems, including dementia. The guide incorporates discussion about different types of services for people with dementia – primary and community care, intermediate care, care for people in the general hospital, specialist mental health services and special groups. It specifically addressed the need to cross organizational and cultural divides in order to effectively respond to people with dementia, including a key message about the need for leadership and champions to implement effective programmes. The report states that:

> The thing that is needed above all else to improve older people's mental health is effective leadership across all health and social care organizations, at all levels. Effective leadership requires a vision of where it is going, a strategy for how to get there and involvement operationally in managing the translation of vision into reality.

(Department of Health 2005b: 23)

To further efforts to integrate aged care and mental health expertise and services to care for people with dementia, the National Institute for Health and Clinical Excellence, working with the Social Care Institute for Excellence, published a joint guideline on dementia (National Collaborating Centre for Mental Health 2006). This ground-breaking document reviewed the evidence on current dementia care practices and provided guidance on establishing joined-up health and social care services for people with dementia and their carers. Taking a care pathway approach, the guideline considers the impact of dementia on the person and their family and friends from the time when they first suspect that there might be a problem, through the assessment and diagnosis process, considering good practice in all aspects of dementia care including end-of-life care. Its holistic approach explicitly includes younger people with dementia and those who have a learning disability and dementia.

Integration of services across systems and within local areas requires a carefully orchestrated collaborative approach that is inclusive and comprehensive. This level of change implementation is more likely to be achieved with a guided or facilitated approach. The next section describes such an approach using a Health and Social Care Change Agent Team (CAT).

Exercise 28.1 The policy context

As part of the integration of services for people with dementia, a local clinic is inviting stakeholders to a meeting to discuss how they will implement the new approach. The meeting begins with local providers expressing their concern about integration. Several, from different disciplines and agencies, are concerned that integration threatens the quality of their services. They are opposed to integration and suggest a way to keep clear boundaries between mental health and older people's services while integrating at a more superficial level.

You are asked to respond to this suggestion, to specify why true integration is a better way to proceed.

What will you say?

The collaborative methodology

The collaborative approach focuses on the experience of service users, carers and frontline staff, enabling them to identify areas for improvement and then develop, test out and monitor small change ideas to see if they are successful. Changes that have brought about improvement are then rolled out across the locality. Initially tested in areas like cancer care and chronic heart disease, a Dementia Services Collaborative was launched in the north-east of England in July 2002. This has been followed by two further collaboratives, a Dementia Collaborative in south-east England and an Older People's Mental Health Collaborative in the West Midlands

The Collaborative Model for Improvement was designed to provide a framework for developing, testing and implementing changes that lead to improvement (Langley *et al.* 1996). In particular it was developed to bring about changes in services where variations existed, recognizing that often the spread of good practice does not happen automatically.

The Collaborative Model for Improvement is based on three fundamental questions:

1   What are we trying to accomplish?

2   How will we know that a change is an improvement?

3   What changes can we make that will result in improvement?

The OPMH collaboratives are a comprehensive way of creating specific service improvements by:

- looking at the service from the service user's point of view
- providing a toolkit for improvement
- dedicating time to the improvement process
- empowering frontline staff to make changes
- creating opportunities for personal and team development
- using networks for shared learning
- providing a structure to continue development and sustain change.

The health and social care change agent team (CAT)[1]

Recognizing the challenges involved in creating integrated health and social care services, a health and social care change agent team (CAT) was created to assist in the implementation process. The CAT was established in 2002 to help health and social care communities tackle the problem of patients who remained in hospital after they were fit for discharge. This was often referred to as delayed transfers of care (DTOCs) or delayed discharges, and was referred to in the media by the rather more provocative term 'bed blocking'. This unhelpful label suggested that the problem lay with the patient, whereas experience showed that the difficulties were usually in the ways in which local organizations worked, or did not work, together. As many of the delayed discharges involved older people with dementia, this particular problem offered an opportunity to try out an integrated approach to problem solving. At the time there was great concern over the high numbers of people, many with dementia, whose discharge from hospital was delayed because services could not be organized to allow their safe return to the community. Patients rarely, if ever, wanted to stay in an acute hospital bed longer than they needed.

In a clear demonstration of how failure to integrate the various aspects of care led to problems for both the recipient and the service system, in systems in which acute hospital care is provided by one organization, community health care by another, and social care by a third organization as there were frequent misunderstandings and ongoing obstacles to working together. Developing an effective, integrated system requires a view that incorporates more than the major players or the representatives who are traditionally at the table. In this instance, the CAT worked across whole systems to identify the barriers and to facilitate changes that would allow more streamlined care. The whole system included: acute hospital care, primary health care and social care, housing, emergency services (ambulance, police and fire services), leisure, transport, lifelong learning, community networks, private and voluntary organizations and many others.

Exercise 28.2   Identifying community stakeholders

You have been asked, as part of your job, to organize a group of stakeholders who might be interested in preventing hospitalizations of people with dementia. One of the first things you need to do is to consider the many risk factors for hospitalization, especially for people with dementia. Then you need to identify the stakeholders who are working in those areas or have some involvement in those services.

Thinking about prevention of hospitalization, who are the community stakeholders you will include in your meeting? Name at least five.

In its first three years, the work of CAT, together with other English Department of Health initiatives reduced the numbers of people whose discharge was delayed from about 5500 in September 1999 to less than 3000. CAT achieved this by working with local health and social care economies to evaluate critically their current service delivery models and identify areas for change. Using a variety of tools, they worked as critical friends alongside commissioners and providers and with agreement from senior management in the key organizations. These key organizations always included all health organizations – primary care trusts and acute hospital trusts – and local authority social services, and also sometimes included, for example, relevant and appropriate independent sector providers, emergency services, housing and other local authority services.

The CAT became involved in helping organizations at many levels, and responded to requests for assistance with the integration of health and social services from many sources. For example, in one local authority in the south of England, a senior social care manager felt that people with dementia in his locality were not always getting the best service. One of the fundamental obstacles to this was that the various services which offer support to people with dementia – principally health services and social care services – were not always as joined up as they might be. In his view, this stemmed from organizational cultures which were greatly distanced and this was embodied in a lack of dialogue between senior managers. The CAT facilitated a half-day meeting of the directors and chief executives of these organizations, together with their senior managers. When asked about the outcomes of the meeting that would make it a success, the manager commissioning the work replied that simply getting the chief officers to sit round the same table in the same room to talk about dementia for a couple of hours would be a significant step forward. While not sufficient in itself, the meeting certainly marked the first step along the road to joining up the services locally.

Process mapping and service redesign – a methodology for effecting change

The CAT found it useful to begin the policy change implementation with a diagnostic phase. This phase begins by building a picture of what is going on within the locality. A key element of this phase is listening to as many views as possible. To achieve this, the CAT arranged interviews with senior managers, usually chief executives and directors, from all the key organizations usually on a one-to-one basis. Interviews allowed participants to present the picture from their point of view and to speak freely and in confidence. Other interviews were conducted in groups, for example, with a community mental health team or with a user or carer forum. This part of the work was quite intensive and done in a short space of time.

Summary reports were prepared and fed back to the senior managers as a group, allowing ample time for discussion. It is important to finish these meetings with an agreed way forward. The strategy used to determine the way forward was to create a process map of the patient/service user journey.

Process mapping

A well-developed exercise to help an organization assess what is working and what is not, is to map the journey of service users in their organizations. This requires both taking stock of the current situation – to map the current journey – and mapping a way to deliver services that seems to make more sense – a service redesign.

Mapping the current journey provides a picture or 'map' of what happens to a service user in the current situation and throws a sharp focus on the bits of the system that are disconnected or make little sense from a patient/service user point of view.

Box 28.1 Case example

CAT were asked to help out a local system where there were high numbers of emergency admissions of people with dementia to acute hospital. This was partly due to the local geography which was rural with a sparse population, making general practitioner cover difficult, especially out of hours. It was also probably partly due to an organizational culture which was averse to risk-taking. The result was a high number of people with dementia on acute wards and difficulty in moving them on, either back to their home or to a care home, when medically fit for discharge. At this point, they were often transferred to the local psychiatric hospital which found its beds full and unable to take emergency mental health admissions. After interviewing the key players in this scenario, the CAT were able to see what was happening. Guided by their experience with other systems and their knowledge of what was working well elsewhere, and their commitment to service integration, the CAT suggested that a liaison psychiatrist should be jointly commissioned. This person could assess and advise on the care and treatment of people with dementia in the acute wards, link with external services to facilitate discharge and provide a teaching service to colleagues and community services to facilitate discharge and/or prevent admissions. This plan was consistent with the new policy of service integration.

Service redesign

The next step in implementing change is to invite key people from all groups involved in the change to work together redesigning services to create a simpler pathway for users. Important aspects of the redesign process include discussion about what is worth retaining from the current situation and what needs to change. This should lead very quickly to the development of an action plan, a projected time for completion of each task or change and a named responsible person for each. Including senior managers in discussions and securing their endorsement early in the process is key.

In many instances, CAT continued their involvement in the process to act as a critical friend during the service redevelopment period, to help maintain the pace if it starts to flag, and to help systems evaluate if they are making a difference.

Box 28.2 Case example

Senior managers in Anyshire invited us to give a presentation to a group of middle managers and practitioners about intermediate care for people with dementia. Intermediate care is defined in the National Service Framework for Older People as:

- responding to or averting a crisis to avoid unnecessary hospital admission

- active rehabilitation following an acute hospital stay to facilitate early discharge

---

- prevent unnecessary admission to long-term residential care

(Department of Health 2001).

In Anyshire, they had refurbished a residential home to provide eight beds which were designated as intermediate care beds for people with dementia. In group discussions following the presentation, it became clear that there had been no discussion to date about how these beds would fit in with other local services. CAT therefore proposed to return for two days of process mapping and service redesign.

On day one, we agreed that we could not map the whole journey of a person with dementia from first signs to end-of-life care. Since we were concerned with intermediate care which aims to prevent admission to hospital or residential care, or facilitate early discharge, we agreed with participants to divide into two groups. One group would consider what currently happens to a person with dementia who reaches a crisis in the community – either they become ill or their carer is unable to provide care for a period of time. The second group considered what currently happens to someone with dementia when they are in hospital and clinically fit to be discharged.

On the second day, we started by reviewing the maps that had been created on day one and discussing which services seemed to meet people's needs well. We then looked at the obstacles to a smoother pathway. Sometimes this meant initiating something simple like a different way of sharing information. In other cases it meant reviewing the inclusion criteria for existing services to ensure that they are accessible to people with dementia. In one or two cases, it meant a more major shift in the organizational culture to facilitate a new way of working. By the end of the day, we had several pieces of flipchart paper covered with an action plan to take the work forward. In the ensuing eight months, we have had contact from time to time with Anyshire to ask how they are getting along, and changes are happening.

It is important to recognize, in undertaking this sort of process mapping, that the work is both physically and emotionally tiring. While it may seem like a golden opportunity for staff to take time away from their usual jobs so that they can critically review their services, it can also feel threatening and uncertain. It may be that, for some people, they have rarely, if ever, been offered this opportunity to think 'outside the box' and they find it hard to engage. The Care Services Improvement Partnership[2] uses a wealth of tools and techniques to support health and social care professionals, people who use services and the people who support them as they work in partnerships to effect change and improve local services.

It has an online directory that brings all of these tools together in an easily accessible, comprehensive resource. The directory aims to stimulate discussion and ideas and provide choices on how to improve services. By bringing together information on a range of methodologies, exercises, icebreakers and energizers, it is intended for everyone. The directory can be found at: http://www.csip.org.uk/resources/directory-of-service-improvement.html

Managed learning networks

Supporting these efforts are regular whole collaborative team meetings where teams can exchange ideas, tell each other what they have been doing and learn from the experiences elsewhere. There are also opportunities for staying in touch via the website and regular newsletters. Extending the collaboration to a wider group was achieved by creating Managed Learning Networks (MLN) in various geographical areas and for different service user groups.

In 2006, one MLN was established for older people's mental health services across the north-west and north-east of England. This has been followed by the launch of a second MLN in the East Midlands. Each of the networks is focused on the implementation of *Everybody's Business: Integrating Mental Health Services for Older Adults – A Service Development Guide* (Department of Health 2005b). The MLN aims to drive forward the implementation of the Service Development Guide by reflecting the priorities and needs of local health and social care communities, while also addressing national priorities and policy directives. Each MLN local team promotes a culture of partnership working, utilizing shared learning and an action learning and problem solving approach to process reform. Teams initially gathered baseline information on services, utilizing current local and regional data. Where necessary, teams process mapped to gather baseline information and conduct gap analysis comparing local service provision with the commissioner's checklist. This was used to inform priorities for the team. Team leaders supplied the MLN with a minimum of one improvement plan bi-monthly, to be shared across the network (www.olderpeoplesmentalhealth.csip.org.uk/managed-learning-networks.html).

At an early meeting of the MLN in the north-west and north-east of England, members agreed to the following expectations:

- to share learning and ideas

- to discuss/debate issues and to problem solve collaboratively

- to innovate and sustain improvements

- to source, record, utilize, evaluate and disseminate examples of practice around the key themes within 'everybody's business'

- to communicate by networking across themes, local teams and individuals ensuring a flow of information across the MLN matrix

- to identify priorities locally in line with key themes and use these as a basis for progression

- to continue to develop as leaders

- to continuously share open and honest feedback within the MLN (www.olderpeoplesmentalhealth.csip.org.uk/managed-learning-networks/member-expectations.html).

A reporting template for improvement work was developed and distributed to MLN members so that details of each improvement initiative can be recorded and sent to all MLN members, to be shared across the MLN and added to the evidence base. At the same time, examples of positive practice, national and local policies and initiatives, relevant research and evidence, service improvement tools, training slides and articles of interest were made available across the network to assist members and their teams in their work.

Exercise 28.3   Including people with dementia in organizational redesign

Look back at the chapters in this book that relate to inclusion of people with dementia in planning and communicating with people who have dementia.

How could stakeholder meetings be designed to include people with dementia in the planning process? Would you invite them to a large meeting?

List three strategies you think would be effective and say why you have selected these strategies.

Conclusion

This chapter has described some of the work of the Care Services Improvement Partnership to help managers, commissioners and providers to reflect critically on their current service configurations and delivery; to consider the options for improvement; and to effect change. This might happen at a strategic level based on a system reform and introducing a cultural shift and new ways of working. Or it might be undertaken by frontline practitioners to make small changes in the presentation and delivery of individual services. There are a number of key issues that are common to all this work and which are crucial to its success:

● People who are using services and their carers should be fully involved in informing the need for change and the development process.

● Strategic change should be developed and delivered across the whole system. Maintaining a position in individual organizations is an obstacle to reforming the system.

● A bottom-up, top-down approach is essential so that the views of all staff, as well as users and carers, are included and everyone feels that they are involved in the process and have a contribution to make.

● Change does not have to be huge – small steps can make a big difference to the way a service is delivered to and received by the user.

● Change is inevitable. It can be perceived as threatening and often leads to a sense of insecurity, but it also offers enormous opportunities to be creative and do things differently.

One of the key outcomes issues facing dementia care, at least in England, has been the challenge of where dementia services should be located and which should be the lead organization. The Department of Health has announced the development of a dementia strategy as a key priority in 2007–08. Leadership and championing will be crucial in developing future dementia services that are fit for purpose and user-centred and led.

Notes

1. The Health and Social Care Change Agent Team is now the National Older People's Programme, part of the Care Services Improvement Partnership.

2. In 2005 eight service improvement teams merged to form the Care Services Improvement Partnership. These included CAT, National Institute for Mental Health in England, Valuing People Support Team, integrated Community Equipment Services and two teams working with children, young people and families, see www.csip.org.uk

Further information

The Department of Health has a web page devoted to policy and guidance in health and social care.

The Care Services Improvement Partnership Older People's Mental Health Managed Learning Networks has a useful website.

References

Audit Commission (2000) *Forget-me-Not*. London: Audit Commission.

Audit Commission (2002) *Forget-me-Not 2*. London: Audit Commission.

Benbow, S. (2006) Report on the NIMHE Ageing and Mental Health Fellowship 2003–2006 (unpublished).

Department of Health (1999) *National Service Framework for Mental Health*. London: Department of Health.

Department of Health (2001) *National Service Framework for Older People*. London: Department of Health.

Department of Health (2005a) *Securing Better Mental Health for Older Adults*. London: Department of Health.

Department of Health (2005b) *Everybody's Business: Integrating Mental Health Services for Older Adults – a Service Development Guide*. Department of Health: London.

Langley, G., Nolan, K., Nolan, T., Norman, C. and Provost, L. (1996) *The Improvement Guide: A Practical Approach to Enhancing Organisational Performance*. San Francisco, CA: Jossey Bass Publishing.

National Collaborating Centre for Mental Health (2006) commissioned by the Social Care Institute for Excellence, and National Institute for Health and Clinical Excellence. *Dementia: a NICE-SCIE Guideline on Supporting People with Dementia and their Carers in Health and Social Care*. London: British Psychological Society and Gaskell.

Index